Andras Gedeon

Science and Technology in Medicine

AN ILLUSTRATED ACCOUNT BASED ON

NINETY-NINE LANDMARK PUBLICATIONS

FROM FIVE CENTURIES

With 1130 Illustrations

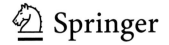 Springer

Andras Gedeon D. Sc.
http://www.scienceandtechnologyinmedicine.com

Library of Congress Control Number: 2005934913

ISBN-10: 0-387-27874-5   e-ISBN 0-387-27875-3
ISBN-13: 978-0387-30171-6

Printed on acid-free paper.

Printed in Singapore   (KYO)

9 8 7 6 5 4 3 2 1

springeronline.com

THIS ENTERTAINING and informative book by Andras Gedeon is about those who contributed science and technology to medicine and it fills an important gap in the history of medicine. Each of the 99 chapters starts with a brief biographical sketch, followed by a description of the scientific or technological discovery. Then the significance is explained clearly, followed by an historical perspective, placing the discovery neatly in the evolution of medicine.

The book will be of value, not only to historians, but also those who wish to illuminate their lectures and speeches with relevant and interesting facts, some of which may be surprising. For example, most associate the name of Doppler with the frequency shift of sound or radar waves. However, Doppler's original paper described the color change associated with a rotating pair of stars in the heavens. Its audible proof for everyone was the frequency change heard when a trumpeter was emitting sound when on a passing train.

Within the various chapters, one finds a smorgasbord of fascinating information on the background of many "modern" medical techniques. For example, mouth-to-mouth resuscitation was in use in the mid 1700s. Electric stimulation was used slightly later to resuscitate subjects with respiratory arrest. Long before the first implanted cardiac pacemaker appeared in 1960, stimulation for cardiac arrest was performed in the late 1800s. These and many other historic tidbits are found in the many very readable chapters.

Each chapter concludes with a perspective that places the discovery nicely in the history of medicine. It tells about the knowledge prior to the discovery, thereby enabling the reader to identify creatively and ingenuity of the discoverer. The perspective does not confine itself to prior medical history; it covers contemporary and prior relevant discoveries in related scientific areas.

The reader will find the book difficult to stop reading. In fact this reviewer found it addicting and it will be found on my bookshelf that contains my most valuable reference books.

MEDICINE IS at the center of human civilization. Medicine is at the cross-roads of science and technology, ethics and philosophy, language and sociology, politics and economy, and many facets more that as a whole determine the nature of our culture. Medicine has arisen from man's existential desire not to be incapacitated by disease, and to escape an untimely early death. Medicine has, in addition, come to be applied not only to improve the quality of human life of those who suffer from illness or malformation, but also to help mankind to transgress the borderlines of its natural habitat and to venture into the deepest oceans and the most distant spheres of the universe. Medicine has been able to reach this capacity because two and a half millennia ago a process was started aiming at making use of the laws of nature for the benefit of humanity.

The beginning of a recognition of natural laws marks the beginning of science and technology. The union of science and technology with health care marks the beginning of medicine as we know it today. It was in the aftermath of the European Renaissance that a new momentum arose in that fruitful development. Increasingly, philosophers, physicians, and scientists drew conclusions from their observations and arranged ever more skillful experiments to test their hypotheses.

The historiography of science has informed us that no direct path leads to truth. Often enough, our view on nature is guided by cultural stimuli rather than by an elusive reality. We cannot even be certain about the relationship between scientific findings and reality. We can be sure, however, of most welcome achievements in the history of medicine that could never even have been thought of without contributions by and the use of science and technology.

Andras Gedeon has provided, in his portrayal of "ninety-nine publications from five centuries", a fascinating panorama of what may be identified as the most decisive "landmarks" in the history of modern medicine. He begins with Albrecht Dürer's book, published posthumously in 1528, as "the first attempt to apply mathematics to the description of the proportions and forms of the human body", and he concludes his list with Michael Phelps' presentation of "a prototype system of a positron emission transaxial tomograph". Within the 450 years separating these two publications, innumerous individual naturalists and research groups have offered their contributions to "science and technology in medicine". For the first three centuries, this has been an all-European endeavor; with the extension of the scientific world view beyond the borders of the European continent, it has become a global effort shared by all who seek to expand knowledge and to adapt human life to ever changing existential conditions.

A listing of the top 99 seminal publications marking the absolute highlights of the influence of science and technology on medicine between the early 16th and the late 20th century should be considered a difficult task. Too many authors come to one's mind that deserve an eternal place in our collective memory. And yet, it is the historian's prerogative to value one against another and to present a personal choice. Andras Gedeon's account represents a most valuable and representative selection, and constitutes a timely record. It is most valuable because it demonstrates the broad international and multidisciplinary foundations of progress in science and technology for the benefit of medicine. It is representative, because it would be difficult to come up with a markedly different list of essential contributions to the progress in medicine as it has been stimulated, in the period under review, by new findings in chemistry, physics, and biology, and by new applications of mathematics and technology. Finally, it is a timely record because, as has happened before, voices are raised nowadays demanding a preference, in medicine, for beliefs over science. It is to be hoped that this book will contribute to a recollection of the multi-faceted scientific and technological origins of today's status of medicine. In addition, it should stimulate young people from all scientific and technological disciplines and in all nations to continue on this path and to further the development of medicine—at the center of civilisation.

Contents

Preface and acknowledgements

FIVE HUNDRED years ago, a young German painter named Albrecht Dürer left his hometown of Nuremberg and started on a journey to Venice, a city at its peak of wealth and influence. Here he met with Luca Pacioli, famed mathematician and theorist of art, and he also got closely acquainted with the first printings of Euclid's geometry and Vitruvius Pollio's classical work on architecture. On his return home, Dürer immersed himself in the study of the spatial representation of objects and specially the form, proportions and movements of the human body. His work "Hierinn sind begriffen vier bücher von menschlicher Proportion", which was published in 1528, just after his death, became the first systematic application of mathematics to the problem of how to create an image of the human body and its movements.

Dürer's study is one of the ninety-nine landmark publications that form the basis of an attempt made in this book to describe the historical progression of important contributions of science and technology to the field of medicine. In each case considered, a summary of the contents of a publication and a short presentation of the author are given. Then the significance of the discovery and its influence on later developments are outlined. Using references to subsequent key advances, the level of knowledge in the field is traced up to modern times. Although necessarily not exhaustive, it is hoped that this approach will highlight the evolution of many important results in science and technology that have played a direct and important role in the progress of medicine over the past five hundred years.

Any selection of topics or specific discoveries is justly subject to criticism. Considering ninety-nine books rather than an even one hundred is intended to be a symbolic invitation to the reader to reflect on how the present framework could be modified according to his or her own knowledge and preferences. Some names and discoveries described here will be well known to many, while others may be unknown to most. Hopefully all readers will find a significant amount of new and interesting information. An equally important ambition of the book is to provide excitement and entertainment by giving a glimpse of the intricate patterns of evolution that have gradually transformed past contributions of science and technology to medicine into what we see around us today.

If all this could, even in the slightest way, further a better understanding of future developments in this multidisciplinary endeavour, then the effort of publishing this book would be more than amply rewarded.

Many individuals and organisations have kindly contributed illustrative material to this book. For a complete list, the reader is referred to the "Image sources and credits" section. The Hagströmer Medico-Historical Library at the Karolinska Institute in Stockholm, the University of Uppsala Library and particularly the Biblioteca Walleriana in Uppsala and the Medical Photographic Library of the Wellcome Library in London have together supplied the bulk of the information used in the book. The competent and always willing help of Gertie Johansson, Harriet Wallman and Clive Coward at these respective libraries is gratefully acknowledged.

Other public organisations that have provided valuable material include the Chemical Heritage Foundation in Philadelphia, the Max Planck Gesellschaft in Berlin, the Science Museum in London, the Deutsches Museum in Munich and in Bonn, the Bibliothèque de l'Académie national de Médecine in Paris, the British Library in London, the Institut fur Geschichte der Medizin der Universität Wien in Vienna, the Universitätsbibliothek in Basel and the University of Pennsylvania Library in Philadelphia.

Assistance and difficult-to-find picture material have been received from several company archives, among which mention should be made of the Carl Zeiss Archiv in Jena, Corning Inc. Archives in Corning, archives at the General Electric Healthcare facility in Stockholm, Merck KGaA in Darmstadt and Siemens Medical Solutions Archives in Erlangen.

I am indebted to several of the prominent scientists mentioned in the book for their generous help, notably professors Mitchell Albert, William Bennett Jr, Per-Ingvar Brånemark, the late Dr Francis Crick, Dr Vinton Cerf, Dr Raymond Damadian, professor Gunnar Fant, Dr Robert Kahn, and professors Paul Lauterbur, Michael Phelps, Peter Wagner and John West.

Additionally, important photographic material and printed matter have been given by Dr Eric Blackwell, Dr Jeffrey Cooper, professors Anna-Liisa Brownell, Håkan Elmqvist and Gert Nilsson and by Lars Forsmark, Brian Högman and Bengt Stånge.

I would like to thank professor Åke Öberg for valuable comments on the draft version of the manuscript and professor Lennart Mathiasson for reviewing the contents of the sections with topics involving chemistry. The sections involving Nobel Laureates have benefited greatly from the expert scrutiny of professor Anders Bárány. I am also indebted to Daniel Gedeon for carefully reading the text from the educated, non-specialist viewpoint. His comments have been most helpful when attempting to make the presentation more easily accessible for the general public.

Book designer Lars E. Pettersson and Magnus Winbladh at Raster Förlag in Stockholm have co-operated to skilfully transform the bare contents into a book presentation with, it is hoped, an appealing form. The steady interest of Beth Campbell at the Springer-Verlag New York Inc. for this book project has been a most appreciated source of encouragement during the work.

Finally, I would like to express my gratitude to the contributing experts, to Ove Hagelin who suggested the Bibliography section and also wrote it in its entirety, to Jeremy Norman for his many helpful comments and suggestions on all aspects of writing and publishing on topics related to the history of science and medicine, to Paul Unschuld for reviewing and commenting on the list of landmark publications and to Leslie Geddes, who not only drew my attention to valuable literature but also, when initially informed about the plan for the book, called the undertaking a "heroic task", thereby cementing my resolve to go through with it.

THE PRACTICE of medicine was considered both an art and a science at least as far back as Hippocrates. The art, intuition, and human considerations required in the practice of medicine may be among the reasons why medicine developed a distinct culture, a distinct educational system, and a distinct literature of its own while it incorporated discoveries from other sciences and technology in the advancement of medical science. Organizing and classifying this distinct medical literature led to the earliest bibliographies of scientific literature, to early knowledge classifications written by physicians that identified the scope of medicine within universal knowledge, to the development of medical libraries, and decades before the Internet, to online indexing and abstracting services that attempted to organize and classify millions of citations covering all medical knowledge. Andras Gedeon's book, *Science and Technology in Medicine*, documents the origins of some of the most significant discoveries in science and technology that were incorporated into medicine. Some of these discoveries were made by physicians and others were not.

Concerning the inevitable difficulties of the practice of medicine, Hippocrates wrote, "Life is short and art is long, occasion fleeting, experience deceptive, and judgment difficult."[1] For millennia before most effective drugs, scientific diagnostic tools, and other elements of modern high-tech medicine, it was often the basic processes of careful observation, and of caring—the art of medicine—that healed the sick as much as any proven remedy. With limited powers to heal, early physicians became acute observers of the processes of life from birth to death, and of the relationship of life to disease. The wide range of ailments which physicians were expected to treat, the complexity of medical experience, and the central importance of medicine to society, may have been elements contributing to the early development of medical schools separate from other educational institutions, to the development of an extensive and distinctive body of medical knowledge, and to

1. Jeremy M. Norman (ed.) Morton's Medical Bibliography, fifth edition, (Aldershot, England: Scolar Press, 1991) 13.

the development of medical libraries separate from other libraries.

Apart from humanitarian considerations, one of the reasons that some physicians may have elected to practice medicine, rather than devote their lives to other scientific work, was that until the growth of industrialization that took place in second half of the nineteenth century the practice of medicine was a primary means by which a person educated in science could earn a living through science rather than by teaching. Prior to the industrial development that occurred in the second half of the nineteenth century, most scientists, other than physicians, were men of inherited wealth, or dependent upon a wealthy patron, or in religious orders. For centuries, the central importance of medicine to society, and the economic independence that the practice of medicine usually brought, made physicians among the best-educated, and among the wealthiest and most respected members of their communities. These factors continued to the reinforcement of medicine's distinct culture.

After the introduction of and spread of printing in the second half of the 15th century, the rapid growth of information inevitably required efforts to organize and classify knowledge. The first science to benefit from these efforts was medicine. The first bibliography on any scientific subject was the French physician, Symphorien Champier's, De medicine claris scriptoribus (c.1506–1507), a bibliography of about 400 works. This was also an early effort at a history of medicine [2]. Later in the sixteenth century, the first great bibliographer and systematizer of knowledge in general was the physician, Conrad Gesner, author of the pioneering Bibliotheca Universalis (1554–55).[3] This listing and classification of 12,000 writings was published when the author was only twenty-nine years old. Among his prolific writings, which ranged from theology to natural history, in addition to medicine and bibliography, Gesner prepared an edition of Galen's writings that included a bio-bibliography of Galen's writings. This was, most probably, the first modern bio-bibliography of any author. The physician, Israel Spach, followed Gesner in producing a universal survey of the knowledge of his time. His Nomenclator scriptorium philosophicorum atque philologicorum (Strassburg, 1598) was called "probably the most important subject bibliography of the 16th century, and a truly amazing summary of contemporary knowledge ... [which] established the method followed by all subsequent bibliographers."[4].

Organizing knowledge, whether it occurred in bibliographies or in the building of book collections in medical libraries, inevitably ran up against the problem of defining medicine as distinct from other sciences, since medicine incorporated information from so many different sciences. In prior centuries, much as

2. Norman, op. cit., 6742.99.

3. Norman, op. cit., 6743

4. Bernard H. Breslauer and Roland Folter, Bibliography, its History and Development (New York: The Grolier Club, 1984) 39. Norman, op. cit., 6743.2.

today, the education of physicians typically included training in general science, such as mathematics and physics, as well as the standard medical curriculum such as anatomy, physiology, botany, pharmacology, chemistry, biology and other topics that we might associate with medicine. As an example of early physicians' background in general science, the first 133 pages of volume one of Albrecht Haller's extensively annotated edition of Herman Boerhaave's guide to the study of medicine, his Methodus Studii Medici (2 vols., Amsterdam, 1751,)[5] contain an annotated bibliography of works pertaining to mathematics and physics. This is a surprisingly comprehensive selection of works in general science that one might not associate with medical training. The author of the original guide, Boerhaave, was a pioneer in chemistry as well as in the teaching of medicine.[6] Having a good education in science, physicians frequently contributed both to the science and technology of medicine and to scientific fields outside the direct purview of medicine. They also willingly applied advances from the non-medical sciences to the science and practice of medicine.

5. Norman, op. cit., 6746.

6. Norman, op. cit., 666.1.

In reviewing the landmark works in Science and Technology in Medicine, and also reviewing the works footnoted "in perspective," I was impressed by how many of the contributions were made by physicians. Conversely it was informative to see how many contributions of scientists trained outside of medicine were applied to medical problems. Because of medicine's distinct culture, and the historic separation of medicine from other sciences, the non-medical origins of some of these contributions may have been forgotten. In addition it is surprising to see how many discoveries that we associate with non-medical science were actually made by physicians.

Among aspects of this book that I find most intriguing are:

As early as Euclid, applications of physics and optics were applied to the study of vision.

What has long been considered the first work of experimental science written in England, De Magnete, a work on electricity and magnetism, was by the physician, William Gilbert.

The French physician Pierre Borel contributed to the discovery of both the microscope and the telescope. Incidentally, he also wrote the first independent bibliography of chemistry and alchemy.

The chemist Joseph Black practiced and taught medicine.

Both Thomas Young and Hermann von Helmholtz, developers of the "Young-Helmholtz" theory of color vision, were trained as physicians. Among his contributions, Helmholtz worked in the "pure" science of physiological optics, and in its clinical applications through his invention of the ophthalmoscope. In addition to deciphering Egyptian hieroglyphics, Thomas Young wrote on the physiology of vision and on medical bibliography, as well as his encyclopedic work, A Course of Lectures on Natural Philosophy and the Mechanical Arts (2 vols, 1807).

The mathematician and physicist, Daniel Bernouilli, whose work on hydrodynamics has applications to fluid flow in the human body, as well as to such subjects aeronautical engineering, was first trained in medicine.

The chemist, Humphrey Davy, was apprenticed to a surgeon and apothecary, and self-educated in chemistry.

The astronomer Johannes Kepler contributed to the study of vision.

Francis Hauksbee, researcher in electricity, and Antoni van Leeuwenhoek, pioneer microscopist, both made their livings in the cloth trade.

Stephen Hales, student of respiratory physiology and blood flow, was a country minister in the village of Teddington.

The chemist Joseph Priestley, a Unitarian minister, published extensively on theology, education, and politics, as well as on subjects in physical science.

Wilhelm Conrad Röntgen's discovery of X-rays was almost immediately adopted by the medical community as the first method of imaging the interior of the human body. A professor of physics, Röntgen never again contributed to medicine.

Also documented in this book are the origins of the parallel development of electronic computing and molecular biology after World War II. These two fields of science and technology brought increasing amounts of mathematics and quantum physics into medicine and biology. Because of the enormous complexity of biological systems in which single protein molecules may contain as many as 10,000 atoms, and the presence of over 100,000 different proteins in the human body, solutions of the structures of proteins, and the study of their intricate interactions were impossible before high speed electronic computers. Prior to electronic computing, humans could not do the calculations for the structures of even very simple non-biological molecules without immense time and effort:

The production of electron density maps for structure analysis involves very heavy calculations on large quantities of numerical data, and the state of the art during the early 1940s was such that the limits of human ability in this area were reached at structures containing not more than about 10 crystallographically distinct atoms. The determination of a 10-atom-type structure involved, in the early 1940s, about six weeks of experimental work followed by anything up to three years of hand computation for a group of human "slaves".[7]

7. Andrew D. Booth, Computers in the University of London, 1945-1962. Quoted in Diana H. Hook & Jeremy M. Norman,

Development of electronic computing in the first decade after World War II opened endless doors in every scientific field. It is estimated that in the operational life of the world's first electronic computer, the ENIAC, from 1945 to the early 1950s, this huge and comparatively slow machine, operating at only 100,000 times the speed of man, performed more calculations than all of mankind had done in the centuries preceding it.[8] By 1960 there were approximately 10,000 mainframe computers operating around the world, of which 6,000 were in the United States. The ability to apply mathematics and quantum physics to biological problems through electronic computing was responsible for endless advances in fields such as medical imaging, pharmacology, bioinformatics and genomics. The first truly useful application of electronic computing to clinical medicine was in medical imaging. The first system of digital imaging applied to medicine was computed tomography. Its inventor, Geoffrey Hounsfield, was an electrical engineer. His work was based to a large extent on the researches on image reconstruction by the mathematician, Alan Cormack.

From the late 1950s medical libraries had to cope with an explosive growth of medical information published in new books and in many new periodicals. This presented an exceptional challenge to the National Library of Medicine in Bethesda, Maryland, which had been chartered since 1879 with the task of indexing and abstracting in the Index Medicus all of medical literature. Faced with an increasingly daunting challenge, NLM was among the earliest institutions to apply electronic computing to problems of information retrieval rather than strictly to the solution of mathematical problems or accounting. Work at NLM and by independent contractors led in the early 1960s to the development of MEDLARS (Medical Literature Analysis and Retrieval System). Using some of this technology, there was the parallel development in the private sector of the first electronic information services such as Lockheed's DIALOG. As a field which incorporated advances from other sciences and technologies throughout its history, it seems fitting that medicine, which invented the bibliography of science, and pioneered in the classification of universal knowledge, also led the way toward online information services—precursors of the virtual library of universal information that is developing on the Internet.

Origins of Cyberspace: A Library on the History of Computing, Networking, and Telecommunications (Novato, CA: historyofscience.com, 2002).

8. Jeremy M. Norman, From Gutenberg to the Internet: A Sourcebook on the History of Information Technology (Novato, CA: historyofscience.com, 2005).

Ninety-nine landmark publications at a glance

1. 1528 DÜRER Mathematics applied to human proportions and to spatial representation of the body.
2. 1575 PARÉ New surgical methods and devices including artificial body parts and prosthesis.
3. 1590 PARACELSUS The introduction of chemistry in medicine, the discovery of the effects of ether.
4. 1603 SANTORIO The first use of quantitative measurements for diagnostics in medicine.
5. 1604 KEPLER The mechanism of image formation and vision correctly explained for the first time.
6. 1614 SANTORIO The first quantitative study of the fluid balance of the body.
7. 1625 SANTORIO Introduction of the quantitative measurement of temperature in medicine.
8. 1652 VAN HELMONT The first time gases are named and the first description of carbon dioxide.
9. 1655 BOREL The first publication describing the compound microscope and its use in medicine.
10. 1665 WREN Introduction of controlled techniques of infusion
11. 1667 HOOKE The first systematic study of the physiology of artificial ventilation.
12. 1680 BORELLI The first study of the mechanics of movements and the heart seen as a mechanical pump.
13. 1684 KIRCHER Early study of the generation and propagation of sound and its medical use.
14. 1684 BOYLE The first work devoted entirely to the biochemistry of blood.
15. 1709 HAUKSBEE Introducing apparatus for studying electrostatics, electric discharges, and light.
16. 1719 LEEUWENHOEK Microscopic investigations leading to many new discoveries in medicine and biology.
17. 1727 HALES The first accurate blood pressure measurement and about gases in chemistry and physiology.
18. 1738 BERNOULLI A theory of gases and fluids, and the first calculation of the work performed by the heart.
19. 1748 JALLABERT The first use of electricity for treatment of paralysis.
20. 1756 BLACK The discovery and properties of carbon dioxide.
21. 1777 SCHEELE The discovery of oxygen and many other new elements and organic acids.
22. 1777 PRIESTLEY The discovery of oxygen, nitrous oxide, nitric oxide, and the composition of water.
23. 1788 KITE The first demonstration of electric resuscitation with artificial ventilation.
24. 1789 LAVOISIER Introducing the modern science of chemistry and the study of oxygen uptake in man.
25. 1791 KEMPELEN The first apparatus for producing speech sounds for letters and words.
26. 1800 VOLTA The invention of the battery and the electric stimulation of hearing.
27. 1800 HERSCHEL Infrared radiation discovered.
28. 1800 DAVY The properties of nitrous oxide and a proposal for its use in surgery.
29. 1806 SERTÜRNER The discovery, isolation and properties of morphine and other alkaloids.
30. 1806 LEGENDRE The first use of a statistical method, the least squares technique, in experimental science.
31. 1819 LAENNEC The invention of the stethoscope and the introduction of auscultation as a clinical tool.
32. 1822 FOURIER A powerful new mathematical method applicable to problems in science and medicine.
33. 1825 LABARRAQUE The introduction of chlorine solutions as a disinfectant.
34. 1827 CIVIALE The development of a new device—the lithotriptor—for crushing bladder stones.
35. 1828 POISEUILLE The mercury manometer introduced for blood pressure measurement.
36. 1835 DUMAS A new theory of chemical reactions leading to the correct formula for chloroform.
37. 1837 MAGNUS The first quantitative blood gas determinations.
38. 1839 DAGUERRE The invention of photography—photomicroscopy—and its early uses in medicine.
39. 1842 LIEBIG The application of organic chemistry to the basic life processes.
40. 1842 DOPPLER The Doppler effect discovered.
41. 1846 HUTCHINSON The invention of the spirometer, and its use for lung function diagnosis.
42. 1848 DU BOIS-REYMOND Exploration of the physiology of electric conduction of nerves and muscles.
43. 1850 HELMHOLTZ The first measurement of the velocity of nerve impulses.
44. 1851 WEBER Blood flow explained using a new wave theory.
45. 1852 HELMHOLTZ The invention of the ophthalmoscope.
46. 1856 FICK The first general overview of the role of physics in medicine.
47. 1858 SNOW The introduction of the scientific approach to anaesthesia.
48. 1858 CZERMAK The invention and introduction of laryngoscopy as a useful clinical tool.
49. 1862 KIRCHHOFF The discovery of spectral analysis for the determination of the chemical elements.
50. 1862 PASTEUR Demonstration of airborne bacteria and the introduction of the germ theory of disease.

51. 1862 HOPPE-SEYLER Haemoglobin discovered and its properties and spectra studied.

52. 1863 MAREY Measurement and registration of the arterial pulse and other physiological parameters.

53. 1866 MENDEL The laws of heredity explained.

54. 1867 LISTER The introduction of antiseptic surgery.

55. 1868 MAXWELL Control theory established as a science.

56. 1870 FICK A new method for measuring the cardiac output.

57. 1871 TRENDELENBURG A new technique and device for intubation and anaesthesia.

58. 1875 VOIT Accurate apparatus for measuring gas exchange to assess the utilisation of foodstuff.

59. 1878 BERT Physiology at high and low pressures. The dissociation curve of oxygen established.

60. 1879 NITZE The invention and development of cystoscopy and related techniques.

61. 1881 KOCH The foundation of the science of bacteriology and modern sterilisation techniques.

62. 1884 ARRHENIUS The explanation of the properties of electrolytes.

63. 1885 VAN'T HOFF A theory for understanding osmotic pressure and chemical equilibrium.

64. 1886 ABBE A new theory and its implementation for much improved optical microscopy.

65. 1887 WALLER The demonstration of electric signals from the skin produced by the beat of the heart.

66. 1889 CURIE The discovery of piezoelectricity and its use in sensors and transducers.

67. 1895 RÖNTGEN The discovery of X-rays.

68. 1896 RIVA-ROCCI The introduction of the modern technique of blood pressure measurement.

69. 1897 THOMSON The discovery of the electron and the development of the Mass-spectroscope.

70. 1898 CURIE The discovery of radioactivity and new radioactive elements.

71. 1902 EINTHOVEN The construction of the modern ECG recorder.

72. 1903 FISCHER The discovery of the hypnotic effects of barbiturates and the study of purines.

73. 1903 TSWETT The invention of the technique of chromatography.

74. 1906 FISCHER The syntheses of amino-acids and peptides.

75. 1910 EHRLICH The foundation of modern chemotherapy, the discovery and clinical use of Salvarsan.

76. 1913 LAUE X-ray diffraction from a crystal observed and explained for the first time.

77. 1914 ABEL Successful dialysis is demonstrated in dogs.

78. 1920 STAUDINGER A theory is proposed for the mechanism of polymerisation, and applied to synthesis rubber.

79. 1922 ASTON The development of masspectrometry and the discovery of the isotopes.

80. 1929 CAROTHERS The invention and production of industrial polymers, particularly polyamide (nylon).

81. 1931 VAN SLYKE The first exhaustive review of clinical chemistry as used in medicine.

82. 1933 ZWORYKIN The invention of the television and the scanning electron microscope.

83. 1938 RUSKA The development of the transmission electron microscope

84. 1941 MARTIN The invention of partition chromatography and gas chromatography.

85. 1945 ECKERT, MAUCHLY ENIAC, the first programmable electronic computer.

86. 1946 KOLFF The introduction of the artificial kidney and other artificial organs.

87. 1951 ENGSTRÖM The first device for volume controlled artificial ventilation suitable for long term treatment.

88. 1953 WATSON, CRICK The structure of the DNA molecule established.

89. 1953 FANT Major advance in electronic speech analysis and synthesis.

90. 1954 EDLER, HERTZ Introducing ultrasound echo cardiography.

91. 1959 ELMQVIST, SENNING The presentation of the first fully implanted pacemaker.

92. 1960 MAIMAN The description of the first LASER and its mode of operation.

93. 1969 BRÅNEMARK Titanium implants in medicine and dentistry.

94. 1971 DAMADIAN Discovery and apparatus for differentiating biological tissue using NMR techniques.

95. 1973 HOUNSFIELD The inventions of X-ray CT-imaging.

96. 1973 LAUTERBUR A new general method of imaging biological tissue exemplified by the MRI technique.

97. 1974 WAGNER, WEST A new method of analysing the ventilation and perfusion conditions in the lungs.

98. 1974 KAHN, CERF A generally useful internet protocol for communication between data networks.

99. 1975 PHELPS The invention of the modern PET imaging technique.

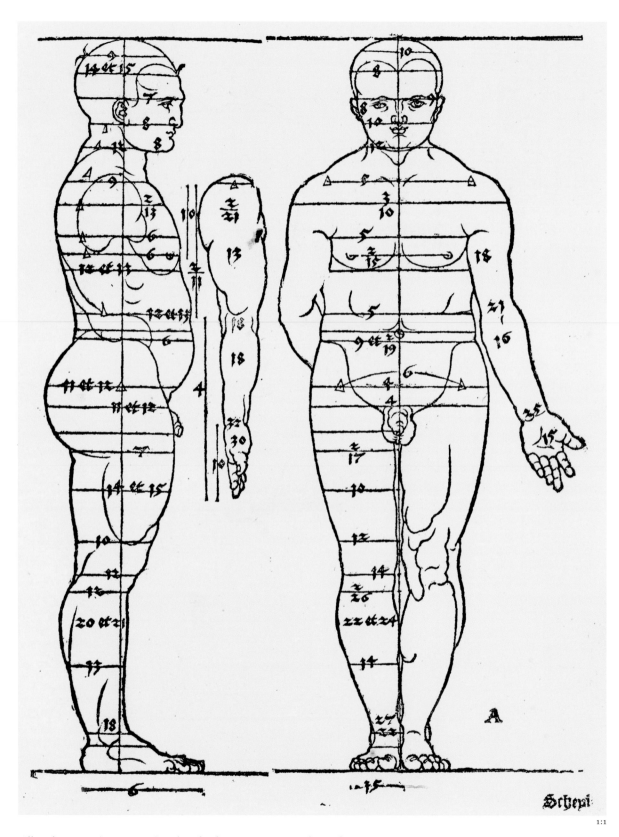

1:1

Albrecht Dürer (1471–1528) makes the first attempt to apply mathematics
to determine the proportions of the human body.

DÜRER was born in 1471 in Nuremberg, where he first studied goldsmithing with his father and then painting with Michael Wolgemut, a leading church painter. As a young man he travelled to Italy, where he was influenced by teachings of Euclid's geometry (1.1) and Vitruvius Pollio's architecture (1.2). His meeting in 1505 with Pacioli, the mathematician and theorist of art, (1.3) also greatly influenced his future work. As an artist he devoted much time to studying perspective and the spatial representation of objects (1.4). All these accumulated insights allowed him to apply mathematical techniques to creating images of the proportions, forms and the motion of the human body. His results were published in 1528 just after his death. The editor of the book, Pirckheimer, was a friend of Dürer, who painted his portrait in 1524.

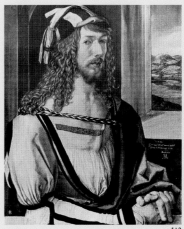

Albrecht Dürer, self-portrait 1498. Dürer was the first artist in Western art to make self-portraits.

Hierinn sind begriffen vier Bücher von menschlicher Proportion.

W. PIRCKHEIMER, EDITOR. NUREMBERG: HIERONYMUS ANDREA FORMSCHNEIDER FOR DÜRER'S WIDOW, 1528.

DÜRER'S PRESENTATION is the first attempt to apply mathematics to the description of the proportions and forms of the human body. These forms, according to Dürer, should be "constructed geometrically or arithmetically and made beautiful by the application of some canon of proportion" (1.5). The book is made up of four separate sections, the last of which is of greatest interest since here, he attempts to treat the movement of bodies in space, a problem involving new, complex and difficult analysis of descriptive spatial geometry. Dürer is believed to be the first to have taken on this challenge (1.5).

IN PERSPECTIVE:
Dürer was a contemporary of Leonardo da Vinci and both made significant advances in producing truthful images of the human body. However, Dürer's systematic approach to finding general mathematical rules to guide this work set him apart and in contrast to the anatomical work of Leonardo da Vinci, Dürer's mathematical treatment of the human form exerted significant influence for centuries. Only fifteen years after Dürer's death, Andreas Vesalius published his famous anatomical work describing the structure of the entire human body (1.6). Although such anatomical atlases grew more and more detailed, accurate and artistic over the following centuries (1.7), it is only with the advances in chemistry (1.8) and as a result the advent of photography (1.9) about three hundred years later, that the imaging of the human body and its motions could be studied with entirely scientific techniques, thereby reaching a significantly higher level of accuracy and sophistication (1.10)

1.1 Euclid. *Elementa geometriæ.* Venice; 1482.
1.2 Vitruvius Pollio M. *De architectura.* Rome; 1486.
1.3 Pacioli L. *De divina Proportione.* Venice; 1509.
1.4 Dürer A. *Underweysung der messung … zu nutz allen kunstlieb haben.* Nuremberg; 1525.
1.5 *Dictionary of Scientific Biography* IV p258. New York; 1970–1990.
1.6 Vesalius A. *De humani corporis fabrica libri septem.* Basel; 1543.
1.7 Bidloo G. *Anatomia humanis corporis & quinque tabulis, per artificiossis.* Amsterdam; 1685.
1.8 Scheele CW. *Sämtliche physische und chemische Werke Vol I, II.* Berlin; 1793. See also #21 Scheele page 120.
1.9 See #38 Daguerre page 202.
1.10 See #52 Marey page 272.

Luca Pacioli (1445–1514) Franciscan friar, mathematician and theorist of art, illustrating a theorem of Euclid.

The first printing of Euclid's Elementa geometria appears in 1482 in Venice.

1:3

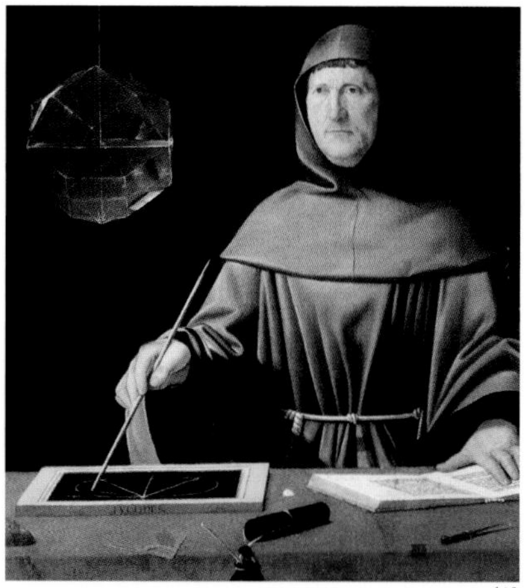

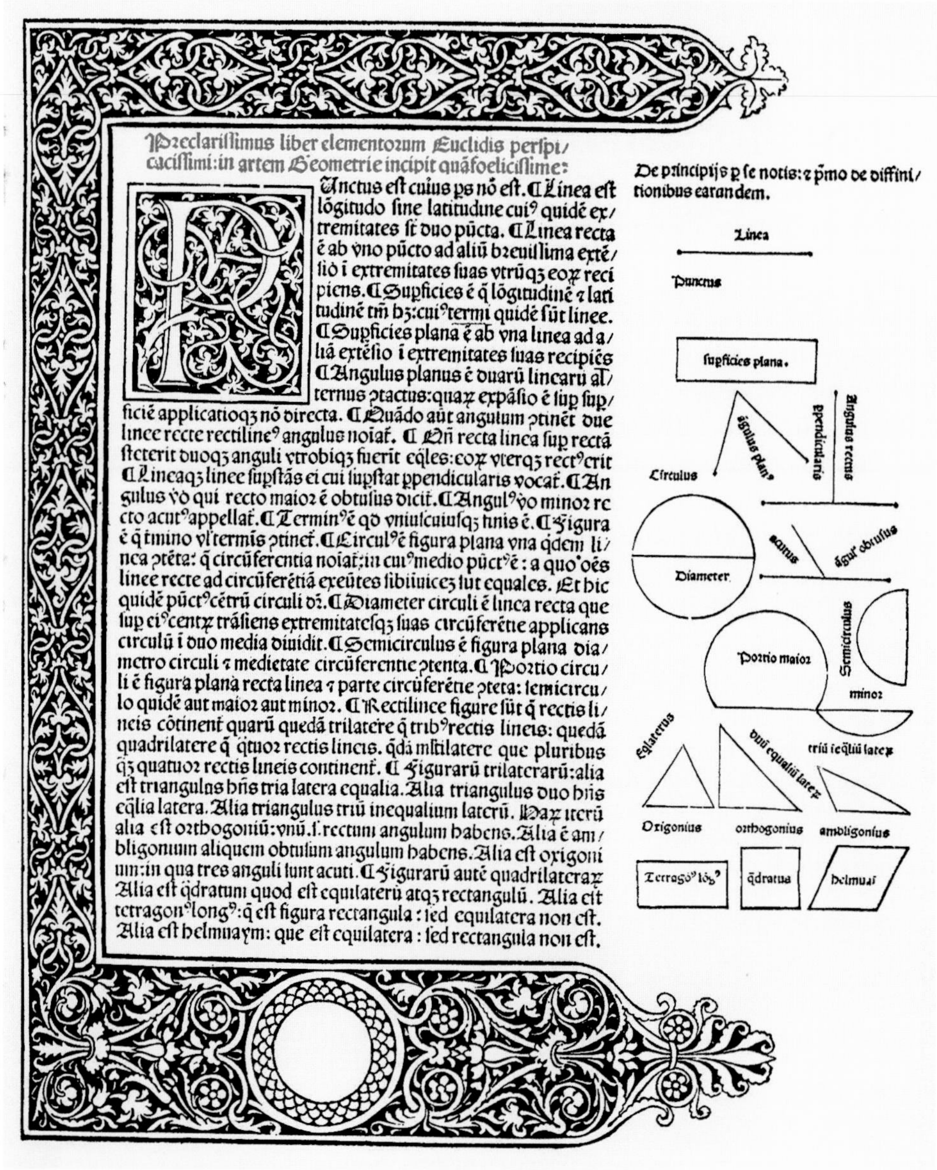

Preclarissimus liber elementorum Euclidis perspicacissimi: in artem Geometrie incipit quafoelicissime:

Punctus est cuius ps nō est. ¶ Linea est lōgitudo sine latitudine cui⁹ quidē extremitates sūt duo pūcta. ¶ Linea recta ē ab vno pūcto ad aliū breuissima extēsio i extremitates suas vtrūq3 eoꝝ recipiens. ¶ Suprficies ē q̄ lōgitudinē ꝛ latitudinē tm̄ hꝫ: cui⁹ termi quidē sūt linee. ¶ Suprficies plana ē ab vna linea ad aliā extēsio i extremitates suas recipiēs ¶ Angulus planus ē duarū linearū alternus ɔtactus: quaꝝ expāsio ē sup suprficiē applicatioq3 nō directa. ¶ Quādo aūt angulum ɔtinēt due linee recte rectiline⁹ angulus noiaṫ. ¶ Qñ recta linea sup rectā steterit duoq3 anguli vtrobiq3 fuerit eq̄les: eoꝝ vterq3 rect⁹ erit ¶ Lineaq3 linee supstās ei cui supstat ppendicularis vocaṫ. ¶ Angulus vō qui recto maior ē obtusus dicit. ¶ Angul⁹ vō minor recto acut⁹ appellaṫ. ¶ Termin⁹ ē qd vniuscuiusq3 finis ē. ¶ Figura ē q̄ tmino vl' termis ɔtineṫ. ¶ Circul⁹ ē figura plana vna q̄dem linea ɔtēta: q̄ circūferentia noiaṫ: in cui⁹ medio pūct⁹ ē: a quo ōes linee recte ad circūferētiā exeūtes sibiīuicē sut equales. Et hic quidē pūct⁹ cētrū circuli dr̄. ¶ Diameter circuli ē linea recta que sup ei⁹ centꝝ trāsiens extremitatesq3 suas circūferētie applicans circulū i duo media diuidit. ¶ Semicirculus ē figura plana diametro circuli ꝛ medietate circūferentie ɔtenta. ¶ Portio circuli ē figura planā recta linea ꝛ parte circūferētie ɔtēta: semicirculo quidē aut maior aut minor. ¶ Rectilinee figure sūt q̄ rectis lineis cōtineṅt quarū quedā trilaterē q̄ trib⁹ rectis lineis: quedā quadrilatere q̄ q̄tuor rectis lineis. q̄dā mltilatere que pluribus q3 quatuor rectis lineis continenṫ. ¶ Figurarū trilaterarū: alia est triangulus hñs tria latera equalia. Alia triangulus duo hñs eq̄lia latera. Alia triangulus triū inequalium laterū. Haꝝ iterū alia est orthogoniū: vnū. s. rectum angulum habens. Alia ē amblygonium aliquem obtusum angulum habens. Alia est oxygonium: in qua tres anguli sunt acuti. ¶ Figurarū autē quadrilateraꝝ Alia est q̄dratum quod est equilaterū atq3 rectangulū. Alia est tetragon⁹ long⁹: q̄ est figura rectangula: sed equilatera non est. Alia est helmuaym: que est equilatera: sed rectangula non est.

De principijs p se notis: ꝛ p̄mo de diffinitionibus earundem.

1:4

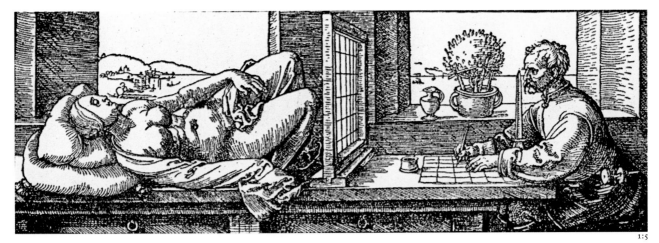

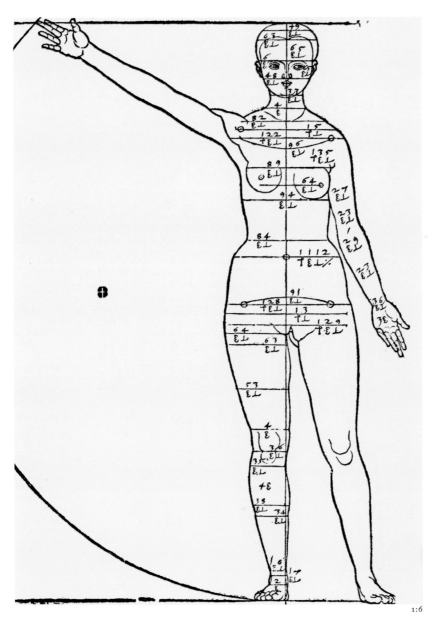

Dürer illustrates how to make a spatial representation of the female body.

The geometrical and arithmetical proportions of the female body. Dürer also attempts to treat the movement of bodies in space, a difficult problem of descriptive spatial geometry.

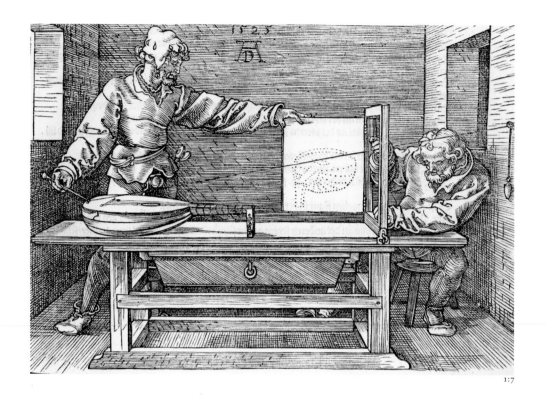

1:7

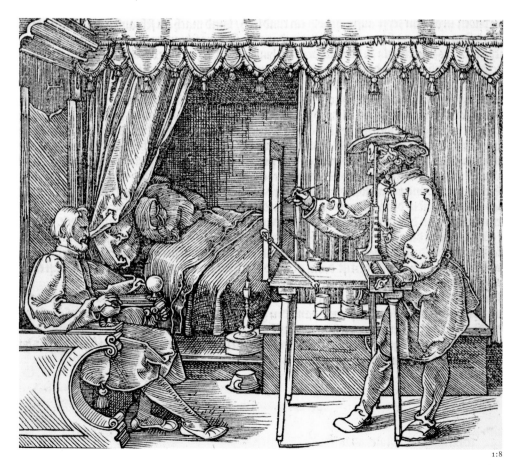

1:8

Dürer's famous illustrations of
geometric methods to reproduce
objects in space.

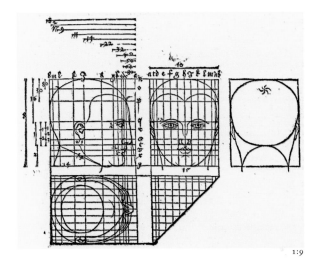

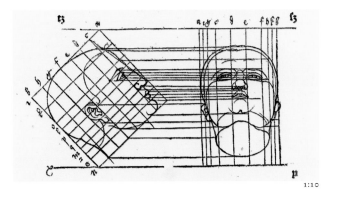

The proportions and projections
of the head and body of a child.

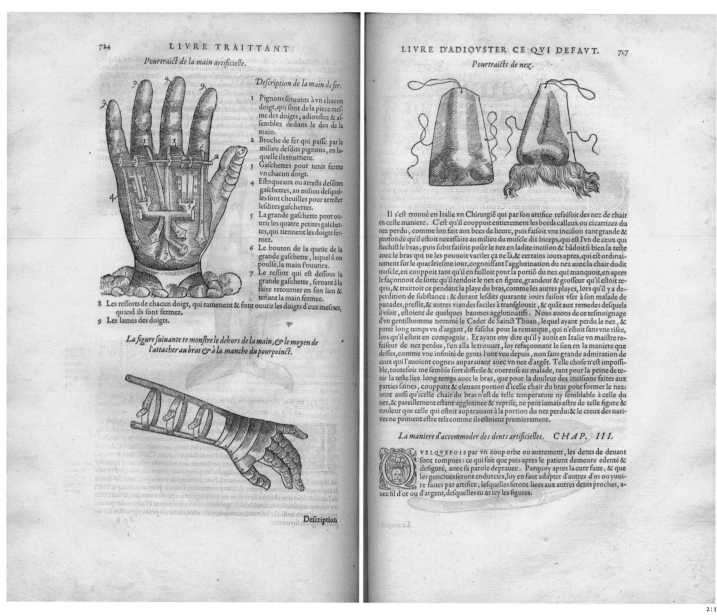

Pourtraict de la main artificielle.

Description de la main de fer.

1 Pignons seruants à vn chacun doigt, qui sont de la piece mesme des doigts, adioustez & assemblez dedans le dos de la main.

2 Broche de fer qui passe par le milieu desdits pignons, en laquelle ils tournent.

3 Gaschettes pour tenir ferme vn chacun doigt.

4 Estoqueaux ou arrests desdites gaschettes, au milieu desquelles sont cheuillez pour arrester lesdites gaschettes.

5 La grande gaschette pour ouurir les quatre petites gaschettes, qui tiennent les doigts fermez.

6 Le bouton de la queüe de la grande gaschette, lequel si on pousse, la main s'ouurira.

7 Le ressort qui est dessous la grande gaschette, seruant à la faire retourner en son lieu & tenant la main fermee.

8 Les ressorts de chacun doigt, qui ramenent & font ouurir les doigts d'eux mesmes, quand ils sont fermez.

9 Les lames des doigts.

La figure suiuante te monstre le dehors de la main, & le moyen de l'attacher au bras & à la manche du pourpoinct.

Description

Pourtraicts de nez.

Il s'est trouué en Italie vn Chirurgië qui par son artifice refaisoit des nez de chair en ceste maniere. C'est qu'il couppoit entierement les bords calleux ou cicatrizez du nez perdu, comme l'on fait aux becs de lieure, puis faisoit vne incision tant grande & profonde qu'il estoit necessaire au milieu du muscle dit biceps, qui est l'vn de ceux qui flechist le bras, puis subit faisoit poser le nez en ladite incision & bãdoit si bien la teste auec le bras qui ne les pouuoit vaciler çà ne là, & certains iours apres, qui est ordinairement sur le quarãtiesme iour, cognoissant l'agglutination du nez auec la chair dudit muscle, en couppoit tant qu'il en falloit pour la portiõ du nez qui manquoit, & apres le façonnoit de sorte qu'il rendoit le nez en figure, grandeur & grosseur qu'il estoit requis, & traittoit ce pendant la playe du bras, comme les autres playes, lors qu'il y a deperdition de substance: & durant lesdits quarante iours faisoit vser à son malade de panades, pressis, & autres viandes faciles à transgloutir, & quãt aux remedes desquels il vsoit, estoient de quelques baumes agglutinatifs. Nous auons de ce tesmoignage d'vn gentilhomme nommé le Cadet de Sainct Thoan, lequel ayant perdu le nez, & porté long temps vn d'argent, se fascha pour la remarque, qui n'estoit sans vne risee, lors qu'il estoit en compagnie. Et ayant ouy dire qu'il y auoit en Italie vn maistre refaiseur de nez perdus, s'en alla le trouuer, luy refaçonnant le sien en la maniere que dessus, comme vne infinité de gents l'ont veu depuis, non sans grande admiration de ceux qui l'auoient cognu auparauant auec vn nez d'argẽt. Telle chose n'est impossible, toutefois me semble fort difficile & onereuse au malade, tant pour la peine de tenir la teste liee long temps auec le bras, que pour la douleur des incisions faites aux parties saines, couppant & eleuant portion d'icelle chair du bras pour former le nez: ioint aussi qu'icelle chair du bras n'est de telle temperature ny semblable à celle du nez, & pareillement estant agglutinee & reprise, ne peut iamais estre de telle figure & couleur que celle qui estoit auparauant à la portion du nez perdu: & le creux des narines ne peuuent estre tels comme ils estoient premierement.

La maniere d'accommoder des dents artificielles.   **CHAP. III.**

VELQVEFOIS par vn coup orbe ou autrement, les dents de deuant sont rompues: ce qui fait que puis apres le patient demeure edenté & desfiguré, auec sa parole deprauee. Parquoy apres la cure faite, & que les gencies seront endurcies, luy en faut adapter d'autres d'os ou yuoire faites par artifice, lesquelles seront liees aux autres dents proches, auec fil d'or ou d'argent, desquelles tu as icy les figures.

Le moyen

The new weapons of the 16th century confronted surgeons with problems unknown to the ancient medical authorities. Ambroise Paré (1510-1590) introduces new methods of wound treatment and designs prostheses for upper and lower extremities as well as artificial noses and eyes of gold and silver. He also constructs a mechanical hand using springs and catches.

PARÉ was born in Laval, France in 1510 and already as a young boy he became apprentice to a barber-surgeon. At the age of twenty-six he became master barber-surgeon and entered military service. For more than three decades he followed the military campaigns of the Wars of Religion, serving King Henry II and later Charles IX and Henry III as the "first military surgeon". His unorthodox methods of wound treatment and his lack of knowledge of Latin (with little formal education the only language he knew was French) put him constantly at odds with the Medical Faculty of the University of Paris, which tried in vain to surpress his writings. Paré was an honest, compassionate person, much liked by his patients. He was deeply religious and had as his motto "I treated him, God cured him".

Les œuvres. Avec les figures & portraicts tant de l'Anatomie que des instruments de Chirurgie, & de plusieurs Monstres.

PARIS: G. BUON, 1575.

IN HIS collected works Paré gives a famous account of how he ran out of boiling oil at the siege of Turin in 1536 and replaced it with an improvised wound dressing made up of egg yolk, oil of roses and turpentine and found it to be superior in reducing infection and promoting wound healing. He opposes cautery for achieving haemostasis and advocates ligature of blood vessels. He also introduces new techniques in obstetrical surgery. In his collected works he describes prostheses of his own design for upper and lower extremities and a hand operated by springs and catches, as well as artificial noses and eyes of gold and silver.

IN PERSPECTIVE:

Paré, just like his contemporaries Vesalius and Paracelsus (2.1), was able to break away from authority and pioneer the developments that would grow strong during the following century. The new weapons of the 16th century confronted surgeons with problems unknown to the ancient medical authorities. However, most of the instruments and techniques available remained similar to those used since Greco-Roman times (2.2)(2.3)(2.4). Major advances first came during the 19th century, when progress in science and technology added new and more sophisticated functionality to surgical instrumentation (2.5). As an example, Middeldorpf introduced galvanocautery in 1854 (2.6). The effect of high frequency currents on tissue was first investigated by d'Arsonval in 1893 (2.7) and the first electrosurgical unit was conceived by de Forest in 1907 (2.8). The development of modern prosthetic engineering is to a large extent based on advances in material science (2.9) and the explosive progress in microelectronics and computers (2.10) during the second half of the 20th century.

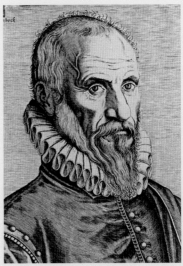

Ambroise Paré at the age of seventy-five.

2:2

2.1 See #3 Paracelsus page 32 and ref. 1.6.
2.2 Milne JS. *Surgical Instruments in Greek and Roman times*. Oxford; 1907.
2.3 Brunschwig H. *Chirurgia*. Strassburg; 1497.
2.4 von Gersdorff H. *Feldbuch der wundarztney*. Strassburg; 1517.
2.5 See #60 Nitze page 310.
2.6 Middeldorpf AT. *Die Galvanokaustik*. Breslau; 1854.
2.7 d'Arsonval A. Action physiologique des courant alternatifs. *Arch Physiol Norm. Path*. 1893;5:401.
2.8 de Forest L. Cautery. U.S.Patent 874,178 Dec. 17; 1907.
2.9 See #78 Staudinger page 400, #80 Carothers page 410 and #93 Brånemark page 480.
2.10 See #85 Mauchley-Eckert page 438.

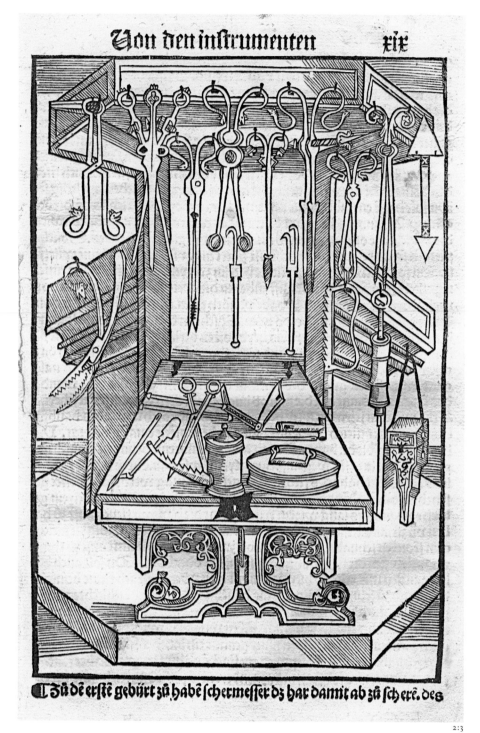

Zů dē erstē gebůrt zů habē schermesser dz har damit ab zů scherē. des

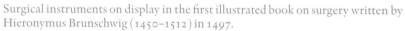

Surgical instruments on display in the first illustrated book on surgery written by Hieronymus Brunschwig (1450–1512) in 1497.

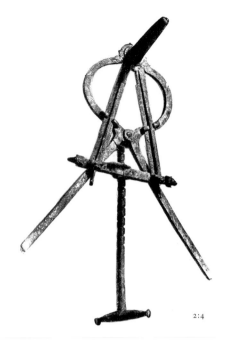

Roman vaginal speculum (top) and a vaginal speculum from 1517 according to von Gersdorff (1455–1529). Although from entirely different epochs, the instruments are strikingly similar.

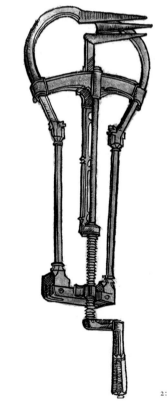

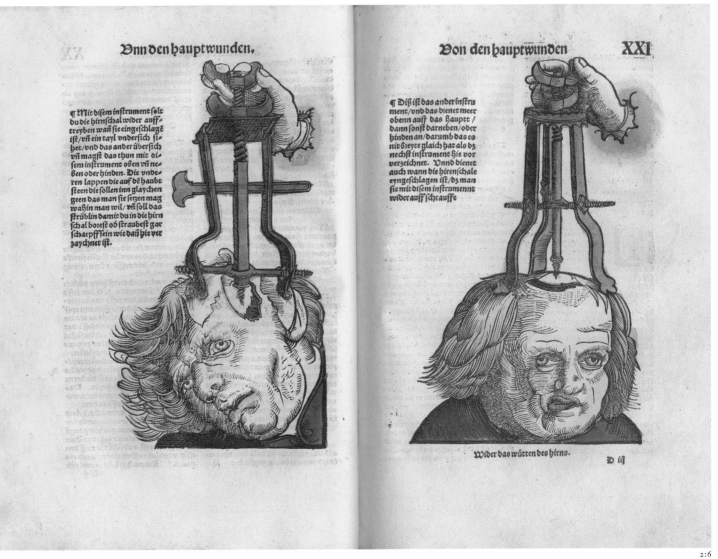

¶ Mit disem instrument solt du die hirnschal wider auff treyben wann sie eingeschlagē ist/vnd ein tayl vndersich si het/vnd das ander übersich vñ magst das thun mit di sem instrumente oben vñ ne ben oder hinden. Die vnde ren lappen die auf dē haubt steen die sollen inn glaychen geen das man sie setzen mag wahin man wil/ vñ soll das ströblin damit du in die hirn schal borest oð straubest gar scharpff sein wie dañ hie ver zaychnet ist.

¶ Diß ist das ander instru ment/vnd das dienet meer obenn auff das Haupt / dann sonst darneben/oder hinden an/darumb das es nit ðreyce glaich hat als ðz nechst instrument hie vor verzeichnet. Vnnd dienet auch wann die hirenschale eyngeschlagen ist/ðz man sie mit disem instrumennt wider auff schrauffe

Wider das wütten des hirns.

D iij

Instrument and method for opening the skull as described in 1517 by von Gersdorff.

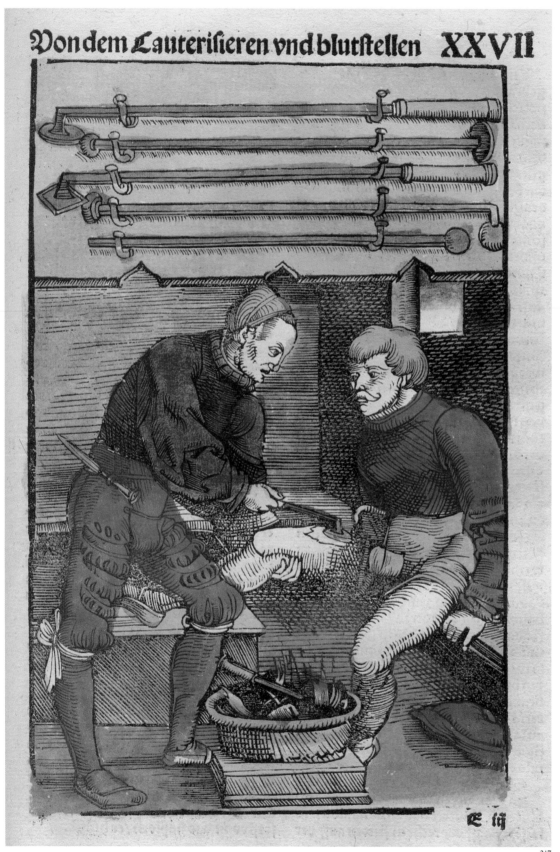

Cauterisation by hot iron in
1517 according to von Gersdorff.

2:7

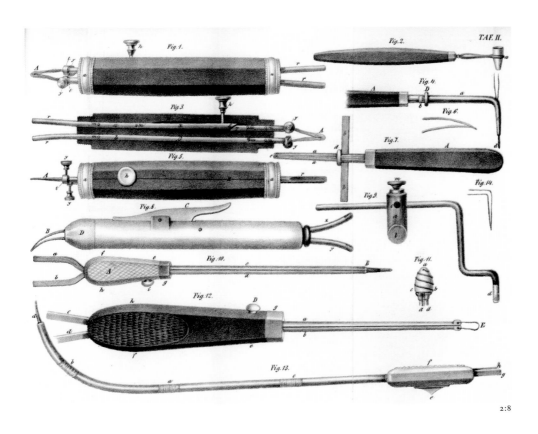

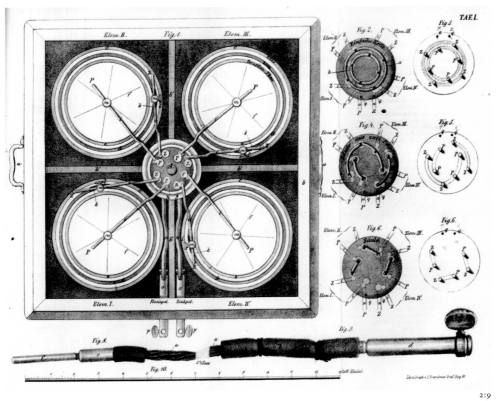

The first instrument for galvanocautery introduced by Albrecht Middeldorpf (1824–1868) in 1854.

Nuhn wissent von dem Embryonato Sulphure im Vitriol vnnd seins gleichen / was Species Vitrioli seindt / als die Salia, das sie alle gar wunderbarlichen Sulphur geben / in dem / so die Corpora Animantata geschieden werden von den Corporibus Embryonatis. Als vom Saltz / vom Salgemmen / von den Speciebus Aluminis, von den Vitriolis, &c. Nuhn aber ein kurtze Regel will ich euch inn gemein geben / das alle Sulphura von den Vitriolatis Salibus, Stupefactiua seindt / Narcotica, Anodyna, Somnifera: Vnnd aber mit einer solchen Proprietet / das an dem orth die Somniferisch arth / so ruwig vnnd so mildt hingeht / daß ohn allen schaden sich abzeucht / nichts auff Opiatische wirckung / als in Iulquiamo, Papauere, Mandragora, &c. sondern gar Mildt / Tugendtlich / ohn all Infectiff. Darumb ich das zum hochsten lob / das ein solch Somniferum Stupefactiuum soll von der Natur selbst Decoquiert sein / Praepariert vnnd Corrigiert. Vnnd dieweil wir Artzt alle sehendt / das die Somnitera viel thundt / vnnd grosse ding thundt / vnnd das aber in den Opiaten ein solchs Gifft ist / das sie nicht zu gebrauchen seindt ohn die gestalt Quintae Essentiae: So sollen wir vnser Zuflucht vnd Verstandt dester mehr setzen hie an das orth / dieweil wir wissen / das viel franckheiten seindt / die ohn Anodyna nicht mögendt geheylt werden / vnnd all jhr Cur in die Anodynen gesetzt seindt von Gott durch die Natur. Darumb bewegt mich dasselbig / diesen Sulphur dester baß zu beschreiben: Wie er gefunde wird / vnnd wie man jhn zu wegen bringet / werdt jhr finden inn den Alchimistischen Processen. Hie sollendt jhr aber wissen von diesem Sulphur / das vnter allen der vom Vitriol am bekanntlichsten ist / das er an jhm selbst Fir ist: Zum andern hatt er ein Suesse / das jhn die Hüner all essen / vnd aber endtschlaffen auff ein Zeit / ohn schaden wieder auffstohndt. Diesen Sulphur sollendt jhr nicht anderst erkennen / dann wo es ist / das ein Kranckheit durch Anodyna soll Curiert werden / das dieser Sulphur thun mag ohn allen schaden / alle Passiones legt er / Sediert ohn schaden alle Dolores, Extinguiert alle Calores, Mitigiert alle grimmige Furnemmen der Kranckheiten: Vnd ist ein Artzney / die in allen dingen soll vorgehn / vnd die Cur / das ist das Confortatiff Quintae Essentiae hernach.

Was

3:1

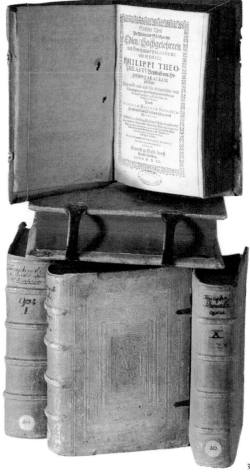

The collected works of Paracelsus (1493–1541), printed around 1590, where he says about ether: "sulphur derived from vitriols and salts is stupefactive, narcotic, analgesic and hypnotic. It acts in a mild and transient way, unlike hyoscyamus, poppy and mandragora." Further down the page he notes: "Chicken will eat it, whereupon they sleep for a moderately long time and wake again without injury."

3:2

PARACELSUS was born in 1493 in Einsiedeln, Switzerland. His early education in mineralogy, botany and natural philosophy was given by his father. Later, he studied under prominent clergy and at Italian universities. He travelled widely but finally settled in Basel where his practice of medicine was initially highly successful. In 1527 he was appointed professor and municipal physician, but the year after he was removed from his duties and expelled from the city because of his extreme views and outrageous behaviour. At the time of his death he was a wandering lay preacher. Paracelsus was a brilliant but highly controversial person who could alienate even his best friends. He was a hard drinker, never short of money, and treated the poor for free while demanding high fees from the rich.

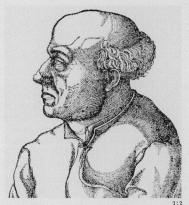

3:3
Theophrastus Bombastus von Hohenheim, also named Paracelsus.

Der Buecher und Schrifften …

IOANNEM HUSERUM. BASEL: C. WALDKIRCH, 1589–1590.

THESE ARE Paracelsus' collected works, based directly on his own writings, in ten volumes. Paracelsus attacks alchemy and traditional medicine based on the four humours (blood, phlegm, yellow and black bile). He rejects the herbal remedies of the ancients (3.1) and introduces compounds of mercury, lead, arsenic, antimony and sulphur in the pharmacopoeia. He directs his therapy against the causes rather than the symptoms of diseases. Paracelsus sees a unity between cosmos and medicine with chemistry as a means of improving practical treatment. He writes on occupational (miners') disease and in the work De Naturalibus Rebus (ca 1540) he reports for the first time the anaesthetic effects of ether (3.2), a substance probably first produced by Cordus (3.3).

IN PERSPECTIVE:
After his death Paracelsus' teachings were widely spread and heatedly debated for about a century. In the end, chemical therapy became increasingly accepted in medicine and his ideas were blended into the move towards chemical physiology, as pioneered by men like van Helmont and Boyle (3.4) His vehement criticism of the ancient authorities foreshadowed the fundamental changes towards a mechanistic approach to science and medicine that took place during the following century (3.5). More than two hundred years after Paracelsus' observations on the effects of ether, Turner recommended sniffing it up the nostrils to combat headaches (3.6). Long first used ether for minor surgery in his dental practice in 1842 (3.7). However, not until his colleague Morton introduced it with the help of Jackson (3.8)(3.9) in the surgical theatre of the Massachusetts General Hospital in 1846 (3.10) did ether gain general acceptance and widespread use.

3.1 Dioscorides P. *De materia medica.* Johannes of Medemblick Colle; 1478. See also *Der Wiener Dioscorides.* Codex Medicus 1,2 Akademische Druck- u Verlagsanstalt: Graz; 1998–1999.

3.2 Paracelsus. *Der Buecher und Schriften.* Vol. VII; 1590. p172.

3.3 Gesner C. *Annotationes in Pedacij Dioscoridis … De Medica Materia.* De artificiosis extractionibus. Strassburg; 1561.

3.4 See #8 van Helmont page 60, #14 Boyle page 88 and #75 Ehrlich page 386.

3.5 See #4 Santorio page 36.

3.6 Turner M. *An Account of the extraordinary medical fluid called Aether.* Liverpool; 1761.

3.7 Long CW. An Account of the First Use of sulphuric Ether … *Southern Med Surg J.* 1849;5(12):705.

3.8 Jackson ChT. *A Manual of Etherization.* Boston; 1861.

3.9 Morton W. *Remarks on the Proper Mode of Administering Sulphuric Ether by Inhalation.* Boston; 1847.

3.10 Bigelow HJ. Insensibility during surgical operations produced by inhalation. *Bost Med Surg J.* 1846; XXXV(16): 309

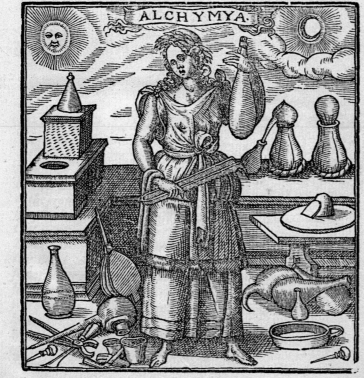

The practife of the new and old phificke, wherein is contained the moft excellent Secrets of Phificke and Philofophie, deuided into foure Bookes. In the which are the beft approued remedies for the difeafes as well inward as outward, of al the parts of mans body : treating very amplie of al diftillations of waters, of oyles, balmes, Quinteffences, with the extraction of artificiall faltes, the vfe and preparation of Antimony, and potable Gold. Gathered out of the beft & moft approued Authors, by that excellent Doctor Gefnerus. Alfo the Pictures and maner to make the Veffels, Furnaces, and other Inftruments thereunto belonging. Newly corrected and publifhed in Englifh, by George Baker, one of the Queenes Maicfties chiefe Chirurgians in ordinary.

ALCHYMYA.

Printed at London, by Peter Short. 1599.

3:4

An early English translation of alchemical texts that includes Conrad Gesner's (1516–1565) description of Cordus's procedure for producing ether: Equal parts of spirit of wine (alcohol) which has been rectified three times and sulphuric acid are allowed to remain in contact for two months, and then the mixture is distilled from a water- or sand-bath; the distillate consists of two layers of liquid of which the upper one is the oleum vitrioli dulce verum or sweet oil of vitriol (ether).

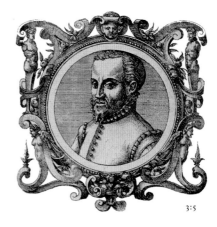

3:5

Valerius Cordus (1515–1544), botanist and apothecary who discovers a method of synthesising ether.

In 1761 Matthew Turner, a surgeon in Liverpool, manufactures and sells ether as an oral remedy for many ailments, i.e. most nervous diseases, gout, rheumatism, pains in the stomach and whooping cough. For headache, however, he recommends it to be snuffed up the nostrils, which gives him a place in the history of inhalation anaesthesia.

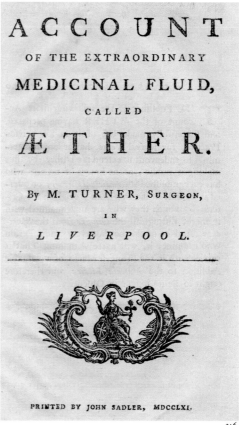

ACCOUNT

OF THE EXTRAORDINARY

MEDICINAL FLUID,

CALLED

ÆTHER.

By M. TURNER, Surgeon,

IN

LIVERPOOL.

PRINTED BY JOHN SADLER, MDCCLXI.

3:6

TO THE

SURGEONS OF THE MASS. GEN. HOSPITAL,

THIS LITTLE WORK IS RESPECTFULLY DEDICATED,

AS AN EVIDENCE

THAT THEIR EARLY AND CONTINUED INTEREST IN THE ADMIN-
ISTRATION OF SULPHURIC ETHER

IS GRATEFULLY APPRECIATED,

BY THEIR

OBT. SERVT.

WM. T. G. MORTON.

3:7

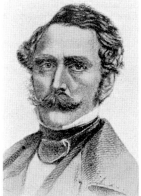

3:9

CHAPTER VI.

ADMINISTRATION OF ETHER BY INHALATION.

How should the Ether be administered?

AT first I made use of a towel, folded into a cone, the interior of which was saturated with ether. This was placed over the nose and mouth loosely, so as to allow the entrance of air all around it, or an opening was left in the apex of the cone. This is a very good method, when chloroform or a mixture of chloroform and ether are employed. I also made use of sponges, placed in a large, short, glass tube, or a funnel, saturated with ether. See my letter of 13th Nov., 1846, published by the French Academy of Sciences. Apparatus for inhaling having been called for, I proposed to make use of a large flask, with a tube loosely fitted to it, and reaching near to a mass of sponges, at its bottom, saturated with ether. I

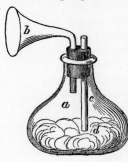

FIG. 2. The first form of Inhaler employed by me.
a. Glass flask, of three pints capacity.
b. Mouth-piece for inhalation of ether vapor.
c. Tube for admission of air and for supplying the sponges with more ether.
d. Sponges, wet with ether.

The air is drawn down the tube c, and over the sponges, wet with ether, which evaporates and mingles with the air, and is then drawn into the lungs through the tube and mouth-piece. A flap of buck-skin, attached to the rim of the mouth-piece, makes the contact over the mouth secure. The air is inhaled and exhaled through the apparatus freely.

3:8

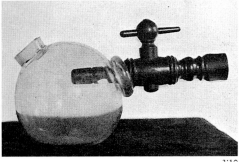

3:10

William Morton (1819–1868), his ether inhaler and a note of gratitude to the surgeons of the Massachusetts General Hospital, published in his account of the first use of ether in 1846.

Charles Jackson's (1805–1880) treatise on ether. Jackson accidentally inhales ether in 1841 and discovers its analgesic property. Later he teaches William Morton chemistry and makes claim to the priority of having discovered the benefit of ether for surgical anaesthesia.

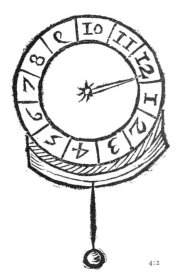

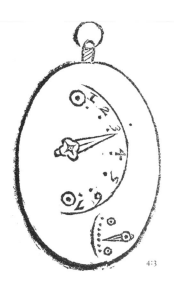

4:2

4:3

METHODI
Vitandorum errorum
Omnium,
QVI IN ARTE MEDICA
CONTINGVNT
Libri Quindecim,

Quorum principia sunt ab auctoritate Medicorum, & Philosophorum principum desumpta, eaq; omnia experimentis, & rationibus analyticis comprobata.

SANCTORIO SANCTORIO
IVSTINOPOLITANO
Medico, & Philosopho
AVCTORE
AD FERDINANDVM
AVSTRIÆ
ARCHIDVCEM SERENISSIMVM,
& inuictissimum.

CVM TRIPLICI INDICE VNO LIBRORVM,
altero Capitum omnium, tertio rerum notabilium.
CVM PRIVILEGIIS.

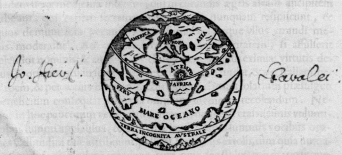

VENETIIS, M·DCIII·
Apud Franciscum Barilettum. N

4:1

Santorio Santorio (1561–1636) introduces quantitative measurements in medicine and describes methods and instruments for measuring the pulse.

SANTORIO was born in Slovenia in 1561, the son of a noble family. After studies of classical languages and literature, he turned to philosophy and medicine, earning his doctorate in 1582. He practised medicine in Croatia and then in Venice, where he made the acquaintance of the physicist Galileo Galilei. With an increasing reputation as a practitioner and supported by the nobility, he was appointed professor of theoretical medicine at the University of Padua. At the end of his second term in 1624 he returned to Venice, where he spent the rest of his life. Santorio was an excellent orator and a popular teacher. He had a cautious, restrained personality and his original ideas were always presented as part of accepted doctrine. With no family and little interest in personal comfort, he amassed a personal fortune during his life.

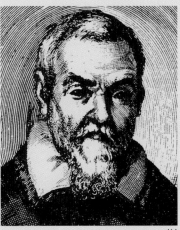

Santorio Santorio   4:4

Methodi vitandorum errorum omnium qui in arte medica contingunt.

VENICE: F. BARILETTUS, 1603.

IN THIS book of practical medicine Santorio describes methods to avoid making mistakes in the art of healing. He introduces the concept of specific, defined disease states and calculates them to be 80,085 in number. More importantly, he says that "number, position and form" greatly influences the living organism and thus deserves study. For this purpose he designs instruments (here for the measurement of the pulse), thereby introducing quantitative measurements in medicine. He summarises his philosophy thus: "One must believe first in one's own senses and in experience, then in reasoning, and only in the third place in the authority of Hippocrates, of Galen, of Aristotle and other excellent philosophers" (4.1)(4.2).

IN PERSPECTIVE:
Santorio was the first exponent of the mechanistic view of the body, which was fully developed by Descartes (4.3), encouraged by the remarkable advances in physics during the 17th century (4.4)(4.5). Also, Boyle's later call for well-defined quantities and concepts in chemistry and his insistence on scientific experiments to verify hypotheses catalysed the change from alchemy to the chemical revolution of Lavoisier (4.6). During the 18th century physiological observations that could not be explained by the mechanical approach gave rise to "vitalism", insisting on living matter containing "sensitive soul" and a "vital force" (4.7). However, by the mid 19th century progress in many branches of science and physiology made it increasingly clear that there was no need to seek explanations based on such an ill-defined notion (4.8)(4.9). During the 20th century the increasing influence of science and technology stimulated (4.10) and greatly empowered the practice of medicine but also gave rise to new dilemmas (4.11).

4.1 Aristotle. *Opera …Venice*; 1482. Collected scientific writings printed in Augsburg 1518.

4.2 Galenus C. *Omnia quae extant opera*. Venice; 1550.

4.3 Descartes R. *De homine figuris*. Leyden; 1662.

4.4 Galilei G. *Discorsi e demonsrazioni matematiche, intorno a due nuoue scienze, …* Leiden; 1638.

4.5 Newton I. *Philosophia Naturalis Principia Mathematica*. London; 1687.

4.6 Boyle R. *The sceptical chymist or chymico-physical Doubts & Paradoxes*. London; 1661. See also #24 Lavoisier page 134.

4.7 Stahl G. *Theoria Medica*. Vera Halle; 1708.

4.8 Bernard C. *Introduction à l'etude de la médecine expérimentale*. Paris; 1865.

4.9 von Helmholtz H. *Das Denken in der Medizin*. Berlin; 1877. Also #42 Du Bois-Reymond page 224.

4.10 Schrödinger E. *What is life?* Cambridge; 1944.

4.11 Reiser SJ. *Medicine and the reign of technology*. Cambridge University Press: Cambridge; 1978. See also #98 Cerf-Kahn page 508.

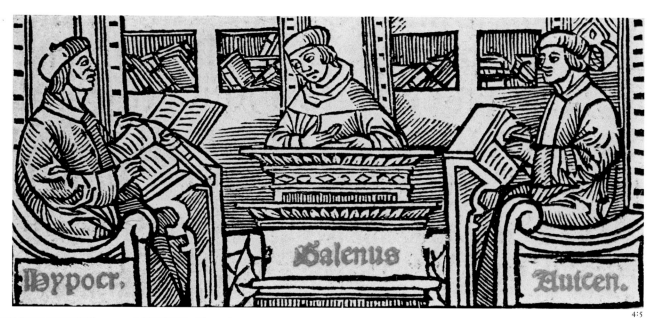

The ancient authorities of medicine, (from left to right) Hippocrates (460–377BC) Galen (130–200AD) and Avicenna (980–1037AD). Their dogma is respectfully challenged by Santorio.

4:5

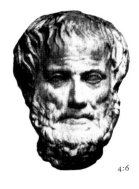

4:6

Aristotle (384–322BC) and his ideas about the location of sensory functions in the brain. Illustration from Aristotle's collected scientific writings printed in the early 16th century.

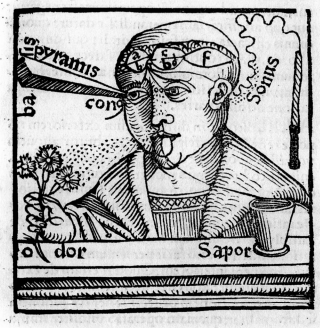

4:7

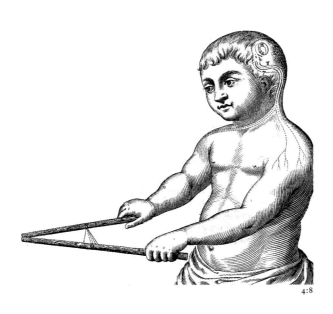

4:8

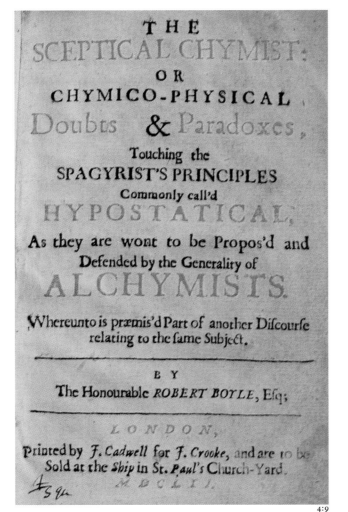

4:9

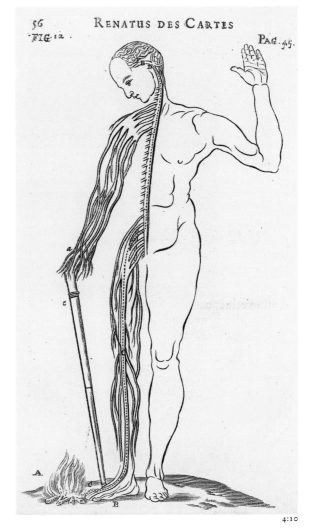

4:10

The location and mechanism of some sensory functions according to René Descartes (1596–1650). Illustrations from what is known as the first book in physiology from 1662, where Descartes attempts to cover all functions of the body.

Title page of Robert Boyle's (1627–1691) important work The Sceptical Chymist, where he insists on the use of clear language, well-defined concepts and scientific experiments to verify any hypothesis. He thereby ushers in the transition from alchemy to the modern science of chemistry.

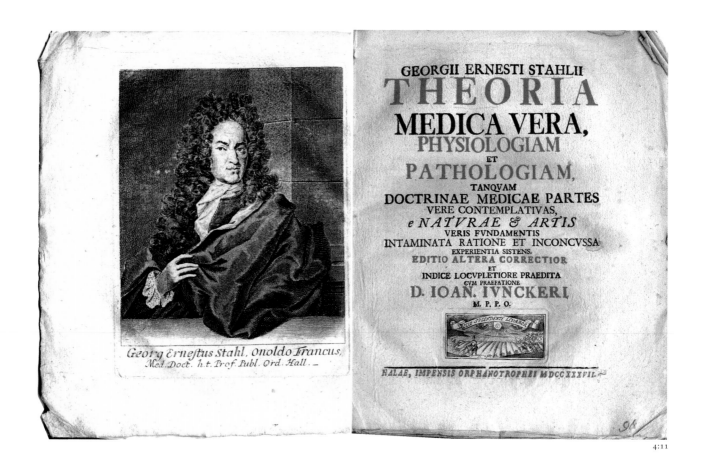

GEORGII ERNESTI STAHLII
THEORIA
MEDICA VERA,
PHYSIOLOGIAM
ET
PATHOLOGIAM,
TANQVAM
DOCTRINAE MEDICAE PARTES
VERE CONTEMPLATIVAS,
e NATVRAE & ARTIS
VERIS FVNDAMENTIS
INTAMINATA RATIONE ET INCONCVSSA
EXPERIENTIA SISTENS,
EDITIO ALTERA CORRECTIOR
ET
INDICE LOCVPLETIORE PRAEDITA
CVM PRAEFATIONE
D. IOAN. IVNCKERI
M. P. P. O.

HALAE, IMPENSIS ORPHANOTROPHEI MDCCXXXVII.

Georg Erneſtus Stahl, Onoldo Francus,
Med. Doct. h.t. Prof. Publ. Ord. Hall.

4:11

Georg Stahl (1660–1734) introduces a new concept, vitalism, to account for many of the shortcomings of the mechanistic view of the human body.

Herman von Helmholtz (1821–1894) (left) and Claude Bernard (1813–1878), leading figures in the scientific movement that during the 19th century greatly advanced knowledge of physiology and made vitalism obsolete.

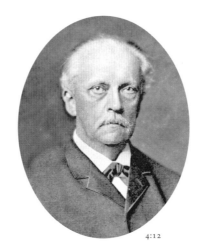

4:12

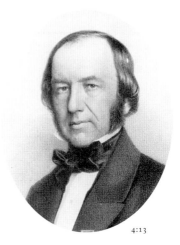

4:13

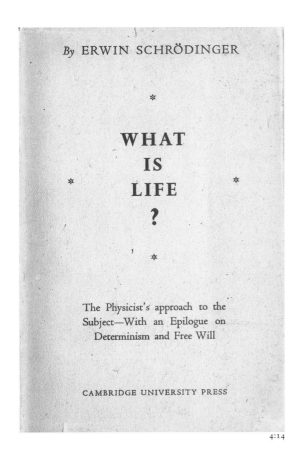

By ERWIN SCHRÖDINGER

✳

**WHAT
IS
LIFE
?**

✳

The Physicist's approach to the
Subject—With an Epilogue on
Determinism and Free Will

CAMBRIDGE UNIVERSITY PRESS

4:14

Erwin Schrödinger (1887–1961), one of the
founders of quantum mechanics, and his influential
book on a physicist's view of what life is. Later, all
three recipients of the 1962 Nobel Prize in medicine,
James Watson, Francis Crick (see #88) and Maurice
Wilkins, testified to how Schrödinger's book turned
their interest towards what later became known as
"molecular biology".

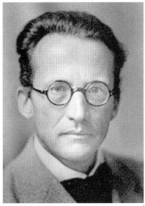

4:16

CONTENTS

4:17

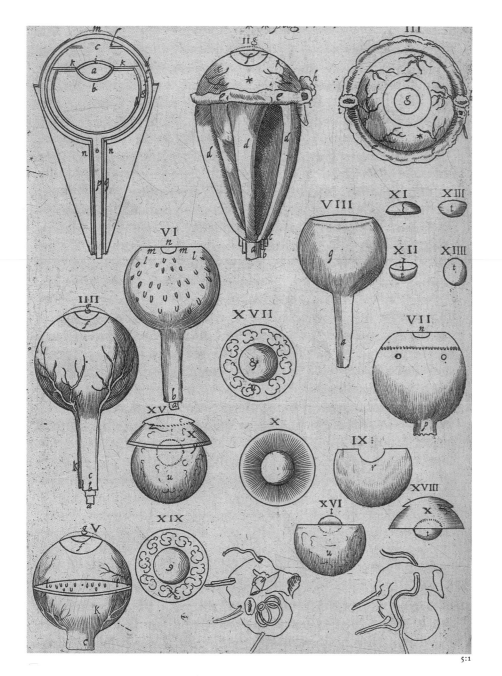

Johannes Kepler's (1571–1630) description of the anatomy of the eye (left) is based on the work of the Arabic scholar Alhazen (965–1039AD) which was available to him as a Latin translation from the 12th century. Below, Alhazen's drawing of the cross section of the eye.

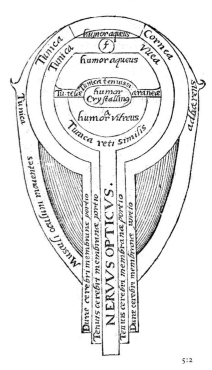

5:1

5:2

JOHANNES Kepler was born in Weil der Stadt in Germany in 1571. His father, a criminally inclined mercenary, left the family when Kepler was seventeen years old. Although intent on becoming a clergyman, Kepler was requested by the University of Tübingen to accept a job in Graz as a school teacher in mathematics. With too few students, his interest first turned to astrology and then to astronomy, setting him off on his famous discoveries of the laws of planetary motion. Kepler was a small, sickly person, restless and eager to distinguish himself. He was deeply religious and believed that God created the universe for order and harmony, and that God's work could be revealed through the tools of mathematics.

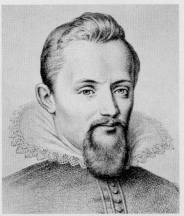

Johannes Kepler   5:3

Ad Vitellionem Paralipomena, quibus Astronomiae Pars Optica traditur.

FRANKFURT AM MAIN: C. MARNIUS & HEIRS OF J. AUBRIUS, 1604.

KEPLER WRITES this treatise (Supplement to Witello, Expounding the Optical Part of Astronomy) after having observed the partial solar eclipse of the year 1600. Using a pin hole camera, he determines the diameter of the moon, which requires a careful analysis of how the image is formed by the light rays. Overcoming the errors of earlier work, Kepler postulates that each point on the object has a corresponding point in the image and that the image point falls on the retina after refraction in the eye. Using the novel concept of "focus" and "pencil of light", Kepler shows that the image on the retina is unfocused and inverted. He also formulates for the first time the photometric inverse-square law.

IN PERSPECTIVE:
Euclid wrote on the reflection and refraction of light and on vision in about 300 B.C. (5.1). The Arabic scholar Alhazen studied lenses and the structure of the eye in about 1000 A.D. and Witelo investigated in around 1270 A.D. what later became known as the sine law of refraction (5.2)(5.3). At about the same time, Bacon studied image formation and suggested the use of convex lenses for magnification (5.4). In 1583 Bartisch published the first book on the equipment and methods of ophthalmology (5.5). Kepler's work, which he developed further after the invention of the telescope (5.6), laid the foundations of the theory of vision and was soon followed by Scheiner's study of the accommodation of the eye (5.7). Eye glasses, first described in 1623 (5.8), have been in use at least since the 14th century (5.9), while contact lenses were introduced by several investigators first in 1888 (5.10). Helmholtz developed a model for colour vision previously introduced by Young (5.11)(5.12) and wrote a classic monograph on physiological optics (5.13).

5.1   Euclid. *Optica & Catoptrica*. Paris; 1557.
5.2   Alhazen – Witelo. *Opticae thesaurus*. Basel; 1572.
5.3   Descartes R. *Discours de la méthod . . .* La Dioptrique. Leyden; 1637.
5.4   Bacon R. *Perspectiva . . .* Frankfurt; 1614.
5.5   Bartisch G. *Ophthalmoduleia. Das ist, Augendienst*. Dresden; 1583.
5.6   Kepler J. *Dioptrice seu demonstratio eorum quae visui & visibilibus propter conspicilla*. Augsburg; 1611. See also #9 Borel page 64.
5.7   Scheiner C. *Oculus hoc est: fundamentum octicum, . . .* Oeniponti, D. Agricola; 1619.
5.8   Daza de Valdes B. *Uso de los Antoios para todo genero de vistas*: . . . Sevilla: por Diego Perez (1623).
5.9   *Beiträge zur Geschichte der Brille*. Carl Zeiss Oberkochen, Marwitz & Hauser Brillenmacher: Stuttgart; 1958.
5.10 Efron N, Pearson RM. Centenary Celebration of Fick's Eine Contactbrille. *Arch Ophtalmol*. 1988;106: p1370, p1373.
5.11 Young T. On the theory of light and colours. *Phil Trans Part 1*; 1802. p12.
5.12 Young T. *A course of lectures on natural philosophy and the mechanical arts*. London; 1807.
5.13 von Helmholtz H. Handbuch der physiologischen Optik. *Allgemeine Encyklopädie der Physik IX Bd*. Leipzig; 1867. See also #45 Helmholtz page 236.

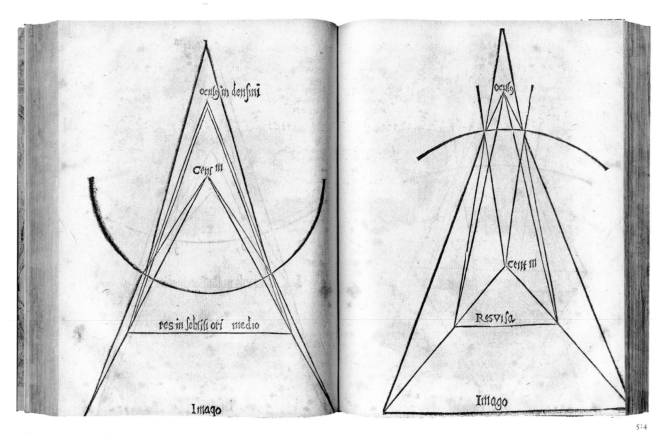

Illustration from the first printing from 1614 of Roger Bacon's (1214–1292) studies of image formation and the function of lenses.

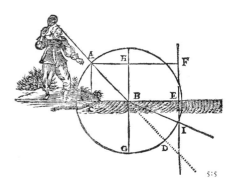

René Descartes (1596–1650) derives the sine law of refraction and applies it to the optics of vision. This treatise forms part of his famous tract introducing new ideas about the proper scientific method.

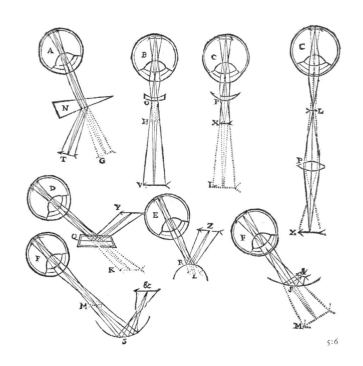

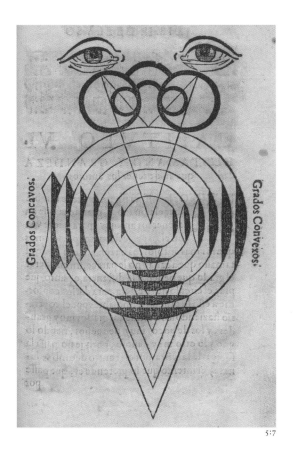

5:7

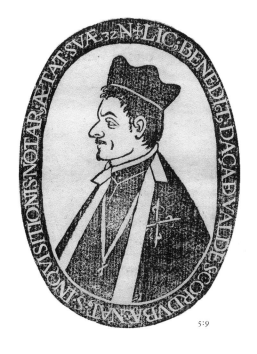

5:9

In 1623 Benito Daza de Valdes (1591–1636) applies, for the first time, advances in optics and in the understanding of vision to the design of eyeglasses.

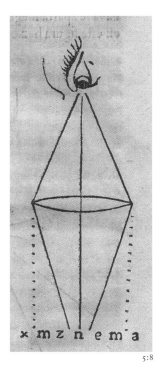

5:8

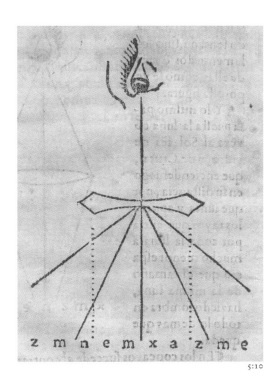

5:10

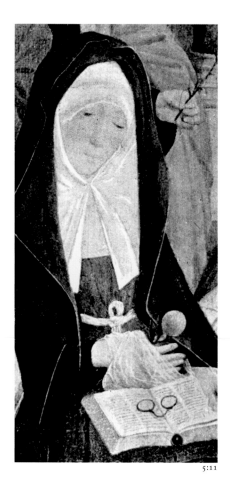

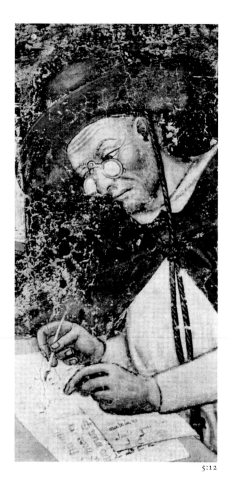

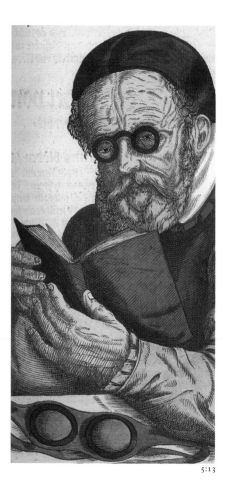

5:11

5:12

5:13

Early representation of eyeglasses (left to right).
The first woman with eyeglasses, from a painting
by Geertgen van Jans, The Holy Family, from
1470. The first man with eyeglasses, fresco showing Cardinal Hugo of Provence from 1352 and
the first book on the equipment and methods of
ophthalmology by Georg Bartisch from 1583.

Different models of eyeglasses from the 18th
century.

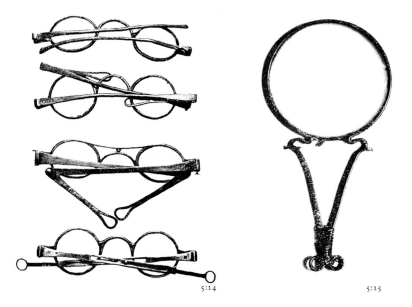

5:14

5:15

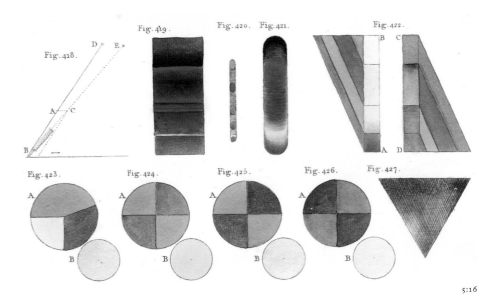

5:16

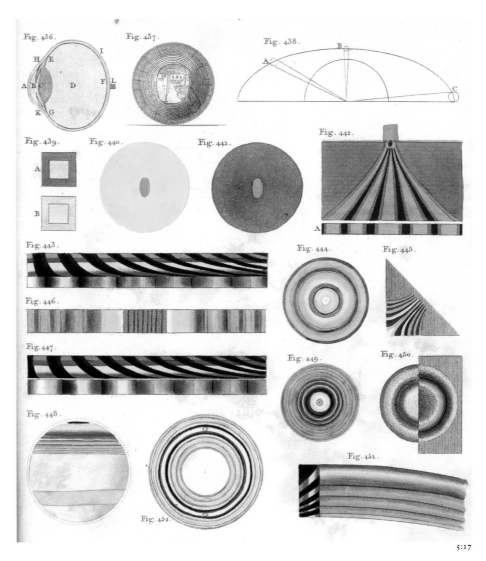

5:17

Illustrations of the nature of colours from Thomas Young's (1773–1829) lectures in 1807. In 1802 Young presents a theory of colour vision that has stood the test of time. It was based on the three fundamental colours red, green and blue and the assumption that corresponding sensitive areas were located in the retina.

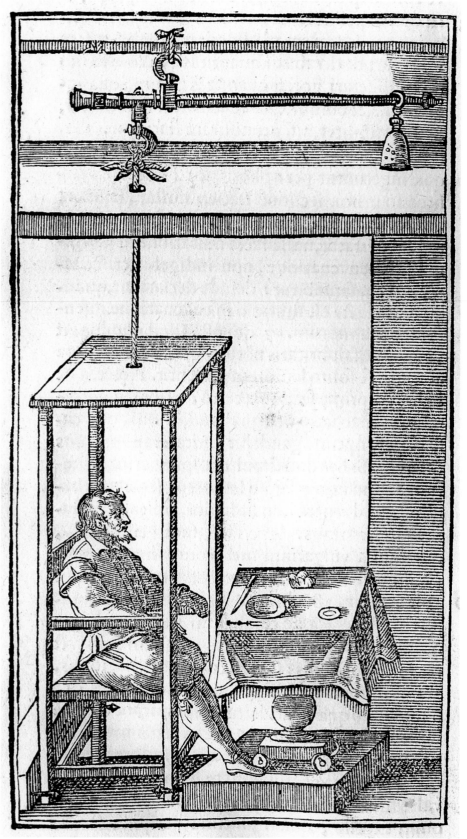

6:1

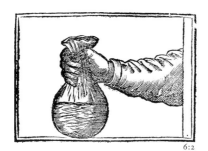

6:2

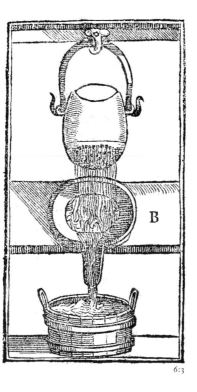

6:3

Santorio Santorio (1561–1636) sitting in the balance that he constructs to determine the net weight change over time after intake and excretion of foodstuffs and fluids. Practical methods used by him to collect and measure excretions are illustrated above.

SANTORIO was born in Slovenia in 1561, the son of a noble family. After studies of classical languages and literature, he turned to philosophy and medicine, earning his doctorate in 1582. He practised medicine in Croatia and then in Venice, where he made the acquaintance of the physicist Galileo Galilei. With an increasing reputation as a practitioner, he was appointed professor of theoretical medicine at the University of Padua. At the end of his second term in 1624 he returned to Venice, where he spent the rest of his life. Santorio was an excellent orator and a popular teacher. He had a cautious, restrained personality and his original ideas were always presented as part of accepted doctrine. With no family and little interest in personal comfort, he amassed a considerable fortune during his life.

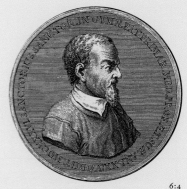

Santorio Santorio   6:4

Ars de statica medica aphorismorum sectionibus septem comprehensa.

VENICE: N. POLO; 1614.

SANTORIO BELIEVES in the traditional teaching that health and disease depend on the balance between the four humours (blood, phlegm, yellow and black bile). However, breaking away from tradition, he insists that this balance must be measured. To do so he constructs a chair scale in which he can determine the daily variations in his own body weight. He finds that a significant part of the excretions occur invisibly through water evaporation from the skin and through breathing (perspiration insensibilis). He also notes the various factors that effect these losses, for instance that they increase due to fever. Santorio reports here his observations together with a series of aphorisms. For almost two centuries this book was considered the most perfect of medical texts and was reprinted many times. (6.1)

IN PERSPECTIVE:
Water loss through the skin and the associated phenomenon of heat loss (6.2) still remains an active field of study in modern times, being of importance in various clinical areas such as surgery, (6.3) treatment of burns (6.4) and in the care of newborn babies (6.5). Two and a half centuries after Santorio's work, Grehant was able to measure the amount of water lost in expired air (6.6). Aschenbrandt soon made more accurate observations and also studied both the heat and moisture conservation and the filtration properties of the nose (6.7). More recently, the investigations of Ingelstedt (6.8) have lead to the development of clinically useful heat moisture exchanging (HME) devices (artificial noses)(6.9). Highly efficient designs incorporating hygroscopic material (6.10) are now widely used to humidify dry respiratory gases in anaesthesia and intensive care. To a large extent these modern devices mimic the intricate functionality of the nose of a camel (6.11).

6.1 Santorio S. *Medica Statica: Beeing the Aphorism of Sanctorius*. Translated by J Quincy London; 1720.

6.2. Thiele FAJ, Senden KG. Relation between skin temperature and the insensible perspiration of the human skin. *J Invest Dermatol*. 1966; 47:307.

6.3 Bauber CD, Clark RG, Howlett P. Insensible water loss in operative patients. *Br J Surg*. 1972;59:300.

6.4 Davies JWL, Lamke L-O, Liljedahl S-O. A guide to the rate of non-renal water loss from patients with burns. *Br J Plast Surg*. 1974; 27:325.

6.5 Levine SZ, Kelly M, Wilson JR. The insensible perspiration in infancy and in childhood II. Proposed basal standards for infants. *Am J Dis Child*. 1930; 39:917.

6.6 Gréhant N. *Recherches physiques sur la respiration de l'homme*. Paris; 1864.

6.7 Aschenbrandt T. *Die Bedeutung der Nase für die Athmung*. Würzburg; 1886.

6.8 Ingelstedt S. Studies on the conditioning of air in the respiratory tract. *Acta Oto-laryng*. 1956; Suppl.131.

6.9 Koch H, et al. A method for humidifying inspired air in posttracheotomy care. *Ann Oto Rhin Laryng*. 1958; 76:991.

6.10 Gedeon A, Mebius C. The Hygroscopic Condenser Humidifier. *Anaesthesia* 1979; 34:1043.

6.11 Schmidt-Nielsen K. Countercurrent Systems in Animals. *Scientific American* 1981; 244(5):118.

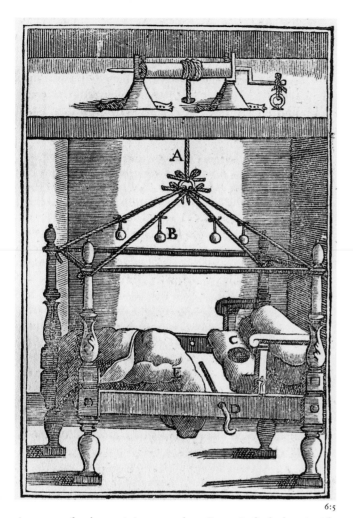

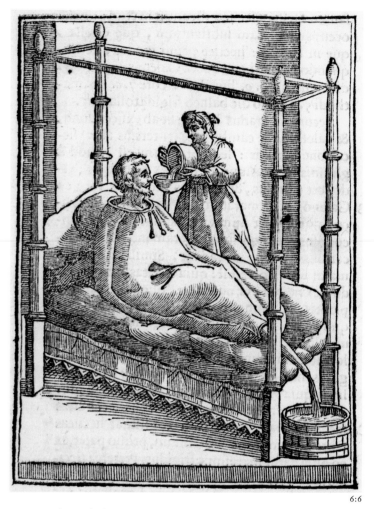

Apparatus for determining water loss. Santorio finds that significant losses occur through the skin and through breathing.

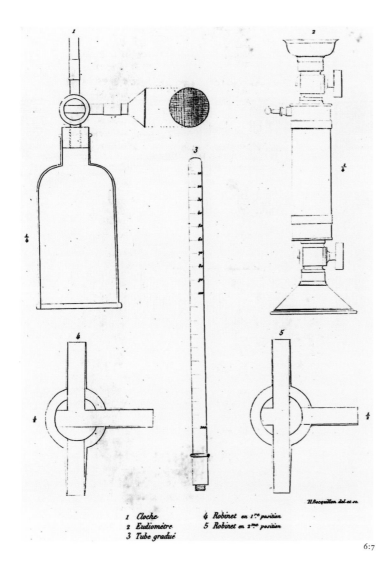

1 *Cloche*
2 *Eudiomètre*
3 *Tube gradué*
4 *Robinet en 1.re position*
5 *Robinet en 2.me position*

6:7

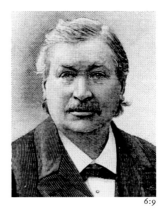

6:9

Nestor Gréhant (1838–1910) makes the first quantitative study of the conditioning of expired gas using the apparatus shown left.

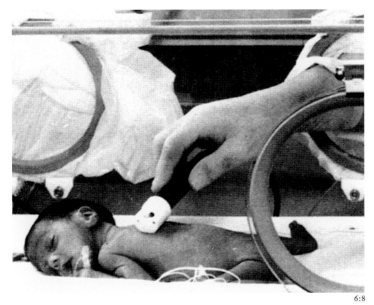

6:8

Modern techniques for measuring evaporative heat and water loss from a new-born using thermistors and capacitive humidity sensors operated in a differential mode.

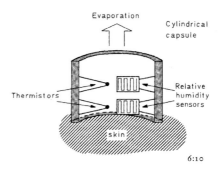

6:10

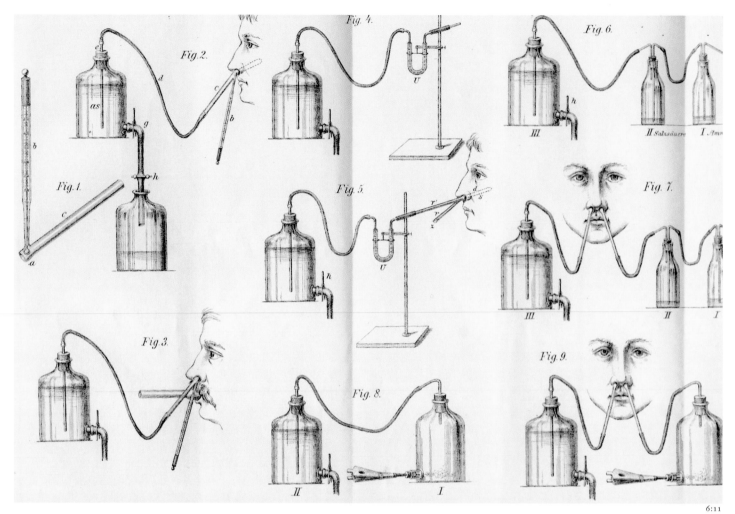

The experiments of Theodor Aschenbrandt in 1886 provide the first quantitative results on both the heat moisture exchanging and the filtrating properties of the nose and the upper airways.

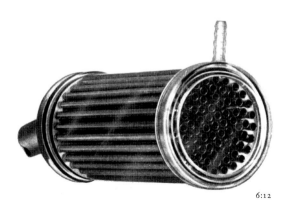

The first heat moisture exchanger apparatus constructed in 1958 for conditioning inspired gas in posttracheotomy care.

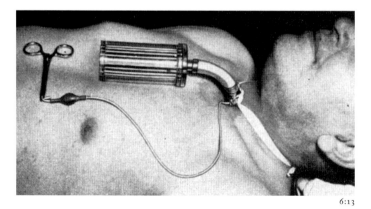

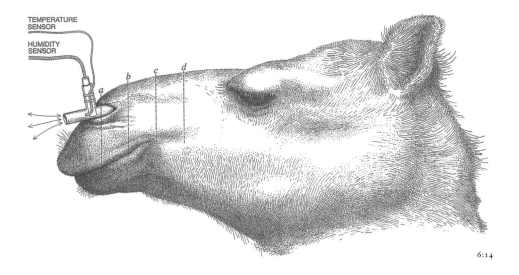

TEMPERATURE
SENSOR

HUMIDITY
SENSOR

6:14

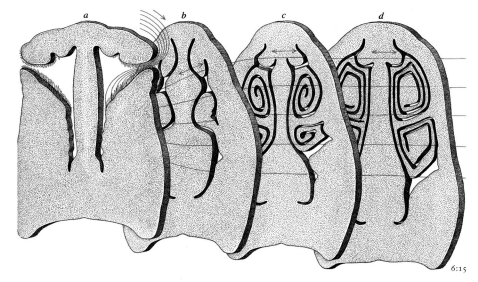

The extremely efficient heat moisture exchange in the nasal cavity of the camel is due to its large surface area and its hygroscopic properties.

6:15

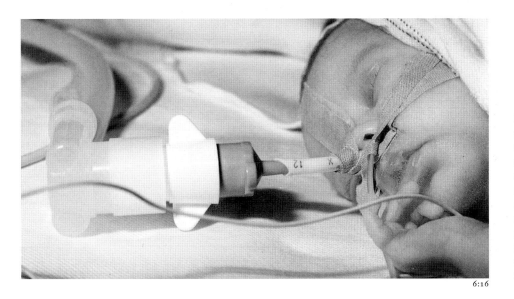

Hygroscopic condenser humidifiers developed during the 1980s operate in a way similar to the nose of the camel and provide humidification in demanding clinical settings. Here a baby is shown breathing through such a device (the white plastic part) when connected to a ventilator in a Neonatal Intensive Care Unit.

6:16

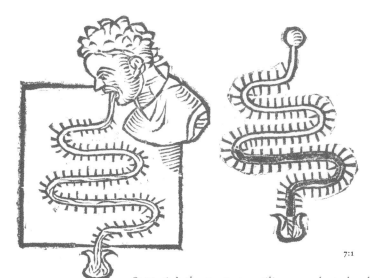

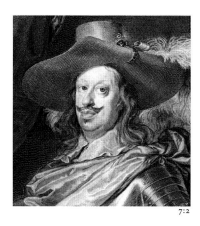

7:1

7:2

Santorio's thermometer utilises a graduated scale for
showing the displacement of a liquid column as the
gas volume changes with body temperature.

Prince Leopold (1617–1675), Duke of Tuscany,
an amateur scientist who in 1657 founds the first
scientific academy, the Accademia del Cimento.

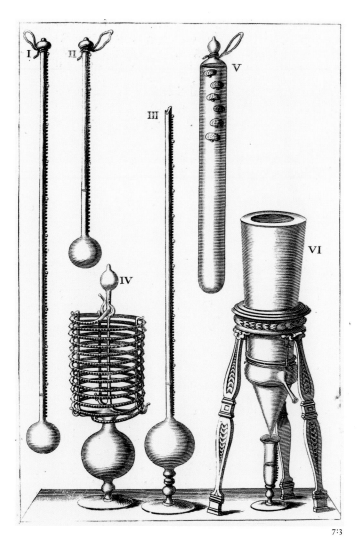

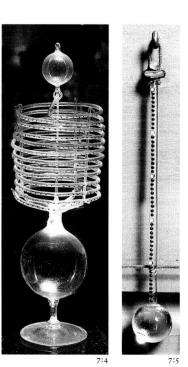

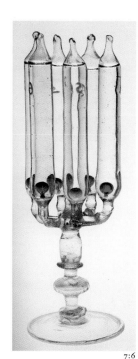

7:4

7:5

7:6

7:3

Apparatus developed by the Accademia del
Cimento. Thermometers of Santorio's
(I–IV) and Galileo's (V) design and a condensation hygrometer (VI). Left, an illustration from 1667, and above the thermometers
as they appear today.

S ANTORIO was born in Slovenia in 1561, the son of a noble family. After studies of classical languages and literature he turned to philosophy and medicine, earning his doctorate in 1582. He practised medicine in Croatia and then in Venice, where he made the acquaintance of the physicist Galileo Galilei. With an increasing reputation as a practitioner, he was appointed professor of theoretical medicine at the University of Padua. At the end of his second term in 1624 he returned to Venice, where he spent the rest of his life. Santorio was an excellent orator and a popular teacher. He had a cautious, restrained personality and his original ideas were always presented as part of accepted doctrine. With no family and little interest in personal comfort, he assembled a considerable fortune during his life.

Commentaria in primam Fen primi libri Canonis Avicennae.

VENICE: J. SARCINA; 1625.

IN ORDER to determine the balance of the "humours" in the body (7.1), Santorio constructed instruments for the measurement of time, air and water flow, humidity and temperature. In this book he describes, for the first time, the principles of construction of these instruments. Although Santorio reveals few details of the designs, some illustrations are provided to explain the methods of measurements. As was his habit, the presentation is integrated with material from established medical doctrine. Here Santorio also comments on the first book of the al-Quanun (Canon of Medicine), written by the Iranian philosopher and physician Ibn Sina (Avicenna) at the beginning of the 11th century.

IN PERSPECTIVE:
The quantitative relationship between the volume and the temperature of a gas utilised in Santorio's thermometer was established two centuries later by Gay-Lussac (7.2). Santorio's devices were further developed during the 17th century, particularly by the members of the first Scientific Academy (Accademia del Cimento) (7.3). Martine evaluated many different temperature scales and he also considered their potential clinical usefulness (7.4). Although Currie put Martine's ideas into medical practice in 1797 (7.5), it remained for Wunderlich to explore the full significance of the temperature changes during illness 1868 (7.6). Farenheit manufactured the first mercury in glass thermometer in 1714 and from the 1820s temperature could also be measured using thermocouples (7.7). Humidity levels were first determined by water condensation (7.3). Hook designed a hygrometer using oat beard and about a century later Saussure developed the hair hygrometer, which remained in use for many years (7.8). Psychrometers using thermocouples in a differential mode (7.9) and thin film capacitive sensors (7.10) have, in more recent times, significantly improved humidity measurements.

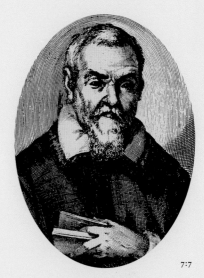

7:7

Santorio Santorio

7.1 See # 6 Santorio page 48.
7.2 Gay-Lussac JL. *Sur la dilatation des gaz et des vapeurs.* Ann de chimie 1802; 43:137.
7.3 *Saggi di natura esperienze fatte nell'Accademia del Cimento.* Florence; 1667.
7.4 Martine G. *Essays Medical and Philosophical.* London; 1740.
7.5 Currie J. *Medical reports, on the effect of water, cold and warm, as a remedy in fever and febrile diseases.* Liverpool; 1797.
7.6 Wunderlich C. *Das Verhalten der Eigenwärme in Krankheiten.* Leipzig; 1868.
7.7 Knowles Middleton WE. *A History of the Thermometer.* Baltimore; 1966.
7.8 Saussure HB. *Essais sur l'Hygrométrie.* Neuchatel; 1783. See also ref. 9.2 for Hook's instrument.
7.9 See ref. 6.8.
7.10 Nilsson GE. On the measurement of evaporative water loss, methods and clinical applications. *Linköping Studies in Science and Technology Dissertations* No 11 Linköping; 1977.

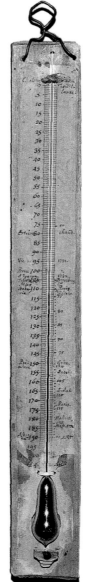

Anders Celsius (1701–1744) and his thermometer (below) and his proposal for a new thermometer scale (right).

Celsius sets the two fixed points of the temperature scale as the boiling and freezing points of water so "one can be sure that several such thermometers, placed in the same air, should always show the same degree …".

Obſervationer om twånne beſtåndiga Grader på en Thermometer.

af AND. CELSIUS.

Thermometrar åro uu förtiden hos oß mycket brukeliga, merendels at hångas på wåggen, antingen til en prydnad, eller ock til at ſe huru mycket wårman til-eller aftager i Kammaren.

De gångbaraſte åro de ſå kallade Florentiſka Thermometrar, ſom kommit in i Swerige från Tyſkland, ock åro alla ſå wida onyttiga, ſom de ej gifwa något wiſt mått på Graderne af wårma eller köld, ock desutan, wid lika wårma, ej wiſa ſamma Grad; hwilket likwål år nödigt, ſå wål wid Meteorologiſka Obſervationers jåmförande ſins emellan, från ſårſkilta orter, ſåſom ock wid åtſkilliga Oeconomiſka ock Phyſicaliſka experimenters anſtållande, hwilka fordra en wiß Grad af wårma.

7:9

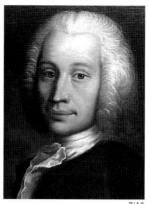

7:10

p. 217

I Fahrenheit	II Florence	III	IV Paris	V D.la Hire	VI Amontons	VII Poleni	VIII D.Reaumur	IX De l'Isle	X Crucquius	XI R.Society	XII Newton	XIII Fowler	XIV Hales	XV Edinburgh

7:8

56

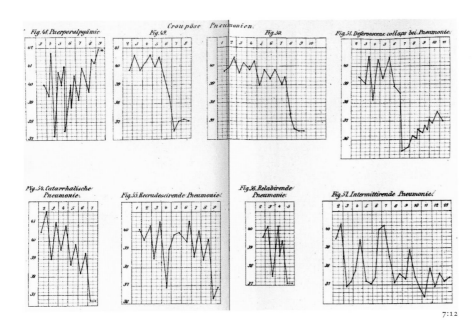

Fig.48.Puerperalpyämie

Croupöse Pneumonien.

Fig.49.

Fig.50.

Fig.51.Deferoscenz collaps bei Pneumonie.

Fig.54.Catarrhalische Pneumonie.

Fig.55.Recrudescirende Pneumonie.

Fig.56.Relabirende Pneumonie.

Fig.57.Intermittirende Pneumonie.

7:12

Carl Wunderlich (1815–1877) explores the significance of temperature changes for diagnosing various diseases. His work establishes the field of clinical thermometry.

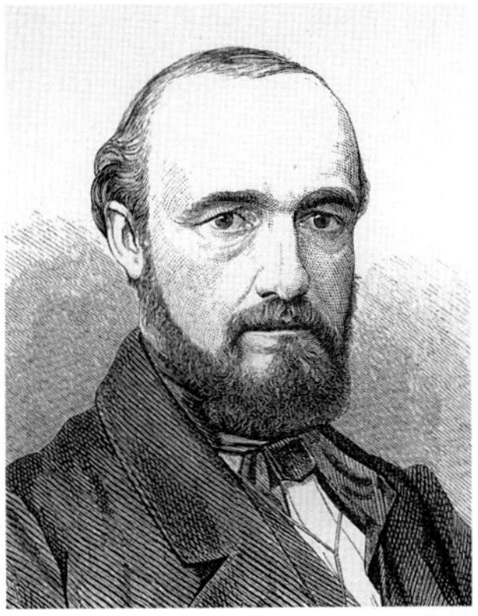

7:13

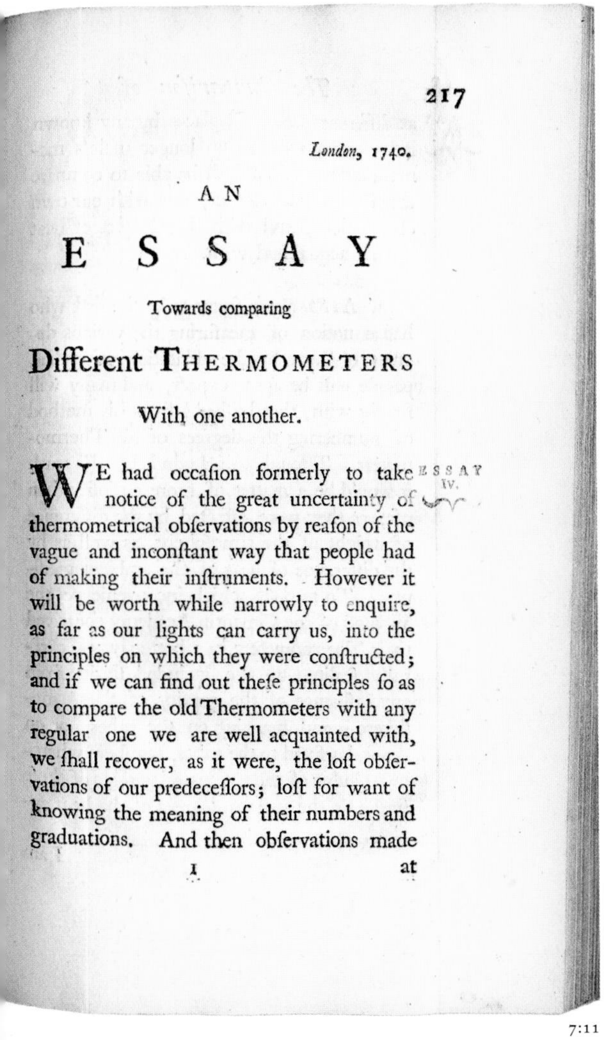

217

London, 1740.

AN

ESSAY

Towards comparing

Different THERMOMETERS

With one another.

WE had occasion formerly to take notice of the great uncertainty of thermometrical obſervations by reaſon of the vague and inconſtant way that people had of making their inſtruments. However it will be worth while narrowly to enquire, as far as our lights can carry us, into the principles on which they were conſtructed; and if we can find out theſe principles ſo as to compare the old Thermometers with any regular one we are well acquainted with, we ſhall recover, as it were, the loſt obſervations of our predeceſſors; loſt for want of knowing the meaning of their numbers and graduations. And then obſervations made

ESSAY
IV.

I   at

George Martine (1702–1741) publishes an essay (left) where he evaluates the many different temperature scales that were in use in the 1740s. He also discusses, for the first time, their use in medicine.

7:11

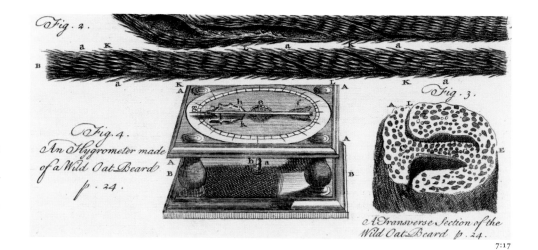

7:17

A century before Saussure's invention (see bottom of this page), Robert Hooke proposes the use of the wild-oat beard for measuring humidity. His description of the function of such a hygrometer is reproduced below.

(see bottom of this page)

THE Beard of a Wild-Oat, cut afunder at the Ends A and B, is reprefented by the two long prickly Figures we are now about to examine.

This little Production of Nature is wonderfully remarkable, on account of its making an exceeding good *Hygrometer*, or Inftrument for difcovering the *Drynefs* or *Moifture* of the Air ; being extremely fenfibly of, and vifibly affected by the leaft Alteration as to thofe Particulars. A Defcription of it muft therefore be an inftructive as well as entertaining Amufement.

Wild-Oat Beard.

7:16

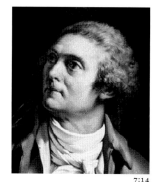

7:14

Horace Saussure (1740–1799) presents his invention, the hair hygrometer. Although not particularly accurate, the principle of this instrument remained in use for almost two centuries.

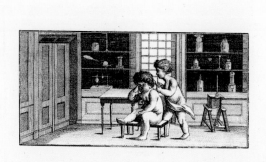

PREMIER ESSAI.
DESCRIPTION
DUN NOUVEL
HYGROMETRE COMPARABLE.

CHAPITRE PREMIER.

STRUCTURE DE L'HYGROMETRE.

§. I. LE cheveu s'alonge quand il s'humecte, & fe contracte ou fe raccourcit quand il fe deffeche. La différence entre le plus grand alongement que puiffe lui donner l'humidité, & la plus grande contraction qu'il puiffe recevoir de la fécherefse

Extenfion du cheveu par l'humidité.

A

7:15

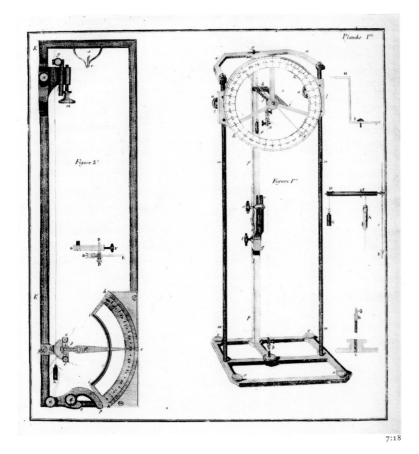

7:18

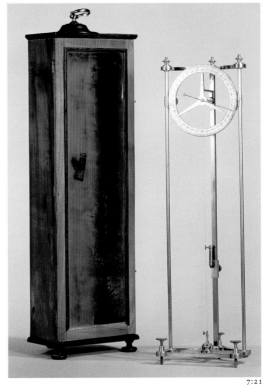

7:21

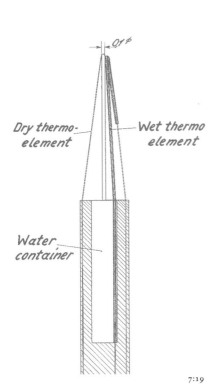

Dry thermo-
element

Wet thermo
element

Water
container

7:19

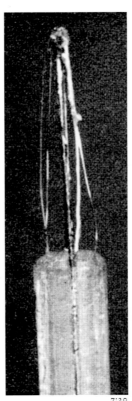

7:20

The hygrometer according to a drawing by Saussure from 1783 (left) and the instrument as it appears today.

Modern methods of hygrometry. Wet and dry thermoelements used differentially (left and middle) and a differential capacitive sensor (below).

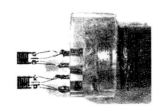

7:22

A Table of the Condensation of the Air.

AA	A	B	C	D	E
48	12	00	Added to 29½ makes	29 2/16	29 2/16
46	11½	01 7/16		30 9/16	30 6/16
44	11	02 13/16		31 5/16	31 12/16
42	10½	04 6/16		33 8/16	33 7
40	10	06 3/16		35 5/16	35 --
38	9½	07 14/16		37 --	36 15/19
36	9	10 2/16		39 5/16	38 7/8
34	8½	12 8/16		41 10/16	41 2/17
32	8	15 1/16		44 2/16	43 11/16
30	7½	17 15/16		47 1/16	46 3/5
28	7	21 3/16		50 5/16	50 --
26	6½	25 3/16		54 5/16	53 10/13
24	6	29 11/16		58 13/16	58 2/8
23	5¾	32 3/16		61 5/16	60 18/23
22	5½	34 15/16		64 1/16	63 6/11
21	5¼	37 15/16		67 1/16	66 4/7
20	5	41 9/16		70 11/16	70 --
19	4¾	45 --		74 5/16	73 11/19
18	4½	48 12/16		77 14/16	77 3/7
17	4¼	53 11/16		82 12/16	82 4/17
16	4	58 2/16		87 14/16	87 7/8
15	3¾	63 15/16		93 1/16	93 3/5
14	3½	71 2/16		100 7/16	99 6/7
13	3¾	78 11/16		107 13/16	107 7/13
12	3	88 7/16		117 9/16	116 8

AA. The number of equal spaces in the shorter leg, that contained the same parcel of Air diversly extended.

B. The height of the Mercurial Cylinder in the longer leg, that compress'd the Air into those dimensions.

C. The height of a Mercurial Cylinder that counterbalanc'd the pressure of the Atmosphere.

D. The Aggregate of the two last Columns B and C, exhibiting the pressure sustained by the included Air.

E. What that pressure should be according to the *Hypothesis*, that supposes the pressures and expansions to be in reciprocal proportion.

8:1

Robert Boyle (1627–1691) proves (compare columns D and E in the table left) that the pressure of a gas is inversely proportional to its volume. (Boyle's law). The title page of this famous publication from 1662 is shown below.

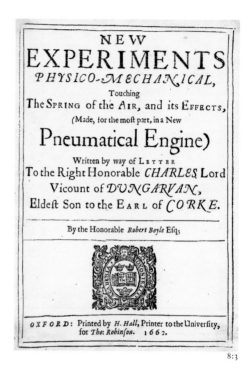

NEW
EXPERIMENTS
PHYSICO-MECHANICAL,
Touching
The SPRING of the AIR, and its EFFECTS,
(Made, for the most part, in a New
Pneumatical Engine)
Written by way of LETTER
To the Right Honorable CHARLES Lord
Vicount of DUNGARVAN,
Eldest Son to the EARL of CORKE.

By the Honorable *Robert Boyle* Esq;

OXFORD: Printed by *H. Hall*, Printer to the University, for *Tho: Robinson.* 1662.

8:3

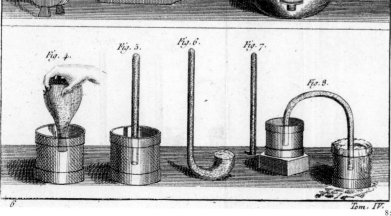

8:2

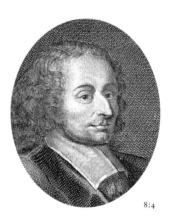

8:4

Blaise Pascal (1623–1662) studies the equilibrium of liquids in a valley and on the top of a mountain and explains the effects of atmospheric pressure.

HELMONT was born in Brussels in 1579, the child of a prominent family. He studied philosophy, geography and law, finally receiving a degree in medicine in 1599. Married into money, he turned down tempting offers of attractive positions and decided to do research of his own rather than as he said "live on the misery of my fellow men" and "accumulate riches and endanger my soul". Some of his writings aroused the wrath of the Theological Faculty of Louvain, but he admitted being in error and escaped with a temporary house arrest. Helmont had a mild personality with a fondness for dreams and visions. Being an occult mysticist who was sceptical to logical thinking, he nevertheless strived to explain the secrets of life in purely chemical terms.

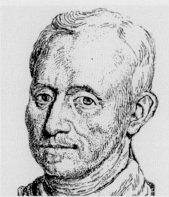

Jean Baptist van Helmont   8:5

Ortus Medicinae. Id est, initia physicæ inaudita.

EDENTE AUTHORIS FILIO, FRANCISCO MERCURIO VAN HELMONT
AMSTERDAM: LOUIS ELZEVIR;1652.

THIS IS the most complete collection of Helmont's medical and alchemical writings. While studying fermentation and combustion of solids, Helmont finds that the smoke produced was specific to the original substance. He calls the escaping smoke "gas" (after "chaos") and identifies several of them, most notably carbon dioxide, which he named "gas sylvestre", meaning "wild", because it tended to break closed glass vessels on expansion. Helmont considers each disease as a specific condition and he looks for causes, including those of psycho-physical origin. He makes advanced observations on asthma, tuberculosis and tissue irritability. He believes fever to be a reaction to irritation and to be beneficial for the healing process.

IN PERSPECTIVE:
Helmont's scientific views are intertwined with his mystical religious metaphysics. His ideas about wound treatment using magnetism inspired Mesmer's teachings of "animal magnetism" during the 18th century (8.1). Mesmerism in turn has left its mark on the modern practices of hypnosis. Strongly influenced by Paracelsus (8.2), Helmont's work represents the transition from alchemy to chemistry as a science, which in the modern sense starts with the work of Lavoisier (8.3).Within three decades of Helmont's death, Pascal had explained the barometric pressure (weight) of air (8.4) and Guericke had developed the first air pump (8.5). Boyle established the quantitative relationship between the volume and the pressure of a gas and also published a critical essay that dealt alchemy a severe blow (8.6). The first microscopic model of gases was presented in 1738 by Bernoulli (8.7) and further developed by Dalton (8.8). The mechanism of breathing and its importance in sustaining life was soon under intense study (8.9) and in 1754 Black prepared and closely examined carbon dioxide for the first time (8.10).

8.1 Mesmer FA. *Memoire sur la Decouverte du Magnetisme Animal.* Geneva & Paris; 1779.
8.2 See #3 Paracelsus page 32.
8.3 See #24 Lavoisier page 134.
8.4 Pascal B. *Traitez de l'équilibre des liqueurs, et de la pesanteur de la masse de l'air.* Paris; 1663.
8.5 Guericke O. *Experimenta Nova (ut vocantur) Magdeburgica De Vacuo Spatio* ... Amsterdam; 1672.
8.6 Boyle R. *New experiments physico-mechanical, touching the spring of the air and its effects.* Oxford; 1662. and ref. 4.6.
8.7 See #18 Bernoulli page 104.
8.8 Dalton J. Experimental essays on the constitution of mixed gases; ... *Mem Lit Phil Soc Manchester* 1802; 5:535. See also ref. 18.6.
8.9 See #11 Hooke page 72.
8.10 See #20 Black page 116.

Otto Guericke (1602–1686) and the
title page of his book from 1672
where he describes the invention of
the air pump, the first electric generator and his experiments on static
electricity.

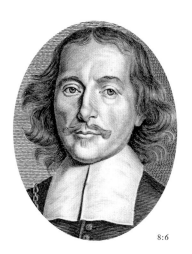

8:6

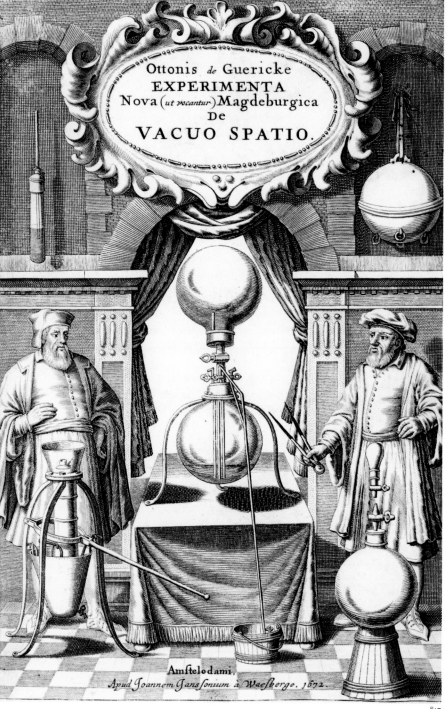

8:7

In 1802 John Dalton (1766–1844) investigates the properties of gas mixtures and establishes the law of partial pressures.

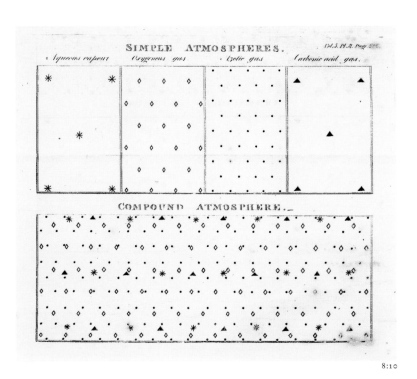

8:10

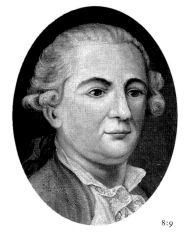

8:8

Illustration of the first kinetic theory of gases proposed in 1738 by Daniel Bernoulli (1700–1782) to explain the basic gas laws.

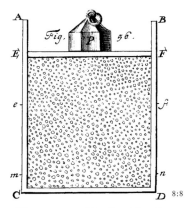

8:9

Franz Mesmer (1734–1815) (portrait above) introduces the idea of "animal magnetism" as a method of healing. Influenced by the ideas of van Helmont, he treats patients with magnets and hypnoses. Initially successful, he is later declared a fraud by a Royal Commission of doctors and academicians in Paris 1794. To the right, an operator puts his patient into a crisis.

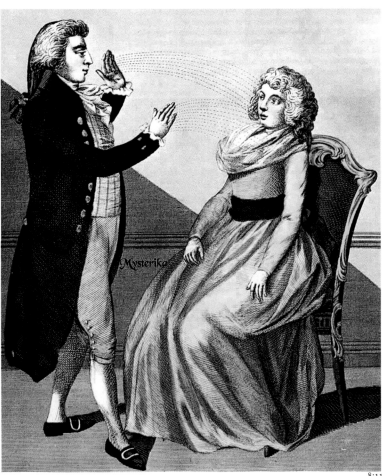

8:11

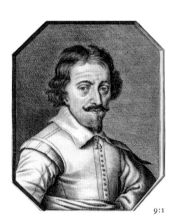

9:1

Zacharias Janssen (1580–1638), the inventor of the compound microscope.

The construction of the compound microscope as explained by Pierre Borel (1620–1671).

Borel reports microscopic observations on the gonorrhoea worm. "A friend of mine observed venomous gonorrhoea on the penis of a soldier. It was a small snaillike infection almost invisible but its progression looks almost like a worm and appeared more pronounced on certain parts of the body. It produced 30 or 40 eggs in the microscope. Small prickly worms appeared from some of these eggs. They were marked to distinguish them from the eggs mentioned above. On compression they produced a milklike liquid."

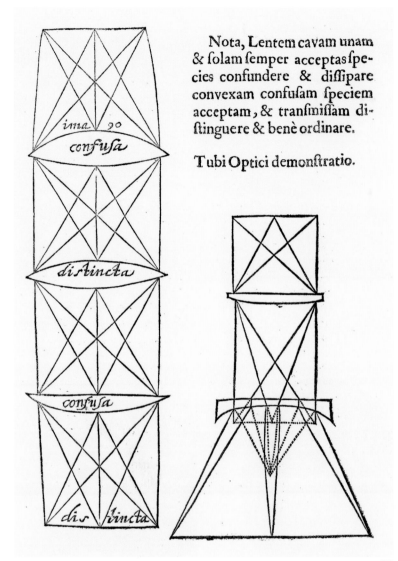

Nota, Lentem cavam unam & folam femper acceptas fpecies confundere & diffipare convexam confufam fpeciem acceptam, & tranfmiffam diftinguere & benè ordinare.

Tubi Optici demonftratio.

9:2

OBSERVATIO LIII
Da Gonorrheæ verme.

IN Gonorrhea virulenta militis, feu in balano ejus, amicus meus obfervavit Infectulum limaciformem, fed ferè invifibilem, quod ejus etiam greffus vel vermium imitabatur, craffefcens in certis corporis locis : 30. autem vel 40. peperit ova in Microfcopio, è quorum quibufdam vermiculi fubtiliffimi, fed hirfuti manabant, punctis autem notata erant & diftincta ova fupradicta. Lac autem quafi refudant fi comprimantur.

9:3

BOREL was born around 1620 in Castres, France, where he practised medicine until 1653, when he moved to Paris and became "médecin ordinaire du roy". He is credited with the first description of brain concussion and is also known to have recommended the use of concave mirrors in the diagnostic examination of the nose and throat (9.1). Borel was an ardent collector of plants, minerals, antiquities and books. He was an energetic man with wide ranging interests and comprehensive knowledge of many subjects. In an effort to establish the priority to certain inventions and scientific discoveries, he published a book which is the first full account of the invention of both the microscope and the telescope.

De vero telescopii inventore, cum brevi omnium conspiciliorum historia … accessit etiam centuria Observationum microcospicarum. /sic/

THE HAGUE: A. VLACQ; 1655–1656.

BOREL DESCRIBES here, for the first time, the discovery and construction of the telescope and the compound (multiple lenses) microscope. He claims that Janssen, a Dutch spectacle maker, invented the microscope sometime during the period 1590–1610. Borel presents evidence to support this claim (which is considered today to be correct) that he had obtained from the Dutch ambassador to France, who had actually seen the compound microscope in 1619. In a separate section of the book dated 1656, Borel also reports one hundred medicophysical observations, some of them illustrated, that he made with such a microscope.

IN PERSPECTIVE:
The compound microscope was soon further developed by Hooke, who used it to study and depict minute details of insects and plants (9.2). At about the same time, van Leeuwenhoek built very good quality single lens microscopes and was able to observe many important biological objects including bacteria, blood cells and spermatozoa for the first time (9.3). The compound microscope evolved into a more practical and frequently used instrument during the 18th century (9.4). In the beginning of the 19th century the technique of chromatic compensation of lenses was fully developed (9.5) and electric light sources for illumination of objects were invented (9.6). Progress was also made in understanding the wave nature of light (9.7) and in examining and improving the properties of optical materials (9.8). Abbe in Germany brought these advances together and developed a new concept for microscopic image formation that lead to superior microscope designs (9.9). In the 20th century, the phase contrast method (9.10), optical coating technologies, new light sources and sophisticated scanning techniques (9.11) have all contributed to making optical microscopy an indispensable tool in many fields of study including medicine.

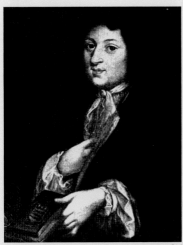

9:4

Pierre Borel, Portrait by J Pauthe 1850 after an original painting now lost.

9.1 *Dictionary of Scientific Biography* Vol. II. New York; 1970–1990. p305.
9.2 Hooke R: *Micrographia: or some Physiological Descriptions of Minute Bodies* … London; 1665.
9.3 See #16 Leeuwenhoek page 96.
9.4 Adams G (the younger). *Essays on the Microscope* …London; 1787.
9.5 Lister JJ. On some properties in achromatic object glasses … *Phil Trans* 1830; 120:187.
9.6 Donne A, Foucault L. *Description du microscope photo-électrique*. Extrait du bulletin de la société d'encouragement pour l'industrie nationale. Paris; 1845.
9.7 Airy G. On the Diffraction of an Annual Aperture. *Phil Mag* 1841; XVIII:1.
9.8 Frauenhofer J. Bestimmung des Brechungs- und Farbenzerstreuungs-Vermögens verschiedener Glasarten … *Denkschriften der k. Akad. d. Wiss. zu München*. 1817; Bd.V.
9.9 See #64 Abbe page 328.
9.10 Zernike F. Das Phasenkontrastverfahren b.d. microscopischen Beobachtung. *Phys Z* 1935; 36:848.
9.11 Pawley JB editor. *Handbook of Biological Confocal Microscopy*. New York: Plenum Press; 1995.

Robert Hooke (1635–1703) introduces the term "cell" when studying the structure of cork. He writes "I could exceedingly plainly perceive it to be all perforated and porous, much like a Honey-comb, but that the pores of it were not regular ... these pores, or cells,... were indeed the first microscopical pores I ever saw ..."

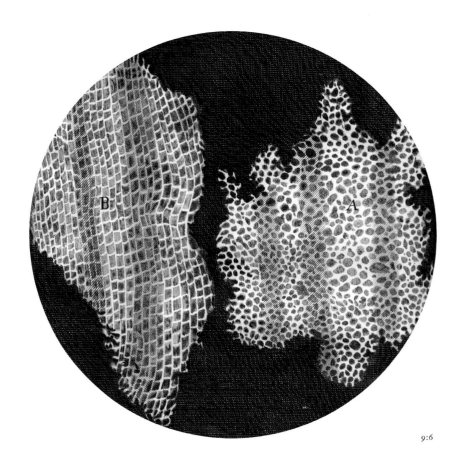

9:6

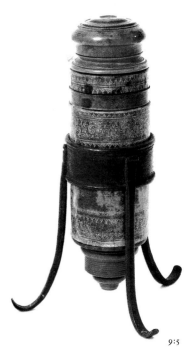

9:5

An Italian 17th century compound microscope as compared to Robert Hooke's famous drawing from 1665 of his own microscope (right).

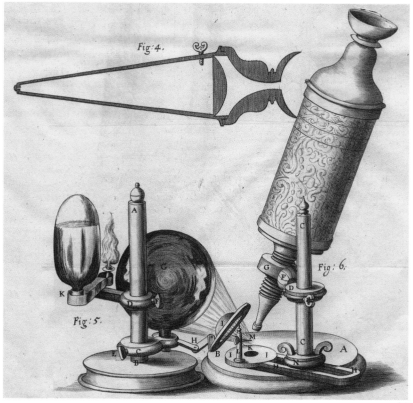

9:7

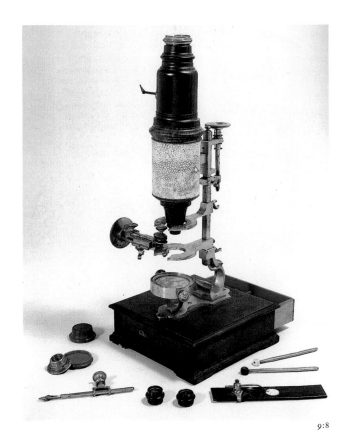

9:8

A century after Hooke's early design, the compound microscope develops into a more sophisticated instrument, as illustrated by this microscope from Augsburg.

Leon Foucault (1819–1868) invents the electric light regulator, a major advance, as these voltaic arc lamps can maintain a strong and steady illumination of the microscope object.

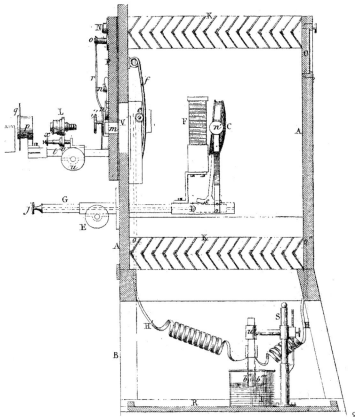

9:9

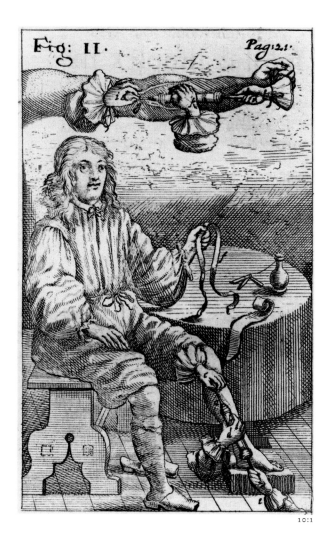

10:1

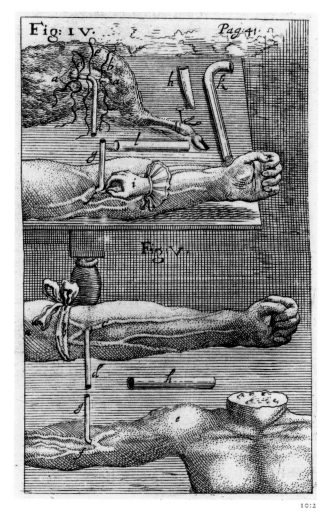

10:2

Infusion and transfusion experiments reported by Johann Elsholtz (1623–1688) in 1665. Infusion (top left) and transfusion from animal to man and from man to man (top right). The best way to perform these procedures is explained in the panels to the right. Because of the death of a patient (probably not due to the procedure), transfusions of blood to human beings were prohibited by law in 1670.

CLYSMATICA NOVA. 41

g. *Tubulus argenteus alter,vena insertus.*
h. *Obturamentum Tubuli, ex penna.*
i. *Manus Chirurgi cutem comprimens.*
k. *Forma Tubuli argentei sine margine , pro Homine.*
l. *Canalis ex penna, utrique Tubulo inserendus.*
   N. *Tubulus* K. in debita maguitudine exprimitur: Tubulorum vero
d. & g. diminuta est proportio.

Fig. V.
Transfusio ex Homine in Hominem.

a. *Brachium mandans.*
b. *Ligatura ipsi injecta.*
c. *Mediana ejus secta.*
d. *Tubulus argenteus insertus , curvatura ad manum versa.*
e. *Brachium recipiens.*
f. *Mediana ipsius secta.*
g. *Tubulus argenteus insertus , curvatura ad cor versa.*
h. *Canalis ex penna, intercedens.*
   N. 1. *Manus Chirurgi cutem comprimentis in utroque brachio scien-*

C 5   501

10:3

CLYSMATICA NOVA. 21

Explicatio notarum in Fig. II.
qua monstratur
Infusio simplex in
Homine.
In crure.
a. *Vena cruralis ramus internus, lanceola apertus.*
b. *Sipho repletus, & Vena insertus.*
c. *Manus Chirurgi sinistra , cutem comprimens.*
d. *Manus Chirurgi dextra , vaginam tenens.*
e. *Manus ministri scapum impellens.*
f. *Vinculum post sectionem remotum.*

In brachio.
g. *Mediana secta.*
h. *Sipho immissus.*
i. *Manus Chirurgi sinistra.*
k. *Manus Chirurgi dextra.*
l. *Manus ministri.*

   Alter. propter febrem venam sibi Medianam aperiri expetebat. Suasi, ut emissa sanguinis sufficiente portione , liquorem praetetea aliquem
B 3   anti-

10:4

W RE N was born 1632 in East Knoyle, England. With a strong family tradition of learning he went to Oxford to study. Here, his many talents for scientific work soon attracted attention. He became a highly skilled demonstrator of anatomy, an exceptional draftsman and, according to Newton, one of the best mathematicians (geometers) of his time. He was appointed professor of astronomy in Oxford 1657 and played a leading role in the formation of the Royal Society of London in 1662, being elected its third president. Knighted in 1673, Wren is best known today as an architect. Among his many achievements in this field is the construction of St Paul's Cathedral in London, where he is also buried.

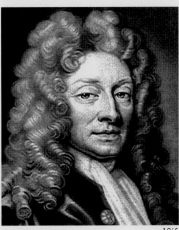

Sir Christopher Wren   10:5

Philosophical Transactions of the Royal Society London. 1665; 1 (December 4):128.

OLDENBURG, THE secretary of the newly formed Royal Society gives "An account of the rise and attempts, of a way to conveigh liquors immediately into the mass of blood" by "the Learned and Ingenious Dr Christopher Wren" and it is observed that the "Noble Benefactor to Experimental Philosophy Mr Robert Boyle" (10.1) ordered the necessary apparatus to be built. In the experiments, which were first attempted 1656 in the home of the French ambassador, Wren ligates the veins of a dog and then introduces a syringe into an opening of the side of the ligature. The syringe is made from animal bladder to which a quill is attached filled with various liquid solutions, most notably one containing opium. He observes that in this case the dog was stupefied but not killed.

IN PERSPECTIVE:
These initial experiments were soon followed by transfusions of blood between animals and also from animals to man. In 1665 Elsholtz performed such experiments (10.2) and soon others followed (10.3)(10.4)(10.5). Because of the death of a patient (probably not due to the procedure), transfusions of blood to human beings were prohibited by law in 1670. At the beginning of the 18th century Anel constructed a syringe similar to those used for rectal injection, but much smaller. In 1853, Pravaz adopted this device to infuse coagulants into the bloodstream (10.6). Together with Wood, who injected opiates (10.7) into joints for pain relief (10.8), Pravaz is credited with having introduced the hypodermic needle into medical practice. Systematic studies of intravenous delivery of anaesthetics for pain relief were reported by Oré in 1875 (10.9). In 1955 Roehr Products Co introduced the "Monoject", the first disposable plastic syringe (10.10) and the prefilled disposable syringe was invented by Murdoch (10.11).

10.1 See #14 Boyle page 88 also ref. 4.6 and ref. 8.6.
10.2 Elsholtz JS. *Clysmatica nova; oder newe Clystier-Kunst.* Berlin; 1665.
10.3 Lower R. The method observed in transfusing the blood out of one animal into another. *Phil Trans* 1666; 1:353.
10.4 Lower R, King E. An account of the experiment of transfusion, practiced upon a man in London. *Phil. Trans* 1667; 2:557.
10.5 Denis J. A letter concerning a new way of curing sundry diseases by transfusion of blood. *Phil. Trans* 1667; 2:489.
10.6 Pravaz CG. Sur un nouveau moyen d'opérer la coagulation du sang dans les artères. *C R Acad Sci* 1853; 36:88.
10.7 See #29 Sertürner page 162.
10.8 Wood A. New method of treating neuralgia by the direct application of opiates to the painful joints. *Edinb Med Surg J* 1855; 82:265.
10.9 Oré PC. *Études cliniques sur l'anesthésie chirurgicale par la méthode des injections de chloral dans les veines.* Paris; 1875.
10.10 Roehr ZM. *Hypodermic syringe.* US Patent 2,728,341 1955. (appl.1951) and *Disposable needle assembly.* US Patent 2,953,243 1960 (appl. 1957).
10.11 Murdoch CA. *Means for use in the administering of drugs, medicines and the like to animals.* US Patent 3,207,157 1965 (appl.1962).

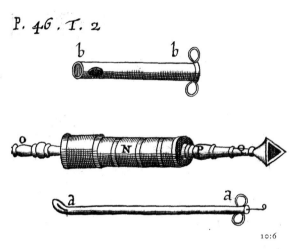

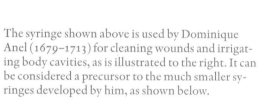

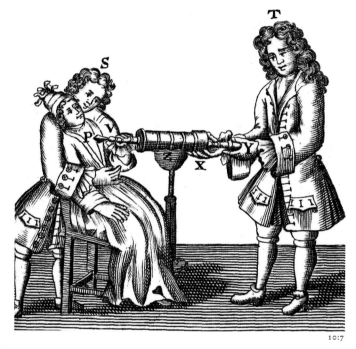

The syringe shown above is used by Dominique Anel (1679–1713) for cleaning wounds and irrigating body cavities, as is illustrated to the right. It can be considered a precursor to the much smaller syringes developed by him, as shown below.

The lachrymal syringe of Anel. It is used to remove obstructions in the canals leading from the eye to the nose to allow the natural progress of tears.

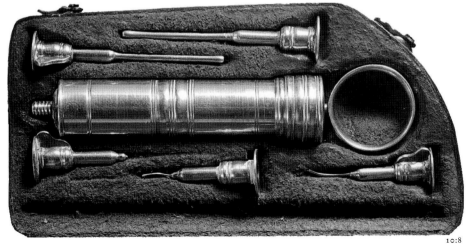

To the right, in 1853 Charles Pravaz (1791–1853) develops a hypodermic needle to inject blood coagulating agents with precision. The picture shows a Pravaz-type glass and silver hypodermic needle from the late 19th century.

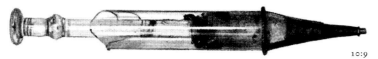

10:9

Above, the original hypodermic needle of Alexander Wood (1817–1884) used to inject opiates into joints for pain relief. Wood shares the credit for introducing the hypodermic needle with Pravaz.

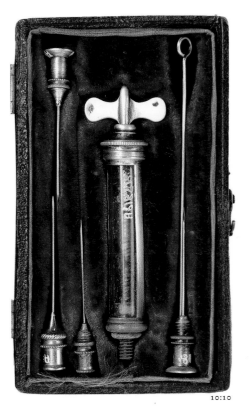

10:10

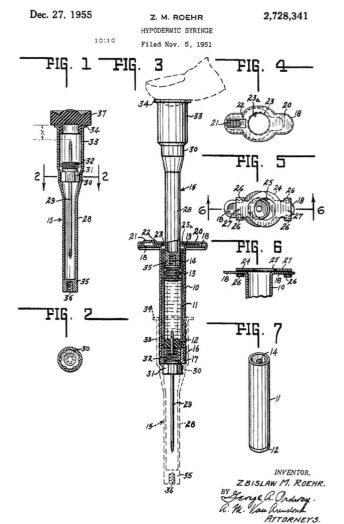

10:11

Dec. 27, 1955   Z. M. ROEHR   2,728,341
HYPODERMIC SYRINGE
10:10   Filed Nov. 5, 1951

Sept. 20, 1960   Z. M. ROEHR   2,953,243
DISPOSABLE NEEDLE ASSEMBLY
Filed July 25, 1957

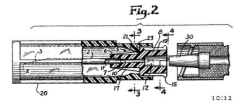

10:12

The patent applications for the first disposable hypodermic syringe (left) and needle assembly (above) invented by Zbislaw Roehr during the early 1950s. The syringe was introduced on the market in 1955 under the name of Monoject.

An Account

Of an Experiment made by M. Hook, of Preserving Animals alive by Blowing through their Lungs with Bellows.

This *Noble Experiment* came not to the Publisher's *hands, till all the preceding Particulars were already sent to the Press, and almost all Printed off, (for which cause also it could not be mentioned among the* Contents:*) And it might have been reserved for the next opportunity, had not the considerableness thereof been a motive to hasten its Publication. It shall be here annexed in the Ingenious* Author *his own words, as he presented it to the* Royal Society, Octob. 24. 1667. *the Experiment it self having been* both *repeated (after a former successful trial of it, made by the same hand a good while agoe)* and *improved the week before, at their* publick Assembly. *The Relation it self followes;*

I Did heretofore give this *Illustrious Society* an account of an Experiment I formerly tryed of keeping a Dog alive after his *Thorax* was all display'd by the cutting away of the *Ribbs* and *Diaphragme*; and after the *Pericardium* of the Heart also was taken off. But divers persons seeming to doubt of the certainty of the Experiment (by reason that some Tryals of this matter, made by some other hands, failed of success) I caus'd at the last Meeting the same Experiment to be shewn in the presence of this *Noble Company*, and that with the same success, as it had been made by me at first; the Dog being kept alive by the Reciprocal blowing up of his Lungs with *Bellowes*, and they suffered to subside, for the space of an hour or more, after his *Thorax* had been so display'd, and his *Aspera arteria* cut off just below the *Epiglottis*, and bound on upon the nose of the Bellows.

And because some Eminent Physitians had affirm'd, that the *Motion of the Lungs* was necessary to Life upon the account of promoting the Circulation of the Blood, and that it was conceiv'd, the Animal would immediately be suffocated as soon as the Lungs should cease to be moved, I did (the better to fortifie my own *Hypothesis* of this matter, and to be the better able to judge of several others) make the following additional Experiment; *viz.*

The Dog having been kept alive, (as I have now mentioned) for above an houre, in which time the Tryal had been often repeated, in suffering the Dog to fall into *Convulsive* motions by ceasing to blow the Bellows, and permitting the Lungs to subside and lye still, and of suddenly reviving him again by renewing the blast, and consequently the motion of the Lungs : This, I say, having been done, and the Judicious Spectators fully satisfied of the reality of the former Experiment; I caused another pair of Bellowes to be immediately joyn'd to the first, by a contrivance, I had prepar'd, and pricking all the outercoat of the Lungs with the slender point of a very sharp pen-knife, this second pair,

Robert Hooke's (1635–1703) account of his ingenious experiments with artificial ventilation of the lungs. Hooke's observations and conclusions are still valid today.

11:1

HOOKE was born in Freshwater on the Isle of Wight in 1653. Even as a boy he demonstrated exceptional skills in constructing ingenious mechanical devices. After formal studies in Oxford he became assistant to Boyle (11.1) and joined the brilliant group of men that founded the Royal Society in 1662. (11.2) As the curator of the experiments at the meetings of the Society he made numerous inventions and original scientific observations. His theory of celestial mechanics and gravitation initiated Newton's own work. Being a friend of Wren (11.2), he also participated in the rebuilding of London after the great fire. Hooke was a difficult, quarrelsome person who engaged in long and bitter fights with his colleagues. A genuine hypochondriac, he lived in a stormy relation with his niece and died at the age of sixty-seven.

Philosophical Transactions of the Royal Society London. 1667; 2 (October 21): 539.

IN THIS treatise entitled "An account of an Experiment made by M. Hook, of Preserving Animals alive by blowing through their Lungs with bellows" Hooke connects a dog with open thorax to two bellows. Using one bellows only he demonstrates repeatedly for an hour that it is "the supply of fresh Air" that keeps the dog alive. Using both bellows, the second to produce permanent positive pressure through rapid pumping, he shows that if the lungs are perforated, a continuous flow of air occurs across it and that this alone is sufficient to keep the dog alive. Thus he proves that "the bare Motion of the Lungs without fresh Air contributes nothing to the life of the Animal".

IN PERSPECTIVE:
Using a pregnant sow, Vesalius was the first to describe the effects of artificial ventilation (11.3). Boyle, assisted by Hooke, had previously shown that animals perish in an enclosed space when air is evacuated (11.4). Mayow found that only a portion of the air is used in respiration, since the gas volume was only reduced by a small fraction on breathing (11.5). He argued that the lungs transferred particles from the air to the blood where they were combusted and gave rise to the temperature of the body. With the discovery of carbon dioxide and oxygen (11.6)(11.7)(11.8), Spallanzani was able to show that oxygen is taken up and carbon dioxide is given off from animals, their tissues and organs (11.9). He also demonstrated that this process is influenced by activity and temperature and by the nature and quantity of food ingested. Quantitative studies of gas exchange and blood gases almost half a century later confirmed his observations (11.10).

11.1 See #14 Boyle page 88.
11.2 See #10 Wren page 68.
11.3 See ref. 1.6 the last chapter.
11.4 See ref. 8.6, p174: A Digression containing some Doubts touching Respiration.
11.5 Mayow J. *Tractatus quinque medico-physici.* Oxford; 1674.
11.6 See #20 Black page 116.
11.7 See #21 Scheele page 122.
11.8 See #24 Lavoisier page 134.
11.9 Spallanzani L. *Mémoires sur la respiration ... traduits en Francais, d'après son manuscrit inédit*, par J. Senebier Geneva; 1803.
11.10 See #24 Lavoisier page 134, #37 Magnus page 196 and #58 Voit page 300.

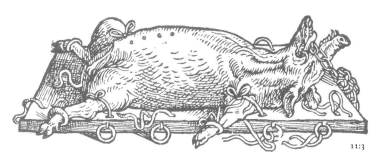

11:3

Andreas Vesalius (1514–1564) describes artificial ventilation for the first time. He writes in 1543: "To proceed: the vivisection I promised a little while ago to describe, you should perform on a pregnant sow or bitch. It is better to choose a sow on account of the voice. For a dog, after being bound for some time, no matter what you may do to it, finally neither barks nor howls, and so you are sometimes unable to observe the loss or weakening of the voice. First, then, you must fasten the animal to the operating table as firmly as your patience and your resources allow, in such a way that it lies upon its back and presents unimpeded the front of its neck and the trunk of its body." Then having pierced "the inner lining of the ribs" Vesalius points out how the lung collapses, though the thorax continues to move just as before. Finally he teaches "But so that life may in some measure be restored to the animal, you must attempt an opening in the trunk of the trachea and pass into it a tube of rush or reed, and you must blow into this so that the lung may expand and the animal draw breath after a fashion; for at a light breath the lung in this living animal will swell to the size of the cavity of the thorax, and the heart take strength afresh and exhibit a great variety of motions."

(540)

pair of Bellows was mov'd very quick, whereby the first pair was always kept full and always blowing into the Lungs; by which means the Lungs also were always kept very full, and without any motion; there being a continual blast of Air forc'd into the Lungs by the first pair of Bellows, supplying it as fast, as it could find its way quite through the Coat of the Lungs by the small holes pricked in it, as was said before. This being continued for a pretty while, the Dog, as I exspected, lay still, as before, his eyes being all the time very quick, and his Heart beating very regularly: But, upon ceasing this blast, and suffering the Lungs to fall and lye still, the Dogg would immediately fall into Dying convulsive fits; but be as soon reviv'd again by the renewing the fulness of his Lungs with the constant blast of fresh Air.

Towards the latter end of this Experiment a piece of the Lungs was cut quite off; where 'twas observable, that the Blood did freely circulate, and pass thorow the Lungs, not only when the Lungs were kept thus constantly extended, but also when they were suffer'd to subside and lye still. Which seem to be Arguments, that as the *bare* Motion of the Lungs *without fresh Air* contributes nothing to the life of the Animal, he being found to survive as well, when they were not mov'd, as when they were; so it was not the subsiding or movelesness of the Lungs, that was the immediate cause of Death, or the stopping the Circulation of the Blood through the Lungs, but the *want* of a sufficient *supply of fresh Air*.

I shall shortly further try, whether the suffering the Blood to circulate through a vessel, so as it may be openly exposed to the fresh Air, will not suffice for the life of an Animal; and make some other Experiments, which, I hope, will throughly discover the *Genuine use of Respiration*; and afterwards consider of what benefit this may be to Mankinde.

FINIS.

11:4

Continuation of Hooke's account of his experiments with artificial ventilation where he concludes that "the bare Motion of the Lungs without fresh air contributes nothing to the life of the Animal." This apparently simple observation was all but forgotten for more than a century.

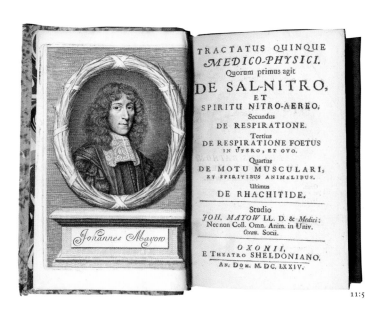

11:5

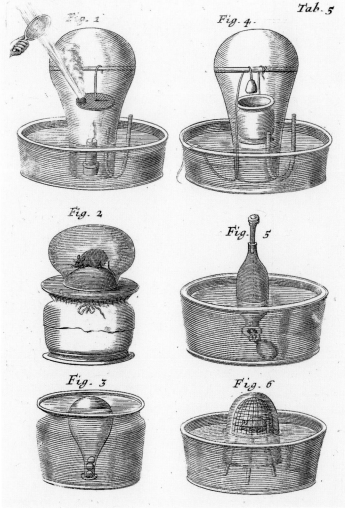

11:6

John Mayow (1645–1679) proves that a certain portion of air is made up of "nitro-aerial" particles (later recognised as oxygen). He finds them to be less abundant in exhaled air but necessary to sustain combustion. He writes in his book from 1674 depicted above, "let a burning candle be placed in water . . . and let an inverted cupping-glass of sufficient height be put over the light and plunged immediately into the water surrounding the light . . . and you will presently see, while the light still burns, the water rising gradually into the cavity of the cupping-glass." Mayow also considers "nitro-aerial" particles as essential for breathing (also for the foetus) and for performing muscular work. His experimental arrangements are shown by the illustrations on the left.

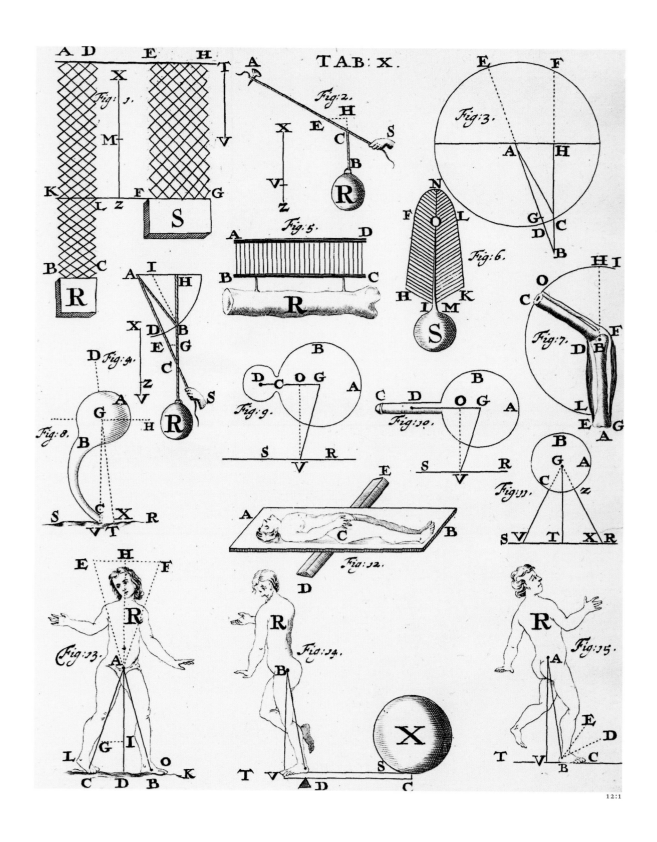

Giovanni Borelli (1608–1679) is the first to apply the new science of mechanics introduced by Galileo Galilei (1564–1642) to physiology. He does this when analysing the movements of the human body and the movements of its muscles.

Borelli was born in Naples in 1608, the son of a Spanish infantryman. Borelli's early years were tumultuous due to the general political turmoil and the private difficulties of his father. As a young man in Rome he made the acquaintance of prominent scientists and patrons of the sciences. Later, when Borelli was professor of mathematics in Pisa, he came to play a leading role in the founding and activities of the "Accademia del Cimento" (12.1). From 1637 he taught mathematics in Messina, Sicily, becoming professor in 1649. The spread of epidemic fevers aroused his interest in anatomy and medicine. He also got involved with politics, one time having a price on his head. Robbed of all his possessions by a servant, he spent the last years of his life in Rome teaching elementary mathematics.

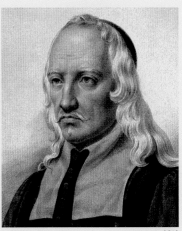

Giovanni Borelli   12:2

De motu animalium.

ROME: A. BERNABO; 1680–1681.

THIS BOOK, which is in two volumes, was published the years following Borelli's death. Its printing was paid for by Queen Christina of Sweden, to which the work is dedicated. The first part deals with the external motions of the animal body due to the interaction of bones and muscles. The second part deals with the internal movements such as respiration and circulation. Here Borelli also considers the origin of the muscle function. He recognises that an explanation entirely based on mechanical concepts is inadequate. He believes that chemical processes and neural stimulation influence the contraction of muscles in general and the heart in particular. His analysis of the working of the heart is based on Harvey's demonstrations (12.2) and a simple hydraulic model.

IN PERSPECTIVE:
In the spirit of the times Borelli conceived the body as a machine to be understood using the new mechanical sciences of Galileo Galilei (12.3) and in doing so he laid the foundations of biomechanics. Borelli was also the first to view the working of the heart as a hydraulic system, an approach soon to be expanded on by Bernoulli (12.4). Strongly influenced by the teachings of Santorio (12.5), Borelli was a keen observer and realised that biomechanics and physics alone could not explain all his observations. He therefore introduced new ideas that would lead to the neurogenic concept of the heart's action and muscular contraction (12.6)(12.7). During the 19th century the physiology of movements and the physics of muscle function were elucidated by the Weber brothers (12.8) and by Fick (12.9), and Marey conducted detailed studies of animal motion using photographic and cinematographic techniques (12.10)(12.11).

12.1 See ref. 7.3.
12.2 Harvey W. *Excercitation Anatomica de motu Cordis et Sanguinis in Animalibus*. Frankfurt am Main; 1628.
12.3 Galilei G. *Discorsi e dimostrazioni ...* Leiden; 1638.
12.4 Borelli GA. *De motu animalium Ed novissima. Johannis Bernouilli meditationes mathematicae de motu musculorum*. Lugduni Bat; 1710.
12.5 See # 4 Santorio page 36.
12.6 Haller A. *Elemanta physiologiae corporis humani*. Lausanne Berne Leiden; 1757–1766.
12.7 Galvani L. *De viribus electricitatis in motu musculari*. Bologna; 1791.
12.8 Weber W, Weber E. *Mechanik der menschlichen Gehwerkzeuge Eine anathomisch-physiologische Untersuchung*. Göttingen; 1836.
12.9 See # 46 Fick page 242 and ref. 46.6.
12.10 Marey E-J. *La machine animale, locomotion terrestre et aérienne*. Paris; 1873.
12.11 Frizot M. *La Chronophotographie*. Beaune (Cote-d'Or); 1984. see also # 52 Marey page 272.

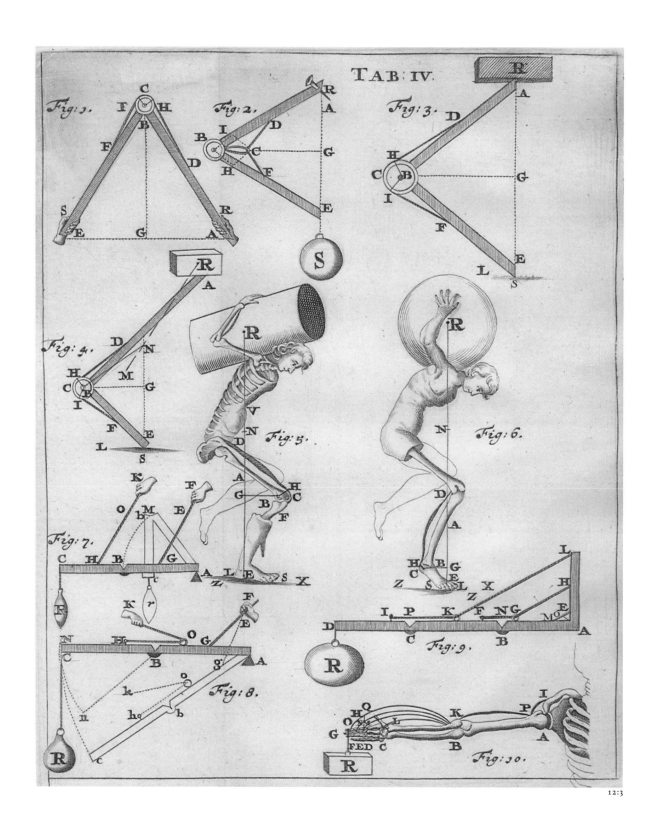

Although Borelli studies muscular control and movement from a mechanical viewpoint (see his diagrams above), he realises that contraction and swelling of the muscles cannot be solely mechanical but must also involve chemical processes.

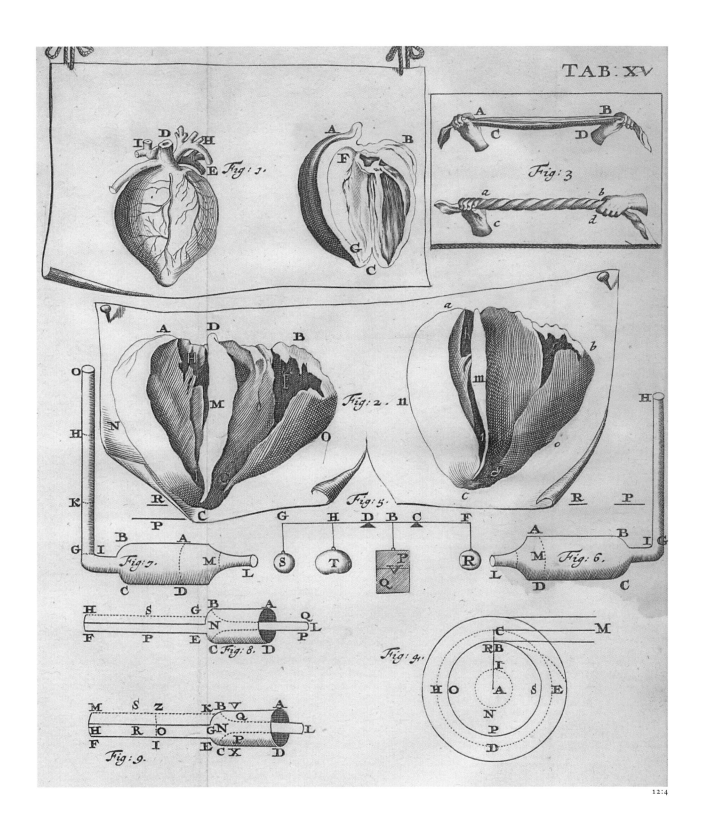

Borelli is the first to argue that the heart beat is a result of a muscular contraction and that the circulatory system can be represented by a simple hydraulic analogue, as illustrated above.

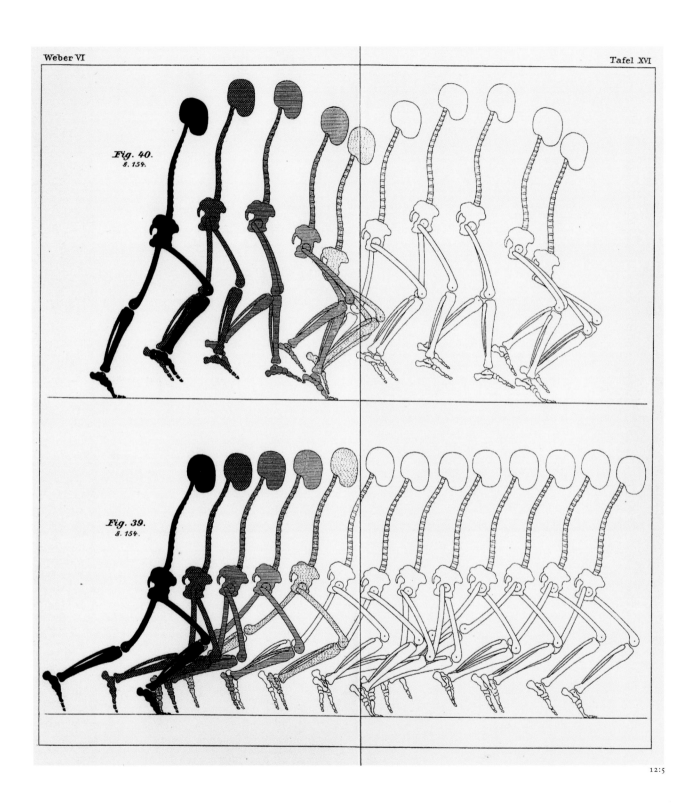

Fig. 40.
§. 154.

Fig. 39.
§. 154.

12:5

In 1836 the brothers Wilhelm Weber (1804–1891) and Eduard Weber (1806–1871) study and visualise the mechanics and physiology of walking.

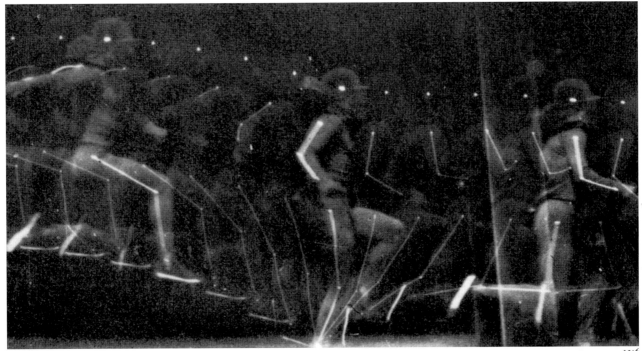

12:6

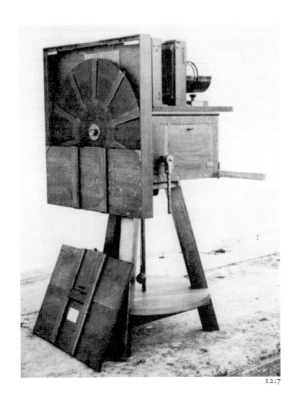

12:7

Etienne Marey (1830–1804) develops new photographic techniques that allow detailed recording and study of rapid motions of animal and man. In one of his experiments a man is running in black cloths with white stripes and dots against a black background (top). Marey's apparatus for taking these pictures, the "chronophotographe" from 1882, is shown on the left.

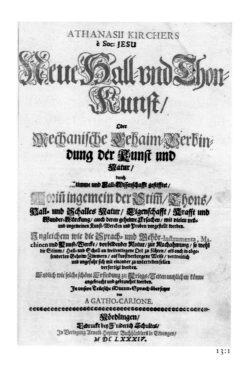

13:1

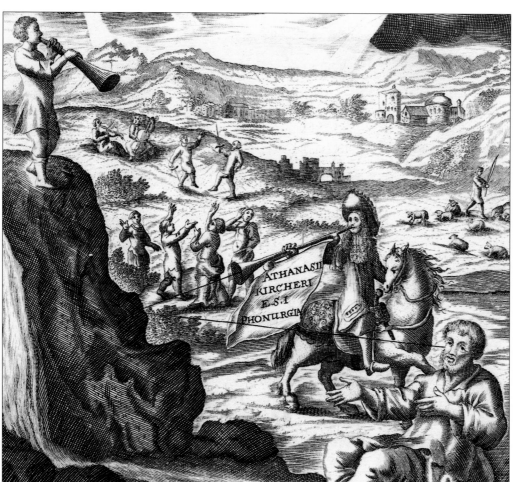

13:2

In 1673 Athanasius Kircher (1602–1680) writes the first book entirely devoted to the nature and properties of sound. The picture above shows the elaborate title page of the German translation of this work. A detail of the frontispiece (left) illustrates some of the observations reported in the book on sound propagation and generations.

KIRCHER was born in Geisa ad Ulster in Germany in 1602. He studied humanities, natural science, mathematics, philosophy, languages and theology and entered the Society of Jesus in 1616. As professor of philosophy and mathematics in Würzburg, he published the first of his forty-four books dealing with his own physico-mathematical experiments on magnetism. His extraordinary variety of interest and education allowed him to write on nearly all fields of the humanities and sciences. In 1633 he settled in Rome and carried out independent studies there for the rest of his life. A polymath, he played a key role during the 17th century in disseminating news about advances in various fields of knowledge, thereby promoting and influencing progress in the sciences and in medicine.

Neu Hall- und Thon-Kunst, oder, Mechanische Gehaim-Verbindung der Kunst und Natur ...

NÖRDLINGEN: F. SCHULTES; 1684.

THIS BOOK, the German translation of Kircher's "New way of making sound" from 1673, is one of the first publications devoted entirely to the study of the nature and properties of sound. Kircher's interest in acoustics arose from his intense study of music, which he believed could provide important understanding and knowledge about the world. As a Jesuit he believed that music could produce strong emotional effects of benefit to the body and soul. For instance, he transcribed the tarantella, music which was customarily played and a dance performed as an "antidote" for the bite of a venomous spider (Apulian tarantula).

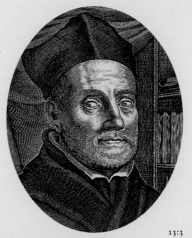

13:3

Athanasius Kircher at the age of seventy-six.

IN PERSPECTIVE:
Kircher was an early microscopist and the first to make medical observations, advancing the idea that microscopic organisms caused infectious disease (13.1). In his main treatise on magnetism and static electricity, "Loadstone or the magnetic art"(13.2), he gave a comprehensive account of the use of magnetism in medicine. Although Boyle had shown (13.3) that sound became extinct in an evacuated space, a more detailed understanding of the nature of sound phenomena was gained only at the beginning of the 19th century, when Young analysed sound propagation and interference phenomena using an analogy with the wave properties of light (13.4) and Chladni demonstrated acoustic resonance patterns in plates (13.5). A decade earlier, Kempelen had investigated the function of the human speech generating organs and built a working mechanical model of them (13.6). With a better understanding of wave phenomena, the mechanism of hearing could be studied in detail (13.7)(13.8). In a major advance Helmholtz combined the physiology of hearing with the science of sound (13.9) and Lord Rayleigh put this science on a rigorous mathematical footing (13.10).

13.1 Kircher A. *Scrutinium physico-medicum contagiosae luis, quae pestis dicitur.* Romae; 1658. See also # 9 Borel page 64.

13.2 Kircher A: *Magnes, sive, de Arte magnetica opus tripartium ...* Cologne; 1643.

13.3 See ref. 8.6 Experiment 27.

13.4 Young T. Outlines of Experiments and Inquiries respecting Sound and Light. *Phil Trans Roy Soc.* 1800; Jan.16.

13.5 Chladni EF. *Die Akustik.* Leipzig; 1802.

13.6 See # 25 Kempelen page 138.

13.7 See # 32 Fourier page 176 and ref. 32.5.

13.8 See # 26 Volta page 144 ref. 26.5 and ref. 26.6.

13.9 von Helmholtz H. *Die Lehre von den Tonempfindungen als physiologische Grundlage für die Theorie der Musik.* Braunschweig; 1863.

13.10 Lord Rayleigh (Strutt J). *The theory of sound.* London; 1878.

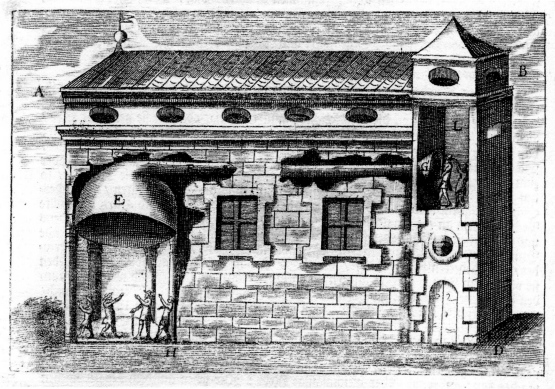

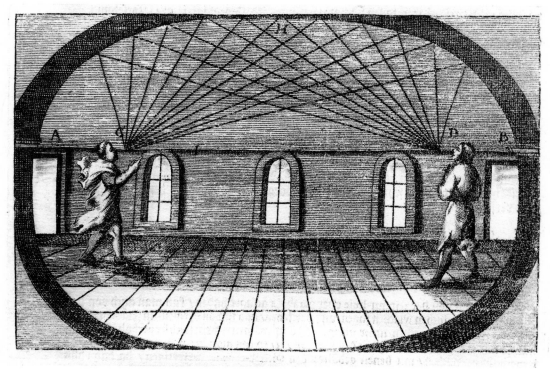

Kircher discusses applications of sound amplification (top), the acoustics of buildings and the phenomenon of echoes.

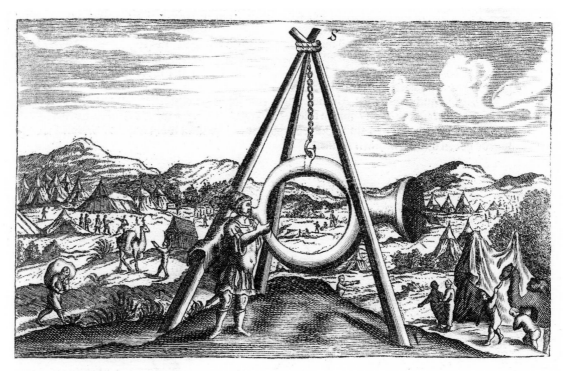

13:6

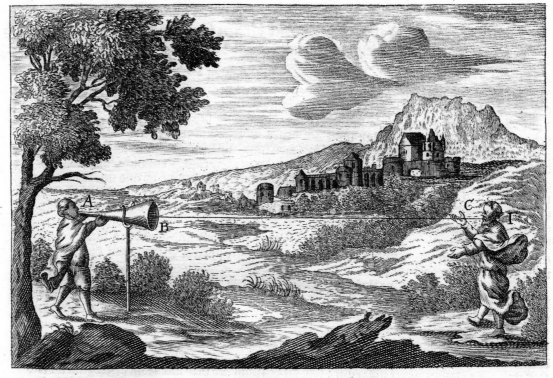

13:7

The big horn used, according to Kircher, by Alexander the Great (356–323BC) to call out to his army (top) and his own (contested) invention, the "speaking trumpet" (below).

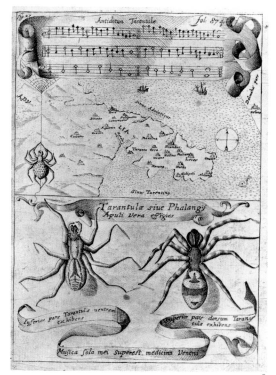

13:8

As a Jesuit, Kircher believes that music has a beneficial effect on both body and soul. He transcribes the tarantella (right), which is commonly played and danced (see picture below) as an "antidote" for the bite of a venomous spider (Apulian tarantula, depicted in the lower left corner of the picture).

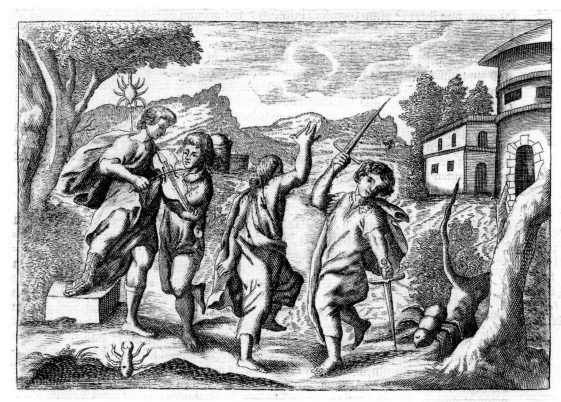

13:9

CAPVT V.

De pestis seminarijs, siue de propagationis conta-
giosæ modo & ratione vberior explicatio.

 X dictis patuit, putrefactionem con-
tagiosam propriè non ex simplici
quatuor elementorum contamina-
tione, sed præterea ex aliena & pe-
regrina qualitatis deleteriæ facultate
superueniente constitutam esse, cu-
ius proprium sit sordidam & foetidam vim in alte-
rum siue per contactum immediatum, siue median-
te fomite transferre, atque adeo idem in alieno & se-
parato subiecto præstare, quod eadem ex insita virtutis suæ efficacia per inspirationem præstitit in priori subiecto; haud secus ac magnes solo ferri contactu
ei vim suam communicat, quàm ferrum sibi insitam
innumeris alijs ferramentis, quamuis à Magnete re-
motissimo spacio dissitum communicare potest;
delectantur enim similia similibus, & ad se inuicem
confluunt, se fouent, se mutuis officijs benignè affi-
ciunt, per reciprocam virium communicationem.
Quemadmodum itaque putredo pestifera siue conta-
giosa non ex primarum qualitatum naturali penua-
rio suæ virtutis & virulentæ efficaciæ robur suscipit;
sed ex abditis naturæ peregrinis Seminarijs foeturam
concipit; ita minimè quoque mirum, tam exoticis
& in-

Pestis specifi-
ca qualitate
inficit corpo-
ra.

13:10

Kircher is the first to apply microscopy to medical research. In
1656 an outbreak of the bubonic plague in Rome turns his interest to the cause of infectious diseases. Two years later he
publishes a famous tract (see the title page on the right) where,
under the heading "A detailed description of the origin of the
plague or the mechanism of its spread", he argues that infection can be carried over through direct contact by microscopic
organisms both between man and when in contact with animals (reproduced in part above).

ATHANASII KIRCHERI
E SOC. IESV
SCRVTINIVM
PHYSICO-MEDICVM
Contagiosæ Luis, quæ PESTIS dicitur.
QVO
Origo, causæ, signa, prognostica Pestis, nec non insolentes
malignantis Naturæ effectus, qui statis temporibus,
cælestium influxuum virtute & efficacia, tum
in Elementis, tum in epidemijs hominum
animantiumque morbis elucescunt,
vnà cum appropriatis remediorum
Antidotis nouâ doctrinâ in
lucem eruuntur.
AD
ALEXANDRVM VII.
PONT· OPT· MAX·

ROMÆ, Typis Mascardi. MDCLVIII.
SVPERIORVM PERMISSV.

13:11

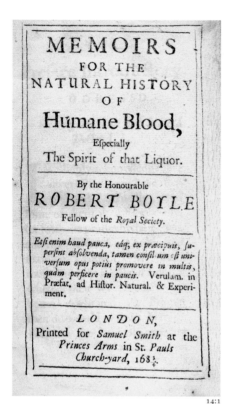

In thirty paragraphs, Robert Boyle (1627–1691) reports on the properties of the human blood. This work can be considered the start of the science of physiological chemistry.

B OYLE was born in Lismore, Ireland, the son of the afflu-ent and influential first Earl of Cork. After private tu-ition, he studied at Eton, in Geneva and later at Oxford. His early interest in astronomy soon yielded to prob-lems in medicine, which led him to chemistry and physics. In 1668 he settled in London and soon turned his house, where his labora-tory was located, into a centre for scientific activities. He was one of the founders and the most prominent member of the Royal So-ciety. A prolific writer on what he called "experimental natural philosophy", he was also a devout, scrupulous man who wrote ex-tensively on "natural theology", that is on the relationship be-tween science and religion.

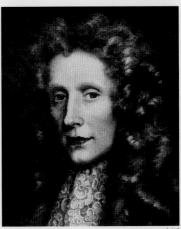

Robert Boyle   14:3

Memoirs for the Natural History of the Human Blood, especially the Spirit of that Liquor.

LONDON: S. SMITH; 1683–1684.

THIS BOOK marks the beginning of physiological chemistry. Boyle describes a large number of experiments on the physical and chemical properties of blood. He investigates its properties when exposed to heat and cold, the density and viscosity of the different components. The behaviour of blood in contact with various chemicals, acids and alkali, is described and an attempt is made to extract gases from it using an air pump (pneumatic engine). Boyle also notes that on contact with air the dark colour of blood turns to a more "pleasant" one. He discusses extensively the many possi-ble uses of blood for medication. The detailed explanations of the concepts and methods used reflect his novel ideas about how to approach a problem in a scientific way (14.1).

IN PERSPECTIVE:
Boyle's work was always original and never dogmatic and it greatly influenced sci-entific thought for almost a century following his death. At the end of the 18th century, better separation techniques allowed Hewson to present the first valid account of the mechanism of blood coagulation (14.2). Davy noted that blood contained carbon dioxide and oxygen (14.3) and Berzelius analysed the separate parts of blood, showing that it contained iron (14.4). Gustav Magnus was the first to measure blood gases in a quantitative way in 1837 (14.5) and soon thereafter Hoppe-Seyler isolated and studied haemoglobin (14.6). The work of Arrhenius on ions in dilute solutions (14.7), steadily improved methods of blood gas analysis (14.8) and the introduction of the pH concept at the beginning of the 20th centu-ry (14.9) all contributed significantly to the development of modern clinical chemistry (14.10). Its central role in the struggle against the polio epidemics in Scandinavia in 1950–1953 (14.11) is one of many examples showing how clinical needs generate technical innovations that in turn further progress in medicine.

14.1 See ref. 4.6.
14.2 Hewson W. *An experimental inquiry into the properties of the blood.* London; 1771.
14.3 See #28 Davy page 156.
14.4 Berzelius JJ. *Föreläsningar i djurkemien Vol. I,* Stockholm; 1806. p130–131. See also ref. 51.3.
14.5 See #37 Magnus page 196.
14.6 See #51 Hoppe-Seyler page 268.
14.7 See #62 Arrhenius page 320.
14.8 Astrup P, Severinghaus JW. *The history of blood gases, acids and bases.* Copenhagen: Munsgaard; 1986.
14.9 See ref. 14.8 Chapter XI.
14.10 See #81 van Slyke page 416.
14.11 See #87 Engström page 450.

156 *The Natural Hiſtory*

The X. (Secondary) Title.

Of the coagulating Power of the Spirit of Humane Blood.

THough the Spirit of Humane Blood, have ſuch a diſſolving power as we have mention'd, in reference to ſome Bodies, yet upon ſome others it ſeems to have a quite contrary Operation. I ſay *ſeems*, becauſe it may be queſtion'd, (and I am not now minded to diſpute it) whether the effect I am going to ſpeak of be a *Coagulation*, properly ſo call'd, that one Body makes of another or a Coalition of Particles fitted, when they chance to meet one another, (in a convenient manner,) to ſtick together. But whatever name ought to be properly given to the thing I am about to ſpeak of, I have found by Tryal purpoſely made, that the

of Humane Blood. 157

the highly rectifyed Spirit of Humane Blood, being well mingled by ſhaking with a convenient quantity, (which ſhould be at leaſt equal) of Vinous Spirits that will burn all away, (for if either of the Liquors be Phlegmatick, the Experiment ſucceeds either not at all, or not ſo well) there will preſently enſue a Coagulation or concretion, either of the whole Mixture, or a great portion of it, into Corpuſcles of a Saline form, that cohering looſly together, make up a Maſs that has conſiſtence enough not to be fluid, though it be very ſoft : and in this form it may remain as far as I have yet tryed, for a good while, perhaps ſeveral weeks, or months at leaſt, if it be kept in a cool place.

14:4

Boyle describes experiments on the coagulation of blood (top) and his early observation of the colour change of blood on oxygenation (below).

Experiment VI.

THe Black or lower part of a Portion of Humane Blood being turn'd uppermoſt, and thereby expos'd to the Air, within half or three quarters of an hour, (ſomewhat more or leſs) acquired by the Contact of it, a pleaſant and florid colour.

14:5

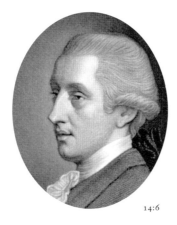

14:6

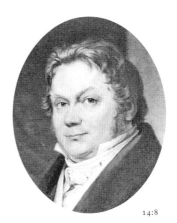

14:8

In a series of reports starting in 1768, William Hewson (1739–1774) describes the discovery of lymphocytes. He also finds fibrinogen to cause the clotting of the blood.

In 1806 Jacob Berzelius (1779–1848) makes the first quantitative determination of the iron content of haemoglobin ("blodets färgämne"). About two decades later he reports an iron content of 0.536% by weight (see below), which is to be compared to the modern value of 0.347%.

XXXII. *Experiments on the Blood, with some Remarks on its Morbid Appearances; by* William Hewson, *F. R. S.*

Read June 14 & 21. 1770.

AS the following Experiments are made on a subject generally thought important, and as the inferences which I have ventured to draw from them seem to explain some appearances in diseases, they will not, I flatter myself, be thought altogether unworthy the attention of this learned Society.

When fresh blood is received into a bason, and suffered to rest, in a few minutes it jellies, or coagulates, and soon after separates into two parts, distinguished by the names of *crassamentum* and *serum.* These two parts differ in their proportions in different constitutions: in a strong person, the *crassamentum* is in greater proportion to the *serum* than in a weak one; and the same difference is found to take place in diseases; thence is deduced the general conclusion, that the less the quantity of *serum* is in proportion to the *crassamentum*, bleeding, diluting liquors, and a low diet, are the more necessary: whilst in some dropsies and other diseases where the

14:7

Undersökning af Blodkakan. 67

af oxblod. Dess färg är roftröd. Michaëlis fann af kalfblodets färgämne ända till 2,2 procent, hvilket dock fynes härröra från ofullkomligt afläzsnande af blodvatten. Af 1,3 del afka, erhällen af 100 del. färgämne ur menniſkoblod, erhöll jag: kolſyradt natron, med ſpår af phosphorſyradt, 0,3, phosphorſyrad kalk 0,1, ren kalkjord 0,2, baſiſk phosphorſyrad jernoxid 0,1, jernoxid 0,5, kolſyra och förluſt 0,1. Ur färgämne af oxblod, ſom ſå trögt låter förvandla ſig till afka, att den ſiſta portion kol måſte medelſt ſalpeter bortbrännas, erhöll jag af 1,0 del afka, återſtod efter 100 del. tort färgämne, phosphorſyrad kalk 0,06, ren kalkjord 0,2, baſiſk phosphorſyrad jernoxid 0,075, jernoxid 0,5, kolſyra och förluſt 0,165. Här faknas alkalihalten, hvilken vid ſalpeterns utlakning bortfördes. Som det phosphorſyrade jernſaltet endaſt genom den analytiſka methoden bildas, ſå förſökte jag att af 100 del. afka af blodets färgämne, på lika ſätt förbrändt med tillfats mot ſlutet af ſalpeter, utfälla jernet utan halt af phosphorſyra, medelſt vätefvafladt ſvafvelammonium, hvarvid jag erhöll 55½ procent jernoxid. Häraf följer ſåledes att blodets färgämne har en jernhalt, ſvarande mot något mer än ½ procent, eller 0,00536 af dess vigt metalliſkt jern, men i hvad form jernet deri finnes är ett problem, ſom vi ännu ej kunnat löſa. Jag ſkall emedlertid anföra det hiſtoriſka om våra bemödanden dertill.

E 2

14:8

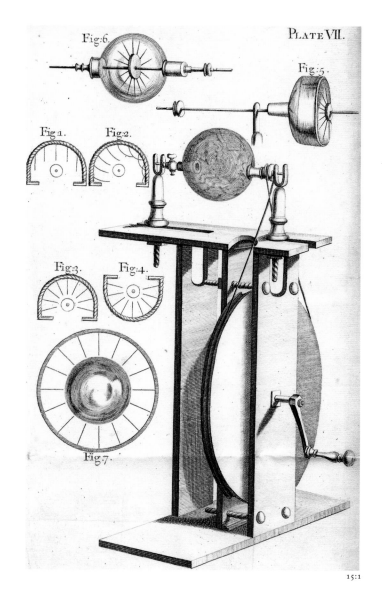

15:1

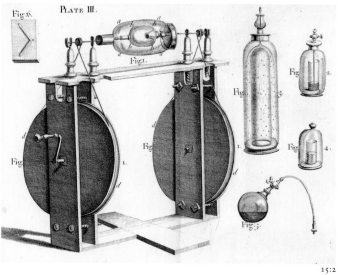

15:2

Two of Francis Hauksbee's (1666–1713) ingenious devices built to generate and study electric charge and discharge. He investigates the light produced by the friction between glass and different materials and when electricity passes through rarefied air.

LITTLE is known about Hauksbee's early life. He was probably born in 1666 in Colchester, worked as a draper and married in 1687. However, by 1703 he was considered an excellent instrument maker and skilled experimenter. Newton, the new president of the Royal Society, invited him to make demonstrations at their weekly meetings. Hauksbee was elected fellow of the Royal Society in 1705. An experimentalist of wide ranging interest, he was not bent on theoretical work or in his own words, echoing those of Newton, he "was not one to amuse himself with vain hypotheses which seem to differ little from romances". A close and fruitful collaboration developed between Newton and Hauksbee and lasted till Hauksbee's death 1713. with Newton often suggesting the experiments and offering possible explanations of the results.

Physico-mechanical Experiments on Various Subjects ...

LONDON: R. BRUGIS; 1709.

IN THIS book, which presents the first systematic experimentation on static electricity, Hauksbee describes his apparatus and observations. The main aim is to understand the origins of light (mercurial phosphorus) previously reported to arise from frictions between glass and mercury. Hauksbee designs ingenious equipment to generate this phenomenon, producing electric charge in various ways and studying the light generated for different materials and different circumstances. In the process he explores the properties of static electricity inside and outside evacuated glass vessels. Hauksbee also investigates capillarity and argues that independent of the material of the capillary tubes, attractive forces over small distances are at play giving rise to some "Universal Establish'd Law of Nature".

IN PERSPECTIVE:

As the Greek word for amber "electron" suggests, static electricity was well know to the ancients (15.1). Gilbert, in his important work on magnetism (15.2), also investigated electrical phenomena and found new materials, notably phosphorus, which were easily charged. Guericke used a rotating sphere of phosphorus to generate static electricity (15.3). Following Hauksbee's work, many electrical machines were built of increasing sophistication and size (15.4)(15.5)(15.6). In a major development, Musschenbroek invented the Leiden jar in 1746. His method of accumulating charge in a glass bottle partially filled with water, as first described by Winkler (15.7), would significantly increase the power of these early machines (15.1). Electric induction of charge between bodies was first practised by Volta in 1775 (15.8) and a sensitive torsion instrument to measure charge was designed in 1785 by Coulomb (15.9). In 1748, Jallabert observed that electricity could be used to stimulate the muscles and was the first to apply it to treating the paralyses of a patient (15.10).

15.1 *Dibner B. Early electrical machines.* Norwalk; 1957.

15.2 Gilbert W. *De magnete, magneticisque corporibus, et de mango magnete tellure.* London; 1600.

15.3 See ref. 8.5.

15.4 Nollet JA. *Essai sur l'Électricité des Corps.* Paris; 1746.

15.5 Watson W. *Expériences et Observations pour servir a l'Explication de la Nature et des Proprietés de l'Électricité.* Paris; 1748.

15.6 von Marum M. *Description d'une Très Grande Machine Électric ...* Haarlem; 1785–1787.

15.7 Winkler JH. *Die Stärke der Electrischen Kraft des Wassers in gläsernen Gefässen, welche durch den Musschenbroekischen Versuch bekannt geworden.* Leipzig; 1746.

15.8 Volta A. *Lettera a Priestley sull'elettroforo perpetuo.* Scelta di Opusculi. 1775; 9:91.

15.9 Coulomb C-A. Construction et usage d'une balance électrique, ... *Mém de l'Acad Sci.* 1785. p569.

15.10 See #19 Jallabert page 110.

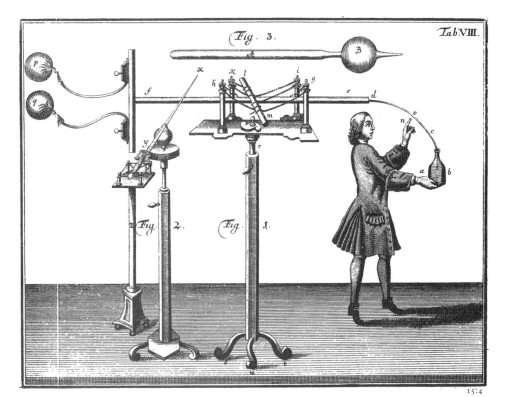

In 1746 Johann Winkler (1703–1770) gives the first description of an experiment with what is known as a Leiden jar (a waterfilled glass jar acting like a primitive capacitor). This device had just been invented by Pieter van Mussenbrook (1692–1761) and greatly enhanced the electric effects produced with early electric machines.

15:4

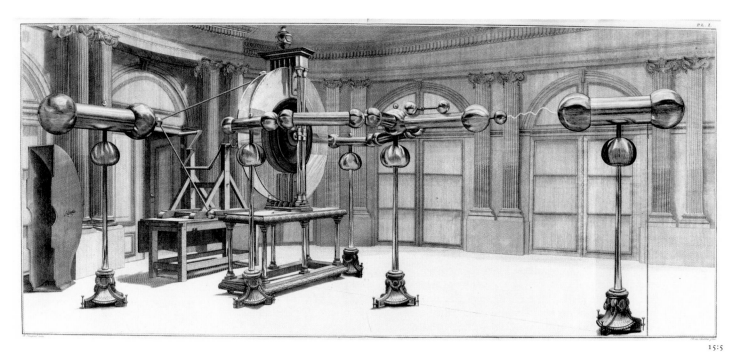

1784 sees Martinus van Marum (1750–1837) build the largest electric machine of the 18th century. The two glass plates are 1.6 m in diameter and the sparks between the brass electrodes can be 0.65 m long.

15:5

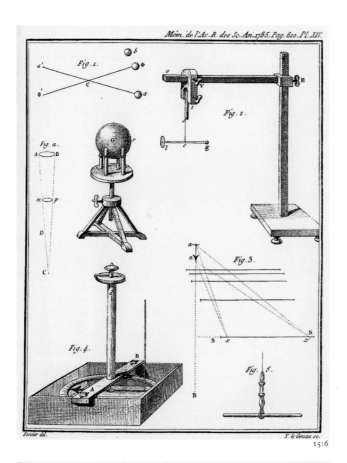

Mém. de l'Ac. R. des Sc. An. 1785. Pag. 610. Pl. XIV.

15:6

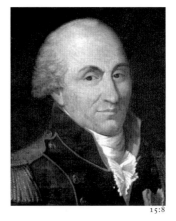

15:8

The construction of a very sensitive torsion balance (see illustrations to the left) allows Charles-Augustin de Coulomb (1736–1806) to measure the electrostatic forces between charged bodies at different distances and to establish what is now called Coulomb's law.

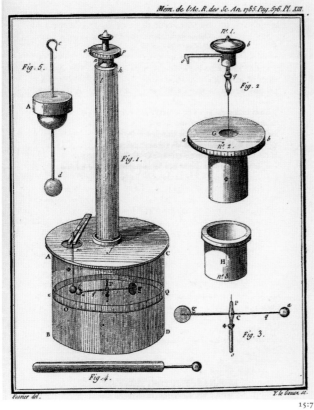

Mém. de l'Ac. R. des Sc. An. 1785. Pag. 576. Pl. XIII.

15:7

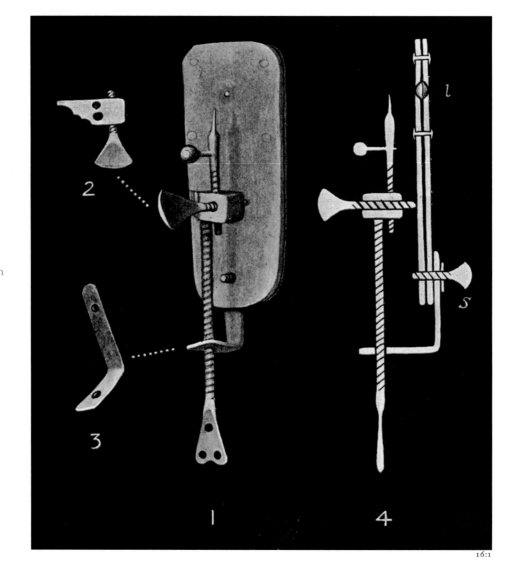

Antoni van Leeuwenhoek
(1632–1723) constructs a
very simple microscope with
high magnification using a
fixed lens ("l") of his own
design and manufacture.
The object under study is
moved using a screw.

16:1

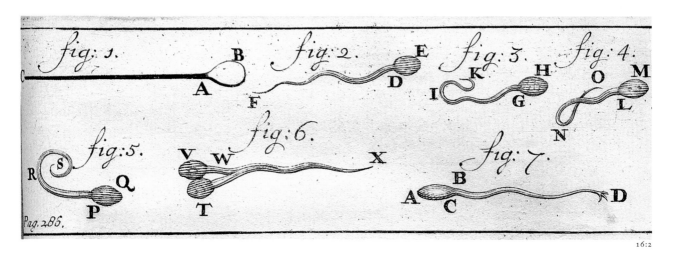

16:2

The first observation of spermatozoa as depicted in Leeuwenhoek's report.

LEEUWENHOEK was born in 1632 in Delft. He died at the age of ninety-one, having spent nearly all of his life in that city. After grammar school, Leeuwenhoek started work first in the cloth trade, then as a shopkeeper and finally as a civil servant. His scientific work began in 1671 and most of his important discoveries were made during the following ten years. The Royal Society elected him a fellow in 1680 and also translated his letters, where he reported his results, into English. His scientific achievements brought him fame and a generous pension. His fellow townsmen called him fondly a "magician" and so many prominent nobility wanted to meet with him that he had to demand introductory letters before seeing them.

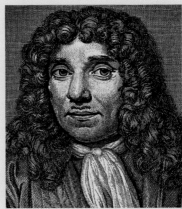

Antoni van Leeuwenhoek   16:3

Opera Omnia. Vol. I–IV.

LEIDEN: J. A. LANDERAK (A. BEMAN); 1719–1722.

LEEUWENHOEK'S COLLECTED work is made up of the 165 letters that he sent to the Royal Society for publication. Grinding his own lenses and using simple, single lens microscopes, he painstakingly observes and documents organic and inorganic structures. His best instrument has a resolving power of ~1 μm at about 500 times magnification, a performance not surpassed for almost two centuries (16.1). Leeuwenhoek's most important findings are in the field of general biology. He studies the spermatozoa of different species and believes that they are the origin of all new life and that fertilisation occurs as a result of its penetration of the egg. Other observations of importance include those on blood corpuscles, capillaries, bacteria and the structure of plants.

IN PERSPECTIVE:
Lacking language skills and unwilling to travel, Leeuwenhoek was rather isolated in his work. Malpighi, an eminent contemporary microscopist and friend of Borelli (16.2), had observed the blood corpuscles already in 1665, but he believed they were fat globules. Malpighi also studied the structure of the lung of a frog and in the process made the first observation of the capillaries in 1661 (16.3)(16.4). This discovery confirmed the theory of circulation of the blood as first proposed by Cesalpino and subsequently demonstrated by Harvey (16.5). About a century later, in patient and careful microscopic studies, Spallanzani made the first observations of mammalian arteriovenous anastomoses. Using a new innovative dissecting microscope (16.6), he was able to follow the development of the circulatory system in a chick embryo (16.7). Whether life originated in the spermatozoa as Leeuwenhoek believed or in the egg as argued by Harvey (16.8) was finally resolved in 1875, when Hertwig demonstrated that fertilisation occurred as a result of a fusion between the two (16.9).

16.1 See #64 Abbe page 328. For the first compound (multiple lenses) microscope see #9 Borel page 64.
16.2 See #12 Borelli page 76.
16.3 Malpighi M. *De pulmonibus observationes anatomicae*. Bologna; 1661.
16.4 Malpighi M. *Opera Omnia*. London; 1686.
16.5 Cesalpino A. *Peripateticarum Quationum Libri Quinque*. Venice; 1571. and ref. 12.2.
16.6 Lyonet P. *Traité anatomique de la chenille, ...* La Haye; 1762.
16.7 Spallanzani L. *De' Fenomeni della Circolazione ...* Modena; 1773.
16.8 Harvey W. *Exercitationes de Generatione Animalium*. London; 1651.
16.9 Hertwig O. *Beiträge zur Kentniss der Bildung Befruchtung und Theilung des tierischen Eies*. Leipzig; 1875.

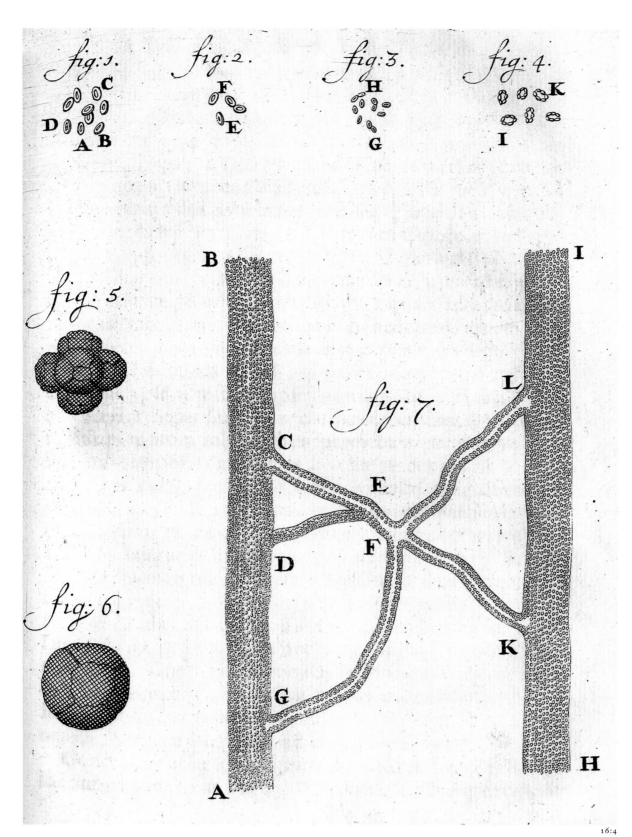

fig: 1.

C
D   B
A

fig: 2.

F
E

fig: 3.

H
G

fig: 4.

K
I

fig: 5.

fig: 6.

fig: 7.

B

C

D

G

A

I

L

E

F

K

H

16:4

The first correct microscopic identification of the red blood corpuscles (in the capillaries) is made by Leeuwenhoek in the year 1700. His illustration of this finding is shown above.

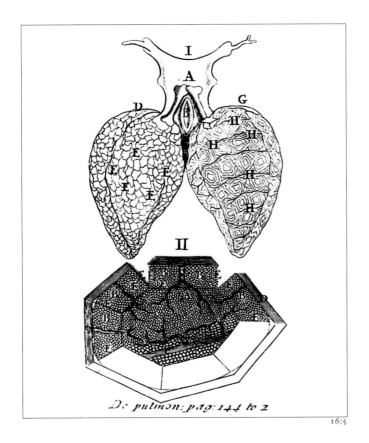

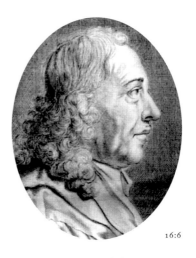

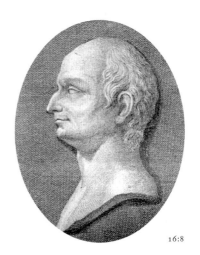

16:6

In 1661 Marcello Malphigi (1628–1694) observes the capillary vascular bed in the lung of the frog. This important discovery eliminates the missing link in William Harvey's (1578–1657) explanation of how blood circulates in the body.

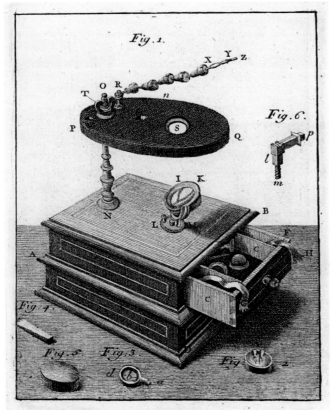

16:7

16:8

Using a newly developed dissecting microscope, Lazarro Spallanzani (1729–1799) painstakingly follows the evolution of chick embryos and observes for the first time mammalian arteriovenous anastomoses (connection between artery and vein).

EXPERIMENT CXVI.

I bored a hole in the side of a large wooden
foffet *a b*, (Fig. 39.) and glewed into it the
great end of another foffet *i i*, covering the
orifice with a bladder valve *r*: Then I fitted a valve *b i*, to the orifice of the iron
fyphon *f f*, fixing the end of the fyphon
faft at *b* into the foffet *a b*: Then by means
of narrow hoops I placed four *Diaphragms*
of flannel at half an inch diftance from each
other, into the broad rim of a fieve, which
was about 7 inches diameter. The fieve was
fixed to, and had a free communication with
both orifices of the fyphon, by means of
two large bladders *i i n n o.*

    The inftrument being thus prepared, pinch-
ing my noftrils clofe, when I drew in breath
with my mouth at *a*, the valve *i b* being
thereby lifted up, the air paffed freely thro'
the fyphon from the bladders, which then
fubfided, and fhrunk confiderably: But when
I breathed air out of my lungs, then the
valve *i b* clofing the orifice of the fyphon, the
air paffed thro' the valve *r* into the bladders, and thereby dilated them; by which
               arti-

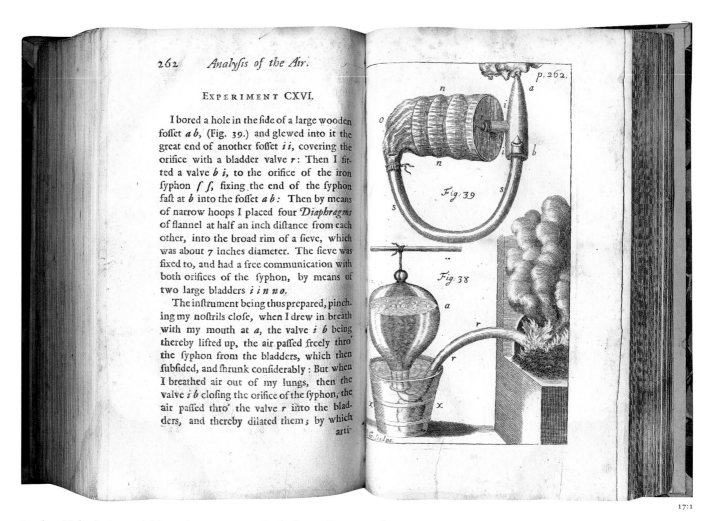

Stephen Hales (1677–1761) introduces a new method of gas collection and storage. He experiments to determine the effects of rebreathing gases and finds that breathing through caustic substances allows longer rebreathing times. Hales' work greatly influences subsequent developments in chemistry and contributes to the discovery of many of the most important medical gases.

H ALES was born into a distinguished family in Bekes-bourne, England, in 1677. He studied at Cambridge, where he was ordained as a deacon in 1709. He then took up residence as minister in the village of Tedding-ton, where he lived the rest of his life. Amid his parish duties he carried out occasional scientific experiments for about twenty years starting in 1713. Although a fellow of the Royal Society, he devoted the last thirty years of his life only to the duties of a country minister. He was serene and cheerful of mind and anxiously guarded the morals of his village. He actively promoted the Gin Act of 1736, which was aimed at "stopping that profusion of spirituous liquors which threaten to ruin the morals and constitution of the common people".

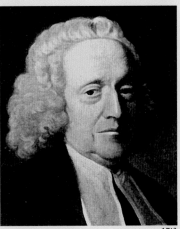

Stephen Hales   17:2

Vegetable Staticks, Statical Essays: containing Hæmastaticks; …

LONDON: W. INNYS, R. MANBY, T. WOODWARD; 1727 AND 1733.

IN THE chapter "Analysis of the Air", Hales presents experiments to determine the amount of air "fixed" to or given off from various bodies. He develops a new method of collecting and storing gas, later to be used by Priestley (17.1), where the gas first passes through water to remove "the acidic spirit". In rebreathing studies he finds that breathing through caustic substances allows much longer rebreathing times. He measures blood pressure by inserting a canula fitted with a long glass tube into the femoral artery of a mare and notes how high the blood rises in the tube. He also manipulates peripheral resistance by injecting among other things brandy and studies the effects on the capillaries, the heart rate and on the blood flow. Aware of Hauksbee's experiments (17.2), Hale speculates that electricity might cause the muscular action of the heart, explaining the forces required to produce the blood pressure observed.

IN PERSPECTIVE:

In 1754, still during Hale's lifetime, Black identified and studied carbon dioxide for the first time (17.3) and before the end of the 18th century many other important medical gases such as oxygen (17.4)(17.1)(17.5), nitrogen, (17.6) and nitrous oxide (17.1)(17.7) were discovered and investigated. The first major improvement in blood pressure measurements after Hale's work was the introduction of the mercury manometer by Poiseuille in 1828 (17.8). This was followed by the invention of sphygmographs (17.9)(17.10), which could display the arterial pulse, and at the end of the 19th century by Riva-Rocci's sphygmomanometer (17.11), which operated according to modern principles. Thus, although just a sideline to his ordinary duties, Hale's scientific studies exerted a profound influence on later developments in medicine.

17.1 See #22 Priestley page 124.
17.2 See #15 Hauksbee page 92.
17.3 See #20 Black page 116.
17.4 See #21 Scheele page 120.
17.5 See #24 Lavoisier page 134.
17.6 Rutherford D. *Dissertatio Inauguralis de Aere Fixo dicto, Aut Mephitico.* Edinburgh; 1772.
17.7 See #28 Davy page 156.
17.8 See #35 Poiseuille page 188.
17.9 Vierordt K. Die *Lehre vom Arterienpuls in gesunden und kranken Zustände, gegrundet auf eine neue Methode der bildlichen Darstellung des menschlichen Pulses.* Braunschweig; 1855.
17.10 See #52 Marey page 272.
17.11 See #68 Riva-Rocci page 350.

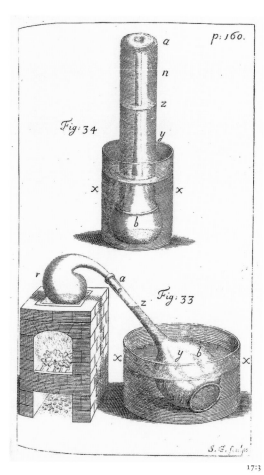

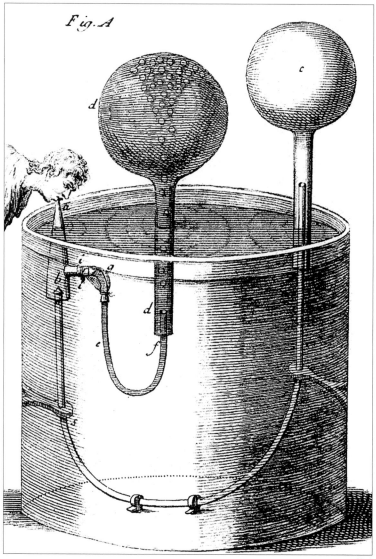

Hales' influential experiments (shown above) that demonstrate that air is "either generated or absorbed" on fermentation (figure 34) and is commonly given off when heating various substances (figure 33).

George Compte de Buffon's (1707–1788) illustration (right) of Hales' simple but ingenious method of determining the quantity of air "destroyed by respiration", that is the difference between oxygen uptake and carbon dioxide elimination during breathing.

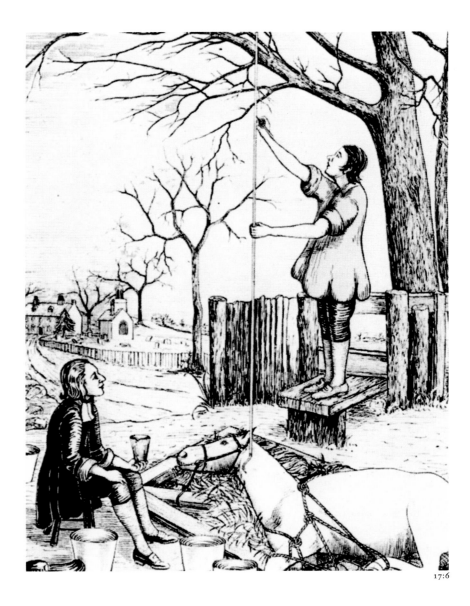

AN ## ACCOUNT

OF SOME

Hydraulick and Hydrostatical Experiments made on the Blood and Blood-Vessels of Animals.

EXPERIMENT I.

1. IN *December* I caused a Mare to be tied down alive on her Back, she was fourteen Hands high, and about fourteen Years of Age, had a *Fistula* on her Withers, was neither very lean, nor yet lusty: Having laid open the left crural Artery about three Inches from her Belly, I inserted into it a brass Pipe whose Bore was one sixth of an Inch in Diameter; and to that, by means of another brass Pipe which was fitly adapted to it, I fixed a glass Tube, of nearly the same Diameter, which was nine Feet in Length: Then untying the Ligature on the Artery, the Blood rose in the
B   Tube

17:5

In a number of pioneering experiments, the first being partly reproduced above, Hales measures the blood pressure and the intrathoracic pressure in animals using his new invention the U-tube manometer. He also gives estimates of the velocity of blood in the arteries, veins and capillary vessels.

Artist view of Hales' experiment on a mare that is partly reproduced above.

17:6

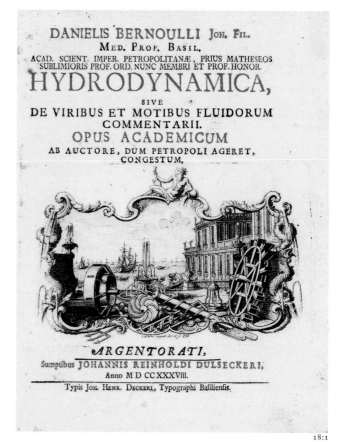

The title page of Daniel Bernoulli's (1700–1782) classical book from 1738, where he introduces the science of hydrodynamics (a word first used here). He derives what came to be called Bernoulli's equation for the steady flow of an incompressible fluid and demonstrates its validity through a number of experiments (some of them illustrated below).

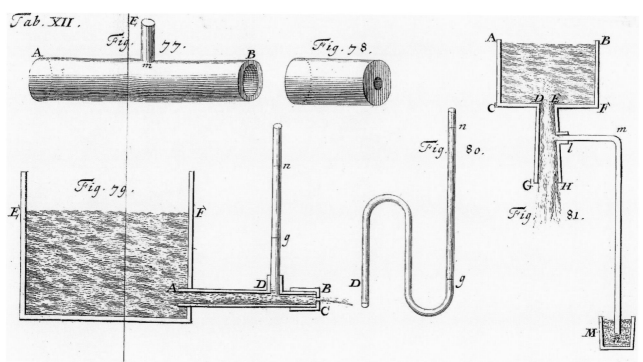

BERNOULLI was born in 1700 in Groningen, where his father Johann was professor of mathematics. First Bernoulli studied medicine in Basel, but under his father's tutoring he soon turned to mathematics and physics. In 1725, Empress Catherine I of Russia invited him to the Imperial Academy of St Petersburg, where he stayed for eight years. Winning the mathematical prize of the Paris Academy ten times, he was appointed professor of physics in Basel in 1750. The Bernoulli family was prone to internal strife. Johann and his brother Jakob I, also a famed mathematician, never got along well and Johann predated his writings about hydrodynamics in an unjust effort to deprive his son Daniel of the priority to his discoveries.

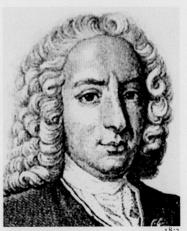

Daniel Bernoulli   18:3

Hydrodynamica, sive de viribus et motibus fluidorum commentarii.

STRASBOURG: J. H. DECKER; 1738.

WITH THIS book Bernoulli names and founds the scientific field of "hydrodynamics". He gives a mathematical treatment of various phenomena related to fluid flow. In chapter IX he analyses the performance of pumps, a study that leads to the first adequate calculation of the work performed by the heart (18.1). In chapter X he considers "elastic fluids", i.e. gases, and he presents the first mathematical model and a kinetic theory of gases. From this theory he deduces the basic gas laws known at that time (18.2) and calculates the relationship between barometric pressure and altitude. Chapter XII deals with stationary fluid flow in tubes and Bernoulli points out that the results obtained (Bernoulli's equation) can also be applied to "the flow of blood in veins and arteries".

IN PERSPECTIVE:

The Bernoulli family was instrumental in the very rapid development of mathematical analysis during the 18th century. Daniel Bernoulli was the first to consistently apply mathematical techniques to physical and physiological problems. The basic laws of the physics of gases were discovered by Gay-Lussac, Avogadro and Dalton at the beginning of the 19th century (18.3)(18.4)(18.5)(18.6). Maxwell was then able to derive a formula for the velocity distribution of particles in a gas, thereby establishing the connection between the microscopic processes and the macroscopic, observable properties (18.7). Poiseuille studied experimentally the flow of different liquids through capillary tubes. He found the law, now named after him, that relates the flow to the pressure, the diameter and the length of the tube and to the viscosity of the liquid (18.8). In 1851 the Weber brothers extended their previous investigation of wave propagation (18.9) to the study of blood flow in the circulatory system (18.10).

18.1 Bernoulli D. "Oratio physiologica de vita " 1737. Reprint of original and German translation Spiess O, Vezár F. *Verhandlungen der Naturforschenden Gesellschaft in Basel* 1940/1941; 52:189.

18.2 See ref. 8.4, 8.6.

18.3 Dalton J. Experimental essays on the constitution of mixed gases; . . . *Mem Lit Phil Soc Manchester* 1802; 5:535. Also see ref. 7.2.

18.4 Gay-Lussac JL. Mémoire sur la combinaison des substances gazeuses, les unes avec les autres. *Mém phys chim Soc d'Arcueil* 1809; 2:207.

18.5 Avogadro A. Essai d'une manière de déterminer les masses relatives des molécule élémentaires des corps . . . *Journal de physique* 1811; 73:58.

18.6 Dalton J. *A New System of Chemical Philosophy.* Manchester; 1827. See also ref. 8.8.

18.7 See # 55 Maxwell page 286 and ref. 55.2.

18.8 Poiseuille JLM. Recherches expérimentales sur le mouvement des liquides dans les tubes de très petits diamètres. *Mém Acad Roy Sci.* 1846; 9:433. See also ref. 35.10.

18.9 Weber EH, Weber W. *Wellenlehre auf Experimente gegrundet . . .* Leipzig; 1825.

18.10 See # 44 Weber page 232.

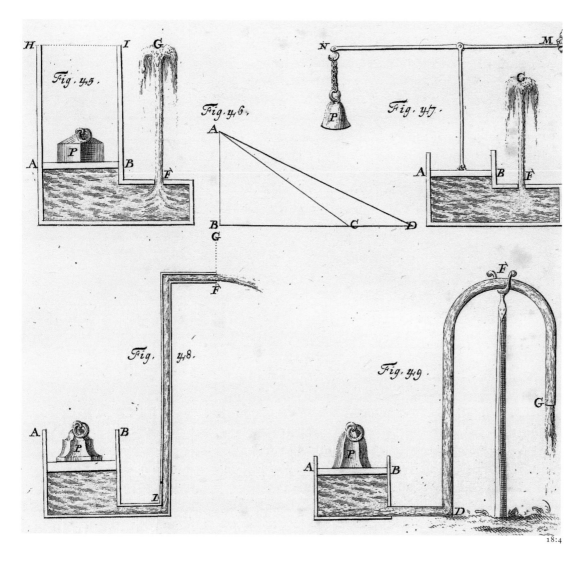

In the ninth chapter of Hydrodynamica Bernoulli deals with "the Motion of Fluids that are Pushed forth not by their own Weight but by an Outside force, and particularly concerning Hydraulic Machines …" (some of the arrangements considered are illustrated to the left). In the introduction to the book he notes, "In Physiology those things that pertain to the motion of liquids in an animal body are already better understood …"

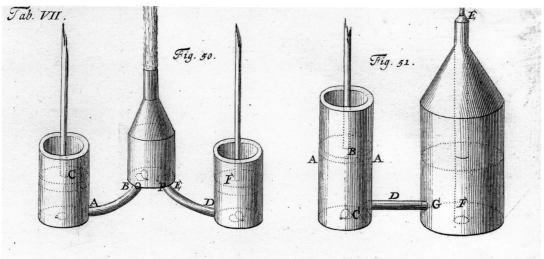

Dicam primo de corde tanquam praecipuo motuum internorum organo: tum aliquod de motu locali subjungam exemplum. methodus autem qua utar tam est facilis, ut omnem calculum tibi consecuturi, si modo animum ad rem istam attendere velitis.

Ponamus singulis cordis pulsibus duas sanguinis uncias ex sinistro cordis ventriculo expelli, et quidem expelli ea velocitate

18:6

qua ad altitudinem duorum pedum sanguis ascendere possit: tum tempore unius horae 4000 pulsus fieri accipiamus. Omnes hae hypotheses statui hominis medio sunt accommodatae: quantitatem sanguinis una systole expulsam docuerunt experimenta innumera: velocitatem colligere maxime licet à decollatis, in quibus aliquando vidi sanguinem ad altitudinem circiteruum pedum supra truncum à corde per carotides fuisse expulsum proptereaque altitudinem à corde numtam facio duorum pedum. numerum denique pulsuum quotidiana confirmat experientia. His igitur positis sequitur à fibris sinistrum cordis ventriculum constringentibus intra spatium unius horae eam vim generari, qua possint 16000 unciae ad altitudinem unius pedis elevari, sive, quod idem est, qua possit una libra ad altitudinem mille pedum evehi. Si deinde dextro ventriculo dimidiam vim tribuamus, dicendum erit, à toto corde singulis horis vim generari vivam, qua possit pondus unius librae et dimidiae ad altitudinem mille pedum elevari. Haec vera est cordis mensura.

18:7

Part of Bernoulli's manuscript of a speech that he delivers at a doctoral dissertation on October 4 1737. Here he explains for the first time how to calculate the work performed by the heart. "I will first speak of the heart as the most important organ of internal movement and then append an example of movement from place to place. The method of which I avail myself here is so simple that you will be able to follow the entire course of the calculation if you will merely direct your attention to it.

We work from the premise that for every single beat of the heart two ounces (0.0624 kg) of blood are expelled from its left chambers at such a velocity that the blood could thereby ascend to a height of two feet (see note below); we further assume 4,000 pulse beats per hour. All these assumptions are appropriate to persons of moderate stature. The quantity of blood expelled by one systole is known from numerous experiments; its velocity may best be obtained on the occasion of a decapitation. Thus I once saw how the blood was cast up approximately a foot above the trunk by the action of the heart through the vessels of the neck and I thereby estimate the height measured from the heart as two feet. Finally, the number of pulse beats is established by daily experience. Given these assumptions we now see that in the period of an hour the muscular fibres that compress the left chambers produce a force capable of raising 16,000 ounces (500 kg) to a height of one foot or, to put it another way, one pound (0.5 kg) to a height of 1,000 feet. If we then ascribe to the right ventricle one half of this force, we may say that in one hour the entire heart produces a force by means of which a weight of 1.5 pounds might be raised to a height of 1,000 feet. This is thus the true measure of the power of the heart."

Note: Bernoulli's calculation gives ~ 6000 m/kg for a 24 hour period which is about 1/3 of the correct value. The main cause for this error is his gross underestimation of the blood pressure, being unaware of the more correct values reported by Stephen Hales a few years before (see #17).

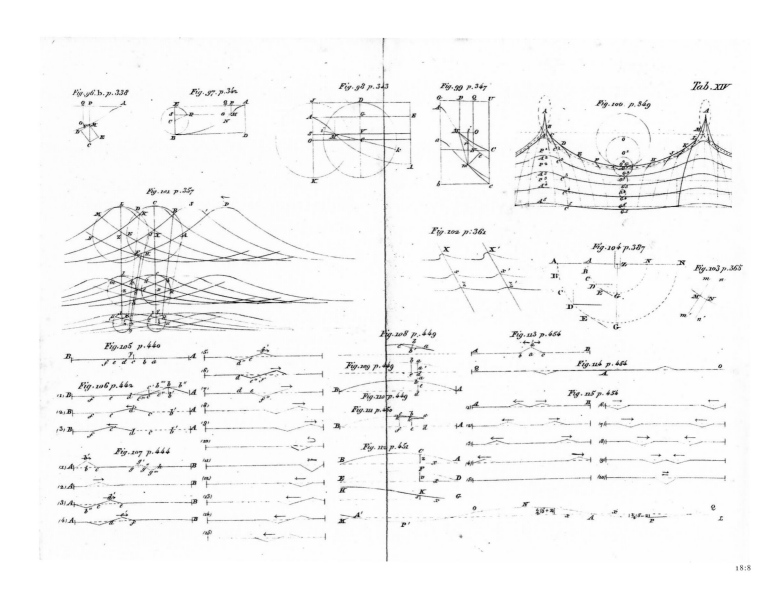

Fig. 96. b. p. 338

Fig. 97. p. 342

Fig. 98 p. 343

Fig. 99. p. 347

Tab. XIV

Fig. 100. p. 349

Fig. 101 p. 357

Fig. 102 p. 361

Fig. 104 p. 387

Fig. 103 p. 365

Fig. 108 p. 449

Fig. 113 p. 454

Fig. 105 p. 440

Fig. 109 p. 449

Fig. 114 p. 454

Fig. 106 p. 442

Fig. 110 p. 449

Fig. 115 p. 454

Fig. 111 p. 450

Fig. 107 p. 444

Fig. 112 p. 451

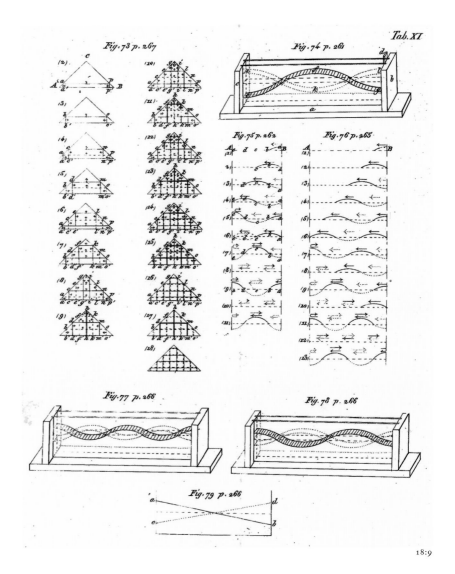

Ernst Heinrich Weber (1795–1878) and his younger brother Wilhelm Eduard Weber (1804–1891) apply the wave theory of sound and light to the hydrodynamic problems of the circulatory system. Their work includes experimental and theoretical investigations of fluid flow in both stiff and elastic tubes.

Jean Jallabert's (1712–1768) account of the first successful use of electricity to reverse paralysis. Initially paralysed on the right side, (below) a locksmith called Nogues is treated with electric shocks every day. After three months he is reported to have regained the full use of his arm (below right).

EXPERIENCES
SUR
L'ELECTRICITÉ,
AVEC
QUELQUES CONJECTURES
SUR LA CAUSE DE SES EFFETS.

PAR MR. JALLABERT

*Professeur en Philosophie Expérimentale &
en Mathématiques, des Sociétés Royales
de Londres & de Montpellier, & de
l'Académie de l'Institut de Bologne.*

A GENEVE,
Chez BARRILLOT & FILS.

M. DCC. XLVIII.

19:1

(127)

JOURNAL
DE QUELQUES
EXPERIENCES
FAITES SUR UN PARALYTIQUE.

§. CLXXXVII. Quelques observations me firent naître l'idée de tenter quel effet l'électricité produiroit sur un paralytique ; & j'avoue que la curiosité de vérifier certains faits eut autant de part à mes premiers essais, que l'espérance de sa guérison.

Le 26. Decembre 1747. le nommé Nogues, maître Serrurier, âgé de 52 ans & d'une complexion assés délicate, vint chez moi. Paralytique du bras droit, il y avoit perdu tout sentiment. Le poignet étoit fléchi vers le côté interne des deux os de l'avant bras; il étoit pendant & sans mouvement. Le pouce, le doigt index, l'auriculai-re

Etat du paralytique, & en particulier de sa main.

19:2

SUR L'ELECTRICITÉ. *133

troit, d'exciter dans tous les muscles qui meuvent l'os du bras les mêmes mouvements convulsifs que j'avois excité dans le deltoïde.

§. CCXXXV. Le 28. Noguès éleva, à la hauteur de plus de 7 piés, un poids de 16 livres attaché à une corde passant sur une poulie fixée au plancher. Et, par le mouvement d'extension du poignet, il jetta avec facilité plusieurs fois de suite une boule. Je mesurai le bras au même endroit que je l'avois deja fait, sa circonférence étoit de plus de 9. pouces.

§. CCXXXVI. Le 29. Mr. Guiot mit par écrit l'état où il avoit trouvé Noguès.

L'embonpoint du bras a beaucoup augmenté, les mouvements du bras, de l'avant-bras, du carpe & des doigts se font avec plus de facilité & de force. J'ai vu le malade empoigner une boule de 4 à 5 pouces de diamètre, & la jetter, en étendant le carpe, à plusieurs pas de distance. Il a aussi élevé par le moyen d'une poulie, en em-poi-

Quatrième rapport de Monsr. Guiot.

I* 3

19:3

J ALLABERT was born in 1712 in Geneva, the son of a preacher who was also professor of mathematics and philosophy. He soon followed in his father's footsteps. First a preacher and then turning his interest to science, he was appointed professor of physics at the age of twenty-five. By 1752 he also held the chair of mathematics and philosophy at the Academy of Geneva. In addition he was made the City Librarian. His main interest was in exploring and explaining the properties of electricity and he had an extensive correspondence with his more famous colleague, l'Abbé Nollet, on these topics (19.1). He also wrote on various meteorological observations.

Experiences sur l'electricité avec quelques conjectures sur la cause de ses effects.

GENEVA: BARRILOT & FILS; 1748.

AFTER A succinct account of what is known about electricity, Jallabert describes his observations on how electricity can stimulate muscles and reverse paralysis. Together with Guiot, a leading surgeon, he examines a locksmith called Nogues, and finds him paralysed on the right side as a result of an accidental blow to the head fourteen years before. The man could not move his arm, he had no sensations in it and he had no control over the fingers of the hand. Holding a Leiden jar (19.2) in his healthy hand and touching it with his paralysed hand, Nogues was treated with electric shocks for over an hour every day. Within two weeks an astonishing improvement in his condition was noted and three months later the patient had regained full use of his arm.

IN PERSPECTIVE:

In 1738 Stuart demonstrated reflex action on a decapitated frog by mechanical stimulation of the medulla spinalis (19.3), but this and Jallabert's observations went largely unnoticed. Instead it was Galvani's experiments with electrical stimulation (19.4) that initiated the controversy that finally led to the breakthrough in the understanding and use of electrical phenomena (19.5). Galvani believed that electricity was generated in the animal tissue ("animal electricity") (19.6) while Volta, experimenting with different metals in contact with tissue, claimed that the current was an external physical phenomenon (19.7). In 1804 Aldini, Galvani's nephew, summarised the observed effects of the galvanic current both on man and on corpses (19.8). The first to study the reactions of nerves to stimuli in a systematic way was Humboldt, who investigated the effects of light, heat, magnetism and electricity (19.9). Subsequently, using much improved instruments and methods, Du Bois-Reymond explored the topic extensively and in depth (19.10). The clinical application of electrical stimulus to the muscular and sensory systems was pioneered by Duchenne de Boulogne (19.11).

19.1 Benguigui I. Théories électriques du XVIIe siècle. *Isis* 1985; 76:442.

19.2 See #15 Hauksbee page 92 and ref. 15.7.

19.3 Stuart A. *Dissertatio de Structura et Motu Musculari.* London; 1738.

19.4 See ref. 12.7.

19.5 Dibner B. *Galvani-Volta A Controversy that led to the Discovery of Useful Electricity.* Norwalk; 1952.

19.6 Compare with #8 van Helmont page 60 and ref 8.1 and #4 Santorio page 36 and ref. 4.7.

19.7 Cavallo T. Some Discoveries Made by Mr Galvani of Bologna with Experiments and Observations on Them. *Phil Trans Roy Soc.* 1793;10:83.

19.8 Aldini J. *Essai théorique et expérimental sur la galvanisme* Vol. 1,2. Paris; 1804.

19.9 von Humboldt A. *Versuche über die gereizte Muskel-und Nervenfaser ...* Vol. 1,2 Berlin; 1797.

19.10 See #42 Du Bois-Reymond page 224.

19.11 Duchenne de Boulogne G. *De l'électrisation localisée et de son application a la physiologie, a la pathologie et a la thérapeutique.* Paris; 1855.

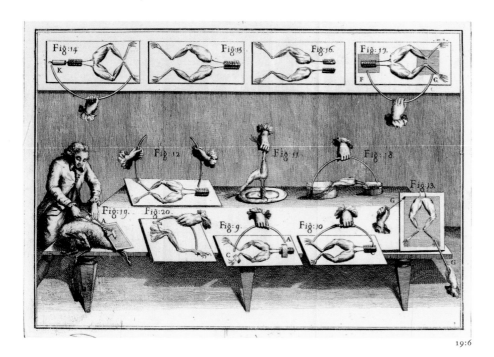

19:6

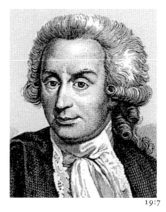

19:7

Luigi Galvani (1737–1798) and his famous demonstration of muscular contractions in frog legs induced by electric discharges.

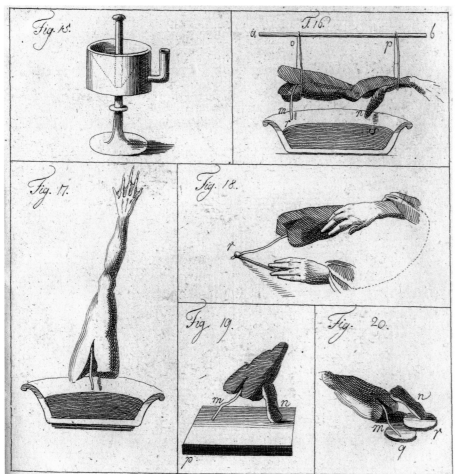

19:5

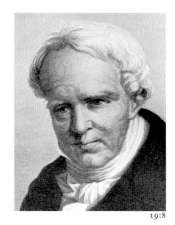

19:8

In 1797 Alexander von Humboldt (1769–1859) reports the first systematic investigation of how different factors such as heat, light, magnetism and electricity affect muscular contractility. The illustration left depicts some of his experiments.

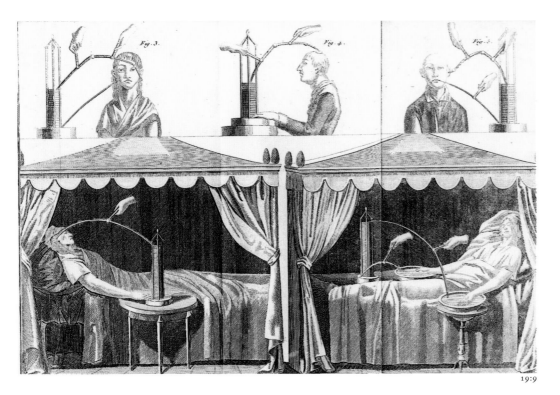

19:9

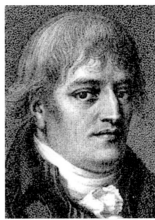

19:11

Giovanni Aldini (1762–1834), a nephew and strong supporter of Galvani, performs electrical experiments on both living persons (top) and corpses (below) and summarises the state of the art in the field of "galvanism" in a book published in 1804.

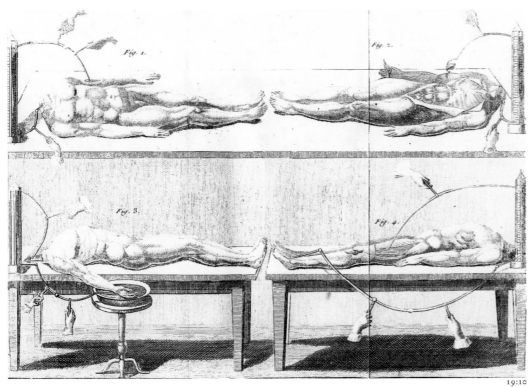

19:10

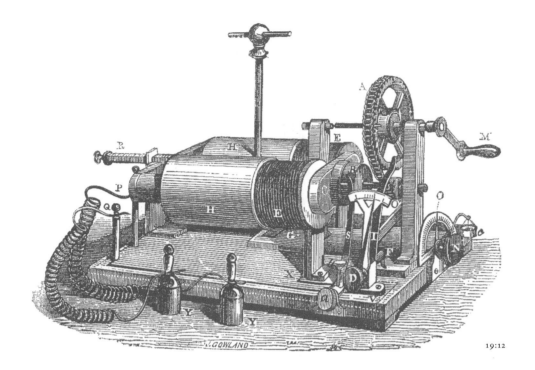

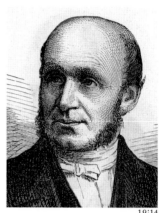

19:14

19:12

In the 1850s Duchenne du Boulogne (1806–1875) develops clinically useful apparatus for electric stimulation. Images show his prototype unit (top) and the final device (below) that he later uses in his pioneering electrophysiologic investigations.

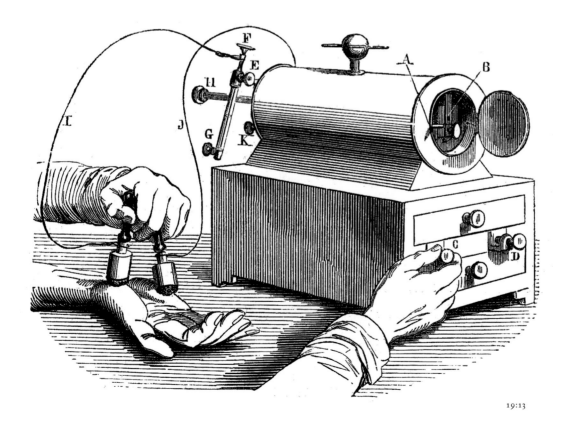

19:13

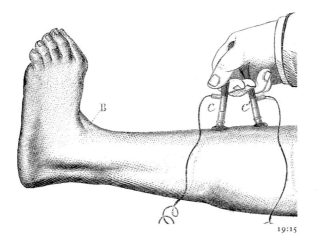

19:15

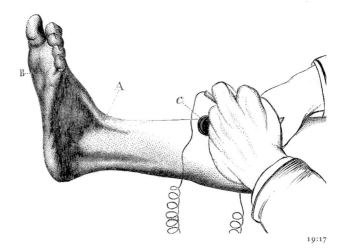

19:17

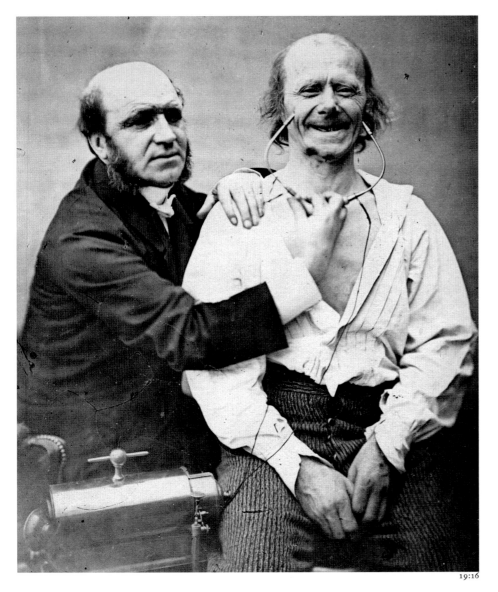

19:16

In an extensive and meticulously documented study that lays the foundation of electrotherapy, du Boulogne describes applications of localised electropuncture either direct (to the muscle) or indirect (to the nerve) (top). He is also among the first to use photography for medical purposes. In his book "The Mechanism of Human Facial Expression", he exposes a test person to facial stimulation using the electrodes (left).

DISSERTATIO MEDICA
INAUGURALIS,
DE
HUMORE ACIDO
A CIBIS ORTO,
ET
MAGNESIA ALBA:
QUAM,
ANNUENTE SUMMO NUMINE,
Ex Auctoritate Reverendi admodum Viri
D. JOANNIS GOWDIE,
ACADEMIAE EDINBURGENAE PRAEFECTI;
NEC NON
Amplissimi SENATUS ACADEMICI consensu,
Et nobilissimae FACULTATIS MEDICAE decreto;
PRO GRADU DOCTORATUS,
SUMMISQUE IN MEDICINA HONORIBUS ET PRIVILEGIIS
RITE ET LEGITIME CONSEQUENDIS,
ERUDITORUM EXAMINI SUBJICIT
JOSEPHUS BLACK GALLUS.
Ad diem 11 Junii, horâ locoque solitis.

EDINBURGI:
Apud G. HAMILTON ET J. BALFOUR
ACADEMIAE TYPOGRAPHOS,
M,DCC,LIV.

20:1

ART. VIII.

Experiments upon Magnesia alba, *Quicklime,
and some other Alcaline Substances ; by*
JOSEPH BLACK, M.D. [*]

PART I.

HOFFMAN, in one of his observations, gives the history of a powder
called *magnesia alba*, which had been long
used and esteemed as a mild and tasteless
purgative; but the method of preparing it
was not generally known before he made it
public [†].

IT was originally obtained from a liquor
called the *mother of nitre*, which is produced
in the following manner :

SALT-PETRE is separated from the brine
which first affords it, or from the water
with which it is washed out of nitrous earths,
by the process commonly used in crystallizing
salts. In this process the brine is gradually
diminished, and at length reduced to a small
quantity of an unctuous bitter saline liquor,
affording

[*] June 5. 1755.
[†] Hoff. op. T. iv. p. 479.

20:2

176 ESSAYS AND OBSERVATIONS

grains. This calcined *magnesia* was dissolved
in a sufficient quantity of spirit of vitriol, and
then again separated from the acid by the addition of an alkali, of which a large quantity is necessary for this purpose. The *magnesia* being very well washed and dryed,
weighed one dram and fifty grains. It effervesced violently, or emitted a large quantity
of air, when thrown into acids, formed a red
powder when mixed with a solution of sublimate, separated the calcarious earths from
an acid, and sweetened lime-water : and had
thus recovered all those properties which it
had but just now lost by calcination : nor
had it only recovered its original properties,
but acquired besides an addition of weight
nearly equal to what had been lost in the fire;
and, as it is found to effervesce with acids,
part of the addition must certainly be air.

THIS air seems to have been furnished by
the alkali from which it was separated by
the acid ; for Dr. *Hales* has clearly proved,
that alkaline salts contain a large quantity of
fixed air, which they emit in great abundance
when joined to a pure acid. In the present
case, the alkali is really joined to an acid, but
without any visible emission of air ; and yet
the

PHYSICAL AND LITERARY. 177

the air is not retained in it : for the neutral
salt, into which it is converted, is the same
in quantity, and in every other respect, as if
the acid employed had not been previously
saturated with *magnesia*, but offered to the
alkali in its pure state, and had driven the
air out of it in their conflict. It seems therefore evident, that the air was forced from
the alkali by the acid, and lodged itself in the
magnesia.

THESE considerations led me to try a few
experiments, whereby I might know what
quantity of air is expelled from an alkali, or
from *magnesia*, by acids.

Two drams of a pure fixed alkaline salt,
and an ounce of water, were put into a Florentine flask, which, together with its contents,
weighed two ounces and two drams. Some
oil of vitriol diluted with water was dropt in,
until the salt was exactly saturated ; which it
was found to be, when two drams, two scruples, and three grains of this acid had been
added. The vial with its contents now
weighed two ounces, four drams, and fifteen grains. One scruple, therefore, and
eight grains were lost during the ebullition,
of which a trifling portion may be water, or
VOL. II.   Z   something

20:3

The title page of Joseph Black's (1728–1799) dissertation (top left), the second part of which deals with the discovery of carbon dioxide. In 1756 he publishes a greatly expanded account of his findings and thereby establishes the foundations of quantitative chemistry. Black, well aware of the work of Stephen Hales more than two decades before, describes quantitative experiments to find out how much gas is expelled from alkalis by acids.

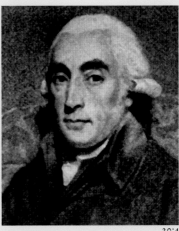

Joseph Black

20:4

BLACK was born in 1728, the fourth of twelve children in the family of a wine merchant of Scots descent living in Bordeaux. At the age of sixteen, he started to study medicine and chemistry at Glasgow University. He received a medical degree in 1754 from the University of Edinburgh with a now historic dissertation (20.1). In 1766, he was appointed professor of chemistry and left all research to devote his time to teaching. His many students testified to his great skill as a teacher, to his pleasant personality and elegant appearance. A bachelor, he enjoyed going to clubs and the company of his friends, among them James Watt, the inventor, and David Hume, the philosopher.

Experiments upon Magnesia Alba, Quicklime, and some other Alcaline Substances. Essays and Observations, Physical and Literary.

EDINBURGH; 1756; 2:157.

THIS TREATISE, an expanded version of the second part of his dissertation (20.1), can be considered as the first quantitative study in chemistry. Black's investigation of magnesium carbonate (magnesia alba) leads him to the discovery that a significant weight loss occurs on heating both magnesium and calcium carbonate, because carbon dioxide (fixed air) is given off in the process. He notes that this new gas puts out fire "as effectually as if it had been dipped in water". He also investigates the reverse reactions, for instance the formation of calcium carbonate (limestone) from calcium hydroxide (quicklime slaked with water) and potassium carbonate (mild alkali). Black discusses the results using a table for the affinities or "elective attractions" of alkaline substances towards acids and fixed air.

IN PERSPECTIVE:
As a medical thesis, Black's aim with the study of magnesium carbonate was to find an efficient substance for dissolving urinary calculi. This ambition failed since magnesium oxide (magnesia usta) turned out to be insoluble in water. Black prepared magnesium carbonate from potassium carbonate (fixed alkali or pearl ashes) and magnesium sulphate (Epsom salt). Black knew (20.2) of Hale's work (20.3) and Hale had stated that potassium carbonate (fixed alkali) "abounds in air". Thus he was not surprised to find that a gas was formed on heating magnesium carbonate. However, his discovery that a gas could combine with a solid and that this gas, carbon dioxide (fixed air), was chemically different from "air" was revolutionary and soon led to the rise of "pneumatic chemistry" (20.4)(20.5)(20.6). The new chemical theories of Lavoisier (20.7) were somewhat reluctantly accepted by Black and in 1790 he wrote to Lavoisier telling him that he had incorporated the new theories in his lectures (20.8)(20.9).

20.1 Black J. *Dissertatio medica inauguralis De Humore Acido a Cibis orto et Magnesia Alba.* Edinburgh; 1754.
20.2 Black J. The main work cited above p176.
20.3 See #17 Hales page 100.
20.4 See #22 Priestly page 124.
20.5 See #28 Davy page 156.
20.6 Keys TE. The Early Pneumatic Chemists and Physicians: Their influence on the Development of Surgical Anesthesia. *Anesthesiology* 1969; 30:447.
20.7 See #24 Lavoisier page 134.
20.8 Thompson T. *History of Chemistry* I. Chapter 9 London; 1830.
20.9 Robinson J. *Lectures on the elements of chemistry.* Edinburgh; 1803.

IT is diffolved in every acid but very flowly, unlefs affifted by heat. The feveral folutions, when thoroughly faturated, are all aftringent with a flight degree of an acid tafte, and they alfo agree with a folution of alum in this, that they give a red colour to the infufion of turnfol.

NEITHER this earth, nor that of animal bones, can be converted into quick-lime by the ftrongeft fire, nor do they fuffer any change worth notice. Both of them feem to attract acids but weakly, and to alter their properties lefs when united to them than the other abforbents.

PART II.

IN reflecting afterwards upon thefe experiments, an explication of the nature of lime offered itfelf, which feemed to account, in an eafy manner, for moft of the properties of that fubftance.

IT is fufficiently clear, that the calcarious earths in their native ftate, and that the alkalis and magnefia in their ordinary condition, contain a large quantity of fixed air, and this

this air certainly adheres to them with confiderable force, fince a ftrong fire is neceffary to feparate it from magnefia, and the ftrongeft is not fufficient to expell it entirely from fixed alkalis, or take away their power of effervefcing with acid falts.

THESE confiderations led me to conclude, that the relations between fixed air and alkaline fubftances was fomewhat fimilar to the relation between thefe and acids ; that as the calcarious earths and alkalis attract acids ftrongly and can be faturated with them, fo they alfo attract fixed air, and are in their ordinary ftate faturated with it : and when we mix an acid with an alkali or with an abforbent earth, that the air is then fet at liberty, and breaks out with violence; becaufe the alkaline body attracts it more weakly than it does the acid, and becaufe the acid and air cannot both be joined to the fame body at the fame time.

I alfo imagined, that, when the calcarious earths are expofed to the action of a violent fire, and are thereby converted into quick-lime, they fuffer no other change in their compofition than the lofs of a fmall quantity of water and of their fixed air. The re-

markable

We have already shewn by experiment, that magnesia alba is a compound of a peculiar earth and fixed air. When this substance is mixed with lime-water, the lime shews a stronger attraction for fixed air than that of the earth of magnesia; the air leaves this powder to join itself to the lime. And as neither the lime when saturated with air, nor the magnesia when deprived of it, are soluble in water, the lime-water becomes perfectly pure and insipid, the lime which it contained being mixed with the magnesia. But if the magnesia be deprived of air by calcination before it is mixed with the lime-water, this fluid suffers no alteration.

If quick-lime be mixed with a dissolved alkali, it likeways shews an attraction for fixed air superior to that of the alkali. It robs this salt of its air, and thereby becomes mild itself, while the alkali is consequently rendered more corrosive, or discovers its natural degree of acrimony or strong attraction for water, and for bodies of the inflammable, and of the animal and vegetable kind; which attraction was less perceivable as long as it was saturated with air. And the volatile alkali when deprived of its air, besides this attraction

attraction for various bodies, discovers likeways its natural degree of volatility, which was formerly somewhat repressed by the air adhering to it, in the same manner as it is repressed by the addition of an acid.

This account of lime and alkalis recommended itself by its simplicity, and by affording an easy solution of many *phænomena*, but appeared upon a nearer view to be attended with consequences that were so very new and extraordinary, as to render suspicious the principles from which they were drawn.

I resolved however to examine, in a particular manner, such of these consequences as were the most unavoidable, and found, the greatest number of them might be reduced to the following propositions:

I. If we only separate a quantity of air from lime and alkalis, when we render them caustic they will be found to lose part of their weight in the operation, but will saturate the same quantity of acid as before, and the saturation will be performed without effervescence.

II. If

Black demonstrates that an "aeriform fluid" that he calls "fixed air" (carbon dioxide gas) is part of such alkaline substances as magnesium alba (magnesium carbonate), lime (calcium oxide), potash (potassium carbonate) and soda (sodium bicarbonate). He summarises that " The above experiments lead us also to conclude, that volatile alkalis, and the common absorbent earths, which lose their air by being joined to acids, but shew evident signs of their having recovered it, when separated from them by alkalis, received it from these alkalis which lost it in the instant of their joining with the acid."

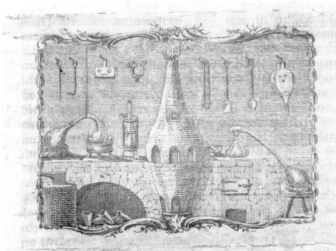

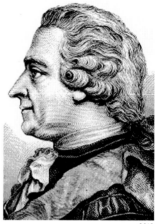

Torbern Bergman (1735–1784), Scheele's teacher and mentor, a talented and multifaceted scientist who did not provide his introduction to Scheele's book (the title page of which is shown on the left) in time and so delayed its publication by almost two years. In the book Carl Wilhelm Scheele (1742–1784) reports the discovery of oxygen and many other important chemical experiments.

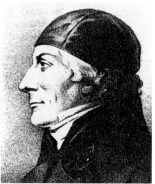

Portrait of Johann Gahn (1745–1818), chemist, mentor and friend of Scheele, to whom this copy of the book is dedicated.

SCHEELE was born in 1742 in Swedish Pomerania. With an elder brother he studied pharmacy at Bauch, a competent apothecary in Gothenburg. He went to Uppsala in 1770 and here he made most of his major discoveries (21.1) under the mentorship of the prominent chemists Gahn and Bergman. In 1775 Scheele was elected a member of the Royal Swedish Academy of Sciences and the same year he moved to the small town of Köping to take over a pharmacy recently inherited by a widow. Despite many flattering invitations from abroad he remained the city pharmacist the rest of his life. Honest and simple in character, Scheele kept himself out of the scientific jealousies and quarrels of his times (21.2). The extensive exposure to toxic chemicals that he synthesised is believed to have contributed to his early death in 1786.

Chemische Abhandlung von der Luft und dem Feuer.

UPSALA, LEIPZIG: M. SWEDERUS; 1777.

THIS BOOK, the publication of which was delayed two years because Bergman did not deliver his promised preface in time, reports ninety-seven experiments, most of them made before 1773, leading to Scheele's discovery of oxygen (fire air). He produces oxygen in different ways, for instance by strongly heating the oxides of mercury and manganese or the carbonates of silver and mercury. The carbon dioxide (aer fixus) produced in the process he removes with an alkali such as potassium hydroxide, leaving pure oxygen. He proves that air freed from carbon dioxide and water vapour consists of oxygen (fire air), which promotes combustion, and nitrogen (foul air) (21.3), which does not.

IN PERSPECTIVE:
Like his contemporary Hales,(21.4) many of Scheele's experiments on gases were motivated by his interest in plant physiology. Scheele discovered seven elements (N, O, Cl, Mn, Mo, Ba, and W), more than any other chemist, and his observation that light darkened silver salts was of fundamental importance in the development of photography (21.5). His highly original work in organic chemistry was truly pioneering. Scheele was the first to prepare many organic acids (citric, lactic, uric, oxalic and tartaric) by first crystallising their salts and then treating these with diluted sulphuric acid. Heating olive oil and the oxide of lead, he found a transparent syrupy liquid, glycerol, a principal component of all fats and oils and a compound still of importance in the modern pharmaceutical industry. Working essentially in isolation and making notes that are difficult to decipher (21.6), Scheele's results became widely known and cited (21.7), mostly through his friend Bergman (21.8).

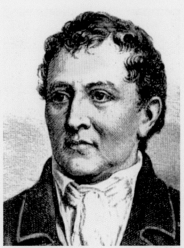

21:4
Carl Wilhelm Scheele (later portrait probably of Scheele after a painting by J Falander).

21.1 See ref. 1.8.
21.2 Wilson G. *The Life of the Honourable Henry Cavendish.* Chapter III London; 1851.
21.3 Nitrogen gas was discovered independently by Daniel Rutherford. See ref. 17.6.
21.4 See #17 Hales page 100
21.5 See #38 Daguerre page 202.
21.6 Boklund U. *Carl Wilhelm Scheele Bruna Boken.* (Brown book) Stockholm; 1961.
21.7 Partington JR. *A History of Chemistry Vol. III.* Mansfield Centre; 1999. p135. Reprint of Ed. 1961–1979.
21.8 See ref. 21.7 p221.

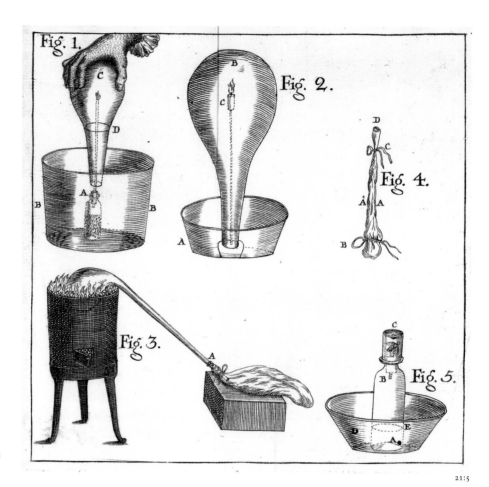

21:5

Apparatus used by Scheele in his experiments.

Some of the chemical symbols and notations used by Scheele in his research notebook.

⊖ *Sal in genere*

✚ *acidum; c.concentratum; d. dilutum*

✚*m. Acidum minerale*

✚⊕ *Acidum Vitrioli*

✚⊕*c. concentratum; d. dilutum*

✚① *Acidum Nitri* ; ✚①⚕*a.n. phlogisticatum*

▽ *Aqua fortis*

✚⊖ *Acidum Salis:* ✚⊖⚧ *a.s. dephlogisticatum*

▽℞ *Aqua Regis*

✚⚒ *Acidum fluoris minerale*

✚✚ *Acidum arsenici*

✚*v. Acidum Vegetabile*

✚⚶ *Acidum tartari*

✚⊕ *Acidum Sacchari*

⊖✚*Sal neutralis*

① *Nitrum*

⊖*c. Sal communis*

⚶*Tartarus; r. ruber; a. albus; p. purus*

⌂ *Borax*

⊖⚹ *Sal ammoniacus*

▽✚*Sal medius terrestris cum acide*

⚵⊕ *Magnesia vitris lata (Sal amarus Anglic.)*

○ *Alumen*

▽⊖ *Sal medius terrestris cum alcali*

⚵⊖ *Alcali volatile magnesia Saturatum*

⚶✚*Sal medius metallicus cum acide*

⊕♀ *Vitriolum cupri (v. Coeruleum.)*

⊕♂ *Vitriolum ferri (v. viride.)*

21:6

122

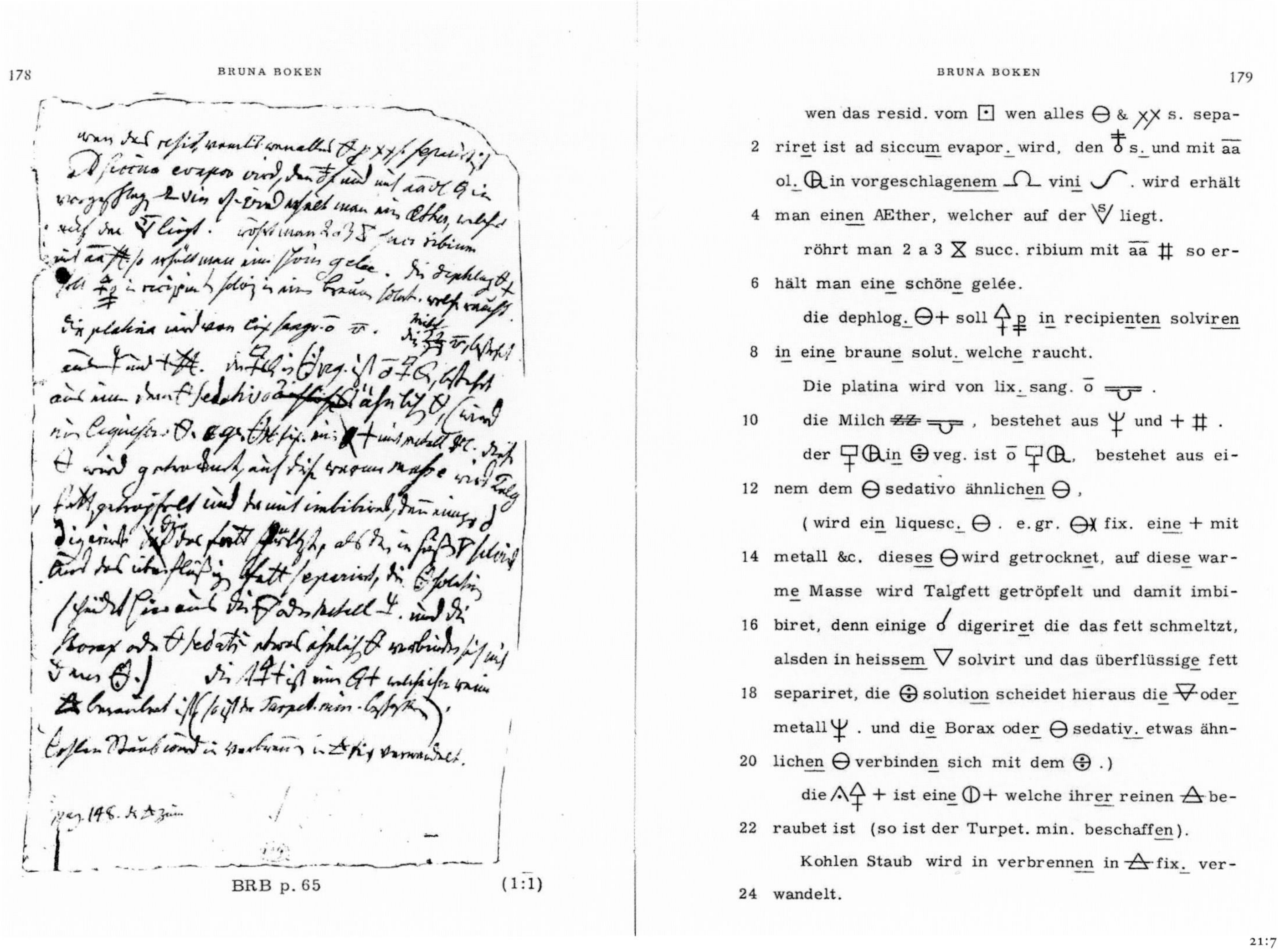

BRB p. 65   (1:1)

wen das resid. vom ⊡ wen alles ⊖ & ✕✕ s. sepa-
2 rir<u>et</u> ist ad siccum evapor. wird, den ⚊ s. und mit a̅a̅
   ol. ⊕ in vorgeschlagen<u>em</u> ♎ vini ♒ . wird erhält
4 man ein<u>en</u> AEther, welcher auf der ⚕ liegt.

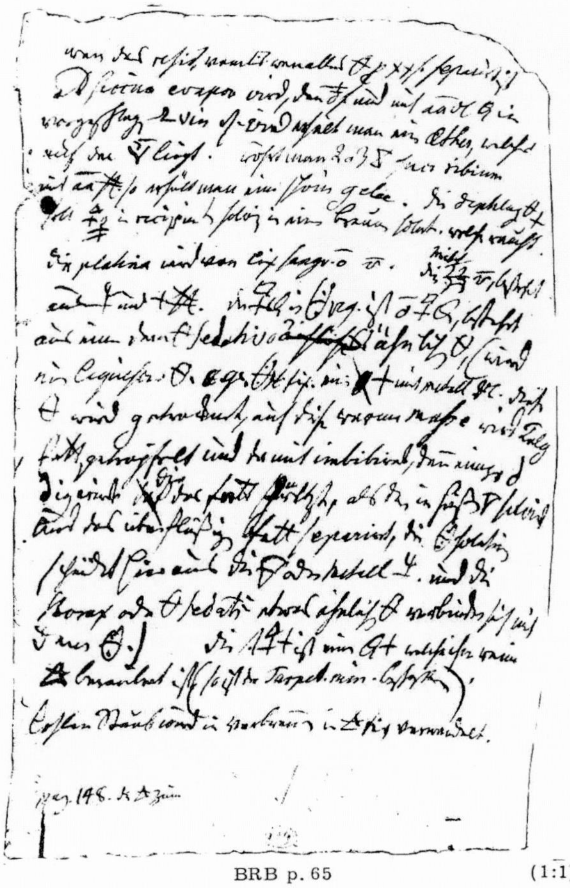

      röhrt man 2 a 3 ✕ succ. ribium mit a̅a̅ ♯ so er-
6 hält man ein<u>e</u> schön<u>e</u> gelée.

      die dephlog. ⊖+ soll ⚷ p in recipient<u>en</u> solvir<u>en</u>
8 in ein<u>e</u> braune solut. welche raucht.

      Die platina wird von lix. sang. o̅ ⎁ .
10   die Milch ≠≠ ⎁ , bestehet aus ♇ und + ♯ .

      der ♀⊕ in ⊖ veg. ist o̅ ♀⊕ , bestehet aus ei-
12 nem dem ⊖ sedativo ähnlich<u>en</u> ⊖ ,

      (wird ei<u>n</u> liquesc. ⊖ . e. gr. ⊖✕ fix. ein<u>e</u> + mit
14 metall &c. dieses ⊖ wird getrock<u>net</u>, auf diese war-
   m<u>e</u> Masse wird Talgfett getröpfelt und damit imbi-
16 biret, denn einige ♂ digerir<u>et</u> die das fett schmeltzt,
   alsden in heiss<u>em</u> ▽ solvirt und das überflüssige fett
18 separiret, die ⊕ solut<u>ion</u> scheidet hieraus die �псⳬ oder
   metall ♇ . und di<u>e</u> Borax oder ⊖ sedativ. etwas ähn-
20 lich<u>en</u> ⊖ verbind<u>en</u> sich mit dem ⊕ .)

      die ⋀⚷ + ist ein<u>e</u> ⊕ + welche ihr<u>er</u> rein<u>en</u> △ be-
22 raubet ist (so ist der Turpet. min. beschaffen).

      Kohlen Staub wird in verbrennen in △ fix. ver-
24 wandelt.

21:7

A page from Scheele's research notes
(shown on the left-hand side above)
and the interpretation of its meaning
(on the right-hand side above). Taking
into account the meaning of the symbols used by Scheele, the text says: "If
the remaining urea from which salts
and crystals have been eliminated is
dried, pulverised and distilled with
equal amount of concentrated sulphuric acid (oleum vitrioli), then one
gets a mixture of alcohol and ether,
with the ether floating on the alcohol."

Joseph Priestley's (1733–1804) focusing lens, which he uses in 1774 to heat mercuric oxide (that is floating on mercury) to produce oxygen for the first time. A later model of this experimental set up is also shown in the photograph.

Antoine Lavoisier (1743–1794) also uses techniques very similar to those of Priestley to produce and study new gases. However, contrary to his contemporaries, he is able to draw far-reaching conclusions from his observations about the nature of the chemical transformations.

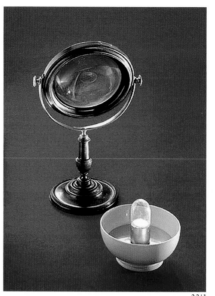

22:1

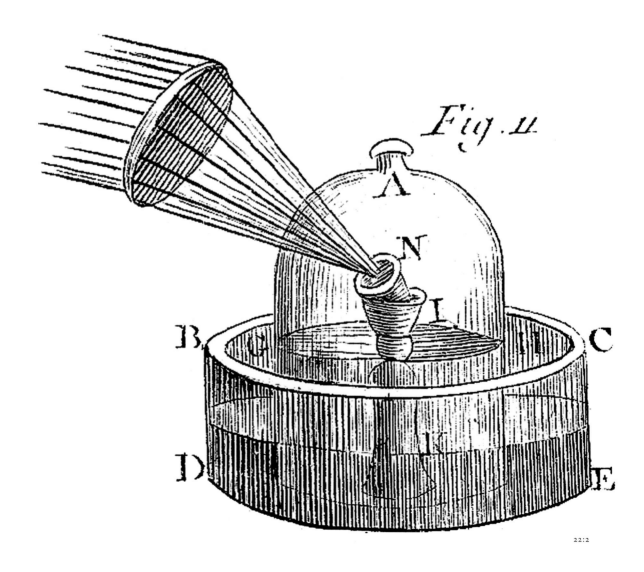

Fig. II

22:2

Born in Birstal Fieldhead in England in 1733, Priestley lost his mother at the age of six and spent his early life with an aunt. He went to local parish schools but also studied a wide range of subjects by himself. He became a preacher, a Unitarian minister, but handicapped by a speech impediment, he turned to teaching and writing. Often dissenting in view, he published extensively on theology, education, science and politics. Priestley's first important scientific paper appeared in 1772 (22.1). He was later persecuted for his stance on religious and political issues (he initially supported the French Revolution) and a mob destroyed his laboratory in Birmingham in 1791. He emigrated to the United States in 1794 and died there ten years later as a friend of president Jefferson.

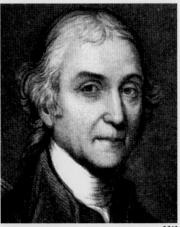

Joseph Priestley

22:3

Experiments and Observations on Different Kinds of Air Vol. I–III.

LONDON: J. JOHNSON; 1774–1777.

IN THESE three volumes Priestley describes his studies on gases, including his discovery of those of major medical interest, oxygen (dephlogisticated air), nitrous oxide (dephlogisticated nitrous gas) and nitric oxide (nitrous air). He prepares oxygen and nitric oxide by heating mercury oxide (mercurius calcinatus) (22.2) and copper nitrate (green precipitate) respectively, using a burning lens. Nitrous oxide is prepared by reacting mercury with a nitric acid solution (spirit of nitre). He identifies sulphur dioxide and ammonia and investigates the role of blood in respiration. Priestley emphasises the need to always use proper equipment in an investigation.

IN PERSPECTIVE:
Priestley's apparatus was simple but he employed it skilfully and followed up his observations with great tenacity. His studies on the effect of plants on gases came to stimulate the discovery of photosynthesis in 1779 (22.3). His interests and methods were greatly influenced by the work of Hales (22.4). He was a true experimentalist with a well equipped laboratory and access to the newly developed eudiometer (22.5) for assessing the quality of an air sample (22.6). Priestley thought that ingenious experimentation would lead to a few basic elements from which all others could be obtained. In consequence, he was vigorously opposed to Lavoisier's new chemical theory (22.7), which allowed for the formation of very many new substances. He expressed the hope that his research into different kinds of air would lead to "applications of great medicinal use". As it appears from the prefaces to the books cited above and some of the letters that Priestley included with his work, he was constantly involved with priority disputes regarding many of his discoveries, such as the discovery of oxygen (22.8) and the constituent elements of water (22.9).

22.1 Priestley J. Observations of different kinds of air. *Phil Trans Roy Soc* 1772; 62:147.
22.2 See also #21 Scheele page 120.
22.3 Ingen-Housz J. *Experiments upon Vegetables, discovering their great Power of Purifying the common Air in the Sun-shine ...* London; 1779.
22.4 See #17 Hales page 100.
22.5 Priestley J. *Experiments and Observations on different kinds of Air.* Vol. III. London; 1774. p380.
22.6 Landriani M. *Richerche fisiche intorno alla salubrità dell'aria.* Milano; 1775.
22.7 See #24 Lavoisier page 134.
22.8 Priestley J. *Experiments and Observations on different kinds of Air.* Vol. II. London; 1774. p304.
22.9 See ref. 21.2.

Marsilio Landriani's (1751–1815) audiometer, which he sends to Priestley for evaluation and which helps Priestley in his investigations of the properties of gases.

Apparatus from Priestley's well-equipped laboratory. His interest in the effect of plants on gases leads directly to the discovery of the mechanism of photosynthesis.

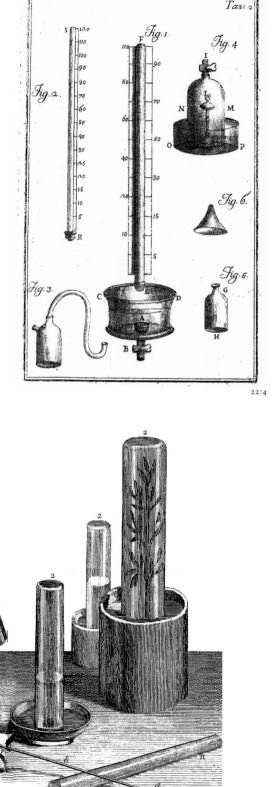

22:4

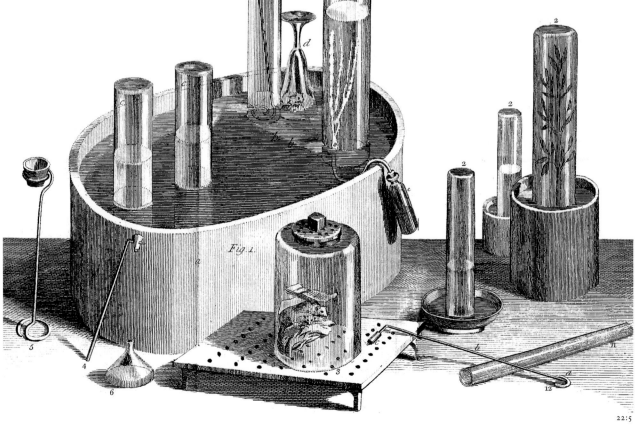

22:5

Priestley prepares nitrous oxide, ammonia, nitrogen dioxide and sulphur dioxide and also studies the role of blood in respiration. He believes that his work will have "applications of great medicinal use."

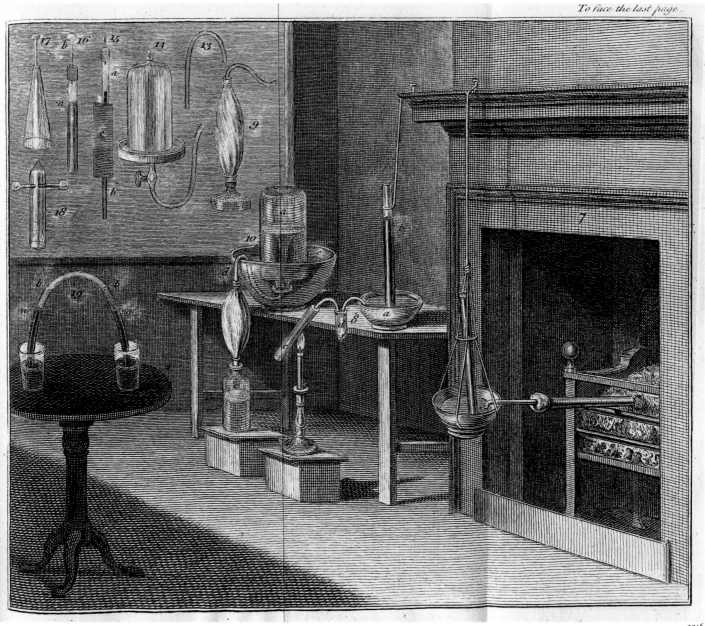

To face the last page.

Charles Kite's (1768–1811) pioneering report on the electric stimulation and conversion of the heart. The equipment he uses is illustrated below.

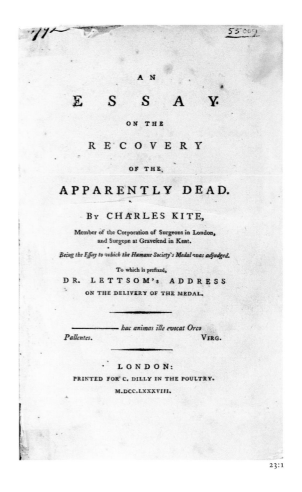

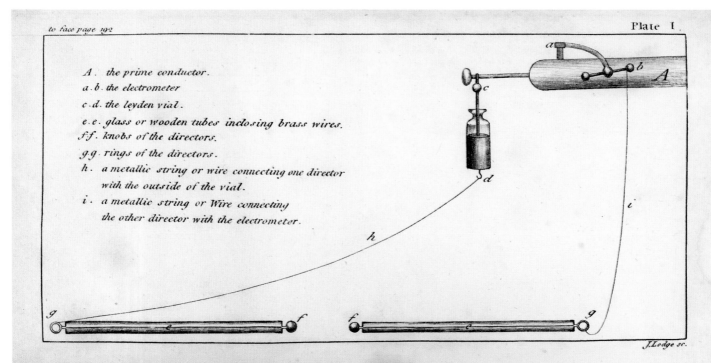

KITE was born in 1768 in the town of Gravesend, England. He practised medicine with great skill and was a member of the Royal College of Surgeons in London. He contributed regularly to the London Medical Journal and published two books, one of them cited below, the other on "select histories of diseases". He died in Gravesend in 1811.

An Essay on the Recovery of the Apparently Dead.

LONDON: C. DILLY 1788.

THIS ESSAY was awarded the silver medal of the Royal Humane Society (23.1). Kite describes the first use of electric shock to revive a three year old child who was assumed dead after falling out of a window. With this report he pioneers later work on the electrical stimulation and conversion of the heart. Kite also emphasises the importance of immediate artificial respiration but believes incorrectly (23.2) that the respiratory movement in itself is responsible for preventing "an apoplexy of the brain". The book also presents a plan for further research on resuscitation and describes apparatus for intubation and for delivering electric shocks.

IN PERSPECTIVE:

In 1744 Fothergill reported with remarkable insight on a successful case of reviving a person by the mouth-to-mouth method (23.3). However, the technique soon fell out of favour, only to be successfully reintroduced about two centuries later. In 1767 a group of wealthy merchants in Amsterdam founded the first society for promoting better methods for "saving drowned persons" (23.4). They offered money to those following recommended procedures and even more money to those successful in resuscitation. Soon, other cities established similar societies, Lille, Vienna, Venice, Copenhagen in 1772, Paris in 1773 and London the following year (23.1). A historic account and updated procedures were published by Herholdt and Rafn in 1796 (23.5). Kite received a silver medal for the work cited above from the Humane Society, while the gold medal was given to Goodwyn, for studies on the importance of ventilation in resuscitation (23.6). Electrical stimulation of the heart was first studied on recently guillotined victims of the French Revolution by Bichat and later by Aldini. (23.7). In 1812 Le Gallois demonstrated the effect of the vagi on the heart and noted for the first time that an area in the medulla controlled breathing (23.8). Rapid progress in measuring techniques led to advances in electrophysiology and in particular to a better understanding of the electrical function of the heart (23.9). This paved the way for techniques of electrical conversion and pacing of the heart and the invention of the ECG (23.10)(23.11).

23.1 The founders Dr W. Hawes and Dr T. Cogan each invited sixteen friends to form the "Humane Society for the recovery of persons apparently drowned" 1774.

23.2 See #11 Hooke page 72.

23.3 Fothergill J. Observation on a Case ... of Recovering a Man Dead in Appearance, by distending the Lungs with Air. *Phil Trans Roy Soc.* 1744–1745. p275.

23.4 Meijer P. Bekendmaaking, *Philosooph* N.86, N.88, N.94 Aug–Oct. Amsterdam; 1767.

23.5 Herholdt JD, Rafn CG. *Forsög til en historisk udsikt over redningsanstalter for drunknede, og underretning om de bedste midler ved hvilke de igen kunne bringes til live.* Copenhagen; 1796.

23.6 Goodwyn E. *The connection of Life with Respiration ...* London; 1788.

23.7 Bichat X. *Recherches physiologiques sur la vie et la mort.* Paris; 1800 and ref. 19.8 Vol.1 p153.

23.8 Le Gallois J. *Expériences sur le principe de la vie, notamment sur celui des movemens du coer, ...* Paris; 1812. See also ref. 44.3.

23.9 Stannius FH. Zwei Reihen physiologischer Versuche. *Arch Anat Physiol wiss Med.* 1852. p85. See also #42 Du Bois-Reymond page 224 and ref 19.11.

23.10 Steiner F. Über die Electropunctur des Herzens als Wiederbelebungsmittel in der Chloroformsyncope. *Arch. klin. Chir.* 1871; 12:748.

23.11 Green T. On death from chloroform; its prevention by galvanism. *Brit Med J.* 1872; 1:552. See also #65 Waller page 334, #71 Einthoven page 366 and #91 Elmquist-Senning page 470.

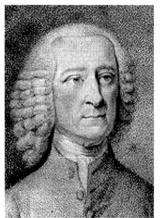

John Fothergill (1712–1780) describes below the first successful revival of a person by the mouth-to-mouth method.

23:3

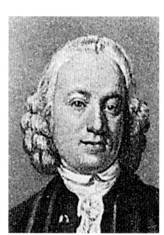

23:5

The announcement of book-seller Pieter Meijer (1718–1781) (whose portrait is shown above), published in Amsterdam in 1767, is shown on the opposite page. Here a generous reward is offered for anybody saving drowned persons. The document also details methods to be used, such as keeping the body warm and dry, sniffing on salt of ammonia, giving alcoholic beverages and blowing air or tobacco smoke into the lungs.

[276]

will be sufficient in this Place: Those who defire an ampler Account may confult the Article itself.

A Perfon fuffocated by the *naufeous Steam* arifing from Coals fet on Fire in the Pit, fell down as dead; he lay in the Pit *between half an Hour and three Quarters;* and was then dragg'd up; *his Eyes ftaring and open, his Mouth gaping wide, his Skin cold; not the leaft Pulfe in either Heart or Arteries, and not the leaft Breathing to be obferved.*

In thefe Circumftances, the Surgeon, who relates the Affair, *applied his Mouth clofe to the Patient's, and, by blowing ftrongly, holding the Naftrils at the fame time, raifed his Cheft fully by his Breath.* The Surgeon *immediately felt fix or feven very quick Beats of the Heart; the Thorax continued to play, and the Pulfe was foon after felt in the Arteries. He then opened a Vein in his Arm; which, after giving a fmall Jet, fent out the Blood in Drops only for a Quarter of an Hour, and then he bled freely.* In the mean time he caufed him to be pull'd, pufh'd, and rubb'd, as much as he could. In one Hour the Patient began to come to himfelf; within four Hours he walked home; and in as many Days returned to his Work.

There were many Hundred People, fome of them of Diftinction, prefent at the Time.

This is the Subftance of the Account; from whence it naturally appears how much ought to be attributed to the Sagacity of the Surgeon in the Recovery of this Perfon. Anatomifts, it is true, have long known, that an artificial Inflation of the Lungs of a dead or dying Animal will put the Heart in Motion, and continue it fo for fome time; yet this is the firft

Inftance

I

23:4

BEKENDMAAKING.

De Bestierders der Maatschappy ter Behoudenis van Drenkelingen, onlangs in Amsterdam opgerecht, hunne menschlievende oogmerken aan alle Ingezetenen der Zeven Provintiën, gaarne zo algemeen als mogelyk willende bekend maaken, hebben goedgevonden door deeze eene korte doch zaakelyke schets derzelven te geeven; terwyl zulks reeds wydloopiger geschied is in *N. 86. N. 88.* en *N. 94* van het weekelyks Blad genaamd de *Philosooph*, in de maanden *Aug., Sept.* en *October* 1767. te *Amsterdam* uitgegeeven.

1. Een ieder, die met goede bewyzen kan aantoonen, een mensch of kind, 't welk zonder eenige beweeging of teken van leeven uit het water is gehaald, door eene goede behandeling weder tot zichzelven gebragt te hebben, zal eene *Premie* genieten, bestaande in zes Gouden Dukaaten, of (indien hy zulks liever heeft) in een Gouden Gedenkpenning, op welken de naam des geenen, die door zyne welaangelegde hulp een ongelukkigen gered heeft, gesteld zal worden;

2. Maar dewyl het meermaalen gebeuren zal, dat 'er meer dan een in de behoudenis eens Drenkelings hebben medegewerkt, zo zal alsdan de *Gedenkpenning* of de zes *Dukaaten* aan hun allen gegeeven worden, om daaromtrent eene billyke schikking onder malkanderen te maaken.

3. Om tot het ontfangen deezer *Premie* gerechtigd te zyn, word alleenlyk eene schriftelyke verklaaring vereischt van twee braave menschen, van onbesproken naam en faam, die geen belang hebben in het trekken van de *Premie*, en, als ooggetuigen, bevestigen dat dezelve aan zoodanig een' Persoon of Persoonen behoort uitgedeeld te worden.

4. Deeze verklaaring moet gebragt of gezonden worden ten huize van den Boekverkooper *Pieter Meijer*, op den Dam te *Amsterdam*; dezelve onderzocht en echt bevonden zynde, zal de uitdeeling der *Premie* een maand na het ontfangen der verklaaring geschieden.

5. By aldien 'er eenige onkosten in een Herberg of ander Huis gemaakt hebben moeten worden, zullen dezelven, mids niet boven de *vier Dukaaten* beloopende, boven de *Premie* voldaan worden, dat zelfs plaats zal hebben 't zy de Verdronkene al of niet gered is, indien men slechts behoorlyk kan bewyzen, dat die onkosten wezenlyk alleen ten nutte van den Drenkeling gemaakt zyn.

6. Een *Genees-* of *Heelmeester* zyn tyd en zorgen tot het herstellen van een Drenkeling aangewend hebbende, en daar voor niet beloond zynde, kan verzekerd weezen dat zulks op eene onbekrompene wyze zal geschieden, 't zy dat de Persoon, omtrent welken hy zyne moeite heeft aangewend, in 't leven behouden is of niet, indien zyne rekening, met behoorlyke bewyzen voorzien, insgelyks aan den Boekverkooper *Pieter Meijer*, word ter hand gesteld.

Voorts mogen wy een ieder verzekeren, dat men hier door geenszins tegen de Wetten der Overigheid zal handelen; dewyl die Wetten, het algemeene best ten doelwit hebbende, toelaaten, niet alleen Drenkelingen uit het water te haalen, maar ook aan dezelven, schoon zy reeds van het leven beroofd schynen, alle behoorlyke middelen tot herstelling te beproeven, zullende, wanneer de aangewende middelen vruchteloos zyn uitgevallen, aan de Ordonnantiën voldaan worden, door het voorgevallene den Gerechte bekend te maaken.

De Beste Middelen die men tot het herstellen van een Drenkeling kan en behoort in 't werk te stellen, gelyk zulks ons reeds, sedert de oprechting deezer Maatschappy, door verscheidene voorbeelden, waar voor de Premie is gegeven, gebleeken is, zyn:

Eerstelyk. Het Blaazen in het *Fondament* (den *Aarsdarm*), door middel van een Tabaks- of andere Pyp, of een Schede van een Mes, waarvan de punt is afgesneeden, of van een Blaasbalg zelve, en hoe spoediger, sterker en aanhoudender dit Blaazen geschied, hoe beter het ook altoos zyn zal. Indien men een brandende Tabakspyp of een zogenaamde Tabaksklisteerpyp (by Monsieur Steitz in de Runstraat te Amsterdam te bekomen) heeft, en dat men dus in plaats van enkele Lucht of Wind den warmen en prikkelenden Rook der brandende Tabak in het Ligchaam op kan blaazen, verdient zulks steeds den voorrang: Dit Blaazen echter in 't algemeen, op de eene of andere der gemelde wyzen, behoort steeds het allereerste werk te zyn, en kan ook altoos zonder eenig tydverzuim overal verricht worden, 't zy op een schuit, op het land aan den kant van 't water, in Steden en Dorpen, op den steenen wal der straaten, of waar ook elders een Drenkeling het eerst wordt nedergelegd, terwyl men inmiddels in de

Tweede plaats, zoodra mogelyk, trachten moet het door en door nat, ja dikwyls reeds yskoud en verkleumd, Ligchaam voorzichtiglyk droog en warm te maaken; ten welken einde wederom verscheidene gemakkelyke middelen meesttyds te vinden of te bekomen zyn; zo als by voorbeeld het warme Hembd en de Onderkleederen van een der omstanders, een of meer wolle Deekens voor 't vuur gewarmd, warme Asch van Bakkers, Brouwers, Zout- of Zeepzieders of van andere Fabrieken, warme Beestevellen, vooral Schaapen-vellen, ja eindelyk de warmte van een maatig vuur, of de koesterende natuurlyke warmte van twee gezonde warme Menschen, zich met den Drenkeling te Bed begeevende; — Terwyl men met het Blaazen en verwarmen van den Drenkeling onverzuimd en teffens voorzichtig bezig is, kan het ook van zeer veel nut zyn, dat het Ligchaam overal, maar voornaamelyk langs den geheelen Ruggengraat van het Hoofd af tot aan het Onderlyf toe, sterk gewreeven word met warme wollen of andere doeken in Brandewyn nat gemaakt, of met veel droog Zout bestrooid. — Men mag ook gerustelyk een doek met Brandewyn nat gemaakt, of eenig sterk vlug Zout, gelyk als de geest van Amoniak-zout is, onder de Neus houden, en de zyden des Hoofds daarmede vryven; — Met de Veer van een Pen in de Keel en Neus te prikkelen, is insgelyks zeer raadzaam; doch Wyn, Brandewyn of eenige andere sterke drank, met wat Zout of iets anders dat prikkelen kan vermengd, in de keel te gieten, behoort nooit eerder te geschieden, dan als men eenig teeken van leven bespeurd heeft; maar inzonderheid kan het ook van zeer veel nut zyn, dat een der omstanderen zynen mond tegen dien des ongelukkigen Drenkelings zettende, en zyn eene Hand de Neusgaaten toehoudende, terwyl hy met de andere Hand op de linker Borst des Drenkelings steunt, deszelfs Longen onmiddelyk tracht opteblaazen, ja wy oordeelen zulks van het eerste oogenblik af aan zo noodig te zyn als het blaazen in den Aarsdarm zelve. Men behoort ook, zo het mogelyk zy, zonder uitstel, alle Drenkelingen te doen Aderlaaten, en best tapt men alsdan het Bloed uit een groote Ader op den Arm, of uit de Strotader zelve af.

Deeze de beste en beproefde Middelen tot herstelling des Levens van Drenkelingen zynde, hoopen en wenschen wy, dat voortaan geene deezer ongelukkigen, gelyk voorheen, *door hen op een Ton te rollen*, *of door hen van Touw onder de Armen door*, *of by de Beenen optehangen, enz.* mishandeld zullen worden, en *dewyl door onervaarnen geene andere Drenkelingen dan alleen die*, *welker ligchaamen reeds duidelyke teekenen van Bederf geeven*, *met zekerheid gezegd kunnen worden inderdaad gestorven te zyn*, vleijen wy ons insgelyks, dat men alle anderen voortaan geene der gemelde Middelen onbeproefd zal laaten; maar ook dat een ieder aan wien eenig ander beproefd middel tot redding der Verdronkenen mogt bekend zyn, zulks edelmoedig aan ons zal opgeven; ja, zo iemand, die het geluk gehad heeft van een Drenkeling te redden, goed mogt vinden ons de *Premie* niet te willen afeischen, verzoeken wy echter van al het voorgevallene tot de redding betrekkelyk, onderricht te worden, om daarvan een goed gebruik te kunnen maaken, wanneer wy zullen goedvinden een verhaal van de door ons beloonde reddingen of andere verrichtingen der *Maatschappy* in 't licht te geeven.

Eindelyk wenschen wy dat hy Gode zal behaagen, door deeze onze pogingen, en de medewerking van anderen, niet alleen het tydelyk maar ook het eeuwig welzyn van veelen onzer Landgenooten en Medemenschen te bevorderen!

Amsterdam, 16 December, 1767.

Te Amsterdam, by PIETER MEIJER, op den Dam.

(Zie bladz. 17)

23:6

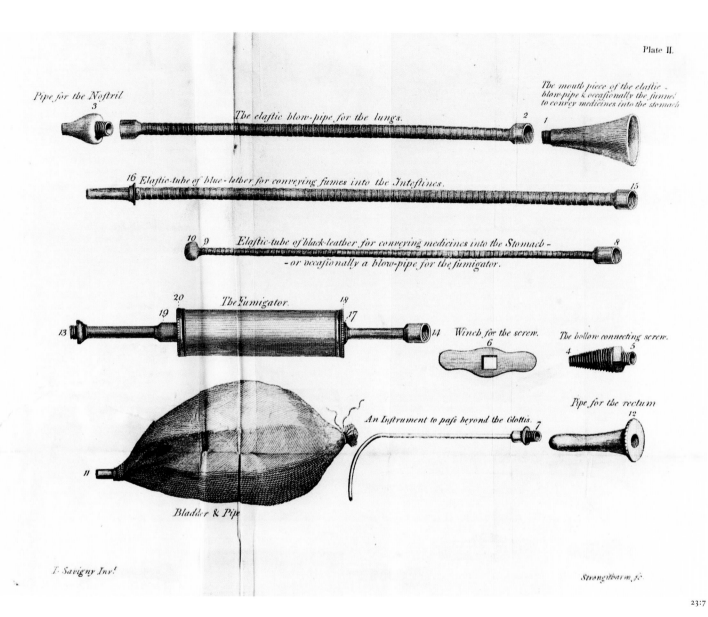

Plate II.

The mouth piece of the elaftic
blow-pipe & occafionally the funnel
to convey medicines into the ftomach

Pipe for the Noftril
3

The elaftic blow-pipe for the lungs.

2

1

16 Elaftic-tube of blue-leather for conveying fumes into the Inteftines.

15

10 9   Elaftic-tube of black-leather for conveying medicines into the Stomach
— or occafionally a blow-pipe for the fumigator.

8

20   The Fumigator.   18
19   17
13   14

Winch for the screw.
6

The hollow connecting screw.
4   5

An Inftrument to pafs beyond the Glottis.
7

Pipe for the rectum
12

11

Bladder & Pipe

T. Savigny Invt.

Strongitharm fc.

23:7

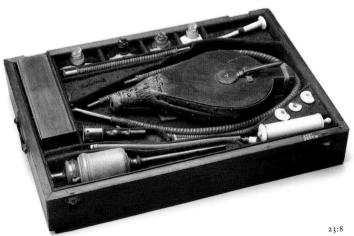

An English resuscitator kit from 1774. The recommended use of this equipment is to revive "Apparently dead" people by blowing tobacco smoke into the lungs or up the rectum.

23:8

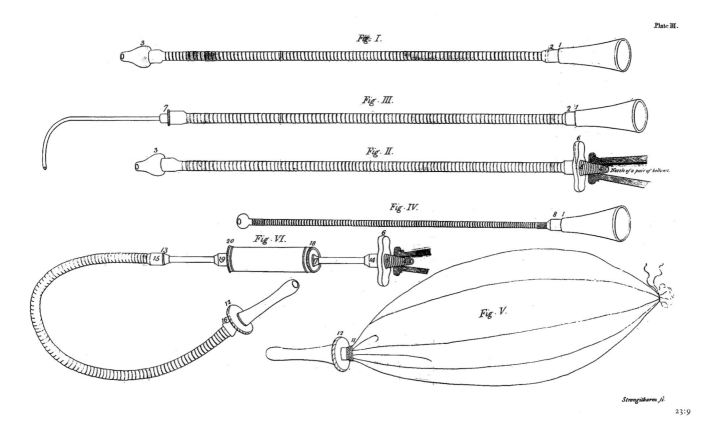

Plate III.

Fig. I.

Fig. III.

Fig. II.

Nozzle of a pair of bellows.

Fig. IV.

Fig. VI.

Fig. V.

Strongitharm sc.

23:9

Above and on the page to the left, illustrations show the intubation sets and bellows to be used for artificial respiration for resuscitation as recommended by Kite.

The apparatus needed to save drowning persons according to Johan Herholdt (1764–1836) and Carl Rafn (1769–1808). They are early to recognise the benefit of oxygen and modify a ventilator apparatus so that it can provide air-oxygen mixtures.

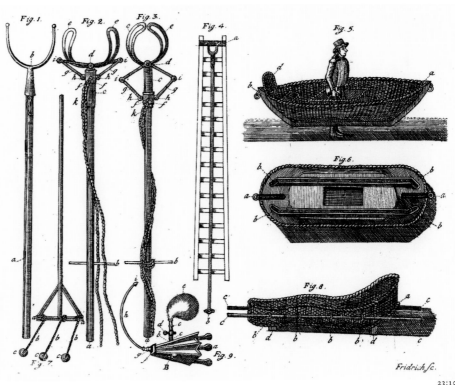

Fig. 1. Fig. 2. Fig. 3. Fig. 4. Fig. 5.

Fig. 6.

Fig. 8.

Fig. 7. Fig. 9.

B

Fridrich sc.

23:10

NOMENCLATURE CHIMIQUE.

MÉMOIRE

Sur la nécessité de réformer & de perfectionner la nomenclature de la Chimie, lu à l'Assemblée publique de l'Académie Royale des Sciences du 18 Avril 1787;

Par M. LAVOISIER.

LE travail que nous présentons à l'Académie a été entrepris en commun par M. de Morveau, par M. Bertholet, par M. de Fourcroy & par moi : il est le résultat d'un grand nombre de conférences, dans lesquelles nous avons été

A

24:1

110 NOMENCLATURE	
Noms anciens.	Noms nouveaux.
Acidum pingue.	Principe hypothètique de Meyer.
Acier.	Acier.
Affinités.	Affinités ou attractions chimiques.
Aggrégation.	Aggrégation.
Aggrégés.	Aggrégés.
Air acide vitriolique.	Gaz acide sulfureux.
Air alkalin.	Gaz ammoniacal.
Air atmosphérique.	Air atmosphérique.
Air déphlogistiqué.	Gaz oxigène.
Air du feu de Schéele.	Gaz oxigène.
Air factice.	Gaz acide carbonique.
Air fixe.	Gaz acide carbonique.
Air gâté.	Gaz azotique.
Air inflammable.	Gaz hydrogène.
Air phlogistiqué.	Gaz azotique.
Air puant du soufre.	Gaz hydrogène sulfuré.
Air putride.	
Air solide de Hales.	Gaz acide carbonique.
Air vicié.	Gaz azotique.
Air vital.	Gaz oxigène.
Airain.	Airain ou alliage de cuivre & d'étain.

24:2

The new chemical nomenclature adopted by Antoine Lavoisier (1743–1794) for his chemical system, which lays the foundation for the modern science of chemistry.

The calorimeter employed by Lavoisier to study the heat produced in chemical reactions and in the metabolic process. With an animal in the centre cage, the amount of melted ice from the double-walled device is taken as the measure of the heat lost from the animal.

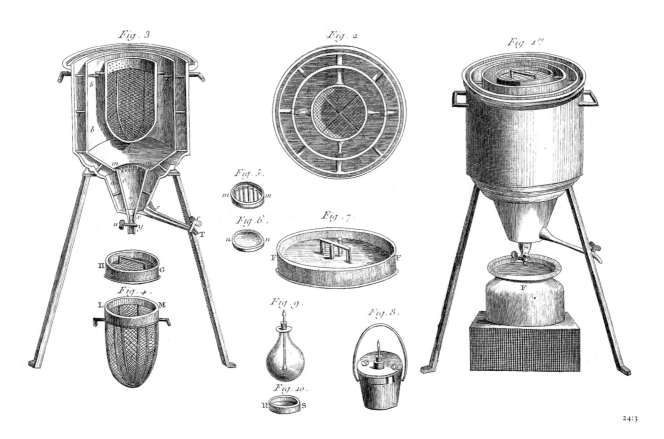

24:3

ORN 1743 in Paris, Lavoisier lost his mother at the age of five and was raised by a loving maiden aunt. He received an excellent basic education at the Collège Mazarin, took a degree in law and soon got captivated by mineralogy, physics and chemistry. Ambitious and extremely energetic and craving public recognition, he entered the Academy of Sciences in 1768, becoming a full member ten years later. Parallel with his extensive scientific work, Lavoisier held many government posts. Liberal in his views, he worked for tax reform, old-age insurance and employment for the poor. He actively supported the French Revolution, but in the wake of the Rein of Terror he was executed on the guillotine 1794. Famed mathematician Lagrange paid tribute to Lavoisier by saying: "It took them only an instant to cut off that head, and a hundred years may not produce another like it". After Lavoisier's death his wife, who was not only his collaborator and illustrator but also his most ardent supporter, collected and published his many unfinished investigations (24.1).

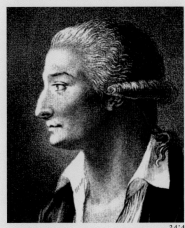

Antoine-Laurent Lavoisier   24:4

Premier Mémoire sur la Respiration des Animaux.

MÉMOIRE DE L'ACADÉMIE ROYALE. PARIS: 1789. P566.

IN THIS study, performed on and written together with Seguin, Lavoisier measures combustion (oxygen uptake) in man. He demonstrates that oxygen (air éminemment respirable or air vital) is taken up in the lungs and that the uptake increases with temperature and during digestion and exercise.

IN PERSPECTIVE:
Lavoisier declared in 1773 that his work would bring about "a revolution in physics and chemistry". He did achieve this by first publishing a new nomenclature for chemistry in 1787 (24.2) and then an account of the results of his extensive experimental investigations in 1789 (24.3). He clarified the role of oxygen in combustion and oxidation and explored the mechanisms of acid formation and water decomposition. Lavoisier also measured combustion and carbon dioxide elimination in animals and, using an ingenious calorimeter, the heat produced due to their metabolism (24.3). Although he was certainly inspired by the work of Hales (24.4) and he may well have known of the discoveries of Scheele, Priestley and Cavendish (24.5)(24.6)(24.7), he worked with great discipline along independent lines of his own (24.8)(24.9). Contrary to other eminent chemists of his time, he was intent on uncovering the basic rules of the chemical reaction. In time the chemical foundation of metabolism was established by Liebig (24.10) and its relation to gas exchange was explored by Pettenkofer and Voit (24.11).

24.1 Lavoisier AL, et al. *Mémoires de Chimie.* Paris; 1803–1805.
24.2 Lavoisier AL, et al. *Méthode de Nomenclature Chimique.* Paris; 1787.
24.3 Lavoisier A-L. *Traité élémentaire de chimie, présenté dans un ordre nouveau et d'après les découvertes modernes.* Paris; 1789.
24.4 See #17 Hales page 100.
24.5 See #21 Scheele page 120.
24.6 See #22 Priestley page 124.
24.7 Cavendish H. Experiments on air. *Phil Trans Roy Soc* 1784; 74:119. See also ref. 21.2.
24.8 Grimaux E. *Lavoisier 1743–1794.* Paris; 1888.
24.9 Guerlac H. *Lavoisier in Dictionary of Scientific Biography VIII.* New York; 1973. p66.
24.10 See #39 Liebig page 208.
24.11 See #58 Voit page 300.

Lavoisier measures gas exchange in man with Madame Lavoisier recording the results at the desk. The subject, the chemist Armand Séguin (1767–1835), is seen in the drawing below performing mechanical work by pressing on a pedal. The drawing on the opposite page shows the same experiment with the subject at rest.

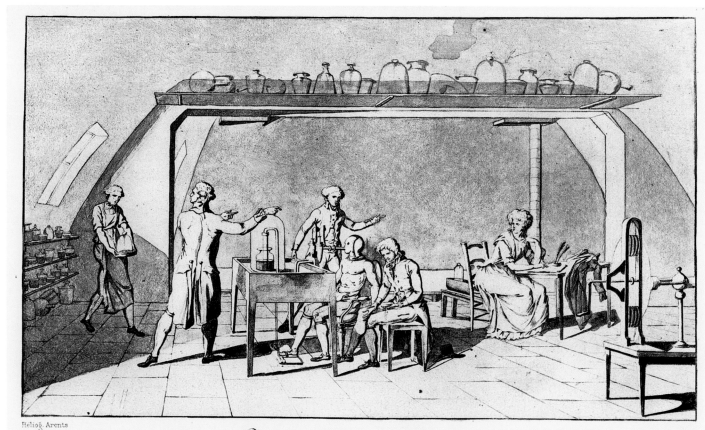

Lavoisier dans son laboratoire

Expériences sur la respiration de l'homme exécutant un travail

Fac-simile réduit d'un dessin de Mme Lavoisier

24:5

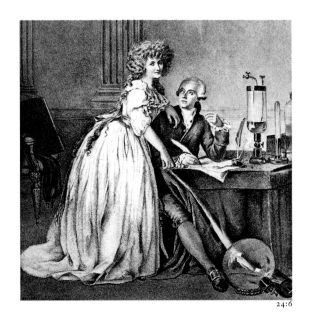

Lavoisier with his wife Marie. Madame Lavoisier is a skilled artist, a competent research assistant to Lavoisier and also manages, despite very difficult times, to publish all of Lavoisier's work that is in progress when he is beheaded during the Rein of Terror of the French Revolution.

24:6

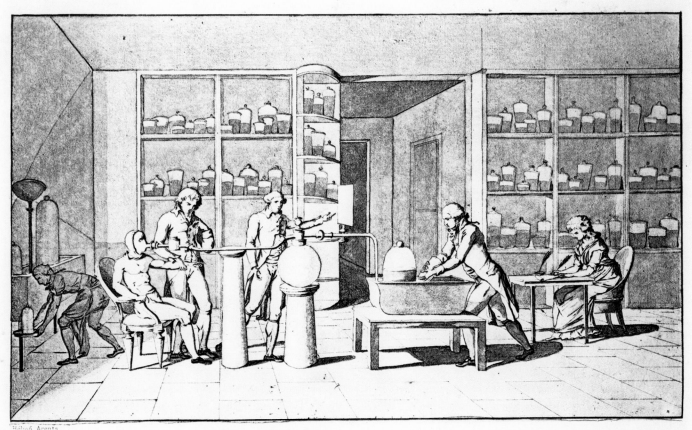

Lavoisier dans son laboratoire
Expériences sur la respiration de l'homme au repos

Fac-simile réduit d'un dessin de Mme Lavoisier

24:7

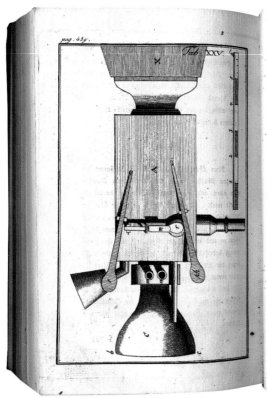

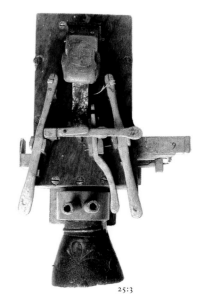

25:1

25:3

Wolfgang Kempelen (1734–1804) describes his apparatus for generating speech sounds of letters and words. The original device as it can be seen today is shown for comparison.

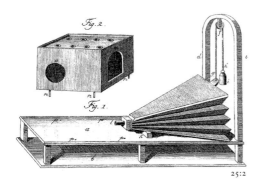

25:2

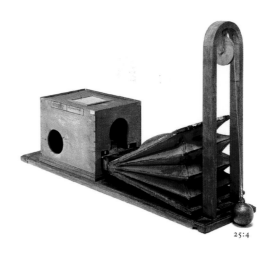

25:4

KEMPELEN was born in Pressburg (Bratislava) in 1734. He studied philosophy and law in Vienna and entered a career as a civil servant. From 1786 he served as a counsellor ("Hofrat") at the office of the Austrian-Transylvanian court. Kempelen had many talents. He constructed bridges and canals, mechanical devices such as pumps and a printing machine for the blind, but he also made landscape engravings and wrote several dramas. He is infamous for a mechanical automaton "the Turk" which was ostensibly a chess-playing machine that could say "Echeck", but in reality a man inside a box manipulated the pieces. From 1770 to the mid 19th century this hoax was a successful illusion, much appreciated by the public (25.1).

Mechanismus der menschlichen Sprache nebst der Beschreibung seiner sprechenden Maschine.

WIEN: J. B. DEGEN; 1791.

KEMPELEN FIRST discusses in general terms the origins of languages and then considers the mechanisms and physiology of speech generation. Finally, he describes a mechanical device that took him twenty years to build and that can produce speech sounds for letters and words. On the nature of language Kempelen argues that human speech and reason are connected and that they develop together over time and he rejects the theory that all languages come from a single (divine) source. He studies the function of the organs of speech and discovers that the cavities over the larynx play the most important role in acoustic articulation. His machine comprises a pressure chamber for the lungs, a vibrating reed for vocal cords, a leather tube, the shape of which helps to produce different vowel sounds, and constrictions controlled by fingers for generating consonants. For plosive sounds he includes movable lips and a hinged tongue.

IN PERSPECTIVE:
Leonardo da Vinci studied the anatomy and mechanism of sound generation in about 1510 (25.2) and almost a century later Casserius first described the vocal and auditory organs in detail (25.3). Kratzenstein, a contemporary of Kempelen, designed acoustic resonators for producing vowel sounds (25.4). In the 1830s Bell investigated the vocal organs (25.5) and Müller studied in a model the function of the vocal cords (25.6). For another century, mechanical models similar to Kempelen's were still the state of the art in synthetic speech generation (25.7)(25.8), but then the first electrical devices were conceived by Dudley (25.9). During the 1950s, fuelled by the rapid progress in electronics and digital computers, artificial speech generation and analysis quickly developed into a highly sophisticated scientific field with many applications (25.10).

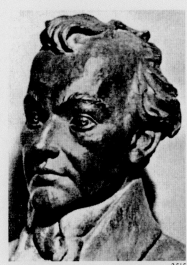

Wolfgang von Kempelen   25:5

25.1 Levitt GM. *The Turk, Chess Automaton.* Jefferson: McFarland & Co; 2000.

25.2 Leonardo da Vinci: *Leonardo on the human body. Drawing 39.* New York:Dover Publications Inc.; 1983.

25.3 Casserius J. *De vocis auditusque organis historia anatomica, tractatibus duobus explicata.* Ferrara; 1600.

25.4 Kratzenstein C. Sur la naissance de la formation des voyelles. *Journal de Physique* 1782; 21:358.

25.5 Bell C. Of the Organs of the Human Voice. *Phil Trans Roy Soc* part II 1832. p299.

25.6 Müller J. *Ueber die Compensation der physischen Kräfte am menschlichen Stimmorgan, …* Berlin; 1839.

25.7 Flanagan J. *Speech Analysis, Synthesis and Perception.* Berlin: Springer Verlag; 1972.

25.8 Cater JP. *Electronically Speaking: Computer Speech Generation.* H. M. Sams & Co.; 1983.

25.9 Dudley H. The Vocoder. *Bell Lab. Records.* December 1939. p122.

25.10 Klatt D. Review of Text-to-Speech Conversion for English. *J Acoust Soc Am* 1987; 82(3): 737 and also #89 Fant page 460.

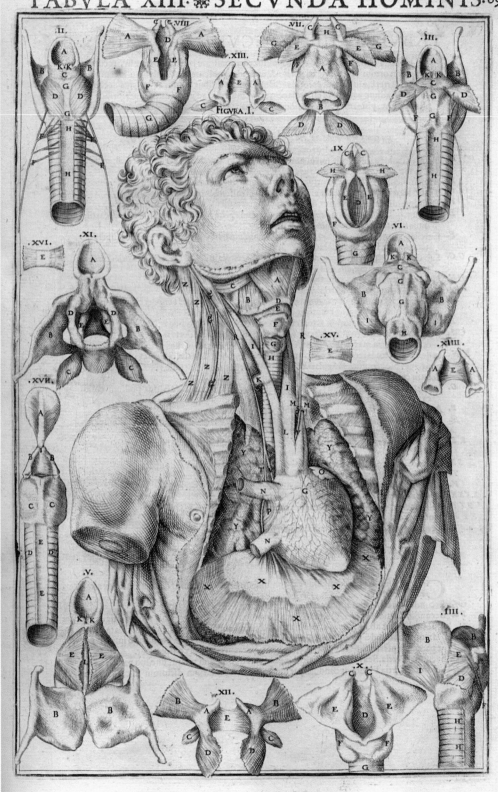

Julius Casserius (1552–1616) publishes the first comparative study of the organs of speech and hearing. His book is also notable because of the accuracy and beauty of the anatomical plates.

25:6

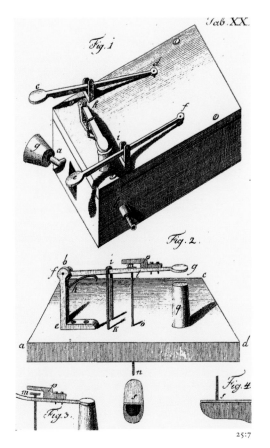

Further details of Kempelen's apparatus as presented in his book and (below), for comparison, the original device as it can be seen today.

25:7

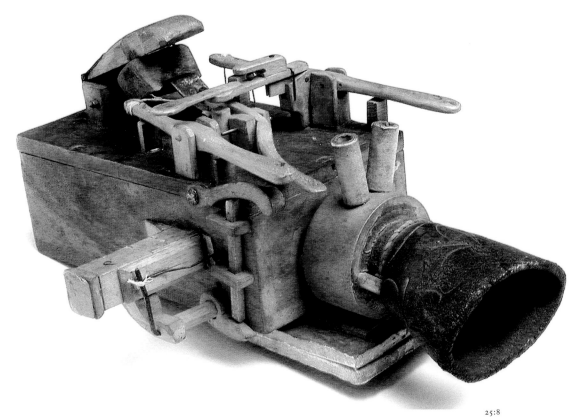

25:8

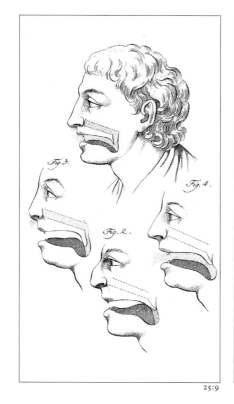

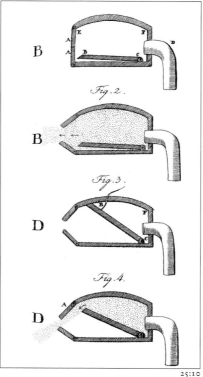

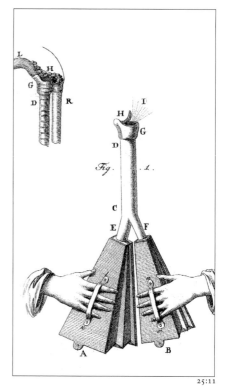

25:9

25:10

25:11

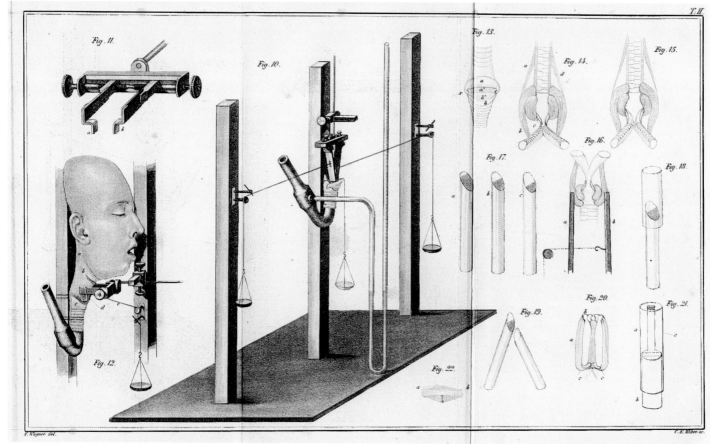

25:12

The top three illustrations on the opposite page show how Kempelen, in order to study the origin of plosive sounds, includes movable "lips" and a hinged "tongue" in his device.

Opposite page below, Johannes Müller (1801–1858) builds a model of the vocal cords and determines the physical conditions for generating specific sounds.

In a major advance, 1939 sees Homer Dudley (1896–1980) introduce the electronic voice analyser and synthesiser, the Vocoder (below). The principle of operation of the first version of this device is shown diagrammatically on the right.

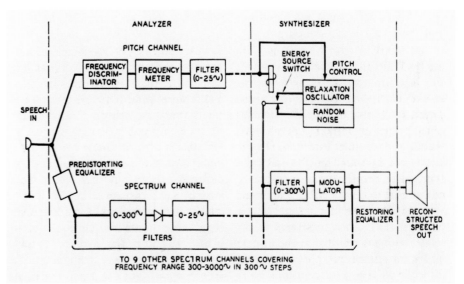

25:13

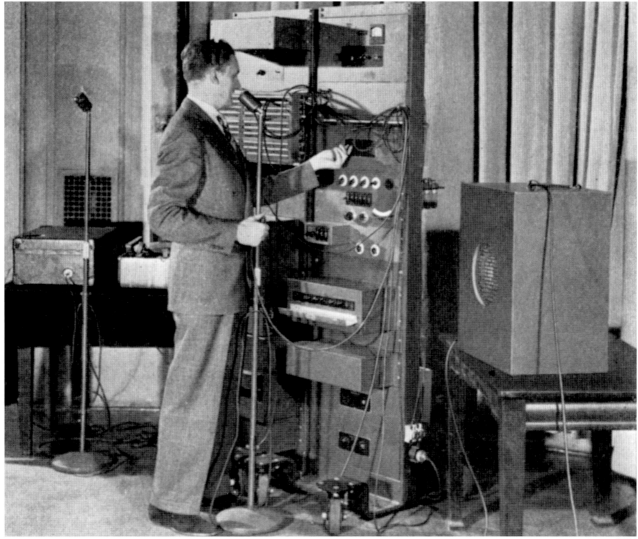

25:14

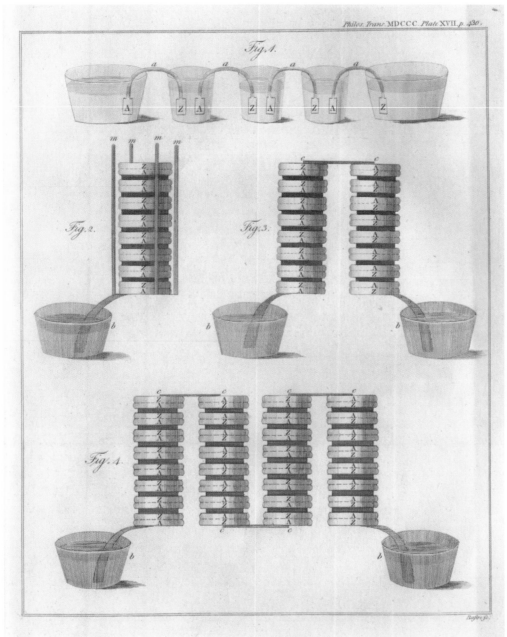

Fig. 1.

Fig. 2.

Fig. 3.

Fig. 4.

Alessandro Volta (1745–1827) invents "the electro-motive" apparatus that produces "endless circulation of the electric fluid" which, he adds, "may appear paradoxical and even inexplicable, but it is no less true and real and you feel it, as I may say, with your hands." Two configurations are discussed, the chain of cups and the stacked plates. The letter A stands for silver plates and Z for Zinc plates.

A Volta stack from around 1800 that is used to dissociate water and other early electro-chemical experiments.

26:1

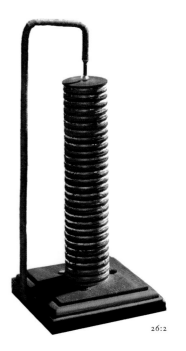

26:2

VOLTA was born in 1745 in Como Italy, the son of a nobleman of small financial means. When his father died in 1752, an uncle sent him to a Jesuit school to study the classics. However, the phenomenon of electricity soon caught his interest. In 1775 Volta invented a new way of accumulating electric charge (the "electrophorus") that brought him recognition. From 1779 and for four decades, he was professor of physics in Pavia and became a member of many learned societies. He travelled widely and corresponded with many contemporary scientists, particularly authorities on electricity (26.1). After his invention of the electric battery in 1800, he devoted the rest of his life to his family and his estate. Volta enjoyed the friendship of Napoleon and other luminaries of his time.

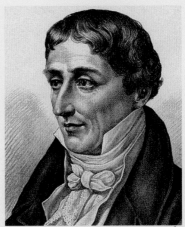

Alessandro Volta   26:3

On the Electricity excited by the mere Contact of Conducting Substances of Different Kinds.

THE PHILOSOPHICAL MAGAZINE. LONDON: SEPTEMBER 1800.

IN THIS letter, Volta describes his discovery of a way to generate a constant electric current (perpetual motion of electric fluid) and explores some of its physical and physiological characteristics. He uses pairs of metals (such as silver and zinc) arranged as a chain of cups (couronne de tasses), each filled with salt water, or as rods (pile) made up by stacking alternating metal plates separated periodically by moistened discs of paper. Volta tests the device on different parts of his body, including his eyes and ears. He feels acute pain, sees flashes of light and hears a crackling, boiling sound. When passing current between his ears he notes "the disagreeable sensation" and "the shock in the brain prevented me from repeating this experiment".

IN PERSPECTIVE:
While Volta believed that his discovery would be "particularly interesting to medicine" and offer "a great deal to occupy the anatomist, the physiologist and the practitioner", his invention also produced fundamental scientific advances, including Oersted's discovery of electro-magnetism (26.2) while lecturing on Volta's pile (26.3) and Faraday's demonstration of electric induction (26.4). Savart determined the frequency sensitivity of the ear (26.5), Duchenne du Bologne and Brenner studied the hearing sensations produced by different electrical stimuli (26.6) and the first audiometer was conceived by Hartmann (26.7). In the 1930s sensitive amplifiers became widely available, introducing a new area in auditory research (26.8). In 1957 the auditory nerve was directly stimulated in a controlled way for the first time by Djourno (26.9). The advances in microelectronics, implanted multiple electrodes and sophisticated methods for speech analysis and recognition have all contributed to the development of the modern, high-performance cochlear implants (26.10)(26.11).

26.1 Nollet (ref. 19.1), Galvani (ref. 19.4), Humboldt (ref. 19.9), Priestley (ref. 22.1), Spallanzani (ref. 16.7), Saussure (ref. 7.8).

26.2 Oersted HC. *Experimenta circa effectum conflictus electrici in acum magneticam.* Copenhagen; 1820.

26.3 Oersted HC. *Laeresaetninger af den nyere Chemie.* Copenhagen; 1820. p15.

26.4 Faraday M. Experimental Researches in Electricity. *Phil Trans Roy.Soc* Part I, 1832. p125.

26.5 Savart F. Sur la sensibilité de l'organe de l'ouie. *Ann Chim Phys* 1830; 44:337.

26.6 Brenner R. *Untersuchungen und Beobachtungen auf die Gebiete der Elektrotherapie.* Vol I,II Leipzig; 1868 and ref 19.11

26.7 Hartmann A. Ueber eine neue Methode der Hörprufung mit Hulfe elektrischer Ströme. *Arch Physiol Leipzig;* 1878. p155.

26.8 Stevens SS, Jones RC. The Mechanism of Hearing by Electrical Stimulation. *J Acoust Soc Am* 1939; 10:261.

26.9 Djourno A, Eyries Ch. Prothèse auditive par excitation électrique a distance du nerf sensoriel a l'aide d'un bobinage inclus a demeure. *La Presse Medicale* 1957; 35:1431.

26.10 Clark GM, Tong YC, Patrick JF. *Cochlear Protheses.* Melbourne: Churchill Livingstone; 1990.

26.11 See #89 Fant page 460 and #85 Eckert-Mauchley page 438 ref. 85.10.

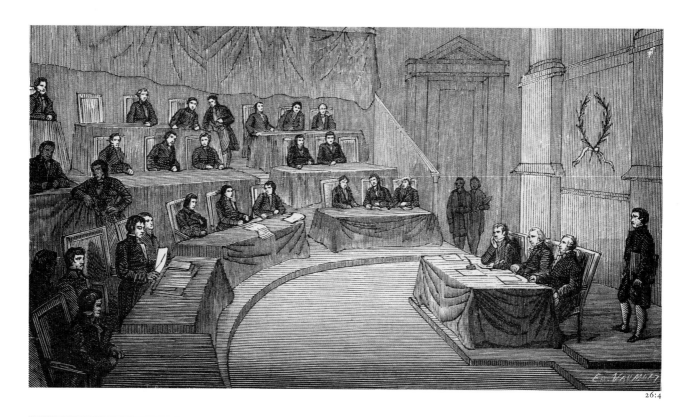

26:4

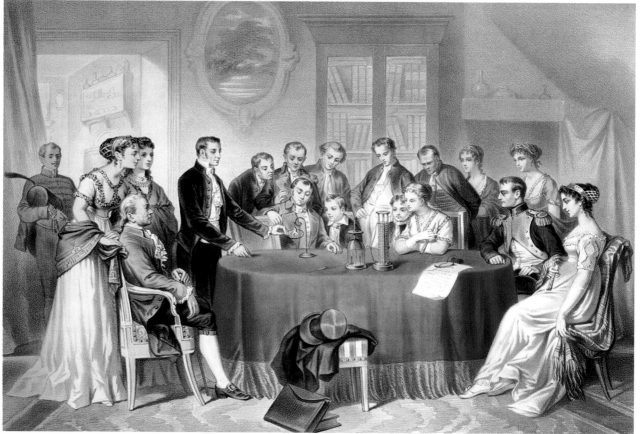

26:5

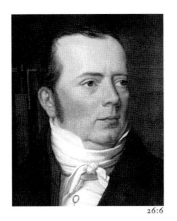

26:6

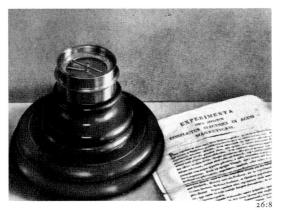

26:8

Hans Christian Oersted (1777–1851) and the magnetic compass used when, in the course of his lecture, he discovers the phenomenon of electromagnetism. Below his lecture notes from 1820 describing how to generate an electric current using a Voltaic pile.

40. Forbinder man flere faadanne til en sammensat electrisk Kjæde, saaledes af f. Er. Zink, Kobber, Vædske, verle med hverandre, og indretter Alt saaledes at det første og det sidste Leed kan sættes i mere eller mindre umiddelbart electrisk Samqvem, saa forstærkes endnu denne Virkning; man seer Zinken ilte sig, og smaae Luftbobler udvikle sig paa Kobberet. Den sammensatte Kjæde kaldes ogsaa efter sin Opfinder og sædvanlige Form Voltas Støtte.

26:9

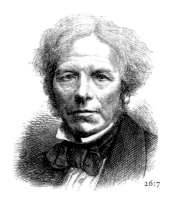

26:7

Michael Faraday (1791–1867) reports his discovery of electromagnetic induction in 1832.

Two accounts of Volta's famous demonstration of his invention for Napoleon Bonaparte. Lecturing at the Academie des Sciences in Paris on 18 November 1800 (top) and in a private setting (below).

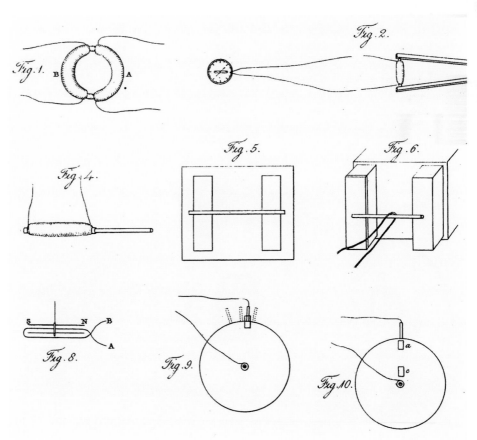

26:10

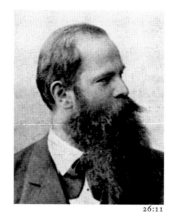

Arthur Hartmann
(1849–1931) conceives
the first audiometer in
1878.

26:11

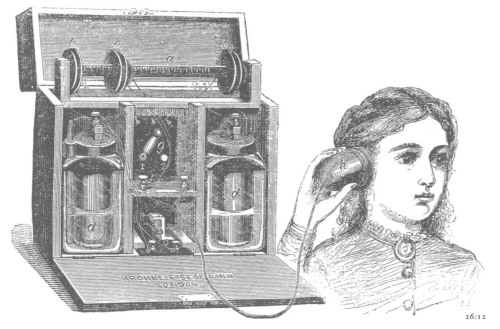

26:12

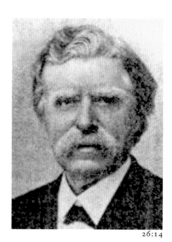

26:14

David Hughes (1831–1900) uses
an induction balance to design
the first practical audiometer,
"the sonometer". The device
and its proper use as taught by
the periodical The Practitioner
in 1880 is shown.

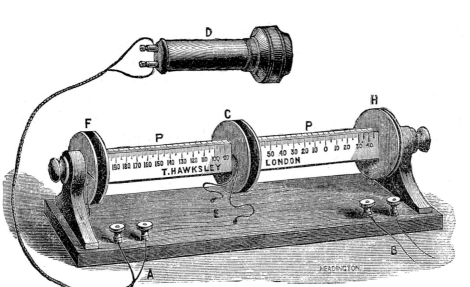

26:13

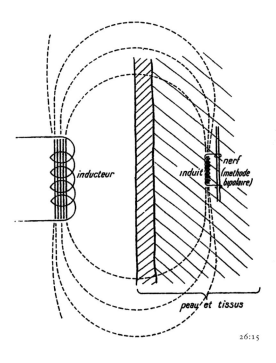

inducteur

induit (methode bipolaire)

nerf

peau et tissus

26:15

PROTHÈSE AUDITIVE PAR EXCITATION ÉLECTRIQUE A DISTANCE DU NERF SENSORIEL A L'AIDE D'UN BOBINAGE INCLUS A DEMEURE

PAR MM.

A. DJOURNO et Ch. EYRIES (Paris)

En 1953, l'un de nous déposait à l'Académie des Sciences un pli cacheté dans lequel, parmi d'autres applications de la méthode des induits (voir La Presse Médicale, t. 65, n° 59, du 3 Août 1957), la possibilité d'agir directement sur le nerf auditif de façon à assurer une prothèse dans les cas où, l'oreille interne étant détruite ou ne fonctionnant plus, tout appareillage acoustique était impossible.

Il entreprenait l'an dernier, après avoir surmonté quelques difficultés techniques, des recherches sur l'animal avec B. Vallancien.

26:17

In 1957 the first controlled study of direct stimulation of the auditory nerve is reported. Electrodes are placed on the nerve during an operation for cholesteatoma (benign tumour). The patient can distinguish differences in pitch in increments of 100 pulses/second and recognises words such as "pappa" "maman" and "allo".

A modern cochlear implant system is made up of the implant with the electrodes and an external part housing the microphone, the batteries, and the microelectronics. The device has advanced speech processing and wireless communication functions. Multi-channel designs with enhanced speech recognition capabilities were first implanted in 1978.

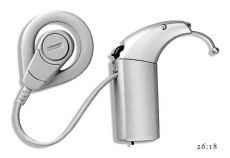

26:18

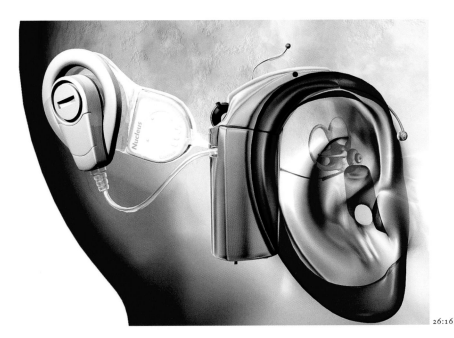

26:16

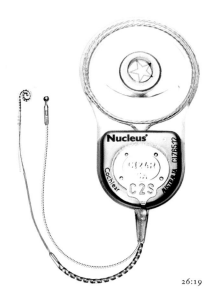

26:19

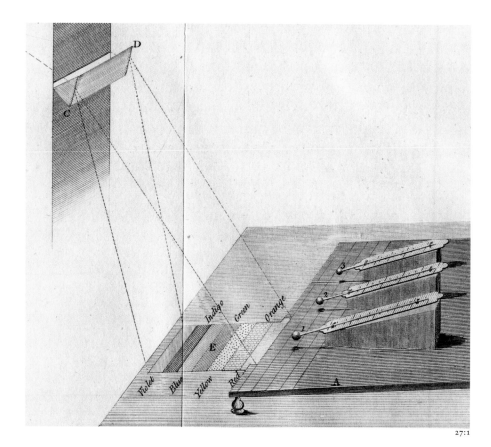

27:1

Wilhelm Herschel's (1738–1822) experiments to measure the effect of heat from the different spectral colours. Different wavelengths of the radiation are allowed to fall on thermometers as a prism is rotated (top) or a focusing mirror is tilted (bottom).

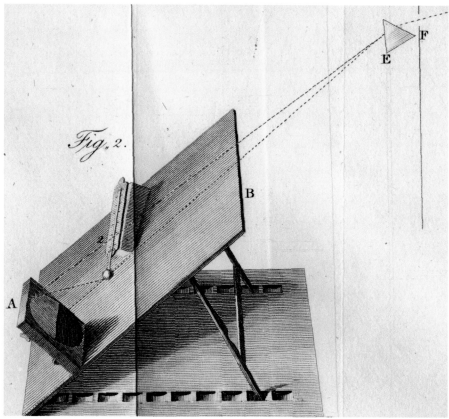

27:2

Herschel was born in Hannover in 1738. As an oboist in his father's regimental band, he visited England in 1756 and fled there a year later when the French occupied Hannover. In the beginning he supported himself by playing and composing music, but soon became obsessed with astronomy, wanting to understand "the construction of the heavens". He learned to design and manufacture large reflecting telescopes superior to all other similar instruments of the time. With his sister Caroline as an assistant, Herschel examined the stars, the moon and the solar system. The discovery of the planet Uranus in 1781 brought him recognition and financial security. He married when he was fifty and his only son John became a prominent scientist and astronomer (27.1). Herschel was knighted in 1816, six years before his death.

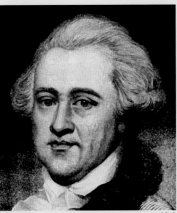

Wilhem Herschel   27:3

Investigation of the Powers of the prismatic Colours to heat and illuminate Objects, …

PHILOSOPHICAL TRANSACTIONS OF THE ROYAL SOCIETY
LONDON. 1800; 1:255.

HERSCHEL REPORTS here on some peculiar observations made while studying the radiation from the sun. Using different combinations of coloured glasses, he says that he "felt the sensation of heat though I had but little light". Studying the phenomena with prisms and thermometers (27.2), Herschel finds that the radiant heat is refrangible but that the maximum heat falls "even beyond visible refraction". Here and in two reports (27.3) immediately following the cited work, he proves that the heat radiation, whether from the sun or from artificial sources, follows the laws of optics as established for light.

IN PERSPECTIVE:

About two decades later, Fraunhofer noted that dark bands appeared when light from the sun passed through a prism (27.4). This observation was explained in 1860 by Kirchoff and Bunsen as the spectra of elements (27.5). Spectroscopy was developed by Vierordt, who also determined the spectral properties of blood (27.6). In the 1970s pulse oximetry evolved into a major clinical tool (27.7) and near infrared spectroscopy was introduced in medical research, particularly for the study of brain function (27.8). Medical imaging with infrared radiation had to await the advent of sufficiently fast and sensitive semiconductor detectors. The first use was for the detection of breast cancer, as suggested by Lawson in 1956 (27.9). The 1970s brought new detector materials, improved optical designs and new applications for diagnosing diseases that directly or indirectly affected the microcirculation of the skin (27.10). More recently, infrared thermography has greatly improved due to advances in microelectronics, detector materials and focal plane array detectors that can produce images quickly, with both high resolution and high temperature sensitivity (27.11).

27.1 See #38 Daguerre page 202 and ref. 38.5.
27.2 See ref. 7.7.
27.3 Herschel W. Experiments on the Refrangibility of the invisible Rays of the Sun. Experiments on the solar, and on the terrestial Rays that occasion Heat. *Phil Trans Roy Soc* Part I 1800. p284, p293
27.4 See ref. 9.8.
27.5 See #49 Kirchhoff page 258.
27.6 Vierordt K. *Die Quantitative Spectralanalyse in ihrer Anwendung auf Physiologie, Physik Chemie und Technologie.* Tubingen; 1876. p59.
27.7 Severinghaus JW. History and recent developments in pulse oximetry. *Scand J Clin Lab Invest* 1993; Suppl. 214:105.
27.8 Jobsis FF. Noninvasive, infrared monitoring of cerebral and myocardial oxygen sufficiency and circulatory parameters. *Science*, 1977; 198:1264.
27.9 Lawson RN. Implication of surface temperatures in the diagnosis of breast cancer. *Can Med Assoc J* 1956; 75:309.
27.10 Cooke ED, Pilcher MF. Thermography in diagnosis of deep venous thrombosis. *Br Med J* 1973; 2:523.
27.11 Keyserlingk JR et al. Infrared imaging of the breast. *The Breast Journal* 1998; 4:245.

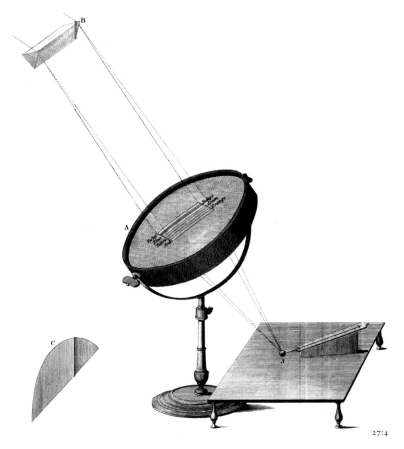

Wilhelm Herschel (1738–1822) discovers the existence of infrared radiation and studies the heating obtained from various sources of radiation.

27:4

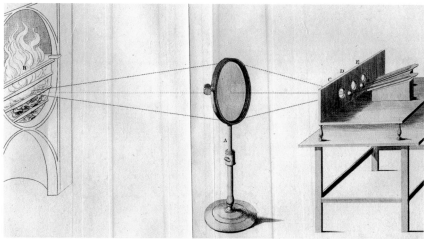

27:5

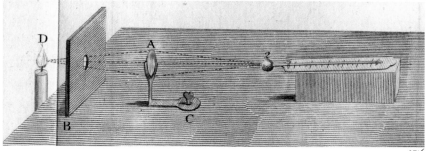

27:6

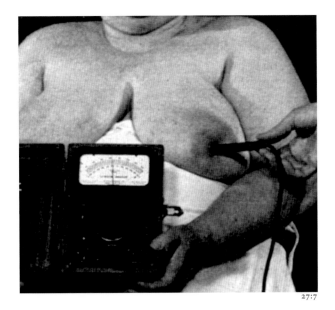

27:7

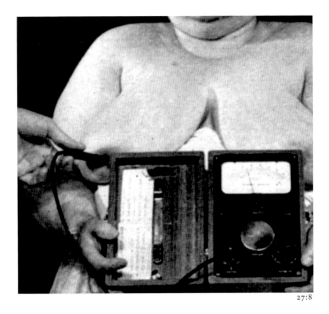

27:8

In 1956 measurement of the skin surface temperature is suggested by Ray Lawson for the diagnosis of breast cancer. The elevated temperature on the left breast demonstrated in the photographs above is indicative of carcinoma.

The Pyroscan device is designated as a high-speed scanner for clinical use in 1964 and produces an image in about 30–180 seconds.

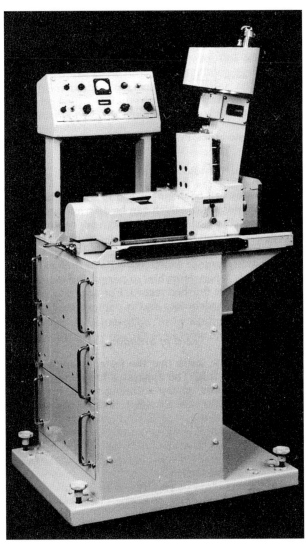

27:9

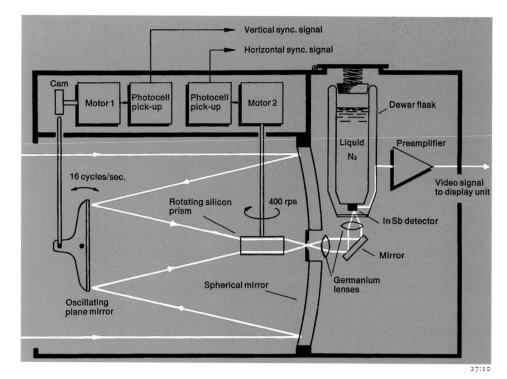

Vertical sync. signal

Horizontal sync. signal

Cam

Motor 1 | Photocell pick-up | Photocell pick-up | Motor 2

Dewar flask

Liquid N₂

Preamplifier

Video signal to display unit

16 cycles/sec.

Rotating silicon prism

400 rps

In Sb detector

Mirror

Germanium lenses

Spherical mirror

Oscillating plane mirror

27:10

A functional diagram of the first commercial infrared scanner that produces 16 frames per second and weighs 17 kg.

The infrared scanner in medical use at the Karolinska Sjukhuset in 1966.

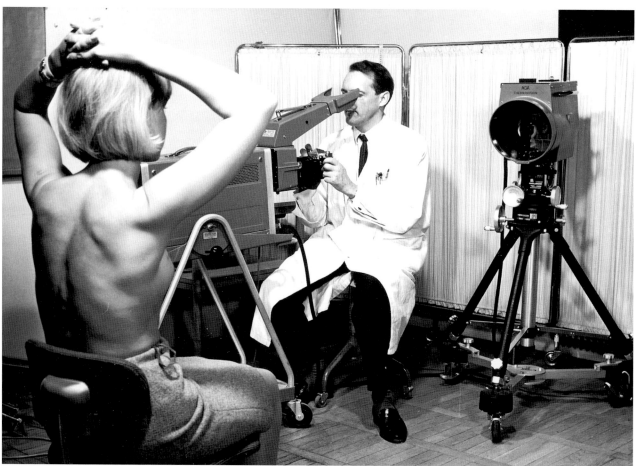

27:11

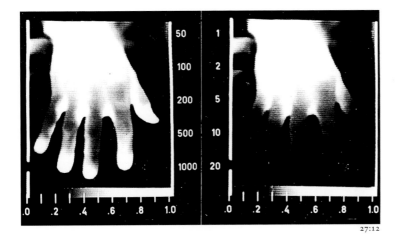

Left, a demonstration of the effect of five minutes of smoking on the circulation in the fingers. Dark areas correspond to lower skin temperature as a result of the reduced peripheral circulation.

Middle, colour images for breast cancer diagnosis from 1978.

Bottom left, an IR-camera from 1974 with a temperature sensitivity of 0.2°C and a weight of 6 kg. Right, a modern battery-operated IR camera with colour display. It has a temperature sensitivity of 0.08°C and a weight of 2 kg.

27:12

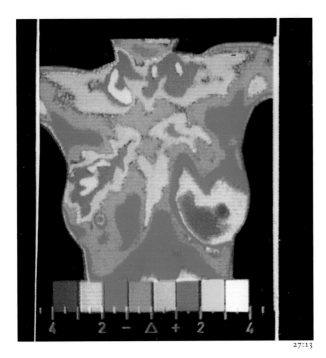

27:13

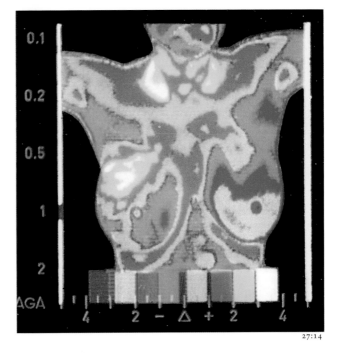

27:14

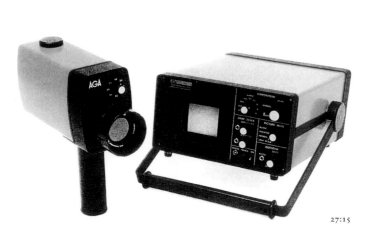

27:15

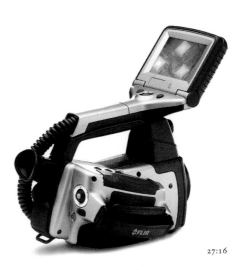

27:16

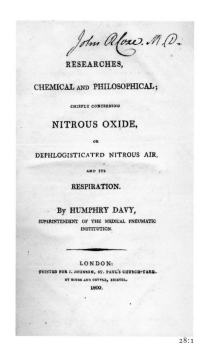

28:1

At the age of twenty-two Humphry Davy (1778–1829) publishes his observations on nitrous oxide. By testing the gas on himself, he notes the alleviation of pain from a wisdom tooth and observes that "it may probably be used with advantage in surgical operations." His comments are, however, overlooked for another forty years. His breathing apparatus is shown below.

MERCURIAL AIR-HOLDER and BREATHING MACHINE.

28:2

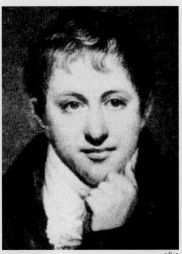

Humphry Davy   28:3

D AV Y was born in Penzance, England, in 1778. On his father's death, at the age of sixteen, he was apprenticed to Borlase, a surgeon and apothecary. He soon embarked on an ambitious self-education programme that included the work of Lavoisier (28.1). In 1798 Davy was appointed superintendent at Beddoes' "Pneumatic Institution", which was set up to explore the therapeutic uses of the new gases (factitious airs) (28.2)(28.3). There, Davy completed his famous study of the properties of nitrous oxide. He was appointed professor of chemistry at the Royal Institution in 1801 and was elected to the Royal Society two years later. Davy was quick to seize on new scientific challenges and opportunities. Accused of arrogance and suffering from a stroke, he spent his last years in unhappy isolation and died in 1829.

Researches, Chemical and Philosophical: chiefly concerning Nitrous Oxide.

LONDON: J. JOHNSON; 1800.

DAVY STARTS his investigation of nitrous oxide by disproving the assertion that it was a contagion (28.4). He experiments on himself and also asks friends to verify his observations. In this way he firmly establishes the pain relieving effects of nitrous oxide. As an example, having an inflamed tooth he notes: "on the day when the inflammation was most troublesome, I breathed three large doses of nitrous oxide. The pain always diminished after the first four or five respirations …". He also suggests that "as nitrous oxide in its extensive operation appears capable of destroying physical pain, it may probably be used with advantage during surgical operation in which no great effusion of blood takes place".

IN PERSPECTIVE:
Davy worked quickly and with great experimental skill and made important discoveries in electro-chemistry, a new field established by Volta's invention of the battery (28.5). The first clinical use of nitrous oxide for pain relief occurred in the dental practice of Wells in 1844 (28.6). Unfortunately, he failed to demonstrate its effect during general surgery, probably due to an inadequate dosage of the gas. The patient woke up in pain and the method was declared a humbug by the surgeons (28.7) and fell quickly into disrepute. However, nitrous oxide was re-introduced as an anaesthetic in dentistry by Colton in 1863 (28.8). The mechanism of the anaesthetic action of nitrous oxide was studied, including at elevated pressures, by Bert (28.9). More widespread use followed due to concerns over the increasing anaesthetic mortality associated with chloroform (28.10) and also as a result of the favourable experiences reported when combining nitrous oxide with oxygen (28.9)(28.11).

28.1 See # 24 Lavoisier page 134.
28.2 See # 22 Priestley page 124.
28.3 Beddoes T, Watt J. *Considerations on the Medicinal Use of Factitious Airs, and on the Manner of Obtaining Them in Large Quatities In two Parts.* Bristol; 1794.
28.4 Mitchill SL. *Remarks on the Gaseous Oxyd of Azote or of Nitrogene, …* New York; 1795.
28.5 See # 26 Volta page 144.
28.6 Keys TE. *The History of Surgical Anesthesia.* Schuman's New York; 1945. p24.
28.7 Wells H. The discovery of etheral inhalation. *The Boston Med. Surg. J.* 1847; 36(15): 298.
28.8 Lyman HM. *Artificial Anaesthesia and Anaesthetics.* New York: William Wood & Co.; 1881. p309.
28.9 See # 59 Bert page 304. See also ref. 28.6 p 73.
28.10 See # 47 Snow page 248.
28.11 Andrews E. The oxygen mixture, a new anaesthetic combination. *Chicago Med. Exam.* 1868; 9:656.

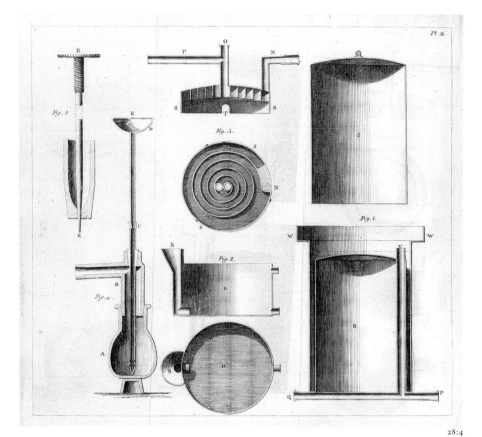

The breathing apparatus invented by James Watt (1736–1819) for the medical use of the newly discovered gases, particularly oxygen. Watt reasoned, "it appears to me, that if it be allowed that poisons can be carried into the system by the lungs, remedies may be thrown in by the same channel."

28:4

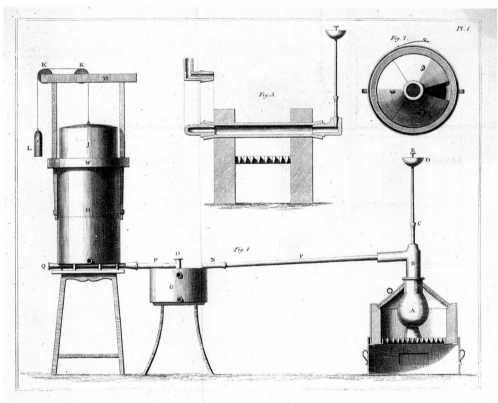

28:5

Thomas Beddoes (1760–1808) establishes the "Pneumatic Institution" near Bristol for curing diseases by inhalation of gases. He and James Watt report good results for many cases of asthma, epilepsy, headache, ulcers, syphilis and other conditions including melancholia. The table below summarises their experience with oxygen therapy.

ANASARCA, GENERAL, AND OF THE LUNGS. ASCITES.

Name.	State in other Respects.	Medicines besides.	What Air.	Circumstances.	Result as to the Disease.	Authority.
7. Mr. G. l.	Dyspeptic : free liver.	Digitalis.	Ox. mod. & ast. lit. dil.	Dyspepsia relieved.	Not cured.	Author, C. 157.
8. Mr. ——		Digitalis.	Ox. nearly pure.	No temporary advantage	Not cured.	Dr. Darwin, A. 76.
8. Mr. Barker.	Free liver.	Many in vain: digitalis.	Ox. mod. dil.	Distress soon removed.	Cure.	Mr. Barr, A. 113.
9. Sir W. Chambers.	Age 75.	Bitters, aperient occas.	Ox. ext. dil.	Dyspnœa removed.	Great ben.	P. N. A. 2.
10. Mary Leucraft.	Ascites.	Crem. tartar.	Ox. mod. dil.	Complexion heightened.	Cure pp.	S. Hill, Esq. A. 7.

ASTHMA, AND DYSPNOEA.

Name.	State in other Respects.	Medicines besides.	What Air.	Circumstances.	Result as to the Disease.	Authority.
11. A Lady.	Spasm. Fit every four days.	None.	Hg. ⅓.	Two short fits in two months.	Consid. ben.	Dr. Ferriar, Vol. II. page 227.
12. J. B——.	Humoral.	None.	Hdc. dil.	Relapsed from imprudence.	Great ben.	Dr. Carmichael, C. 101. A. 82.
13. Mr. ——.	Humoral.		Ox.	Inhaled but once.	Much ease.	Dr. Ferriar, C. 82.
14. Mr. T——.	Humoral.	Tonics in the day, opium at night.	Ox. ext. dil. in the forenoon, and hg. dil. in the evening.	The disease appeared aggravated six weeks by the dil. ox. when exhibited alone.	Cure pp.	Dr. Thornton, C. 77.
15. Lady.	Dyspnœa.	Tonics. Aperients occas.	Ox. mod. dil.	Walks up stairs with less dyspnœa after the inhalation.	Imperfect trial.	Dr. Thornton, C. 18.
16. Rev. Dr. ——.	Fit every night, ending in expectoration.	Emetics. Aperients occas. and tonics.	Ox. ext. dil.	Strength and appetite increased.	Cure pp.	Mr. Townsend, G. 398.
17. Mrs. Barrett.	Spasmodic.	Tonics. Aperients occas.	Ox. ext. dil.	Complexion heightened.	Cure pp.	P. N. A. 25.
18. Mr. ——.	Humoral.	Tonics.	Ox. ext. dil.	General health established.	Much ben.	Mrs. Barrett, A. 26.
19. B. Clopton, Esq.	Spasmodic.	None.	Ox. ext. dil.	Strength, and spirits, improved.	Cure pp.	P. N. A. 48.
20. Mrs. Barker.	Orthopnœa.	Tonics.	Ox. ext. dil.	Cancer less indurated.	Cure pp.	Mr. Barker, A. 23.
21. A Lady.	Humoral.	Aperients.	Ox. mod. dil.	Immediate relief.	Cure pp.	Mr. Phipps, A. 70.

28:7

Method and equipment from the 1870s for the administering nitrous oxide. Below, delivering the gas to the patient from a bag. On the top of the opposite page, inhalers designed for patient connection.

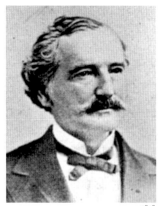

28:8

Gardner Colton (1814–1898) pioneers the medical use of nitrous oxide. In 1863 he introduces it in dental practice, where it quickly becomes highly popular.

Joseph Clover (1825–1882) is a pioneer and an eminent designer of equipment for the delivery of inhalation anaesthetics. One of his early apparatus for combined ether and nitrous oxide administration is shown on the opposite page.

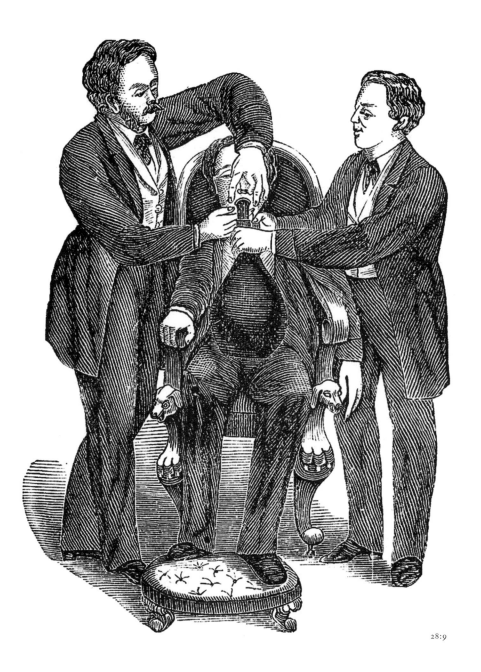

28:9

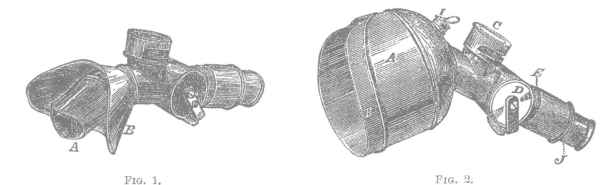

FIG. 1.   FIG. 2.

Codman & Shurtleff's Inhalers for Nitrous Oxide.

FIG. 1.—Inhaler for Nitrous Oxide Gas : A, hard-rubber mouth-piece ; B, metallic hood.

FIG. 2.—A, metallic hood ; B, flexible rubber hood, projecting from within the metallic face-piece ; C, exhaling-valve ; D, two-way stop-cock ; I, packing, through which a silk cord passes ; E, sliding-joint, where J is detached to connect the ether-reservoir ; J contains the inhaling-valve.

28:10

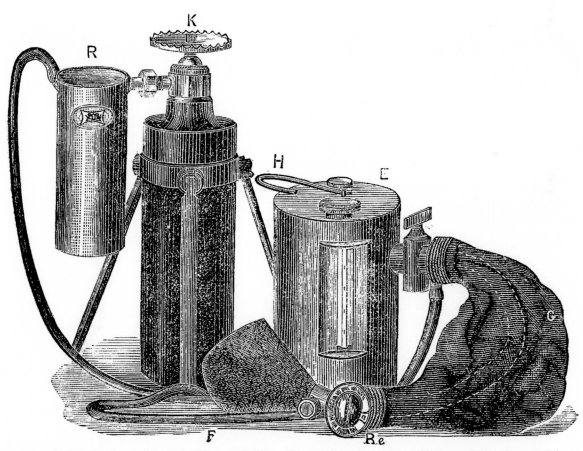

Clover's Inhaler for Ether and Nitrous Oxide: E, container for ether ; F, face-piece ; G, caoutchouc bag traversed by a tube, for the direct transmission of ether vapor. By a proper arrangement the vapor can be combined in the bag with nitrous oxide from the receiver R, K. Re, regulator.

28:11

In 1806 Friedrich Sertürner (1783–1841) reports his discovery of morphine ("opium acid") as the active substance of opium (left). Five years later, his discovery largely ignored, he argues for the proper use and medical benefits of morphine in the paper shown below.

47

III.

Darſtellung

der reinen Mohnſäure *) (Opiumſäure)

nebſt einer

chemiſchen Unterſuchung des Opiums

mit

vorzüglicher Hinſicht auf einen darin neu entdeckten Stoff und die dahin gehörigen Bemerkungen.

Vom

Herrn Sertürner in Paderborn.

Im Journale der Pharmazie 13ten Bandes machte ich einige Bemerkungen über die beſondern Eigenſchaften des im Handel vorkommenden Opiums, welche mir nach den bis jetzt bekannten Beſtandtheilen deſſelben unerklärbar waren; auch äußerte ich zugleich, daß jene

*) Dieſes ſcheint mir der angemeſſenſte Name zu ſeyn, weil ich ſie bis jetzt in keinem andern Vegetabil als dem Mohne gefunden habe.

29:1

99

Ueber

das Opium

und

deſſen kryſtalliſirbare Subſtanz.

Vom

Herrn Apotheker Sertürner,

in Eimbeck.

Man hat an mehreren Orten mit der kryſtalliſirbaren Subſtanz des Opiums Verſuche in arzneylicher Hinſicht angeſtellt, und alle treffen in ihrem Urtheil dahin zuſammen, daß dieſe Subſtanz ſelbſt auf ſchwache Perſonen keine Wirkung äußere; dies befremdet mich um ſo mehr, da ſowohl Desrosne als ich, was dieſen Punkt des Opiums betrifft, übereinſtimmen *). Hätte

G 2   man

*) Wahrſcheinlich hat der Verfaſſer auch hierüber Erfahrungen geſammelt — denn einzig nur dieſe können entſcheiden. Ich muß aufrichtig geſtehen, alle die mir bekannten ſprechen nicht für die Wirkſamkeit dieſes Stoffes. Man ſehe auch Pagen=

29:2

SERTÜRNER was born in Neuhaus in 1783, one of six children in a family of Austrian descent. His father worked as an engineer and inspector for the prince-bishop of Padeborn. After the father's death in 1798, Sertuner was apprenticed to the court apothecary Cramer. In 1803 he passed with distinction his examination for the title assistant apothecary and embarked on his study of opium. He moved to the town apothecary of Einbeck in 1806 and, still as an assistant, he published an extensive account of his findings on morphine that about a decade later caught the attention of the world. In 1820 he took over the town pharmacy of Hameln. He was happily married there and had six children. A good father, honest and pleasant in character, Sertürner was a hypochondriac and at the end of his life also suffered mental disturbances.

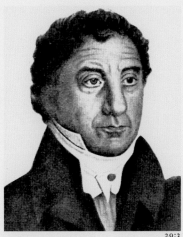

Friedrich Sertürner

29:3

Darstellung der reinen Mohnsäure (Opiumsäure) nebst einer chemischen Untersuchung des Opiums.

JOURNAL DER PHARMACIE. LEIPZIG: J. B. TROMMSDORF; 1806; 14:47.

SERTÜRNER REPORTS on his extensive investigation of "opium acid". In fifty-seven different tests he isolates the sleep inducing factor (schlafmachenden Stoff, Principium somniferum) of opium and elucidates its properties. He identifies nine different constituents of opium and by testing the substances in different ways, including on a dog, he finds the active part to be a crystalline material that he calls vegetable alkali. He predicts that other plants may also yield useful active pharmacological substances.

IN PERSPECTIVE:

Opium (Papaver somniferum) has a long history in medicine. Theophrastus' treatise on botany ca 300 BC (29.1), Celsus' encyclopaedia of all medical knowledge ca 30 AD (29.2) and Avicenna's influential collected writings ca 1000 AD, (29.3) all give details on the preparation and use of opium. However, at the end of the 18th century the medical effects of opium extracts were still unpredictable and so investigators looked for the pure, active component of the plant (29.4). The French apothecary Derosne almost succeeded in isolating it, having prepared narcotine (Salt of Derosne) in 1803 (29.5). Sertürner reported his first observations in 1805 (29.6), but all his writings went largely unnoticed until 1817 after he had published an extension of his previous work (29.7)(29.8) and introduced the word morphium (after Morpheus, the Greek god of sleep) for the active substance (29.8). In 1821 Magendie introduced the new family of alkaloid chemical compounds into medical practice (29.9). It was soon noticed that the effect of morphine increases when administered intravenously (29.4), but this method became available in practice only after the invention of the hypodermic needle (29.10).

29.1 Theophrastus: *De Plantis, De causis plantarum*. Venice; 1465.
29.2 Celsus C. De medicina Florence; 1478. See also ref. 3.1.
29.3 Avicenna: Canon medicinæ. Milan; 1473. See also #7 Santorio page 54.
29.4 Krömeke F. Friedrich Wilh. *Sertürner, der Entdecker des Morphiums*. Jena; 1925. p5.
29.5 Derosne C. Mémoires sur l'opium. *Ann. Chim.* 1803; 45:257.
29.6 Sertürner FW. Säure im Opium, Nachtrag zur Charakteristik der Säure im Opium. Auszuge aus Briefen an den Herausgeber. *J der Pharm* 1805;13:229.
29.7 Sertürner FW. Über das Opium und dessen kristallisirbare Substanz. *J der Pharm* 1811; 20:99.
29.8 Sertürner FW. Ueber eins der furchterlichsten Gifte der Pflanzwelt, ... *Ann. der Phys* 1817; 27:192.
29.9 Magendie F: *Formulaire pour la préparation et l'emploi de plusieurs nouveaux médicaments, tels que la noix vomique, la morphine ...* Paris; 1821.
29.10 See ref. 10.8 and #10 Wren page 68.

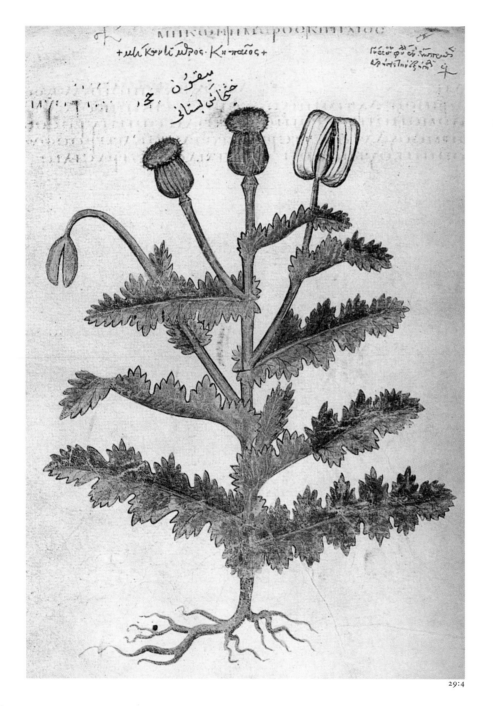

29:4

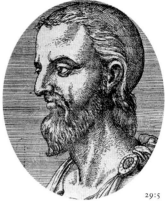

29:5

Dioscorides Pedanius (c. 40–90 AD) summarises in five books, called De Materia Medica, the preparation and properties of about 600 plants. Most of them he ascribes significant medical value.

Opium (papaver somniferum) as depicted in the oldest extant illustrated manuscript of Dioscorides' work, from 512 AD.

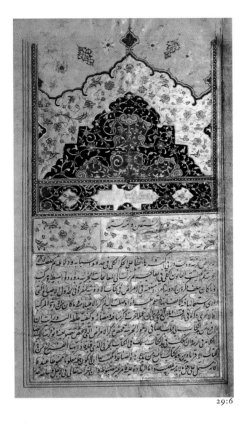

29:6

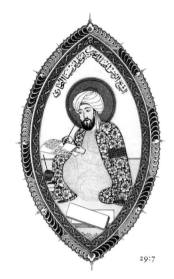

29:7

Avicenna (Ibn sina) (980–1037), philosopher, scientist and physician who writes a highly influential medical text called The Canon of Medicine (the introductory page is shown left), where he says that "it is desirable to produce a deeply unconscious state, so as to enable the pain to be born" and that the most powerful of the stupefacients is opium.

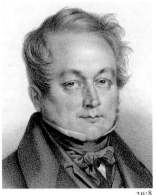

29:8

Francois Magendie (1783–1855) introduces morphine and other alkaloids (such as quinine, atropine and strychnine) into medical practice in 1822. The illustration shows a chapter on morphine from the first American edition of his book in 1824.

---

32   MORPHINE AND THE

[Mr. Brande has lately given the following estimate of the relative proportions of the ultimate elements of morphine :

Carbon 72.00
Nitrogen 5.50
Hydrogen 5.50
Oxygen . . . . . . 17.
                    ‾‾‾‾‾‾
                    100   k]

ACTION OF MORPHINE ON MAN AND ON ANIMALS.

Pure morphine being but little soluble, would scarcely seem to form the narcotic part of opium.[l] Nevertheless, direct experiment has abundantly proved that such is the fact. For example, even the weak dose of a quarter of a grain, or half a grain (gr. .205, or 0.41 troy) of morphine, dissolved in oil, produces effects very markedly narcotic; but this narcotic power becomes very manifest when the morphine is combined with acids; because the salts of mor-

k [Journal of Science, &c. No. 32.]
l It must be recollected that morphine does not exist free in opium. It is united to the meconic acid, and is thus in the state of a salt of morphine. Should not the meconate be made and tried, it being the natural preparation ?—Tr.

SALTS OF MORPHINE.   33

phine are more soluble than the morphine itself.[m]

I employed the acetate, the sulphate, and the hydrochlorate, of morphine, as remedies, nearly three years ago; and found that these salts afford all the advantages which we can expect to meet with in opium, without having any of its inconveniences.[n] As my first trials showed that the hydrochlorate was less useful than the acetate and sulphate, I soon discontinued my researches on that salt. Perhaps it would be well were they resumed.

MORPHINÆ ACETAS.

Acetate of Morphine.

This salt is formed by combining directly, in an evaporating dish, acetic acid and morphine, and letting the mixture slowly evaporate to dryness. The difficulty of obtaining it crystallized, on account of its extreme deliquescence, renders it necessary to adopt this mode of preparation.[o]

m See MM. Orfila and Magendie's experiments on this subject in the Nouveau Journal de Médecine, tom. i. p. 123.—Tr.
n Nouveau Journal de Médecine, Paris, 1818.
o The acetate of morphine crystallizes in soft silky prisms, which are very soluble; the sulphate,

29:9

APPENDICE.

Sur la Méthode des moindres quarrés.

Dans la plupart des questions où il s'agit de tirer des mesures données par l'observation, les résultats les plus exacts qu'elles peuvent offrir, on est presque toujours conduit à un système d'équations de la forme

$$E = a + bx + cy + fz + \&c.$$

dans lesquelles a, b, c, f, &c. sont des coëfficiens connus, qui varient d'une équation à l'autre, et x, y, z, &c. sont des inconnues qu'il faut déterminer par la condition que la valeur de E se réduise, pour chaque équation, à une quantité ou nulle ou très-petite.

Si l'on a autant d'équations que d'inconnues x, y, z, &c., il n'y a aucune difficulté pour la détermination de ces inconnues, et on peut rendre les erreurs E absolument nulles. Mais le plus souvent, le nombre des équations est supérieur à celui des inconnues, et il est impossible d'anéantir toutes les erreurs.

Dans cette circonstance, qui est celle de la plupart des problêmes physiques et astronomiques, où l'on cherche à déterminer quelques élémens importans, il entre nécessairement de l'arbitraire dans la distribution des erreurs, et on ne doit pas s'attendre que toutes les hypothèses conduiront exactement aux mêmes résultats ; mais il faut sur-tout faire en sorte que les erreurs extrêmes, sans avoir égard à leurs signes, soient renfermées dans les limites les plus étroites qu'il est possible.

De tous les principes qu'on peut proposer pour cet objet, je pense qu'il n'en est pas de plus général, de plus exact, ni d'une application plus facile que celui dont nous avons fait usage dans les recherches précédentes, et qui consiste à rendre

Adrien-Marie Legendre (1752–1833) conceives the method of least squares, the first mathematical technique for evaluating experimental results that is based on statistical considerations.

30:1

Adrien-Marie Legendre

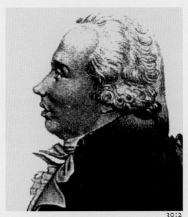

Adrien-Marie Legendre

30:2

LEGENDRE was born into a prosperous Parisian family in 1752. He studied mathematics and physics and defended his thesis in 1770 at the Collège Mazarin. In 1782 he won the mathematics prize of the Berlin Academy and three years later he was admitted to the French Academy. The small fortune that allowed him to do his research full-time was swept away by the French Revolution. A tireless worker, he put his finances in order little by little with the help of his wife. Legendre's timid nature and competition from his even more brilliant fellow mathematicians Laplace and Lagrange made his carrier advance slowly. However, in 1813 he replaced Lagrange at the Bureau de Longitude and remained there till his death two decades later.

Nouvelles Méthodes pour la Détermination des Orbites des Comètes; avec un Supplément. Appendice sur la Méthode des Moindres Quarrés.

PARIS: COURCIER; 1806.

IN THIS treatise dealing with the calculation of the orbits of comets, Legendre announces the method of least squares. The question of how to combine observations to confront theoretical predictions on celestial mechanics had been one of great significance for a long time (30.1) and it had occupied Legendre's mind for some years (30.2). Legendre applies here his new technique to observations made to determine the length of the meridian quadrant through Paris. His presentation, "one of the clearest and most elegant introductions of a new statistical method in the history of statistics" (30.3), gained rapid and widespread acceptance.

IN PERSPECTIVE:
Legendre's work introduced statistical methods in the evaluation of the observations of experimental science. In 1809 Gauss showed that under certain assumptions observational errors had a normal (Gaussian) distribution (30.4). His claim to have used the least squares principle of Legendre since 1795 led to animosities since, as was often his habit, he did not publish his results but just wrote them down in his notebook (30.5). Laplace immediately incorporated Gauss' results into his own research on the so-called central limiting theorem (30.6)(30.7), thereby giving the least squares method and the normal distribution of the error around the mean a more solid probabilistic base. Studying heredity and the propagation of character from generation to generation, Galton developed intuitive methods of dealing with statistical outcomes when many factors, each normally distributed, are at play (30.8). He introduced the concepts of variance and regression (30.9) and made statistical techniques generally useful in many new fields such as medicine and the social sciences. Subsequently Galton's results were put on a sound mathematical footing by Edgeworth (30.10).

30.1 Stiegler SM. *The History of Statistics The Measurement of Uncertainty before 1900.* Cambridge: The Beknap Press, Harvard University Press; 1998.
30.2 See ref. 30.1 p56.
30.3 See ref. 30.1 p13.
30.4 Gauss CF. *Theoria Motus Corporum Coelestium.* Hamburg; 1809.
30.5 See #32 Fourier page 176.
30.6 See ref. 30.1 p136 and p139.
30.7 Laplace P. *Oevres completes de Laplace (1878–1912)* Vol 12. Paris; 1898. p349.
30.8 Galton F. Typical laws of heredity. *Nature* 1877; 15:492, 512, 532.
30.9 See ref. 30.1 p293–299.
30.10 See ref. 30.1 p300.

minimum la somme des quarrés des erreurs. Par ce moyen, il s'établit entre les erreurs une sorte d'équilibre qui empêchant les extrêmes de prévaloir, est très-propre à faire connoître l'état du système le plus proche de la vérité.

La somme des quarrés des erreurs $E^2 + E'^2 + E''^2 + $ &c. étant

$$(a + bx + cy + fz + \&c.)^2$$
$$+ (a' + b'x + c'y + f'z + \&c.)^2$$
$$+ (a'' + b''x + c''y + f''z + \&c.)^2$$
$$+ \&c. \, ;$$

si l'on cherche son *minimum*, en faisant varier x seule, on aura l'équation

$$o = \int ab + x\int b^2 + y\int bc + z\int bf + \&c.,$$

dans laquelle par $\int ab$ on entend la somme des produits semblables $ab + a'b' + a''b'' + $ &c. ; par $\int b^2$ la somme des quarrés des coëfficiens de x, savoir $b^2 + b'^2 + b''^2 + $ &c., ainsi de suite.

Le *minimum*, par rapport à y, donnera semblablement

$$o = \int ac + x\int bc + y\int c^2 + z\int fc + \&c.,$$

et le *minimum* par rapport à z,

$$o = \int af + x\int bf + y\int cf + z\int f^2 + \&c.,$$

où l'on voit que les mêmes coëfficiens $\int bc$, $\int bf$, &c. sont communs à deux équations, ce qui contribue à faciliter le calcul.

En général, *pour former l'équation du* minimum *par rapport à l'une des inconnues, il faut multiplier tous les termes de chaque équation proposée par le coëfficient de l'inconnue dans cette équation, pris avec son signe, et faire une somme de tous ces produits.*

On obtiendra de cette manière autant d'équations du *minimum*, qu'il y a d'inconnues, et il faudra résoudre ces équations par les méthodes ordinaires. Mais on aura soin d'abréger tous les calculs, tant des multiplications que de la résolution, en n'admettant dans chaque opération que le nombre de chiffres

Continuation of Legendre's text. Starting on the previous page he writes, "Of all the principles which can be proposed for that purpose, I think there is none more general, more exact, and more easy of application, than that of which we made use in the preceding researches, and which consists of rendering the sum of squares of the errors a minimum. By this means, there is established among the errors a sort of equilibrium which, preventing the extremes from excerpting an undue influence, is very well fitted to reveal that state of the system which most nearly approaches the truth."

30:3

$$\frac{d\nu}{dr}\,\varphi'\,\nu + \frac{d\nu'}{dr}\,\varphi'\,\nu' + \frac{d\nu''}{dr}\,\varphi'\,\nu'' + \text{etc.} = 0$$

$$\frac{d\nu}{ds}\,\varphi'\,\nu + \frac{d\nu'}{ds}\,\varphi'\,\nu' + \frac{d\nu''}{ds}\,\varphi'\,\nu'' + \text{etc.} = 0$$

Hinc itaque per eliminationem problematis solutio plene determinata deriuari poterit, quamprimum functionis φ' indoles innotuit. Quae quoniam a priori definiri nequit, rem ab altera parte aggredientes inquiremus, cuinam functioni, tacite quasi pro basi acceptae, proprie innixum sit principium triuium, cuius praestantia generaliter agnoscitur. Axiomatis scilicet loco haberi solet hypothesis, si quae quantitas per plures obseruationes immediatas, sub aequalibus circumstantiis aequalique cura institutas, determinata fuerit, medium arithmeticum inter omnes valores obseruatos exhibere valorem maxime probabilem, si non absoluto rigore, tamen proxime saltem, ita vt semper tutissimum sit illi inhaerere. Statuendo itaque $V = V' = V''$ etc. $= p$, generaliter esse debebit $\varphi'(M - p) + \varphi'(M' - p) + \varphi'(M'' - p) +$ etc. $= 0$, si pro p substituitur valor $\frac{1}{\mu}(M + M' + M'' + \text{etc.})$, quemcunque integrum positiuum exprimat μ. Supponendo itaque $M' = M'' = $ etc. $= M - \mu N$, erit generaliter, i. e. pro quouis valore integro positiuo ipsius μ, $\varphi'(\mu - 1)N = (1 - \mu)\varphi'(-N)$, vnde facile colligitur, generaliter esse debere $\frac{\varphi'\Delta}{\Delta}$ quantitatem constantem, quam per k designabimus. Hinc fit $\log\varphi\Delta = \frac{1}{2}k\Delta\Delta + \text{Const.}$, siue designando basin logarithmorum hyperbolicorum per e, supponendoque Const. $= \log\varkappa$,

$$\Delta\varphi = \varkappa e^{\frac{1}{2}k\Delta\Delta}$$

Porro facile perspicitur, k necessario negatiuam esse debere, quo Ω reuera fieri possit maximum, quamobrem statuemus $\frac{1}{2}k = -hh$; et quum per theorema elegans primo ab ill. Laplace inuentum, integrale $\int e^{-hh\Delta\Delta}\,d\Delta$, a $\Delta = -\infty$ vsque ad $\Delta = +\infty$, fiat $= \frac{\sqrt{\pi}}{h}$, (denotando per π semicircumferentiam circuli cuius radius 1), functio nostra fiet

$$\varphi\Delta = \frac{h}{\sqrt{\pi}}\,e^{-hh\Delta\Delta}$$

178.

Functio modo eruta omni quidem rigore errorum probabilitates exprimere certo non potest: quum enim errores possibiles semper limitibus certis coërceantur,

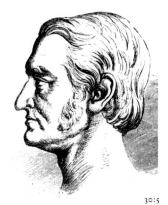

Carl Friedrich Gauss (1777–1855) derives the "Gaussian" or "Normal" distribution of the error in a single observation, assuming that the most probable value is given by the arithmetic mean of the observed values.

SUPPLÉMENT AU MÉMOIRE

SUR LES

APPROXIMATIONS DES FORMULES

QUI SONT FONCTIONS DE TRÈS GRANDS NOMBRES.

Mémoires de l'Académie des Sciences, Ire Série, Tome X, année 1809; 1810.

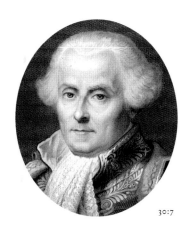

Pierre-Simon Laplace (1749–1827) incorporates the results of Gauss and Legendre into his own research on what is called The Central Limit Theorem, thereby giving the least squares method a solid probabilistic base.

J'ai fait voir, dans l'article VI de ce Mémoire, que, si l'on suppose dans chaque observation les erreurs positives et négatives également faciles, la probabilité que l'erreur moyenne d'un nombre n d'observations sera comprise dans les limites $\pm \frac{rh}{n}$ est égale à

$$\frac{2}{\sqrt{\pi}} \sqrt{\frac{k}{2 k'}} \int dr \, e^{-\frac{k}{2 k'} r^2};$$

h est l'intervalle dans lequel les erreurs de chaque observation peuvent s'étendre. Si l'on désigne ensuite par $\varphi\left(\frac{x}{h}\right)$ la probabilité de l'erreur $\pm x$, k est l'intégrale $\int dx \, \varphi\left(\frac{x}{h}\right)$ étendue depuis $x = -\frac{1}{2}h$ jusqu'à $x = \frac{1}{2}h$; k' est l'intégrale $\int \frac{x^2}{h^2} dx \, \varphi\left(\frac{x}{h}\right)$ prise dans le même intervalle; π est la demi-circonférence dont le rayon est l'unité, et e est le nombre dont le logarithme hyperbolique est l'unité.

Supposons maintenant qu'un même élément soit donné par n observations d'une première espèce, dans laquelle la loi de facilité des erreurs soit la même pour chaque observation, et qu'il soit trouvé égal à A par un milieu entre toutes ces observations. Supposons ensuite qu'il soit trouvé égal à A $+ q$ par n' observations d'une se-

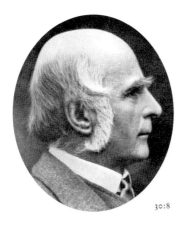

30:8

Illustration of the intuitive method used by Francis Galton (1822–1911) to obtain the statistical outcomes when many factors, each normally distributed, are at play. Studying the transmission of hereditary traits, he introduces the concepts of variance and regression.

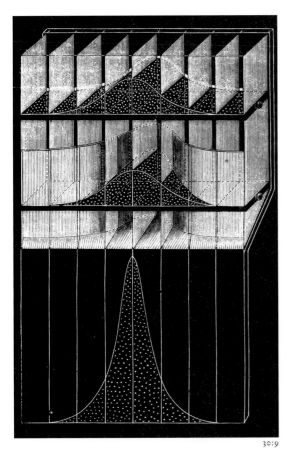

30:9

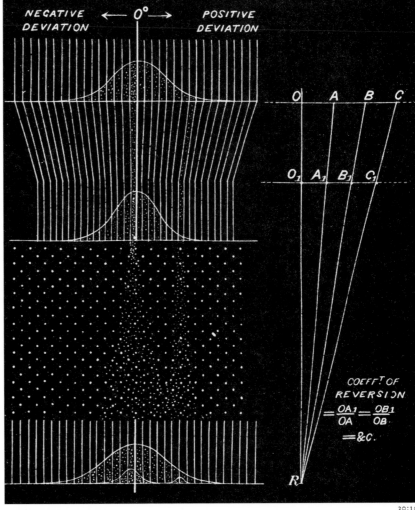

30:10

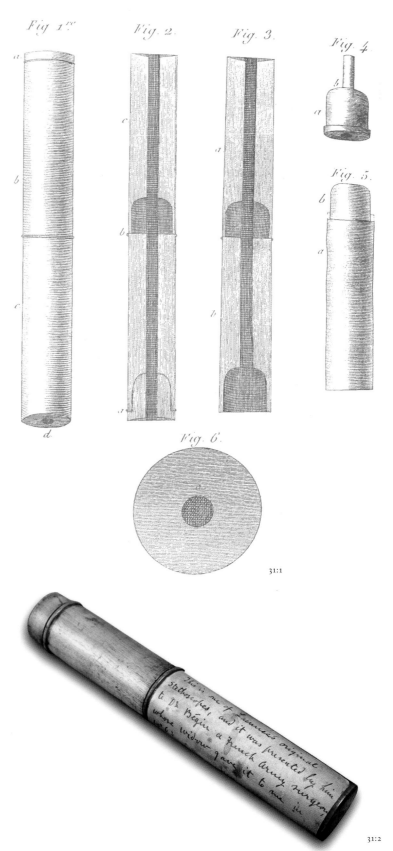

Fig. 1ᵉʳ   Fig. 2.   Fig. 3.   Fig. 4.

Fig. 5.

Fig. 6.

31:1

31:2

René Laennec (1781–1826) describes his invention, the stethoscope (right), with his own device shown below. The picture of Laennec listening with his ear against the chest of a patient at the Necker Hospital is from about 1816, the year when the invention was made.

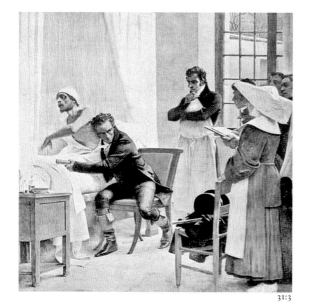

31:3

LAENNEC was born in Quimper, France in 1781. Due to the early death of his mother he was raised by an uncle, a physician in Nantes. As a young boy he assisted in taking care of the sick in the city's hospitals. Bent on classical studies and on playing the flute, he nevertheless went to Paris to study medicine under Corvisart (31.1). Presenting a thesis in 1804, he was first a private practitioner and later a physician at the Neckar Hospital. Here he became interested in the diseases of the chest, which led to his invention of the stethoscope in 1816. Later many honours came to him, including membership of the Académie de Médecine. Laennec was of poor health all his life, suffering from asthma, headaches and dyspepsia. He succumbed to tuberculosis, a disease he so effectively diagnosed, in 1826.

René Laennec   31:4

De l'auscultation médiate ou traité du diagnostic des maladies des poumons et du coeur, fondé principalement sur ce nouveau moyen d'exploration.

PARIS: J. A. BROSSON, J. S. CHAUDÉ; 1819.

LAENNEC DESCRIBES how to diagnose diseases of the lungs and the heart using auscultation. He also announces the invention of the stethoscope, a tube of cedar wood that could amplify the sounds, thereby making his "médiate" auscultation superior to the traditional "immediate" auscultation when placing the ear directly on the chest. Using precise terminology, Laennec correlates different sounds from the chest with different organs and their diseases as established by later autopsy findings.

IN PERSPECTIVE:
Hippocrates (around 400BC) recommended shaking patients (succussion) and listening to the sound coming from their chests. In a major advance Auenbrugger who, like Laennec, had a strong interest in music, introduced chest percussion, the tapping on the chest with a finger and used the sounds for diagnostic purpose (31.1)(31.2). However, his work went unnoticed for nearly half a century, until Corvisart translated it into French, adding much explanatory material from his own experience (31.1). Piorry modified and improved on the design of the stethoscope and introduced the pleximeter, a plate that when placed on the chest was struck with a percussor, an arrangement that replaced Auenbrugger's finger tapping (31.3). The auscultation technique, although difficult to master, became widely accepted after Skoda introduced a new improved sound classification system based on physical acoustics and a simplified terminology (31.4). The binaural stethoscope was introduced in the 1850s and soon after the invention of the telephone (31.5), Stein could develop the sphygmophone, a stethoscope fitted with an electric microphone (31.6). Defining the usefulness and limitations of auscultation remains an active area of study (31.7)(31.8)(31.9)(31.10).

31.1 Auenbrugger L. *Nouvelle méthode pour reconnaître les maladies internes de la poitrine par la percussion de cette cavité*. Ouvrage traduit du latin et commenté par J. N. Corvisart Paris; 1808.

31.2 Auenbrugger L. *Inventum novum ex percussione humani ut signo abstrusos interni pectoris morbos detengendi*. Wien; 1761.

31.3 Piorry PA. *De la percussion médiate et des signes obtenue à l'aide de ce nouveau moyen d'exploration, dans les maladies des organes thoraciques et abdominaux*. Paris; 1828.

31.4 Skoda J. *Abhandlung über Perkussion und Auskultation*. Vienna; 1839.

31.5 Bell AG. *Telegraphy*. US Patent 174.465 March 1876.

31.6 Stein S. Das Sphygmophone, ein neuer electro-telephonischer Apparat zur diagnose der Herz- und Pulsbewegungen. *Berl Klin Wochsch* 1878; 49:723.

31.7 Osmer JC, Cole BK. The stethoscope and roentgenogram in acute pneumonia. *South Med J* 1966; 59:75.

31.8 Loudon R, Murphy RLH. Lung sounds (state of the art). *Am Rev Respir Dis* 1984; 130: 663.

31.9 Stevenson LW, Perloff JK. The limited reliability of physical signs for estimating hemodynamics in chronic heart failure. *JAMA* 1989; 261:884.

31.10 Melbye H. Bronchial airflow limitation and chest findings in adults with respiratory infection. *Scand J Prim Health Care* 1995; 13:261.

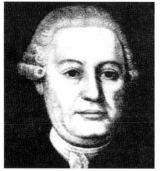

31:5

Leopold Auenbrugger (1722–1809) discovers the diagnostic value of chest percussion, possibly as an analogy to the thumping of wine casks to determine their fullness, a procedure that was practised by his father, who was an innkeeper. His "Inventum Novum", published in 1761, is one of the great medical classics.

LEOPOLDI AUENBRUGGER

MEDICINÆ DOCTORIS
IN CÆSAREO REGIO NOSOCOMIO NATIONUM
HISPANICO MEDICI ORDINARII.

INVENTUM NOVUM

EX

PERCUSSIONE THORACIS HUMANI
UT SIGNO

ABSTRUSOS INTERNI
PECTORIS MORBOS
DETEGENDI.

LABORE ET FAVORE.

VINDOBONÆ,

TYPIS JOANNIS THOMÆ TRATTNER, CÆS. REG.
MAJEST. AULÆ TYPOGRAPHI.

MDCCLXI.

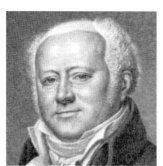

31:7

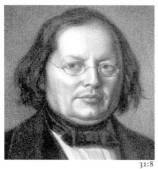

31:8

31:6

Forty-seven years after its first publication, Jean-Nicholas Corvisart (1755–1821) (centre portrait) translates Auenbrugger's work into French and adds many new clinical observations of his own. This work instantly establishes percussion as an important diagnostic modality.

Joseph Skoda (1805–1881) improves the terminology and the sound classification system of the percussion technique, which makes the method easier to teach and to use in the clinics.

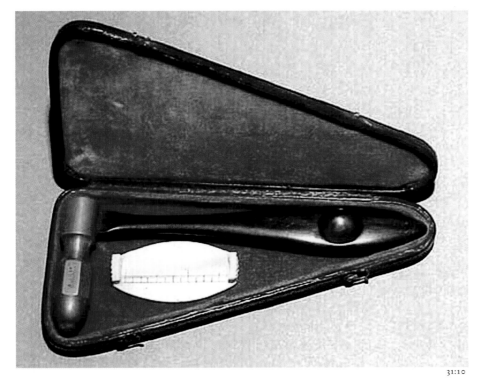

31:10

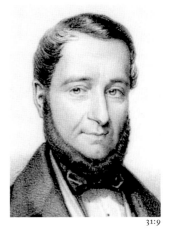

31:9

In 1826 Adolph Piorry (1794–1879) invents the percussor and the pleximeter. The pleximeter plate is placed against the chest and struck by the percussor.

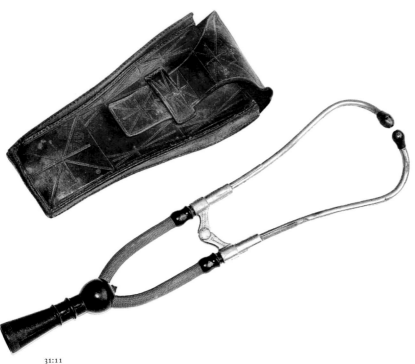

31:11

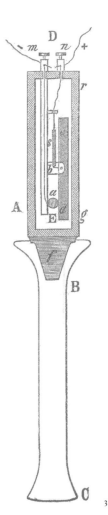

31:12

George Camman (1804–1863) constructs the first practical binaural stethoscope in around 1855. The device shown is from the 1870s.

With the development of telephone technology, sensitive microphones became available. In 1878 S. Stein connects such a microphone to a stethoscope. The image shows his "Sphygmophone", which allows electric registrations of the pulse and the heart sounds.

THÉORIE
DU MOUVEMENT DE LA CHALEUR
DANS LES CORPS SOLIDES (1),

PAR M. FOURIER.

Et ignem reguat numeri. (PLATO.)

I.

Exposition.

1. LES effets de la chaleur sont assujettis à des lois constantes que l'on ne peut découvrir sans le secours de l'analyse mathématique. L'objet de cet ouvrage est d'exposer les lois de l'équilibre et du mouvement de la chaleur, et d'en

(1) Ce Mémoire est la copie littérale de la pièce déposée aux archives de l'Institut le 28 septembre 1811, et qui a été couronnée dans la séance publique du 6 janvier 1812. *Il n'a été fait aucun changement au texte de cette pièce.* Elle contient tous les principes fondamentaux d'une nouvelle branche de la physique-mathématique : il était nécessaire d'exposer ces principes avant de publier les recherches entreprises depuis par l'auteur sur le même sujet.

1819.   24

32:1

DES MATIÈRES.   533

Numéro de l'article. | Numéro des pages.

21.

$$\frac{1}{4}\pi z = e^{-\frac{1}{2}\pi x}.\cos.\left(\frac{1}{2}\pi y\right) + \frac{1}{3}e^{-\frac{3}{2}\pi x}.\cos.\left(\frac{3}{2}\pi y\right)$$
$$+ \frac{1}{5}e^{-\frac{5}{2}\pi x}.\cos.\left(\frac{5}{2}\pi y\right) + \frac{1}{7}e^{-\frac{7}{2}\pi x}.\cos.\left(\frac{7}{2}\pi y\right) + \text{etc.}$$

281.   z est la température fixe du point de la barre dont les coordonnées sont x et y.

281.   Développement d'une fonction arbitraire φx en série de sinus d'arcs multiples.

Dans l'équation

$$\varphi x = a\sin.x + b\sin.2x + c\sin.3x + d\sin.4x + \text{etc.},$$

on détermine les coefficiens a, b, c, d, etc., en éliminant les inconnues dans un nombre infini d'équations du premier degré.

On obtient ainsi l'équation :

22.

$$\frac{1}{2}\pi\varphi x = \varphi\pi\left[\sin.x - \frac{1}{2}\sin.2x + \frac{1}{3}\sin.3x - \frac{1}{4}\sin.4x + \text{etc.}\right]$$
$$- \varphi''\pi\left[\frac{1}{1^2}\sin.x - \frac{1}{2^2}\sin.2x + \frac{1}{3^2}\sin.3x - \frac{1}{4^2}\sin.4x + \text{etc.}\right]$$
$$+ \varphi^{iv}\pi\left[\frac{1}{1^3}\sin.x - \frac{1}{2^3}\sin.2x + \frac{1}{3^3}\sin.3x - \frac{1}{4^3}\sin.4x + \text{etc.}\right]$$
$$- \varphi^{vi}\pi\left[\frac{1}{1^4}\sin.x - \frac{1}{2^4}\sin.2x + \frac{1}{3^4}\sin.3x - \frac{1}{4^4}\sin.4x + \text{etc.}\right]$$
$$+ \text{etc.}$$

Par exemple le développement de la fonction $e^x - e^{-x}$ donne la série :

299.

$$e^x - e^{-x} = \frac{e^\pi - e^{-\pi}}{\frac{1}{2}\pi}\left(\frac{\sin.x}{1+\frac{1}{1}} - \frac{\sin.2x}{2+\frac{1}{2}} + \frac{\sin.3x}{3+\frac{1}{3}} - \frac{\sin.4x}{4+\frac{1}{4}} + \text{etc.}\right)$$

299.   On peut donner à l'équation générale de l'article 22 la forme suivante :

23.

$$\frac{1}{2}\pi\varphi x = \sin.x\int(dx\varphi x\sin.x) + \sin.2x\int(dx\varphi x\sin.2x)$$
$$+ \sin.3x\int(dx\varphi x\sin.3x) + \text{etc.}$$

32:2

"The effects of heat are subject to immutable laws that cannot be discovered without recourse to mathematical analysis. The object of this work is to expound the laws of the equilibrium and movement of heat." With this declaration Jean Fourier (1768–1830) introduces a new mathematical technique of singular utility in science and medicine that is now named after him. The sine series expansion of a function shown below is taken from his publication from 1822 and demonstrates the application of his method.

Illustration of Fourier's experimental arrangement to study heat propagation across thin slabs (the object of study is to be placed at c-c in the figure).

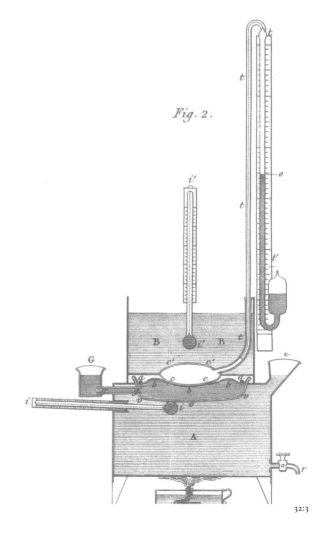

Fig. 2.

32:3

Jean Baptiste Fourier

FOURIER was born in 1768 in Auxerre, France. By the age of nine he had lost both his parents and he was sent to a military school, where his talent for mathematics was discovered. He played an active role during the French Revolution and was arrested during the Terror, barely escaping with his life. He was teaching mathematics at the École Polytechnique when in 1798 he was asked to join Napoleon's Egyptian campaign. Napoleon, recognising the outstanding diplomatic and administrative skills of Fourier, appointed him to several important posts. After Napoleon's fall Fourier, who was previously only a part-time scientist, devoted all his time to mathematics. In 1822 he became secretary of the Académie des Sciences and the following year a member of the Royal Society. He died in 1830 from a disease contracted during his stay in Egypt.

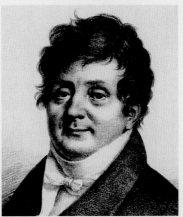

Jean Baptiste Fourier

Théorie Analytique de la Chaleur.

PARIS: F. DIDOT, PÈRE ET FILS; 1822.

FOURIER PRESENTS his analysis of how heat diffuses in bodies of different shapes and under various boundary conditions. As an example, combining great analytical skill and physical intuition, Fourier solves the problem of determining the temperature distribution in the semi-infinite strip that is uniformly hot at one end and uniformly cold along the sides. The mathematical techniques used to solve the partial differential equations involved imply that an algebraic function can be represented over a finite interval by trigonometric expansions.

IN PERSPECTIVE:

Fourier started to work on heat diffusion around 1807. In 1805 Gauss had already used trigonometric expansions for interpolation in orbital calculations (32.1) but as was often the case (32.2), his results remained unpublished for a long time (32.3). An early application of Fourier analysis to temporally varying functions were Ohm's theory of the galvanic element (32.4) and his work in acoustics (32.5). Spatial Fourier transform analysis applied to data from a Michelson interferometer led in the 1960s to the development of high resolution spectroscopy (32.6). Also, for decades structural determinations of complex molecules important in medicine have invariably relied on X-ray diffraction data analysed with spatial Fourier methods (32.7)(32.8). Because of the overwhelming computational burden posed by many of these applications, rapid progress would have been impossible without advances in computer technology (32.9) and new numerical methods, most notably the Fast Fourier Transform (FFT) algorithm (32.10). The FFT technique is also central in modern medical imaging such as MRI (32.11). Fourier said: "Profound study of nature is the most fertile source of mathematical discoveries". History shows that his mathematical discovery has been remarkably useful in the study of nature and in medicine.

32.1 Heideman MT, Johnson DH, Burrus CS. Gauss and the History of Fast Fourier Transform. *Arch Hist Exact Sci* 1985; 34:265.
32.2 See #30 Legendre page 166.
32.3 Gauss CF. Nachlass, Theoria Interpolationis Methodo Nova Tractata. In: *Carl Friedrich Gauss Werke* 3 Göttingen; 1866. p265.
32.4 Ohm GS. *Die galvanische Kette, mathematisch bearbeitet.* Berlin; 1827.
32.5 Ohm GS. Über die Definition des Tones ... *Ann Phys Chem* 1843; 59:513. See also ref. 13.9
32.6 Connes J. Reserches sur la spectroscopie par la transformation de Fourier. *Rev d'Optique Théor Exp* 1961; 40: 41 and p116,p171, p231 see also #49 Kirchhoff page 258.
32.7 See #76 Laue page 390 and #88 Watson-Crick page 456.
32.8 Booth AD. *Fourier technique in X-ray organic structure analysis.* Cambridge: Cambridge University Press; 1948.
32.9 See #85 Eckert-Mauchly page 438.
32.10 Cooley JW, Tukey JW: An algorithm for machine calculation of complex Fourier series. *Mathematical Computation* 1965; 19:297. See also ref. 32.1
32.11 See #96 Lauterbur page 498 and ref. 96.5.

An Algorithm for the Machine Calculation of Complex Fourier Series

By James W. Cooley and John W. Tukey

An efficient method for the calculation of the interactions of a 2^m factorial experiment was introduced by Yates and is widely known by his name. The generalization to 3^m was given by Box et al. [1]. Good [2] generalized these methods and gave elegant algorithms for which one class of applications is the calculation of Fourier series. In their full generality, Good's methods are applicable to certain problems in which one must multiply an N-vector by an $N \times N$ matrix which can be factored into m sparse matrices, where m is proportional to $\log N$. This results in a procedure requiring a number of operations proportional to $N \log N$ rather than N^2. These methods are applied here to the calculation of complex Fourier series. They are useful in situations where the number of data points is, or can be chosen to be, a highly composite number. The algorithm is here derived and presented in a rather different form. Attention is given to the choice of N. It is also shown how special advantage can be obtained in the use of a binary computer with $N = 2^m$ and how the entire calculation can be performed within the array of N data storage locations used for the given Fourier coefficients.

Consider the problem of calculating the complex Fourier series

$$(1) \qquad X(j) = \sum_{k=0}^{N-1} A(k) \cdot W^{jk}, \qquad j = 0, 1, \cdots, N-1,$$

where the given Fourier coefficients $A(k)$ are complex and W is the principal Nth root of unity,

$$(2) \qquad W = e^{2\pi i/N}.$$

A straightforward calculation using (1) would require N^2 operations where "operation" means, as it will throughout this note, a complex multiplication followed by a complex addition.

The algorithm described here iterates on the array of given complex Fourier amplitudes and yields the result in less than $2N \log_2 N$ operations without requiring more data storage than is required for the given array A. To derive the algorithm, suppose N is a composite, i.e., $N = r_1 \cdot r_2$. Then let the indices in (1) be expressed

$$(3) \qquad \begin{aligned} j &= j_1 r_1 + j_0, & j_0 &= 0, 1, \cdots, r_1 - 1, & j_1 &= 0, 1, \cdots, r_2 - 1, \\ k &= k_1 r_2 + k_0, & k_0 &= 0, 1, \cdots, r_2 - 1, & k_1 &= 0, 1, \cdots, r_1 - 1. \end{aligned}$$

Then, one can write

$$(4) \qquad X(j_1, j_0) = \sum_{k_0} \sum_{k_1} A(k_1, k_0) \cdot W^{jk_1 r_2} W^{jk_0}.$$

Received August 17, 1964. Research in part at Princeton University under the sponsorship of the Army Research Office (Durham). The authors wish to thank Richard Garwin for his essential role in communication and encouragement.

297

The introduction in 1965 of the Cooley-Tukey algorithm (known as the Fast Fourier Transform, FFT) greatly increases the speed of calculations and thereby the usefulness of the Fourier methods.

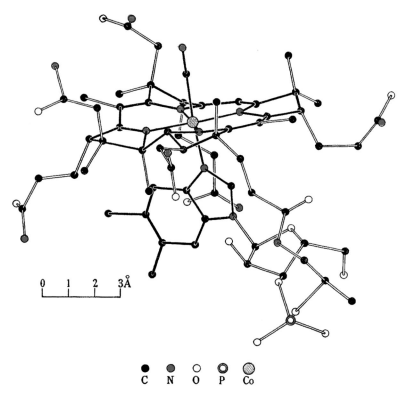

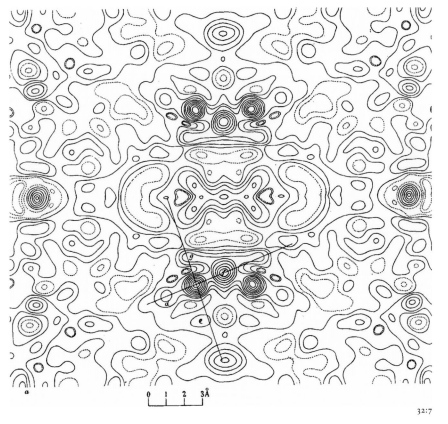

FIGURE 18. Atomic positions in the molecule of vitamin B_{12}. These are derived from the positions found in the air-dried crystals seen in projections on the b plane.

32:6

The atomic positions (left) and the chemical structure of vitamin B_{12} (below right).

The electron density map of air-dried vitamin B_{12} crystals, obtained in 1957 by Dorothy Hodgkin (1910–1994) using spatial Fourier analysis of X-ray diffraction data. This is one of the first of the complex molecular structures of importance in biology and medicine that is determined using Fourier techniques (see #76).

(III)

32:8

32:7

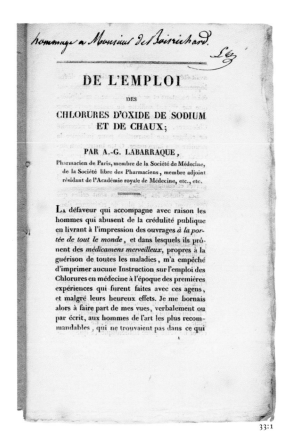

Antoine Labarraque (1777–1850) discovers the disinfecting effects of sodium hypochlorite.

In the introductions (left) he writes, " The disfavour that rightly accompanies those people who abuse the credulity of the public by furnishing the impression of works within the grasp of Everyman in which they extol marvellous medicaments fit to cure any disease prevented me from publishing a Monograph on the employment of chlorides in medicine at the time of the first experiments on these agents, despite their beneficial effects."

The beginning of the instructions of use published by the Parisian police authority is reproduced below and reads, "Repeated experiments have demonstrated that chloride of lime dissolved in water has the property of disinfecting the air and significantly slowing putrefaction."

(4)

PRÉFECTURE DE POLICE.

Paris, le 19 octobre 1825.

Nous, Conseiller d'État, Préfet de Police,
Vu le Rapport du Conseil de Salubrité, duquel il résulte que des expériences multipliées, faites successivement dans diverses localités et notamment à la Morgue, ont démontré l'efficacité de l'emploi du Chlorure de chaux comme moyen de désinfection d'après les procédés du sieur *Labarraque*, pharmacien à Paris, rue Saint-Martin, n°. 69 ,

Avons arrêté ce qui suit :

ARTICLE PREMIER.

Il sera établi des appareils désinfectans de l'invention du sieur *Labarraque*, à la Morgue et chez chacun des Commissaires de Police ci-après désignés, etc., etc.

(5)

INSTRUCTION sur la Manière de se servir du Chlorure de Chaux d'après le procédé indiqué par le sieur LABARRAQUE *, pharmacien.*

Des expériences réitérées ont démontré que le Chlorure de chaux étendu dans l'eau a la propriété de désinfecter l'air et de ralentir d'une manière sensible la putréfaction.

L'emploi de ce procédé peut devenir utile dans une foule de circonstances, on se bornera, dans la présente Instruction , à en faire l'application aux deux cas les plus fréquens.

Il sera facile , par analogie, de se servir du même procédé toutes les fois que l'on croira à propos d'y recourir.

Levée et Inspection d'un Cadavre.

Avant d'approcher d'un cadavre en putréfaction , il faudra se procurer un baquet, dans lequel on mettra une voie d'eau (24 litres), on versera dans cette eau un flacon (un demi-kilogramme) de Chlorure de chaux et l'on remuera bien le mélange.

LABARRAQUE was born in Oléron, France, in 1777. He studied at an apothecary in St-Jean-de-Luz and later in Montpellier for Chaptal, a professor of chemistry and also a prominent industrialist who owned and directed large chemical factories. Labarraque moved to Paris and working as a pharmacist, he proved that a sodium hypochlorite solution (eau de Labarraque) was an effective disinfectant. First used in slaughterhouses, in 1823 the Paris police officially adopted his method of disinfecting for handling corpses and latrines (33.1). The method was soon used in morgues, dissecting rooms and also in clinical work, where it was applied to hospital infections, gangrenes and ulcerations. In 1825 Labarraque was awarded the 3,000-franc prize of Baron Montyon by the Academy of Sciences. In later life Labarraque actively promoted public health issues. He died in Paris in 1850.

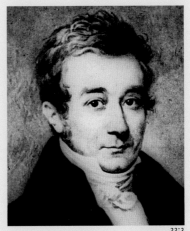

Antoine-Germain Labarraque 33:3

De l'emploi des chlorures d'oxide de sodium et de chaux.

PARIS: L'AUTEUR, HUZARD; 1825.

IN THE very beginning of this privately printed account of the uses of sodium hypochlorite solutions for disinfecting, Labarraque states that he did not publish his first successful medical experiences with chlorine solutions out of fear of being counted among charlatans with miracle cures. He then reprints the instructions for the Parisian Préfecture de Police on how to use the disinfectant and gives a number of examples of its use both in public health and in specific medical cases.

IN PERSPECTIVE:
Chlorine was discovered by Scheele in 1774 (33.2) and first used as a bleaching agent (potassium hypochlorite or Javelle water) by Berthollet and Chaptal (33.3). De Morveau found hydrochloric acid effective in removing the smell from rotting corpses and he designed an apparatus for disinfecting purposes which produced a "gradual discharge of oxygenated muratic acid gas" (chlorine) (33.4). Interestingly, just as Labarraque announced his discovery, Sérullas found another important disinfectant, iodoform (33.5). Semmelweis demonstrated the benefits of disinfectants for antisepsis, by ordering hand-wash with chlorinated lime (calcium oxide, calcium hydroxide complexes with chlorine) before examining patients in a maternity ward (33.6)(33.7). In a major advance Lister, prompted by Pasteur's discovery of airborne contagion (33.8), introduced carboxyl acid (phenol) into operative practice, thereby ushering in a new era in surgery (33.9). Hypochlorite solutions are strongly alkaline and thus irritant to the skin. In 1915 Dakin therefore introduced boric acid as a buffer (Dakin's solution) (33.10). Hypochlorite solutions remain the core of many modern disinfecting products and chlorine is still widely used for water treatment due to its high efficiency and ease of application.

33.1 Labarraque A-G. *Ordonance du préfet de police, en date du 19 octobre 1823, prescrivant l'emploi du chlorure de chaux* ... Paris; 1825.

33.2 See #21 Scheele page 120.

33.3 Partington JR. *The History of Chemistry*. Vol. III Mansfield Centre; 1999. p497, p557.

33.4 De Morveau G. *Traité des moyens de désinfecter l'air, de prévenir la contagion, et d'en arrêter les progrès*. Paris; 1805.

33.5 Sérullas GS. Mémoire sur l'iodure de potassium l'acid hydriodique et sur un composé nouveau de carbone, d'iode et d'hydrogène. *Ann Chim Phys* 2 sér. 1822; 20:163.

33.6 Skoda J. Ueber die von Dr Semmelweis entdeckte wahre Ursache ... *Sitz. d. kaiserl. Akad. Wiss. math. nat* 1849; 8:168.

33.7 Semmelweis IP. *Die Aetiologie, der Begriff und die Profylaxis des Kindbettfiebers*. Pest; 1861.

33.8 See #50 Pasteur page 264.

33.9 See #54 Lister and also ref. 73.4 on phenol.

33.10 Dakin HD. On the use of certain antiseptic substances in the treatment of infected wounds. *Br Med J* 1915; 2:318.

33:4

In the first years of the 19th century Louis Guyton de Morveau (1737–1816) discovers that hydrochloric acid is effective in removing smell from rotting corpses. He designs apparatus, both stationary and portable, that produce a "gradual discharge of oxygenated muratic acid" (chlorine).

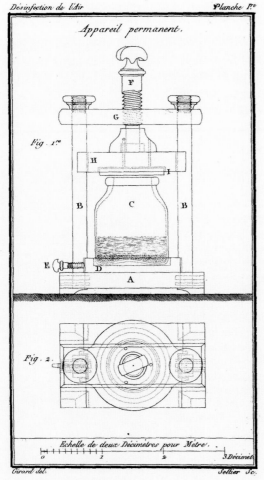

33:5

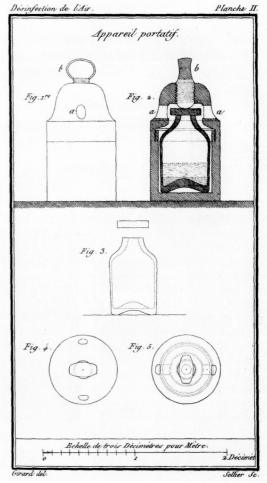

33:6

In 1847 Ignaz Semmelweis (1818–1865) introduces disinfectants for antisepsis by ordering hand-wash with chlorinated lime for the doctors and nurses of a maternity clinic in Vienna. The result is a dramatic drop in patient mortality, as demonstrated by the last column of the table from his book, first published in 1861.

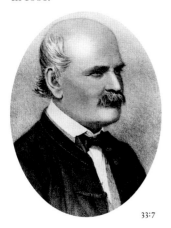

33:7

Jahr	Gebärende	Todte	Percent-Antheil	Gebärende	Todte	Percent-Antheil
1829	2141	34	$1._{59}$	3012	140	$4._{64}$
1830	2288	12	$0._{52}$	2797	111	$3._{97}$
1831	2176	12	$0._{55}$	3353	222	$6._{62}$
1832	2242	12	$0._{53}$	3331	105	$3._{15}$
				Trennung des Gebärhauses in zwei Abtheilungen.		
				I. Abtheilung: Klinik für Schüler und Schülerinnen.		
1833	2138	12	$0._{57}$	3737	197	$5._{29}$
1834	2024	34	$1._{67}$	2657	205	$7._{71}$
1835	1902	34	$1._{78}$	2573	143	$5._{55}$
1836	1810	36	$1._{98}$	2677	200	$7._{47}$
1837	1833	24	$1._{30}$	2765	251	$9._{09}$
1838	2126	45	$2._{11}$	2987	91	$3._{04}$
1839	1951	25	$1._{23}$	2781	151	$5._{04}$
1840	1521	26	$1._{70}$	2889	267	$9._{05}$
				I. Abtheilung: Klinik für Aerzte.		
1841	2003	23	$1._{14}$	3036	237	$7._{07}$
1842	2171	21	$0._{96}$	3287	518	$15._{08}$
1843	2210	22	$0._{99}$	3060	274	$8._{09}$
1844	2288	14	$0._{61}$	3157	260	$8._{02}$
1845	1411	35	$2._{48}$	3492	241	$6._{08}$
1846	2025	17	$0._{83}$	4010	459	$11._{04}$
				Einführung der Chlorwaschungen im Mai 1847 an der Abtheilung für Aerzte.		
1847	1703	47	$2._{75}$	3490	176	$5._{00}$
1848	1816	35	$1._{92}$	3556	45	$1._{27}$
1849	2063	38	$1._{84}$	3858	103	$2._{06}$
In 66 Jahren	141903	1758	$1._{21}$	153841	6224	$4._{04}$

33:8

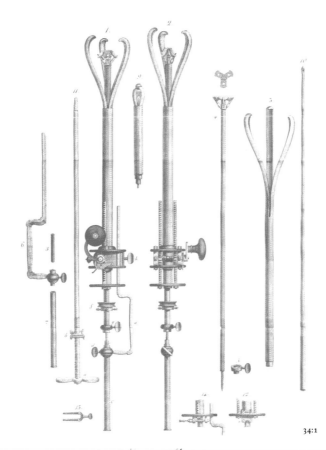

Jean Civiale (1792–1867) improves the technique of lithotrity. He invents instruments that can be introduced into the bladder trans-urethally (as shown below) to drill into and then crush the stone. In this way, the painful lithotomy operations can be avoided.

34:1

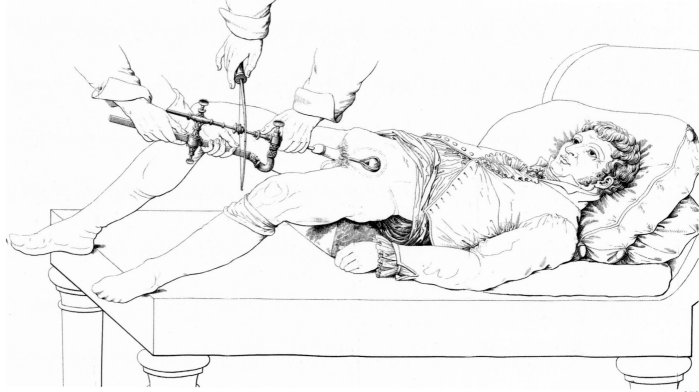

34:2

CIVIALE was born in Thiézac, France, in 1792 to peasant parents. He studied medicine in Paris from 1817 under the direction of Dupuytren, famed professor of clinical surgery at the Ecole de Médecine. After a short spell as a physician in Brioude, he returned to Paris to devote the rest of his carrier to urology and specially to find improved techniques for the removal of bladder stones (lithotrity) without having to resort to a painful operation (lithotomy). His first success in a clinical case in 1824 started a bitter controversy about the priority to the procedure (34.1). Civiale was a poor lecturer but an excellent writer. He wrote extensively on topics in urology and founded his own department specialising in lithotrity at the Necker Hospital. He performed more than 3,000 procedures and amassed a considerable fortune. On his death in 1867 he left a significant part of it to his department.

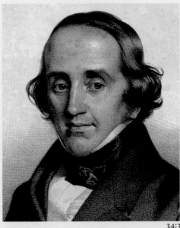

Jean Civiale   34:3

De la Lithotritie, ou broiement de la pierre dans la vessie.

PARIS: BÉCHET JEUNE; 1827.

THIS WORK is an extension of a shorter communication published by Civiale the year before. Here Civiale describes his technique of lithotrity and presents arguments to defend his theories and method against its critics. At the end of the book Civiale includes a report to the l'Académie Royale des Sciences summarising an independent investigation of Civiale's claim of priority to lithotrity.

IN PERSPECTIVE:
Celsus wrote on lithotomy (about 30 AD) and the Arabic surgeons Al Razi (about 900 AD) and Albucasis (about 1000 AD) can be considered as originators of the field of lithotrity, since they developed special instruments and a drilling technique for crushing the stone (34.2)(34.3). Paré devoted ten chapters in his work (34.4) to the removal of kidney stones, but significant improvements in instrumentation and procedures came only in the early 19th century through the work of Civiale and his detractor Leroy d'Etoilles (34.5). Later Bigelow (34.6) introduced lithotripsy (litholapaxy), the crushing of the stone, followed at once by the washing out of the fragments. Early studies in the generation (34.7) and effects of acoustic shock waves led to the first laboratory, non-contact destruction of a kidney stone (34.8). Soon in vivo research followed (34.9) and culminated in the first clinical use of extracorporeal shock wave therapy (ESWT) in man in 1980 (34.10). Concerns about the safety of this technique have recently led to studies suggesting that shock waves could also be useful as a therapeutic modality in orthopaedic disease (34.11).

34.1 von Kern V. Bemerkung über die neue, von Civiale und le Roy verübte Methode, die Steine in der Harnblase zu zermalen und auszuziehen. Wien; 1826. See also the landmark publication of Civiale cited below.

34.2 Spink MS, Lewis IL. *Albucasis on surgery and instruments*. London: Wellcome Institute of the History of Medicine; 1973. See also ref. 29.2.

34.3 Ellis H. *A History of Bladders Stone*. London: Blackwell Scientific Publications; 1969.

34.4 See #2 Paré page 26 also The Collected Works of Ambroise Paré. Lib. 17 chapt. 34–44 Transl. T. Johnson London; 1634.

34.5 Leroy d'Etoilles JJ. *Histoire de la lithotritie, précédée de réflexions sur la dissolution des calculs urinaires*. Paris; 1839.

34.6 Bigelow HJ. Lithotrity by a single operation. *Am J med Sci* 1878; 75:117.

34.7 Eisenmenger W. Eine elektromagnetische Impulsschallquelle zur Erzeugung von Druckstössen in Flussigkeiten und Festkörpern. In: *Proc. 3-rd Int. Congr. Acoustics*; 1961 Amsterdam: Elsevier; 1962. p326.

34.8 Haeusler E, Kiefer W. Anregung von stosswellen in flussigkeiten durch hochgeschwindigkeitswassertropfen. *Verh D Physikal Gesell* 1971; 6:786.

34.9 Chaussy C, et al. The use of chock waves for the destruction of renal calculi without direct contact. *Urol Res* 1976; 4:175.

34.10 Chaussy C, Brendel W, Schmiedt E. Extracorporeally induced destruction of kidney stones by shock waves. *Lancet* 1980; 2:1265.

34.11 Haupt G. Use of extracorporeal shock waves in the treatment of pseudarthrosis, tendopathy and other orthopedic diseases. *J. Urol.* 1997; 4:158.

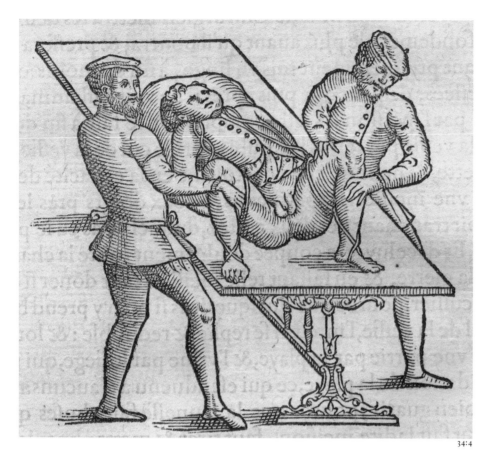

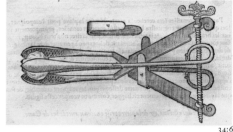

Preparation for the removal of kidney stones and a device for crushing the stone, as described by Ambroise Paré in 1575. (see #2)

34:4

34:6

Henry Bigelow (1818–1890) invents an instrument that, after crushing the stone, also flushes it out. The picture shows his lithotrite and evacuator for litholapaxy from c. 1880.

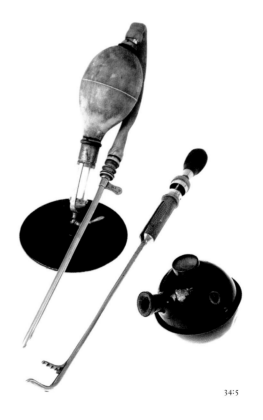

34:5

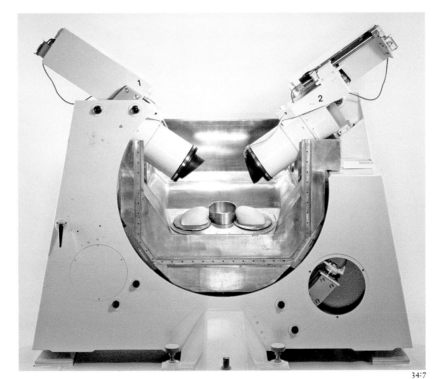

The first device, the "Nierenlithotripter HM1" built in 1982 for extracorporeal shock wave therapy. The technique of crushing stones with focused acoustic waves is introduced in 1976 by Christian Chaussy and collaborators.

A modern lithotripter using electrohydraulic shock wave technology.

34:7

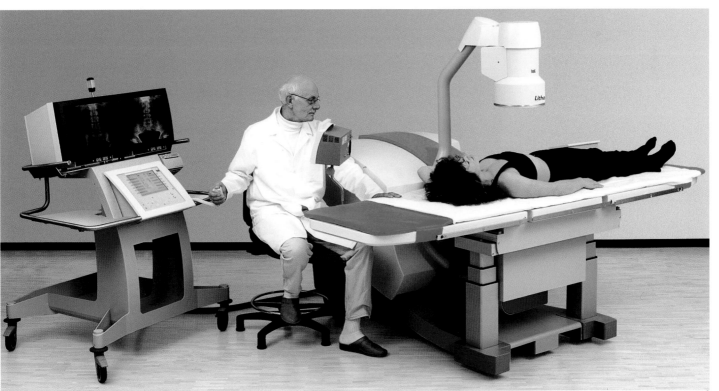

34:8

Jean Léonard Poiseuille's (1797–1869) doctoral thesis from 1828. He invents the "hémo-dynamometer", which introduces the use of mercury in a manometer. He studies the variation of blood pressure with breathing and the distension of the arteries due to the pulse.

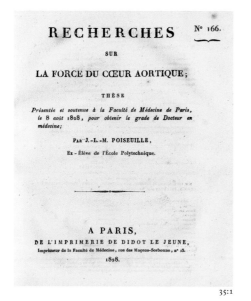

35:1

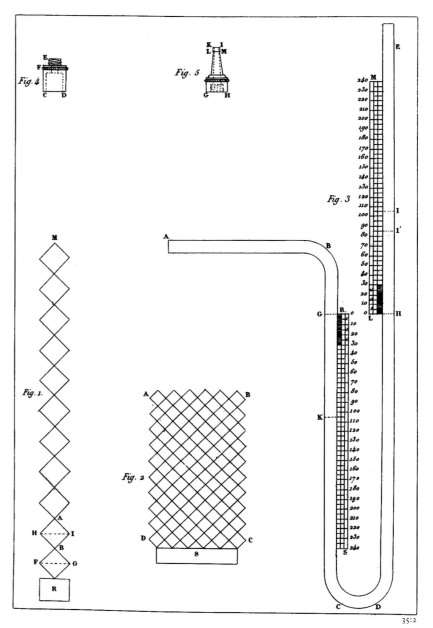

35:2

POISEUILLE was born in Paris in 1797, the son of a carpenter. He studied at the École Polytechnique and received his degree as doctor of medicine in 1828 by presenting the thesis cited below. His research in physiology won him the Montyon medal (35.1) four times and in 1842 also membership of the Académie de Médecine. He wrote a number of reports for the Académie on physiological topics and was also one of the editors of the "Dictionnaire de médecine usuelle" from 1849. In 1860 Poiseuille was appointed inspector of the primary schools in Paris. He died in his native city in 1869.

Recherches sur la force du coeur aortique.

THÈSE. PARIS: DIDOT JEUNE; 1828.

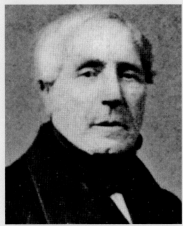

Jean Léonard Poiseuille

35:3

AFTER A short historic introduction of previous work on the pumping effect of the heart, citing the work of Borelli (35.2), Kreill (35.3) and Hales (35.4), Poiseuille describes his device (hemodynamometer) and method for measuring blood pressure. He introduces the use of a mercury manometer and employs potassium carbonate to prevent coagulation of the blood. Poiseuille finds that the blood pressure rises and falls with expiration and inspiration and he is also able to measure the distension of the artery due to the arterial pulse.

IN PERSPECTIVE:
Poiseuille's work represents a major advance in blood pressure measurement. A further improvement was made in 1847 by Ludwig, who attached a float to the surface of the mercury and arranged this to write on a drum at constant rotation (35.5). The first recording showing the respiratory effects on arterial pulsation were made this way. The slow response of this system was recognised as a problem by Vierordt who, using Weber's wave analysis of the blood flow in the arteries (35.6), conceived the first sphygmograph in 1855 (35.7). This delicate device worked by exerting a direct mechanical counter-pressure on the artery. Vierordt's concept was soon developed by Marey (35.8) into a device that was compact enough to be attached to the forearm for clinical use. Poiseuille's thesis work cited above led him also to investigations of fluid flow in the capillaries. He determined the influence of temperature on the flow of various liquids with an accuracy of about 0.5% within modern values. Together with Hagen (35.9), Poiseuille established the dependence of the flow on the driving pressure, the diameter and the length of the tube and on the viscosity of the fluid (35.10). This relation, which is named after him, is fundamental in all hydrodynamic considerations of the circulatory system.

35.1 See #33 Labarraque page 180.
35.2 See #12 Borelli page 76.
35.3 Kreill J(ames). *Tentamina medico-physica, ad quasdam quastiones,quae oeconomiam animalem spectant, accommodata.* London; 1718.
35.4 See #17 Hales page 100.
35.5 Ludwig C. Beiträge zur Kentniss des Einflusses der Respirationsbewegung auf den Blutlauf im Aortensysteme. *Arch Anat Phys wiss Med.* 1847. p242.
35.6 See #44 Weber page 232.
35.7 See ref. 17.9.
35.8 See #52 Marey page 272.
35.9 Hagen GH. Ueber die Bewegung des Wassers in engen cylindrischen Rohren. *Ann Phys Chem* 1839; 46:423.
35.10 Poiseuille JL. Recherches expérimentales sur le mouvement des liquides dans les tubes de très-petits diamètres. *C R Acad Sci* 1840; 11:961, p1041, p1841 and *C R Acad Sci* 1841; 12:112.

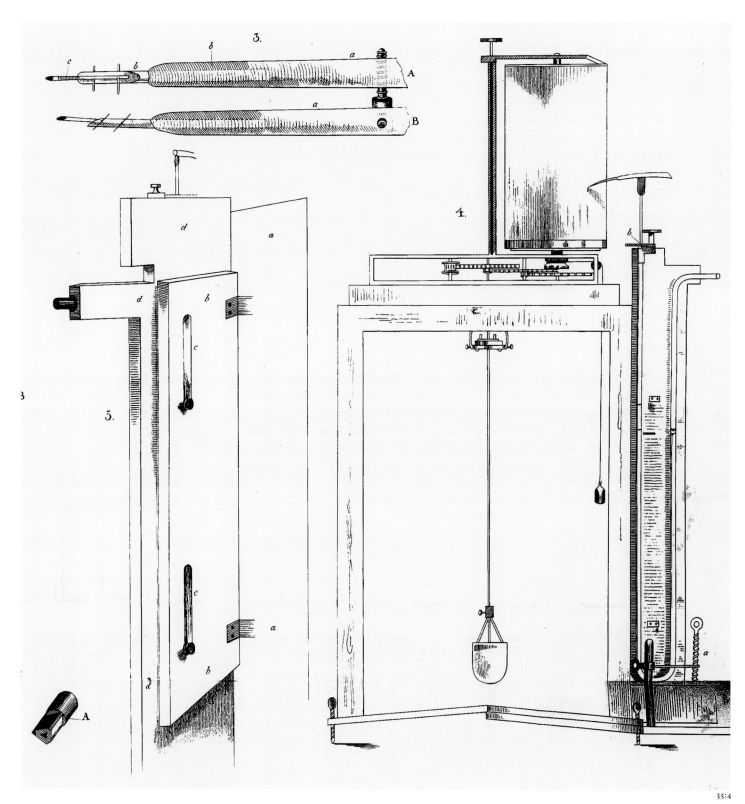

In 1847 Carl Ludwig (1816–1895) places a float on the surface of
the mercury manometer and arranges a stylus to write on a drum
at constant rotation. In this way he makes the first registrations of
the effect of breathing on blood pressure.

35:4

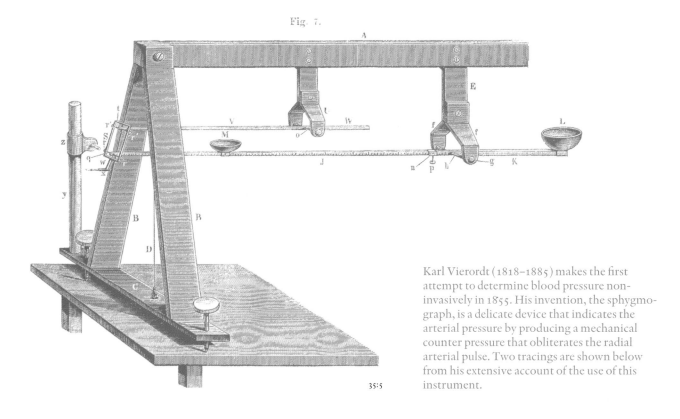

Fig. 7.

35:5

Karl Vierordt (1818–1885) makes the first attempt to determine blood pressure non-invasively in 1855. His invention, the sphygmograph, is a delicate device that indicates the arterial pressure by producing a mechanical counter pressure that obliterates the radial arterial pulse. Two tracings are shown below from his extensive account of the use of this instrument.

Fig. 32. (XXII 2 a. Fr. 77.) Gangräna pulmonum.

Tafel A.

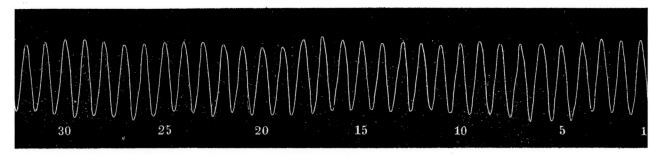

Fig. 34. (XXIV 1. a. Fr. 99.) Morbus cordis.

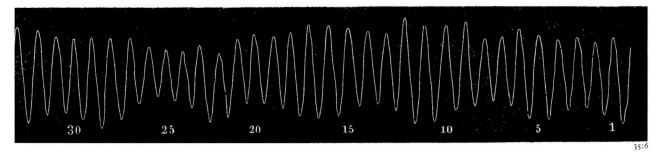

35:6

RECHERCHES

DE

CHIMIE ORGANIQUE,

RELATIVES

A L'ACTION DU CHLORE SUR L'ALCOOL.

LOI DES SUBSTITUTIONS OU MÉTALEPSIE.

Par M. J. DUMAS.

Lu à l'Académie des Sciences, le 13 janvier 1835.

Dans un mémoire que j'ai eu l'honneur de communiquer récemment à l'Académie, je suis revenu, ainsi que je l'avais annoncé, sur la question des éthers, et j'ai ajouté quelques arguments à ceux qui nous avaient déterminés autrefois à publier sur ces corps une théorie qui a soulevé tant de discussions, qu'on peut s'étonner qu'elle ait pu résister à des attaques si vives et si répétées.

Je craindrais d'abuser des moments de l'Académie, en lui retraçant l'histoire de ce point de la science, avec les détails circonstanciés qui seraient nécessaires pour rendre à chacun ce qui lui appartient. Je me bornerai donc à préciser ici les idées qui ont apparu successivement.

pyro-acétique. La préparation s'exécute comme avec l'alcool ; mais, ainsi que l'observe M. Liebig, on en obtient bien davantage.

Le produit purifié par l'acide sulfurique, comme dans le cas précédent, a été soumis ensuite à l'analyse.

0,699 matière ont fourni 0,260 d'acide carbonique, et 0,061 d'eau. Ces résultats donnent en centièmes :

Carbone 10,29
Hydrogène 0,97
Chlore 88,74
$$\overline{100,00}$$

Tous ces résultats s'accordent entre eux, et s'accordent fort bien aussi avec les résultats calculés d'après la formule $C^4 H Ch^3$; celle-ci donnerait en effet :

C^4 76,52   10,24
H 6,25   0,83
Ch^3 663,96   88,93
$$\overline{746,73 \qquad 100,00}$$

Ces résultats s'accordent également bien avec ceux qui seraient tirés de la même formule, relativement à la densité de la vapeur. On a, en effet,

C^4 . . . . . . $= 0,8432$
H . . . . . . $= 0,0688$
Ch^3 . . . . $= 7,3150$
$$\frac{8,2270}{2} = 4,113.$$

A new way of looking at chemical reactions is proposed by Jean Baptiste Dumas (1800–1884) in 1835. His substitution theory and careful measurements allow him to determine the correct formulas for many new organic substances, including (as is shown above) that of chloroform $CHCl_3$.

DUMAS was born in Alais, France, in 1800. As a teenager he wanted to join the Navy, but he soon turned to science and was apprenticed to an apothecary. In 1816 he left for studies in Geneva. On the recommendation of Humboldt (36.1), who noted his talent, he went to Paris in 1823 to set up a small chemical laboratory and to lecture at the École Polytechnique. In 1832 he was elected a member of the Academy of Sciences, becoming its permanent secretary in 1868. Dumas was a brilliant teacher and as professor of organic chemistry at the École de Médecine and at the Sorbonne he trained a generation of distinguished French chemists. He had a mild, generous personality, always looking for a compromise to resolve problems. After the Revolution in 1848 he became politically active and as president of the Paris Municipal Council he oversaw the transformation and modernisation of the city.

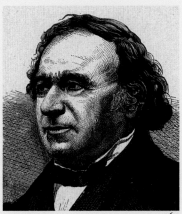

Jean Baptiste Dumas   36:3

Recherches de chimie organique relative à l'action du chlore sur l'alcool. Loi des substitutions ou métalepsie.

LU À L'ACADÉMIE DES SCIENCES 1835. PARIS: F. DIDOT; 1835.

HERE DUMAS introduces a new way of looking at organic chemical reactions. His substitution or exchange (métalepsie) theory sets up rules for how hydrogen is replaced in reactions by an equivalent number of moles of another substance such as a halogen. Using this concept, Dumas is able to determine the proper composition of the newly discovered substances and gives them the now accepted names chloroform, bromoform and iodoform (36.2).

IN PERSPECTIVE:
The disagreements and animosities between the three leading chemists of the 1830s, Dumas, Liebig (36.3) and Berzelius arose not only from different scientific viewpoints but also from different personalities and to some extent due to nationalistic feelings (36.4). Dumas' theory of substitution initiated the downfall of the established dualistic (electronegative or acid versus electropositive or alkaline) chemical system of Berzelius (36.5). In 1831, within a few months, a substance later called chloroform by Dumas was independently discovered by Guthrie (36.6), Soubeiran (36.7) and Liebig (36.8). In 1847 Flourens demonstrated in animal studies that chloroform and ether had similar anaesthetic effects (36.9). At the same time in Edinburgh, Simpson with the help of Waldie, a chemist, was looking for anaesthetics for use in midwifery that did not have the unpleasant smell of ether, an agent that had just been introduced with great success for surgical anaesthesia (36.10). At the first clinical use of chloroform, Simpson reports that Dumas happened to be present and "was, in no small degree, rejoiced to witness the wonderful physiological effects of a substance with whose chemical history his own name was so intimately connected" (36.11).

36.1 See ref. 19.9 for an important work of Alexander von Humboldt.
36.2 See ref. 33.5 and ref. 36.6–36.8.
36.3 See #39 Liebig page 208.
36.4 Partington JR. *A History of Chemistry*. Vol. III Chapter. XI Mansfield Centre: Martino fine books; 1999.
36.5 Berzelius JJ. *Lärobok i kemien*. Vol. 1–6 Stockholm; 1812–1830.
36.6 Guthrie S. New mode of preparing a spirituous solution of Chloric Ether. *Am J Sci and Arts* 1832; 21:64 and p405 and On pure Chloric Ether. *Am J Sci and Arts* 1832; 22:105.
36.7 Soubeiran E. Recherches sur quelques Combinaisons du Chlore. *Ann Chim Phys* 1831; 48:113.
36.8 Liebig J. Ueber die Verbindungen welche durch die Einwirkung des chlors auf Alkohol, Aether, ölbildendes Gas und Essiggeist entstehen. *Ann der Pharm* 1832; 1:182.
36.9 Flourens P. Chloro-forme. *Arch Gen de Med* 4 ser. 1847; 13:549.
36.10 See #47 Snow page 248.
36.11 Simpson JY. Account of a New Anaesthetic Agent as substitute for sulphuric Ether in Surgery and Midwifery. *Comm Medico-Chirurgical Soc Edin*. Edinburgh; 1847. 10th November.

Recherches *sur quelques Combinaisons du Chlore,*

Par M. E. Soubeiran.

(Communiqué par l'auteur.)

Des nombreuses combinaisons entre le chlore et l'oxigène que la théorie chimique fait prévoir, les suivantes sont seules connues :

Protoxide de chlore.	2 vol. chlore	+1 vol. oxigène.
Deutoxide de chlore.	1 vol.	+2 vol.
Acide chlorique....	2 vol.	+5 vol.
Acide oxichlorique..	2 vol.	+7 vol.

36:4

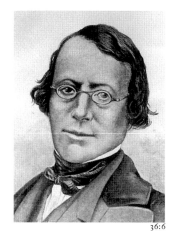

36:6

In 1831 Eugène Soubeiran (1793–1858) prepares chloroform, a substance he calls incorrectly "éther bichlorique".

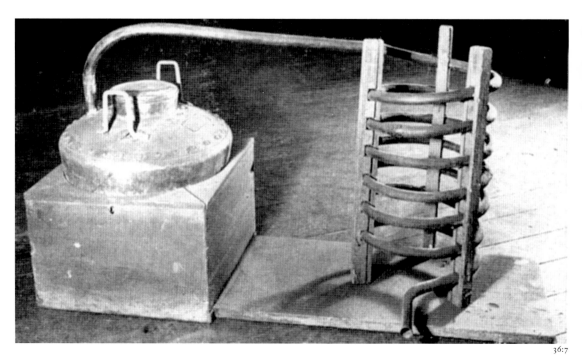

36:7

Art. VI.—*New mode of preparing a spirituous solution of Chloric Ether;* by Samuel Guthrie, *of Sackett's Harbor, N.Y.*

Mr. Editor—As the usual process for obtaining chloric ether for solution in alcohol is both troublesome and expensive, and as from its lively and invigorating effects it may become an article of some value in the *Materia Medica*, I have thought a portion of your readers might be gratified with the communication of a cheap and easy process for preparing it. I have therefore given one below, combining these advantages with unerring certainty in the result.

At the same time as Soubeiran, Samuel Guthrie (1782–1848) also prepares chloroform, but from whiskey (he had no alcohol) and chlorinated lime. He uses the equipment shown above and calls the new compound chloric ether or sweet whiskey.

36:5

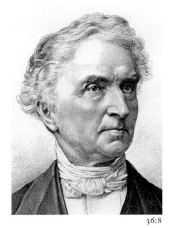

36:8

Justus von Liebig (1803–1873), independently of Soubeiran and Guthrie, synthesises chloroform, also in 1831. He calls the substance chloral.

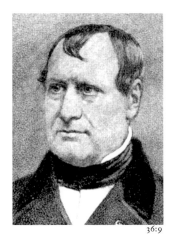

36:9

Marie Flourens, (1794–1867) discovers the anaesthetic effects of chloroform. This is communicated in a very short note in April 1847 (right) saying, "Monsieur Flourens has tried a new substance going by the name of chloro-form. After some minutes, an animal subjected to its vapours is completely anaesthetised. These phenomena have proven to be the same as in anaesthesia with sulphuric or hydrochloric ether."

Ueber die Verbindungen, welche durch die Einwirkung des Chlors auf Alkohol, Aether, ölbildendes Gas und Essiggeist entstehen;

von

Justus Liebig.

Die Bildung und Zusammensetzung des ölartigen Körpers, welcher durch die Einwirkung des Chlors auf Alkohol entsteht, hat neuerdings die Aufmerksamkeit mehrerer Chemiker beschäftigt.

36:10

M. Flourens a essayé un corps nouveau connu sous le nom de *chloro-forme*. Après quelques minutes, l'animal soumis à l'inhalation de ces vapeurs a été tout à fait éthérisé. Les phénomènes ont été les mêmes que dans l'éthérisation par l'éther sulfurique ou chlorhydrique.

36:11

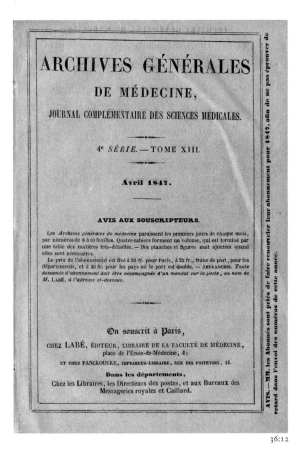

36:12

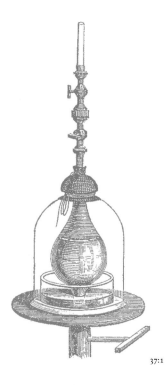

37:1

Gustav Magnus (1802–1870) reports the first quantitative determination of blood gases. He injects blood samples of horses into a mercury funnel and extracts the blood gases by repeatedly applying negative pressure using the equipment shown left. As appears from his table below, he finds the arterio-venous difference to be positive for oxygen and negative for carbon dioxide. He calculates the carbon dioxide balance over the lungs assuming a value for the cardiac output and so uses (in reverse), for the first time, what later became known as Fick's principle (see #56).

	Cubikcentimeter.		
Blut von ein. Pferde	125 gaben 9,8 Luft	{	5,4 Kohlensäur. 1,9 Sauerstoff 2,5 Stickstoff
Venöses Blut von demselben Pferde, am 4. Tage, nach der Entziehung des arteriellen aufgefangen	205 - 12,2 -	{	8,8 Kohlensäur. 2,3 Sauerstoff 1,1 Stickstoff
Dasselbe Blut	195 - 14,2 -	{	10,0 Kohlensäur. 2,5 Sauerstoff 1,7 Stickstoff
Arterielles Blut von einem sehr alten, aber gesund. Pferde	130 - 16,3 -	{	10,7 Kohlensäur. 4,1 Sauerstoff 1,5 Stickstoff
Dasselbe Blut	122 - 10,2 -	{	7 Kohlensäur. 2,2 Sauerstoff 1 Stickstoff
Venöses Blut von demselben alten Pferde nach 3 Tagen aufgefangen	170 - 18,9 -	{	12,4 Kohlensäur. 2,5 Sauerstoff 4,0 Stickstoff
Arterielles Blut v. einem Kalbe	123 - 14,5 -	{	9,4 Kohlensäur. 3,5 Sauerstoff 1,6 Stickstoff

37:2

MAGNUS was born in Berlin in 1802, the son of a wealthy merchant. After private studies in mathematics and natural sciences, he received his doctorate at the University of Berlin in 1827. He then spent a year in Stockholm working in the laboratory of Berzelius, who became his lifelong friend and mentor. Magnus returned to Berlin as a lecturer in chemistry and technology. He was appointed professor of technology and physics at the University of Berlin in 1845, a post he held the rest of his life. His main research interest initially lay in the field of chemistry, but later his attention turned increasingly to problems in physics, where he conducted significant experimental work in many areas.

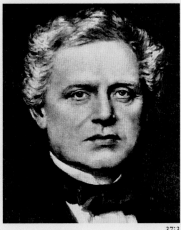

Gustav Magnus   37:3

Ueber die im Blute enthaltenen Gase, Sauerstoff, Stickstoff und Kohlensäure.

ANNALEN DER PHYSIK UND CHEMIE. LEIPZIG: 1837; 40:583.

IN THIS paper Magnus determines the oxygen, nitrogen and carbon dioxide content of the arterial and venous blood of horses. He introduces blood into mercury in a funnel and, by repeatedly applying negative pressure, he liberates the gases from the blood. The mercury seal maintains the anaerobic conditions when transferring the gases to a eudiometer (37.1) for analysis. Magnus finds a positive arterio-venous difference for oxygen and a negative difference for carbon dioxide. From this he concludes that carbon dioxide is added not in the lungs but during circulation. He also calculates the balance of carbon dioxide, assuming values for the cardiac output and carbon dioxide elimination and the measured arterio-venous difference. This is the first use of what later came to be called Fick's principle (37.2).

IN PERSPECTIVE:
Boyle showed back in 1662 that significant amounts of gas could be liberated from blood using an air pump and Davy had observed that blood contains both oxygen and carbon dioxide (37.3). Magnus' work led to a long controversy regarding whether combustion took place during circulation as argued by Magnus and Pfluger (37.4) or at least partially in the lungs as argued by Ludwig (37.5). The matter was settled by a series of papers by Marie and August Krogh in 1910, showing that no other process than diffusion took place in the lungs (37.6)(37.7). The specific oxygen binding capacity of blood was discovered by Meyer in 1857 and soon after haemoglobin was isolated and studied by Hoppe-Seyler (37.8). At the beginning of the 20th century Barcroft and Haldane improved the methods of blood gas analysis (37.9)(37.10). The clinical importance of measuring blood gases during the 1950s polio epidemics motivated the subsequent development of modern blood gas electrode technology (37.11).

37.1   See #22 Priestly page 124 and ref. 22.6.
37.2   See #56 Fick page 290.
37.3   See ref. 8.6 and #28 Davy page 156.
37.4   Pfluger E. Zur Gasometrie des Blutes. *Zbl Med Wiss* 1866; 4(20):305.
37.5   Ludwig C. Zusammenstellung der Untersuchungen über Blutgase. *Z k k Ges Ärtzte in Wien* 1865; 1:145.
37.6   Krogh A. On the mechanism of the Gas-Exchange in the Lungs. *Skand Arch Physiol* 1910; 23:248.
37.7   Krogh A, Krogh M. On the tension of gases in the arterial blood. *Skand Arch Physiol* 1910; 23:179.
37.8   Meyer L. *Die Gase der blutes*. Inaugural-dissertation Medicinische Fakultät Würzburg. Göttingen; 1857. See also #51 Hoppe-Seyler page 268.
37.9   Barcroft J. *The respiratory function of the blood*. Cambridge; 1913.
37.10 Haldane JS. *Methods of Air Analysis. 2nd ed.* London; 1918. See also ref. 81.5.
37.11 Severinghaus JW, Astrup P, Murray JF. Blood Gas Analysis and Critical Care Medicine. *Am J Respir Crit Care Med* 1998; 157:S114. See also ref. 14.8 and #87 Engström page 450.

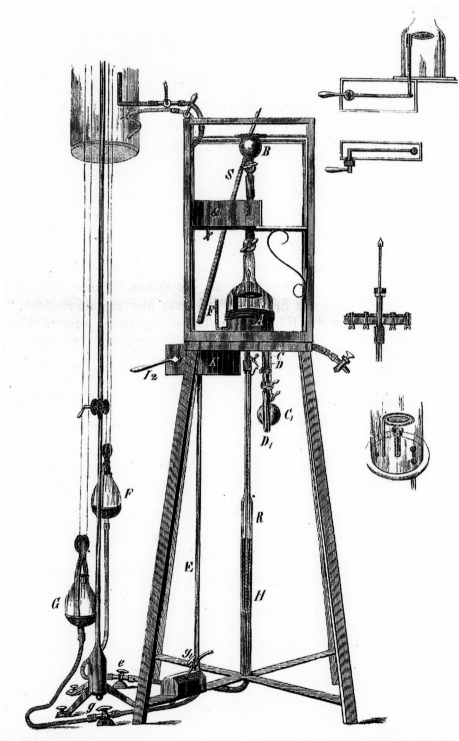

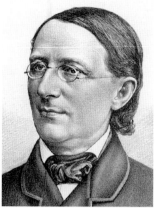

37:5

Carl Ludwig (1816–1895) and
his improved blood gas apparatus. Ludwig argues, in opposition to Magnus, that at least
some of the combustion of oxygen takes place in the lungs.

He is eventually proven
wrong in 1910 by the research
of August Krogh (1874–1949).

37:4

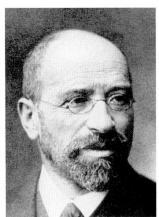

37:6

Nathan Zuntz (1847–1920) constructs an ingenious apparatus (right) with which he can sample simultaneously the arterial and venous blood of horses. The skill of his experimental work allowed him to obtain accurate cardiac output values that have stood the test of time.

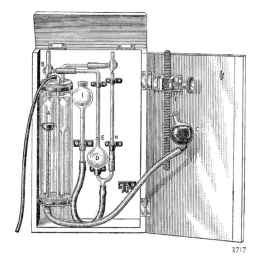

37:7

In 1898 John Haldane (1860–1936) introduces improved techniques and equipment for gas analysis that make it possible to measure oxygen and carbon dioxide concentrations down to 0.005%. His methods remain a cornerstone of respiratory gas analysis for almost half a century.

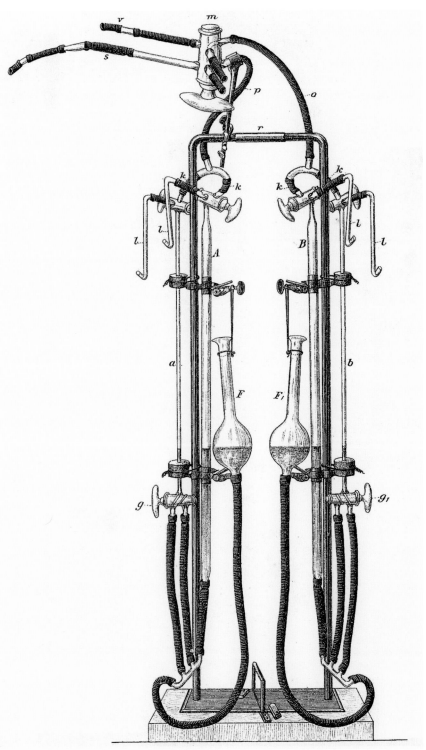

37:8

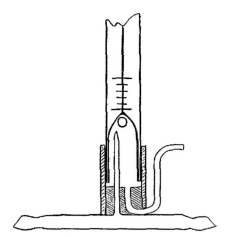

Fig. 1. Micro-tonometer, to be inserted into a blood-vessel of an animal.

37:9

Krogh's micro-tonometer (above) is used to make accurate blood gas determinations in vivo, without the need to extract blood samples.

August and Marie Krogh (1874–1943) study the simultaneous variation of the alveolar carbon dioxide and oxygen tension with time. Their results conclusively show that diffusion alone can adequately explain the gas exchange process in the lung.

Tonometric experiments.

No.	Time	Total tension mm	Gases in tonometer CO$_2$ %	O$_2$ %	
1	2·30—2·55	− 10	4·1	15·3	Determinations of total tension not very reliable
2	2·55—3·20	− 10	4·5	14·5	
3	3·25—3·45	− 10	3·9	14·9	
4	3·50—4·17	− 15	3·4	15·9	
5	4·22—4·57	− 30	3·4	15·4	

Tensions calculated.

Time	Tension of CO$_2$ in Bifurcation	Alveoli	Blood	Tension of O$_2$ in Bifurcation	Alveoli	Blood	
2·49	—	3·8	—	—	17·0	—	Determinations of alveolar tension unreliable
2·52	4·1	—	—	16·5	—	—	
2·55	—	—	4·1	—	—	15·1	
3·14	—	3·8	—	—	17·2	—	
3·17	4·3	—	—	16·4	—	—	
3·20	—	—	4·5	—	—	14·3	
3·25	—	3·9	—	—	16·7	—	
3·43	—	3·8	—	—	16·8	—	
3·45	—	—	3·9	—	—	14·7	
3·46	3·8	—	—	17·0	—	—	
4·15	—	3·6	—	—	17·3	—	
4·17	—	—	3·3	—	—	15·6	
4·19	3·3	—	—	17·6	—	—	
4·56	3·1	—	—	17·9	—	—	
4·57	—	—	3·3	—	—	14·8	

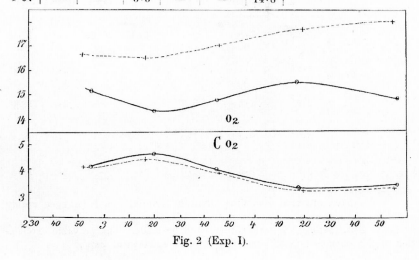

Fig. 2 (Exp. I).

37:10

A functional diagram of the first prototype unit from 1958 (shown below) of the electrode technology developed by Richard Stow and John Severinghaus for the measurement of blood carbon dioxide tensions. A membrane, permeable for carbon dioxide, separates the blood or gas to be analysed from the silver-silver chloride electrodes.

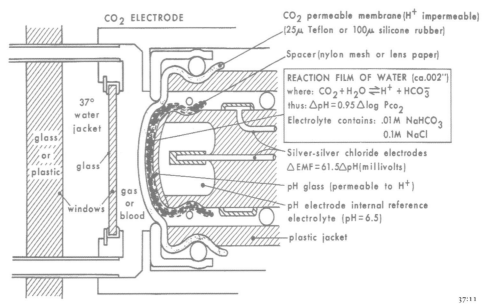

CO$_2$ ELECTRODE

CO$_2$ permeable membrane (H$^+$ impermeable) (25μ Teflon or 100μ silicone rubber)

Spacer (nylon mesh or lens paper)

REACTION FILM OF WATER (ca.002")
where: $CO_2 + H_2O \rightleftharpoons H^+ + HCO_3^-$
thus: $\Delta pH = 0.95 \Delta \log P_{CO_2}$
Electrolyte contains: .01 M NaHCO$_3$
    0.1 M NaCl

Silver-silver chloride electrodes
$\Delta EMF = 61.5 \Delta pH$ (millivolts)

pH glass (permeable to H$^+$)

pH electrode internal reference electrolyte (pH = 6.5)

plastic jacket

37° water jacket

glass or plastic

glass

windows

gas or blood

37:11

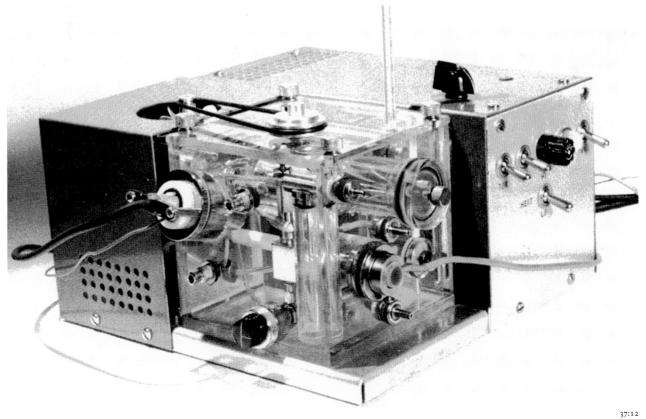

37:12

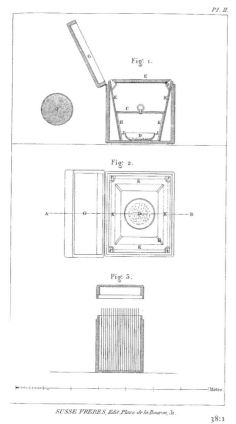

SUSSE FRERES, Edit. Place de la Bourse, 31.

38:1

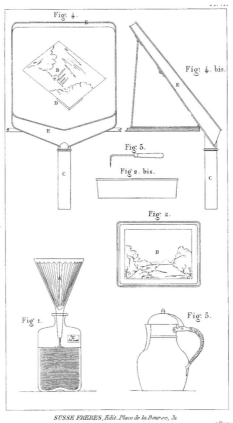

SUSSE FRERES, Edit. Place de la Bourse, 31.

38:3

Louis Daguerre's (1787–1851) presentation of the practical procedures involved in his new "Daguerréotype" process for creating permanent photographic images.

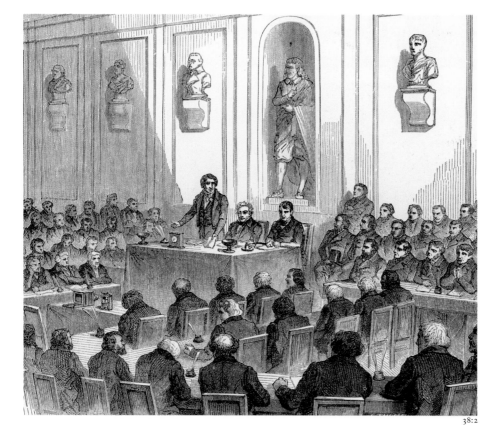

38:2

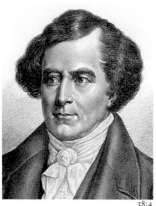

38:4

Francois Arago (1786–1853), a physicist and an influential member of the Chamber of Deputies in Paris, is a staunch supporter of Daguerre. He is shown left announcing the new invention of the photographic process in front of the French Academie des Sciences on 10 August 1839.

AGUERRE was born in Cormeilles-en-Parisis in 1787. Showing talent for drawing, he was apprenticed in 1803 to a scene-painter at the Paris Opera. In 1822 he met with instant success when establishing the Diorama, a "magical" picture show that created illusions of reality by using printed screens and special light effects. In 1829, Daguerre entered into partnership with the impoverished Niépce, to develop his invention "heliography", a slow and impractical process that nevertheless could create permanent pictures on coated pewter plates. In 1835 Daguerre accidentally discovered an efficient way of developing the latent photographic image and two years later a method to fix the image. Arago, physicist and influential member of the Chamber of Deputies, announced the discoveries in 1839 (38.1), unleashing "daguerreotypomania" around the world. The French government promptly purchased the rights to the process and granted Daguerre a generous life pension.

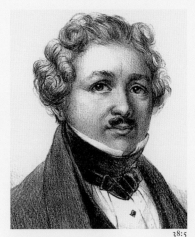

Louis Jaques Daguerre   38:5

Historique et description des procédés du Daguerréotype et du Diorama.

PARIS: LEREBOURS ET SUSSE FRÈRES; 1839.

DAGUERRE GIVES here a practical but rather superficial guide to the "Daguerréotype" process. Niepce's description from 1829 of the heliographic technique is also reprinted, together with Daguerre's explanation of the differences between the two methods. Included are also the reports of the special committees (the political, led by Arago and the scientific, led by Gay-Lussac) that were appointed to evaluate the new technology.

IN PERSPECTIVE:
The basic mechanism of photographic registration, the light sensitivity of silver salts, was discovered by Scheele (38.2). The use of a portable "camera obscura" that also plays a central role in the early developments of photography was conceived by Hooke 1694 (38.3). Although Daguerre, thanks to his influential ally Arago, quickly received due recognition for his work, able scientists and inventors other than Niepce, such as Bayard, Herschel and Talbot, also made significant contributions (38.4)(38.5) and by the time of Daguerre's death in 1851 the wet-colloid process of Archer was about to overtake the dominant position of the Daguerreotype (38.4). Only a few weeks after the appearance of the book cited above, Donne and Foucault etched daguerreotypes of microscopic images using nitric acid and made paper prints from the engraved plate that Donne used in his medical courses at the Charité Clinic in Paris (38.6). Duchenne de Boulogne and Darwin used photography to study the facial expressions in various physiological and emotional states (38.7)(38.8) and Charcot made extensive use of photography to differentiate hysteria from epilepsy (38.9) and to document the faces and other physical characteristics of patients with neurological diseases (38.10).

38.1 Arago DF. *Rapport de M Arago sur la Daguerréotype.* Lu à la séance de la Chambre des Députés le 3 juillet 1839. Paris; 1839.
38.2 See #21 Scheele page 120.
38.3 Derham W. *Philosophical Experiments and Observations of the late Eminent Dr Robert Hooke London*; 1726. p295. See also #11 Hooke page 72.
38.4 Gernsheim H. *The History of Photography.* London: Thames Hudson; 1969.
38.5 Herschel JF. On the chemical action of the rays of the solar spectrum on preparations of silver and other substances, ... *Phil Trans* 1840; 1:1.
38.6 Donne A, Foucault L. *Cours de Microscopie complémentaire des études médicales ...* Paris; 1844–1845.
38.7 Duchenne de Boulogne G. *Méchanisme de la physionomie humaine, ...* Paris; 1862.
38.8 Darwin C. *The expression of emotions in man and animals.* London; 1872.
38.9 Charcot J-M. *Iconographie Photographie de la Salpetriere,* 3 vols. Paris; 1877–1880.
38.10 Charcot J-M. *Nouvelle Iconographie de la Salpetriere,* 28 vols. Paris; 1888–1918.

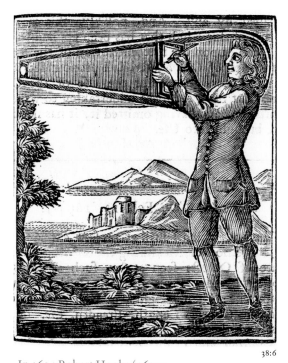

38:6

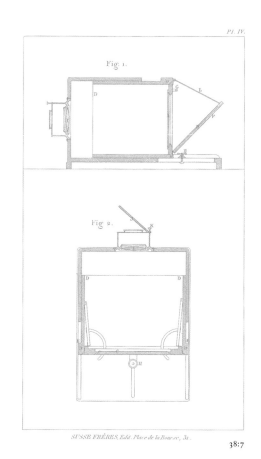

PL. IV.

Fig. 1.

Fig. 2.

SUSSE FRÈRES, Edit. Place de la Bourse, 31.

38:7

In 1694 Robert Hooke (1635–1703) conceives the portable camera obscura, an apparatus that he calls a "Picture-Box". He recommends it to be used with advantage during travel.

Daguerre's drawings of his camera (top right) and a picture of a camera from 1839.

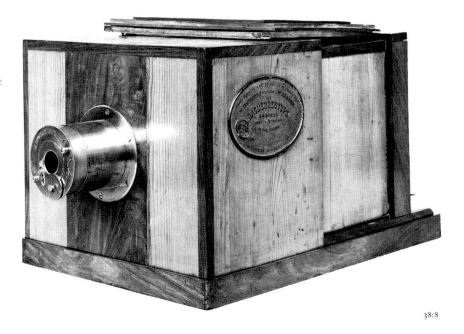

38:8

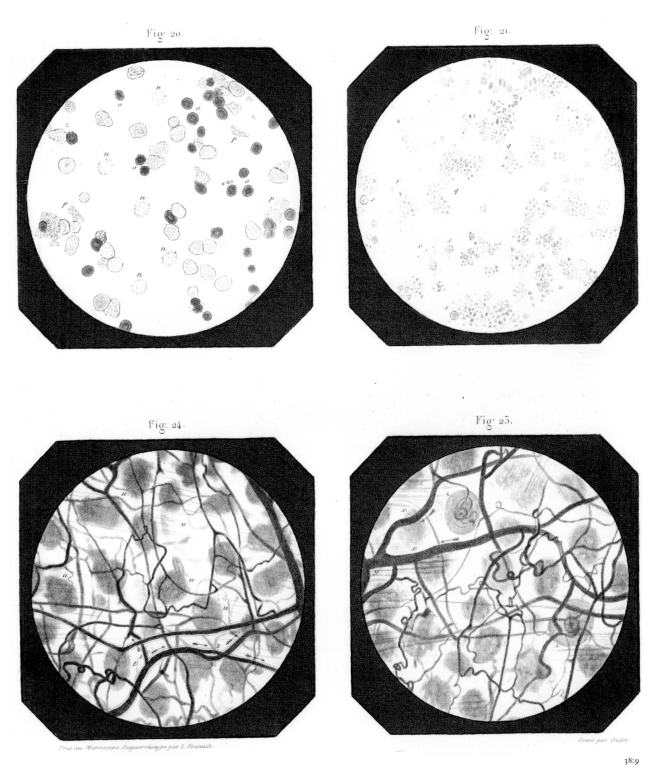

Fig. 20. Fig. 21.

Fig. 24. Fig. 25.

Pris au Microscope Daguerréotype par L. Foucault.

Gravé par Oudet.

38:9

The first photographic registrations for medical purposes of an image taken through a microscope. These pictures are printed using plates that are etched daguerreotypes of microscopic images. They show blood cells (top) and blood circulation in the tongue of a frog (bottom). Only a few weeks after the public announcement of Daguerre's invention, these pictures are incorporated at the Charité Clinic in Paris in a course on microscopy in medicine.

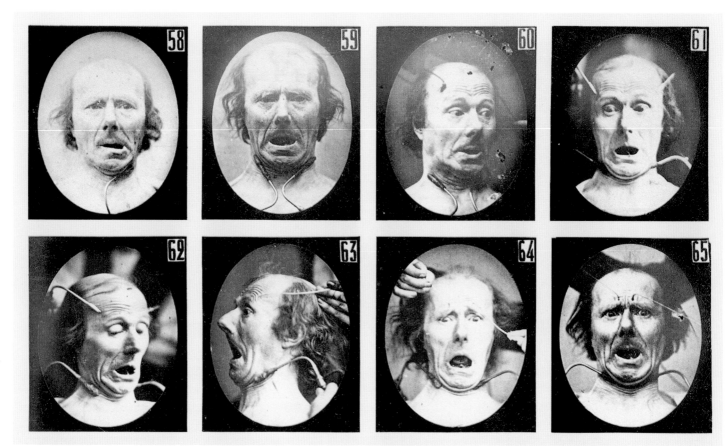

38:10

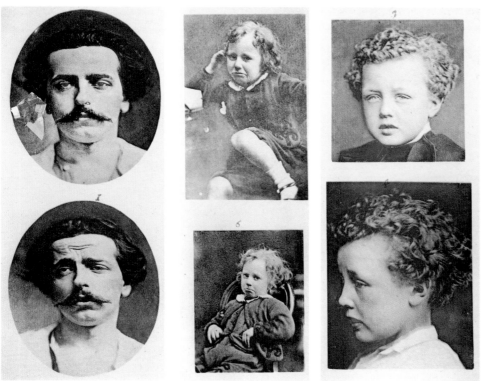

In 1862 Duchenne de Boulogne (1806–1875) uses photography to document the expressions produced when applying electrical stimulation to facial muscles.

A decade later Charles Darwin (1809–1882) makes photographic records of the facial expressions associated with different emotional states in man and also in animals.

38:11

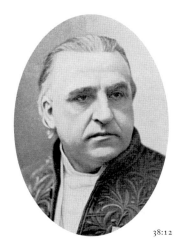

38:12

For four decades, starting in the 1870s, Jean-Martin Charcot (1825–1893) makes extensive photographic documentation of hysteria, epilepsy and the facial and the physical characteristics of patients with neurological diseases.

Patient with cerebral atrophy and epilepsy (right).

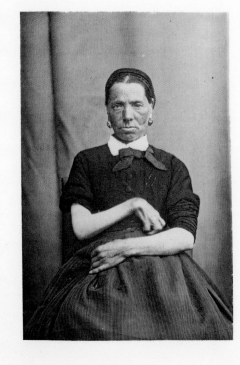

Planche I.

ATROPHIE CÉRÉBRALE : ÉPILEPSIE PARTIELLE

HÉMIPLÉGIE DROITE

38:14

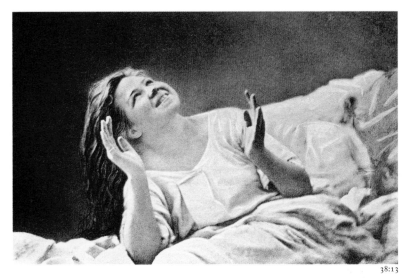

38:13

Patient feeling ecstatic and threatened.

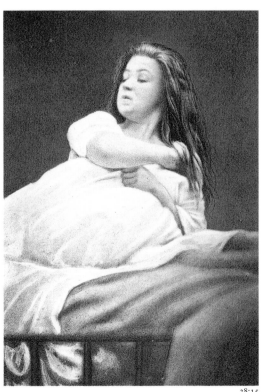

38:15

Rheinweinen), in denen das zur Löslicherhaltung der Harn=
säure nothwendige Alkali fehlt.

Bei Thieren, welche größere Mengen Wasser genießen,
wodurch die schwerlösliche Harnsäure in Auflösung erhalten
wird, so daß der eingeathmete Sauerstoff darauf wirken
kann, finden wir im Harn keine Harnsäure, sondern Harn=
stoff. Bei Vögeln ist als Secretionsproduct die Harnsäure
vorherrschend.

Wenn wir zu 1 Atom Harnsäure 6 Atome Sauerstoff und
4 Atome Wasser hinzutreten lassen, so zerlegt sie sich in
Harnstoff und Kohlensäure

$$1 \text{ At. Harnsäure } C_{10} N_8 H_3 O_6$$
$$4 \text{ » Wasser} \quad\Big\}\Big\{\quad 2 \text{ At. Harnstoff } C_4 N_8 H_{16} O_4$$
$$6 \text{ » Sauerstoff} \qquad H_8 O_{10} = 6 \text{ » Kohlensäure } C_6 \qquad O_{12}$$
$$\overline{C_{10} N_8 H_{16} O_{16}} \qquad\qquad \overline{C_{10} N_8 H_{16} O_{16}}$$

34. Der Harn der Gras freffenden Thiere enthält keine
Harnsäure, wohl aber Ammoniak, Harnstoff und Hippursäure,
oder Benzoesäure. Bei einem Hinzutreten von 9 Atomen
Sauerstoff zu der empirischen Formel ihres Blutes, fünf
mal genommen, haben wir darin die Elemente von 6 Atomen
Hippursäure, 9 At. Harnstoff, 3 At. Choleinsäure, 3 At.
Wasser und 3 At. Ammoniak; oder wenn wir uns denken,
daß während der Metamorphose dieses Blutes 45 Atome
Sauerstoff hinzutreten, so haben wir 6 At. Benzoesäure,
13½ At. Harnstoff, 3 At. Choleinsäure, 15 At. Kohlen=
säure und 12 At. Wasser.

$$5 (C_{48} N_{12} H_{73} O_{15}) + 90 = C_{240} N_{60} H_{350} O_{84} =$$

$$=\begin{cases} 6 \text{ At. Hippursäure } 6 (C_{13} N_2 H_{16} O_5) = C_{108} N_{12} H_{96} O_{30} \\ 9 \text{ » Harnstoff } 9 (C_2 N_4 H_8 O_2) = C_{18} N_{54} H_{72} O_{18} \\ 3 \text{ » Choleinsäure } 3 (C_{38} N_2 H_{66} O_{11}) = C_{114} N_6 H_{198} O_{53} \\ 3 \text{ » Ammoniak } 3 (N_2 H_6) = N_3 H_{18} \\ 3 \text{ » Wasser } 3 (H_2 O) = H_6 O_5 \end{cases}$$
$$\overline{C_{240} N_{10} H_{390} O_{84}}$$

oder

$$5 (C_{48} N_{12} H_{73} O_{15}) + O_{45} = C_{240} N_{60} H_{390} O_{120} =$$

$$=\begin{cases} 6 \text{ At. Benzoesäure } 6 (C_{14} \quad H_{10} O_5) = C_{84} \quad H_{60} O_{18} \\ 27/2 \text{ » Harnstoff } 27 (C \quad N_2 H_4 \quad O) = C_{27} N_{54} H_{108} O_{27} \\ 3 \text{ » Choleinsäure } 3 (C_{38} N_2 H_{55} O_{11}) = C_{114} N_6 H_{193} O_{55} \\ 15 \text{ » Kohlensäure } 15 (C \quad O_2) = C_{15} \quad O_{30} \\ 12 \text{ » Wasser } 12 (H_2 O) = H_{24} O_{12} \end{cases}$$
$$\text{Summa} \quad C_{240} N_{60} H_{390} O_{120}$$

35. Verfolgen wir zuletzt die Metamorphose der Gebilde
in dem Foetus der Kuh und betrachten wir das im Blute der
Mutter zugeführte Protein als den Stoff, welcher eine
Umsetzung erleidet oder erlitten hat, so ergiebt sich, daß
2 At. Protein ohne Hinzutreten von Sauerstoff oder einer
fremden Substanz die Elemente enthalten von 3 At. Al=
lantoin, 4 At. Wasser und 1 At Choloidinsäure, (Kinds=
pech, Meconium??).

$$2 \text{ At. Protein} = 2(C_{48} N_{12} H_{72} O_{14}) + 2 \text{ At. Wasser} = C_{96} N_{24} H_{148} O_{30} =$$

$$=\begin{cases} 3 \text{ At. Allantoin } 3 (C_8 N_8 H_{12} O_6) = C_{24} N_{24} H_{35} O_{18} \\ 1 \text{ » Choloidinsäure} \qquad C_{72} \quad H_{112} O_{12} \end{cases}$$
$$\overline{C_{96} N_{24} H_{148} O_{30}}$$

39:1

Justus von Liebig (1803–1873) is the
first to investigate systematically the
chemical foundation of the life
processes. He studies and classifies the
constituents of foodstuffs and attempts to explain nutrition, metabolism, heat generation and respiratory
gas exchange in chemical terms.

The famous "Kali-Apparat" of Liebig
from 1837. His equipment and
method for improved, standardised
organic elemental analysis soon becomes one of the cornerstones of subsequent research in organic chemistry.

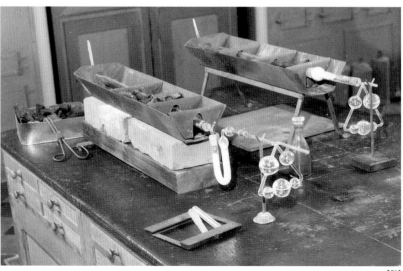

39:2

L IEBIG, the son of a drug and paint salesman in Darmstadt, was born in 1803. Failing in school, he concentrated his efforts on chemical experiments. After taking a degree at Erlangen 1822 he went to study in Paris. He stayed there for only two years, but studying under Gay-Lussac (39.1) left a lifelong impression on his work. Humboldt, recognising Liebig's talent (39.2), recommended him for a position in Giessen. Here, from 1825 as professor, he built up a large world-renowned chemical laboratory and established a system of teaching and research that became the forerunner of present day academic institutions. Liebig was kind-hearted but had a sharp pen and used it freely to criticise opponents. He had many bitter quarrels but bore no grudges and when in error, he was able to admit it after some time.

Die organische Chemie in ihrer Anwendung auf Physiologie und Pathologie.

B RAUNSCHWEIG: V IEWEG F & S OHN ; 1842.

L IEBIG OUTLINES some of the key chemical processes of the basic organic functions. He discusses respiration and nutrition, metabolism, heat generation and the motion of the body in chemical terms. Liebig divides food into plastic (protein, nitrous substances) and respiratory (non-nitrous fats and carbohydrates). He argues that the first type is for building up organs and for generating energy and the second type accounts for the generation of heat. At the end of the book Liebig presents chemical formulas and analytical results in support of his theories. Aware of the complexity of the topic, Liebig expresses the hope that the most important result of his book will be to open up new directions for research.

IN PERSPECTIVE:

In 1840, after making formidable contributions to all aspects of organic chemistry (39.3)(39.4) and wary of the acrimonious controversies particularly with Dumas (39.3), Liebig decided to look for applications for the new knowledge in chemistry (39.5). Studies of the composition of plants led him to an interest in physiology. Liebig's cited work had its roots in the experiments of Lavoisier (39.6), but more directly in the early work on "animal chemistry" of Berzelius (39.7) and in Magendie's studies demonstrating the importance of protein in the food supply of mammals (39.8). By synthesising disparate facts, Liebig was able to cast new light on the role of organic chemistry in the life processes. The ageing Berzelius, to whom Liebig affectionately dedicated the book, called it "armchair physiology" but Bischoff, Voit and Pettenkofer, who all later conducted important work on the metabolism of different foodstuffs (39.9)(39.10), acknowledged the seminal impact of Liebig's book.

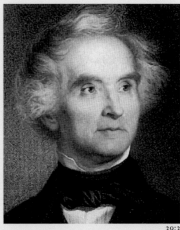

Justus von Liebig   39:3

39.1 See ref. 7.2, ref. 18.4 for important works of Gay-Lussac.

39.2 See #36 Dumas page 192 and ref 36.1.

39.3 See #36 Dumas page 192.

39.4 Partington JR. *A History of Chemistry*. Vol. III Chapter X. Mansfield Centre: Martino fine books; 1999.

39.5 von Liebig J. *Die Organische chemie in ihrer Anwendung auf Agricultur und Physiologie*. Braunschweig; 1840.

39.6 See #24 Lavoisier page 134.

39.7 See ref. 14.4.

39.8 Magendie F. *Précis élémentaire de physiologie*, 2 vols. Paris; 1816–1817.

39.9 Bischoff T, von Voit C. *Die Gesetze der Ernährung des Fleischfressers durch neue Untersuchungen festgestellt*. Leipzig; 1860.

39.10 Pettenkofer MJ, von Voit C. Untersuchungen über die Respiration. *Ann Chem Pharm* 1862/1863; Suppl 2:52.

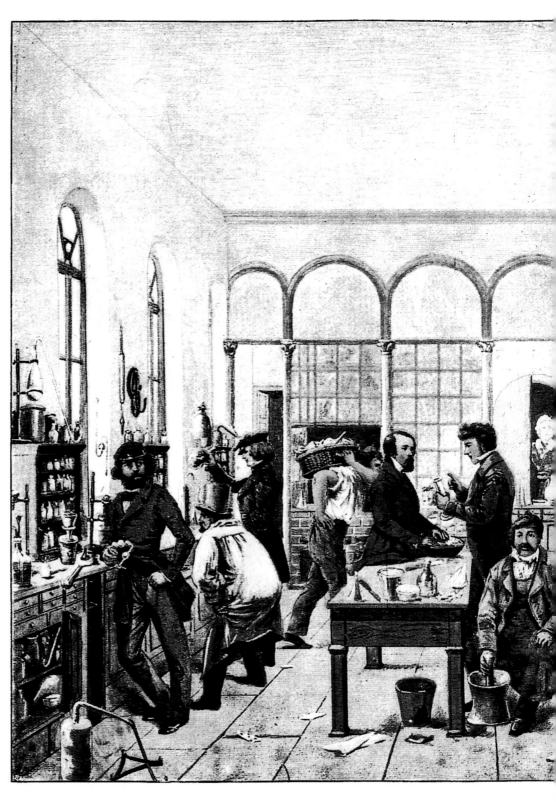

Liebig's world-renowned chemical laboratory in Giessen around 1840. Here he builds up a method of teaching and research that becomes a forerunner of present day academic institutions.

Juſtus Liebigs chemiſches Laboratorium a

(Erbaut vom Univerſitäts

Nach einer gleichzeitigen

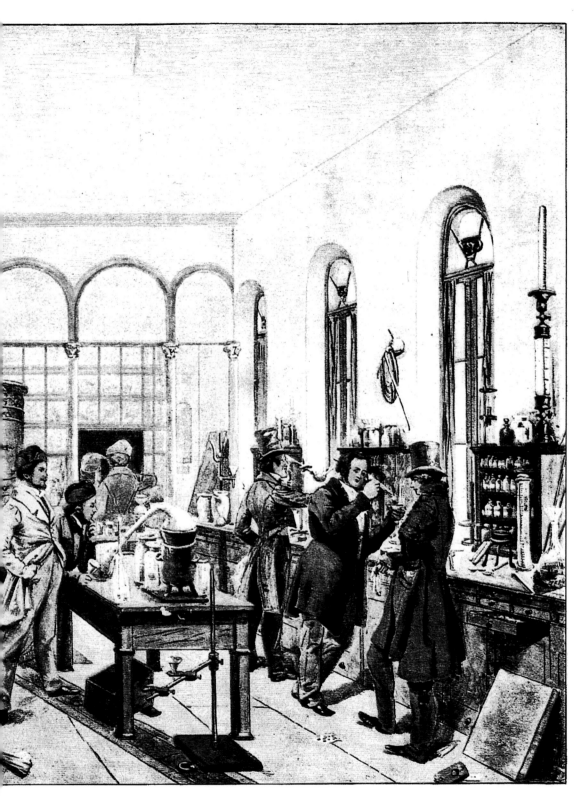

Seltersberg zu Gießen um das Jahr 1840.

Hofmann im Herbst 1839.)

von Wilhelm Trautschold.

39:4

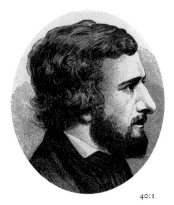

40:1

Hypolite Fizeau (1819–1896)
independently discovers the
"Doppler effect" for sound
and predicts its existence also
for light sources.

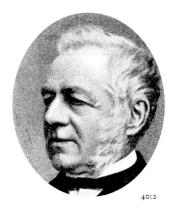

40:2

In 1845 Christophorus Buys
Ballot (1817–1890) proves
Doppler's theory for sound
waves using trumpeters on a
train between Amsterdam
and Utrecht.

pour M. Arago.

Ueber das
farbige Licht der Doppelsterne
und einiger anderer
Gestirne des Himmels.

Versuch einer das Bradley'sche Aberrations-Theorem als inte-
grirenden Theil in sich schliessenden allgemeineren Theorie.

Von

Christian Doppler,

Professor der Mathematik und praktischen Geometrie am technischen Institute und ausserordentl. Mitglied der
königl. böhm. Gesellschaft der Wissenschaften.

*Comparez
Comptes rendus
T. XVI p. 404
Abbé Moigno
p 1183.*

(Aus den Abhandlungen der k. böhm. Gesellschaft der Wissenschaften (V Folge, Bd. 2)
besonders abgedruckt.)

Prag, 1842.
In Commission bei Borrosch & André.

*Comparez les expériences acoustiques faites [...] obtenir
de fer par le Doct.[?] Ballot d'Utrecht
[...] la fausse Théorie de de Doppler
[...] rapport [...] Poggendorf Annalen T. 66 p 321 a 351.*

40:3

The title page of Johann Christian Doppler's (1803–1853)
landmark treatise, where he suggests that double stars show
different colours because they revolve around one another
and so one is moving towards the observer and the other
away from him. As appears from the inscriptions, Doppler
sent this copy of his work to Alexander Humbold (see #19),
a scientist of wide-ranging interests, who later passed it on to
his friend Francois Arago (see #39) with a suggestion to compare the results with the work of Buys Ballot (see above left).

DOPPLER was born in 1803 in Salzburg. Talented in mathematics, he studied at the Polytechnique Institute in Vienna. In 1835, his intent to emigrate to America was abandoned when he was offered a position as professor of mathematics and practical geometry at the State Secondary School in Prague. From 1841 he held the same chair at the State Technical Academy and in 1850 he was named director of the Physical Institute at the University of Vienna. Doppler's health was always poor and he died of a lung disease during a trip to Venice in 1853.

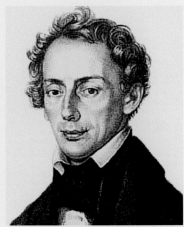

Johann Christian Doppler 40:4

Ueber das farbige Licht der Doppelsterne und einiger anderer Gestirne des Himmels.

PRAG: BORROSCH & ANDRÉ; 1842.

DOPPLER PROPOSES that the different colour tones of double stars that revolve around one another could be explained by the notion that the wavelength of light would be shifted as a result of the different relative motion of the two stars compared to the observer. He gives the correct formula for the magnitude of this shift and points out that the phenomenon should also be applicable to sound propagation. Several incorrect examples given by Doppler in support of his theory do not detract from the importance of his discovery.

IN PERSPECTIVE:
Ballot, using trumpeters on a train, proved Doppler's theory for sound in 1845 (40.1). Fizeau independently discovered the "Doppler shift" of light and gave the proper explanation of it. He was the first to determine in a laboratory the absolute value of the speed of light and also its value in a moving medium (40.2). In 1964, following the invention of the LASER (40.3), optical Doppler techniques were able to be developed for the measurement of fluid movement and flow (40.4). About a decade later the technology was applied in medicine, first to the blood flow in the retinal vessels (40.5) and then to the microcirculation in a finger and other parts of the body (40.6)(40.7). In the late 1950s Satomura showed the feasibility of using the Doppler effect in ultrasonic waves for diagnostic purposes (40.8) and within a decade continuous-wave Doppler ultrasound devices had been developed for use in peripheral and arterial vessel studies (40.9)(40.10), in cardiology (40.11) and in obstetrics (40.12). The first pulsed ultrasound Doppler technique appeared in 1969 (40.13) and could differentiate between different moving targets.

40.1 Ballot B. Akustische Versuche auf der Niederländischen Eisenbahn nebst gelegentlichen Bemerkungen zur theorie des Hrn Prof Doppler. *Ann Phys Chem* 1845; 66:321.

40.2 Fizeau MH. Sur le hypothèses relatives a l'éther lumineux. *Ann Chim Phys* 3ser. 1859; 57:385.

40.3 See #92 Maiman page 474.

40.4 Yeh Y, Cummins HZ. Localized fluid flow measurements with an He-Ne laser spectrometer. *Appl Phys Letters* 1964; 4:176.

40.5 Riva C, Ross B, Benedek GB. Laser Doppler measurements of blood flow in capillary tubes and retinal arteries. *Invest Ophtalmol* 1972; 11:936.

40.6 Stern MD. In vivo evaluation of microcirculation by coherent light scattering. *Nature* 1975; 254:56.

40.7 Öberg PÅ, Shepherd AP, editors. *Laser-Doppler Blood Flowmetry (Developments in Cardiovascular Medicine DICM 107)*. Kluwer Academic Publisher; 1990.

40.8 Satomura S. Ultrasonic Doppler Method for the Inspection of Cardiac Functions. *J Acoust Soc Am* 1957; 29:1181. See also ref. 90.11.

40.9 Rushmer RF, Baker DW, Stegall HF. Transcutaneous Doppler flow detection as a non-invasive technique. *J Appl Physiol* 1966; 21:554.

40.10 Gosling RG, King DH. Arterial assessment by Dopplershift ultrasound. *Proc Roy Soc Med* 1974; 67:447.

40.11 Lube M, Safarov Yu, Yakimenkov LI. Ultrasonic Detection of the Motions of Cardiac Valves and Muscles. *Sov Phys Acoust* 1967; 13:59.

40.12 Johnsson WL, et al. Detection of Fetal Life in Early Pregnancy with an Ultrasonic Doppler Flowmeter. *Obst Gyn* 1965; 26:305. See also ref. 90.8.

40.13 Wells PN. A range-gated ultrasonic Doppler system. *Med. & Biol. Eng* 1969; 7:641.

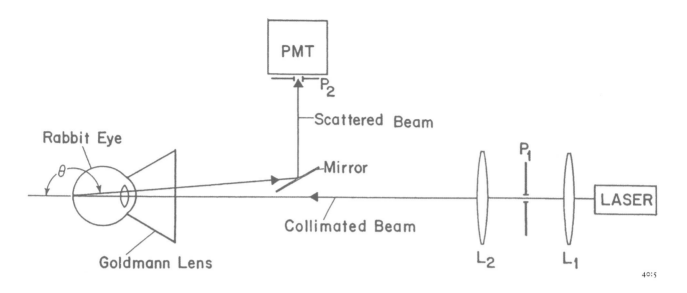

PMT

P$_2$

Scattered Beam

Rabbit Eye

θ

Mirror

Collimated Beam

Goldmann Lens

P$_1$

L$_2$

L$_1$

LASER

40:5

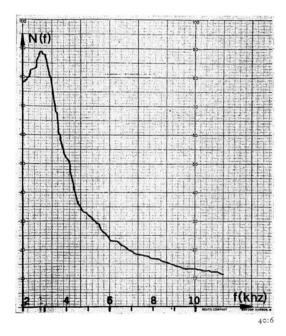

N(f)

f(khz)

40:6

The first laser Doppler measurements for medical purposes are made on blood flow in the retinal arteries of rabbits in 1972. The experimental setup (top diagram) and the power spectrum of the scattered light from the retinal arteriole (left) are shown.

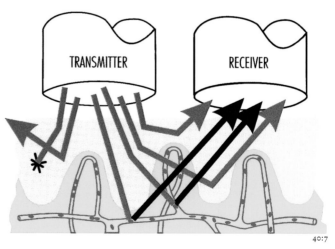

TRANSMITTER

RECEIVER

40:7

The principle of laser Doppler measurements of microvascular tissue perfusion.

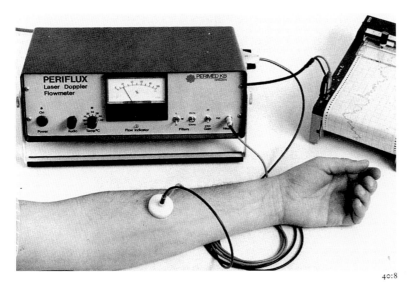

40:8

An instrument for microvascular tissue perfusion measurements from the early 1980s.

Modern laser Doppler perfusion imaging system showing peripheral circulation in the hand and in the heart during and after coronary by-pass surgery.

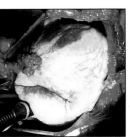

The human heart at rest during coronary by-pass surgery.

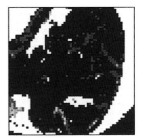

Virtually no myocordial perfusion before release of coronary vessel clamp.

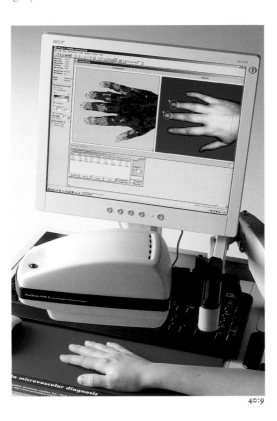

40:9

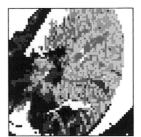

A map of myocordial perfusion following release of coronary vessel clamp.

40:10

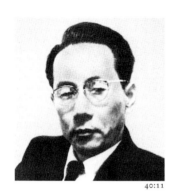

40:11

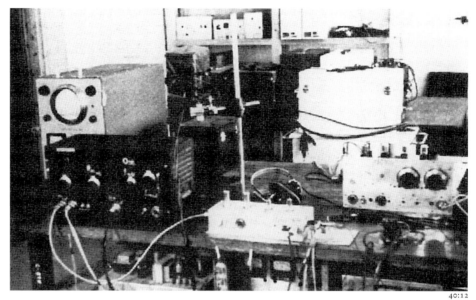

40:12

Shigeo Satomura (1919–1960) pioneers the use of ultrasound Doppler techniques for medical diagnostics. The photograph shows his original equipment from the late 1950s at the Osaka University. His transducer and the registrations obtained by him from cardiac motions are shown below.

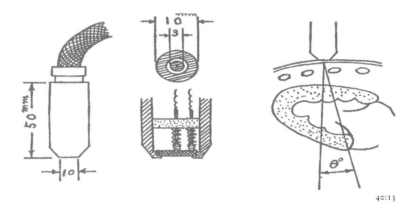

40:13

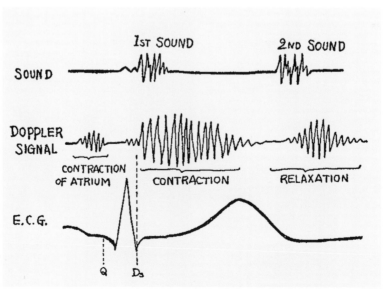

40:14

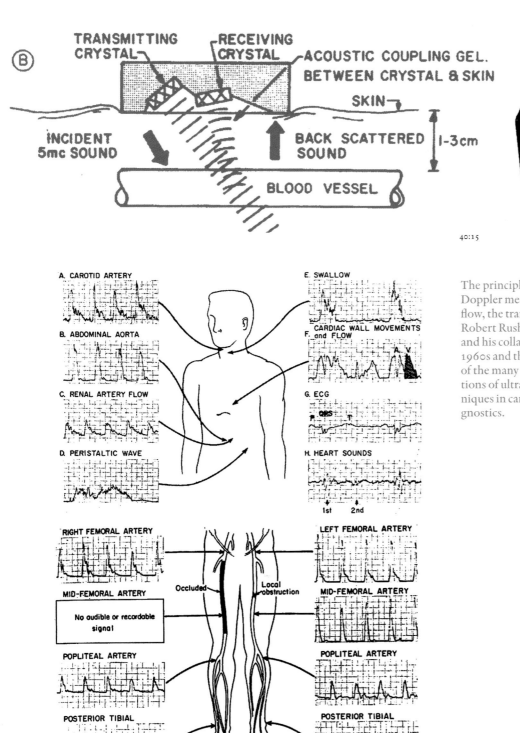

B

TRANSMITTING CRYSTAL

RECEIVING CRYSTAL

ACOUSTIC COUPLING GEL. BETWEEN CRYSTAL & SKIN

SKIN

INCIDENT 5mc SOUND

BACK SCATTERED SOUND

1-3cm

BLOOD VESSEL

40:15

A. CAROTID ARTERY

B. ABDOMINAL AORTA

C. RENAL ARTERY FLOW

D. PERISTALTIC WAVE

E. SWALLOW

CARDIAC WALL MOVEMENTS
F. and FLOW

A.V.

G. ECG

QRS

H. HEART SOUNDS

1st   2nd

RIGHT FEMORAL ARTERY

MID-FEMORAL ARTERY

No audible or recordable signal

POPLITEAL ARTERY

POSTERIOR TIBIAL

Occluded

Local obstruction

LEFT FEMORAL ARTERY

MID-FEMORAL ARTERY

POPLITEAL ARTERY

POSTERIOR TIBIAL

DORSALIS PEDIS ARTERY

Right
No signal

Left
Faintly audible

40:16

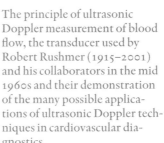

40:17

The principle of ultrasonic Doppler measurement of blood flow, the transducer used by Robert Rushmer (1915–2001) and his collaborators in the mid 1960s and their demonstration of the many possible applications of ultrasonic Doppler techniques in cardiovascular diagnostics.

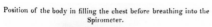

Position of the body in filling the chest before breathing into the Spirometer.

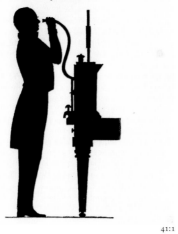

41:1

In 1846 John Hutchinson (1811–1861) invents a spirometer and demonstrates that it offers a "precise and easy method of detecting disease" of the lungs. The illustrations show his apparatus and the recommended way of using it when standing.

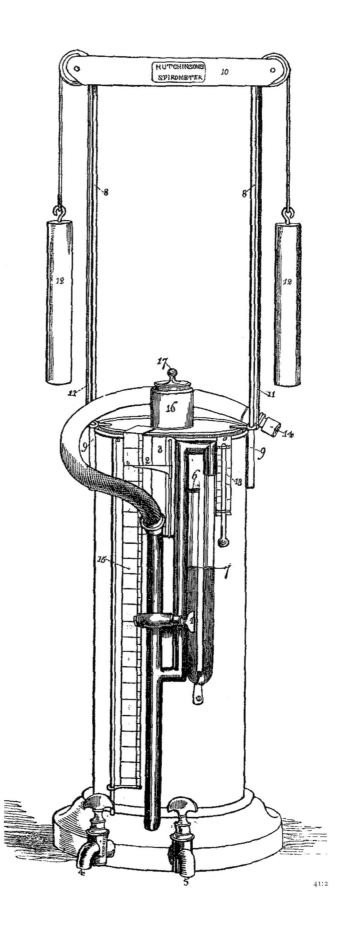

41:2

HUTCHINSON was born in Newcastle upon Tyne in 1811. His early interest was mechanical engineering, but later he studied medicine. In 1836 he began working as a physician to the Britannia Life Assurance Company (41.1) and became a Fellow of the Statistical Society 1842. He married in 1840 and had three children, but left his family in 1852 and emigrated to Melbourne, Australia. Here gold deposits had been discovered and Hutchinson was caught up in the "gold fever" (41.2). In 1855 he reappeared in Australia as a consulting physician, but six years later he left for Fiji, where he soon developed dysentery and became "careless of himself and fell into intemperate habits" and died of "the combined effects of disappointment, disease and the absence of all comforts" (41.2).

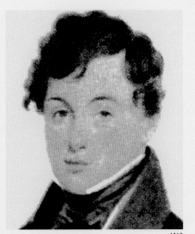

John Hutchinson   41:3

On the Capacity of the Lungs, and on the Respiratory Functions, with a View of establishing a Precise and Easy Method of detecting Disease by the Spirometer.

MEDICO-CHIRURGICAL TRANSACTIONS. ROY MED CHIR SOC, LONDON. 1846; 29:137.

AFTER A short historic introduction, Hutchinson explains what the "vital capacity" of the lung is. Then in seven chapters and more than two hundred paragraphs he describes in detail a spirometer of his own design and the measurements of the vital capacity of more than two thousand individuals made with this instrument. He studies the influence of the size of the thorax, the subject's height, weight, age, and sex and also the effect of phthisis, the fibrotic complication of tuberculosis that reduces vital capacity by destroying lung tissue.

IN PERSPECTIVE:
Lavoisier, Beddoes, Watt and Davy all used gasometers to study respiration (41.3). However, Hutchinson's device was a significant advance over previous equipment and more importantly his extensive and systematically collected measurements established spirometry as a diagnostic method. In 1864 Gréhant was the first to study the gas composition of the expired volume in relation to the gas distribution in the lungs (41.4) and a few years later Speck built much improved spirometers for measuring gas exchange in man during exercise (41.5). In 1904 Tissot's design (41.6)(41.7) reduced the resistance to breathing and made the excursion of the bell of the device proportional to the volume change. His device became the "gold standard" in spirometry for more than half a century. Hutchinson's concept of vital capacity is still very much in use today (41.8). In 1980 a study of more than 5,200 men over thirty years of age showed vital capacity to be a useful predictor of pulmonary disease and cardiac failure (41.9).

41.1 Spriggs EA. John Hutchinson, the inventor of the spirometer—his North Country background, life in London and scientific achievements. *Med History* 1977; 21:357.

41.2 Gandevia B. John Hutchinson in Australia and Fiji. *Med.History* 1977; 21:365.

41.3 See #24 Lavoisier page 1364 and #28 Davy page 156 and ref.28.3.

41.4 See ref. 6.6 and ref. 37.7 also #97 Wagner-West page 504.

41.5 Speck C. Untersuchungen über Sauerstoffverbrauch und Kohlensäureausathmung der Menschen. *Schriften Ges Beförd. gesam Naturwiss zu Marburg Cassel*; 1871:10 See also #58 Voit page 300 and ref. 58.4.

41.6 Tissot J. Nouvelle méthode de mesure et d'inscription du débit et des mouvements respiratoires. *J Physiol Path Gén* 1904; 6:688.

41.7 Tissot J. Nouvelle méthode de mesure et d'inscription du débit et des movements respiratoires de l'homme et des animaux. *Trav l'Assoc Inst Marey* Vol II 1910. p231.

41.8 Petty TL. John Hutchinson's mysterious machine revisited. *Chest* 2002; 121:219S.

41.9 Kanel WB, et al. The value of measuring vital capacity for prognostic purposes. *Trans Assoc Life Insur Med Dir Am* 1980; 64:66.

30.—The persons I have examined may be arranged as follows :—

Sailors (merchant service)	121
Fire Brigade of London	82
Metropolitan police	144
Thames ditto	76
Paupers	129
Mixed class (artisans)	370
First Battalion Grenadier Guards . . .	87
Royal Horse Guards (Blue)	59
Chatham recruits	185
Woolwich Marines	573
Pugilists and wrestlers	24
Giants and dwarfs	4
Pressmen . 30 } Printers . . .	73
Compositors . 43 }	
Draymen	20
Girls	26
Gentlemen	97
Diseased cases	60
Total number . .	2130

41:4

164.—Q.—Table of the Comparison of Healthy and Diseased Cases.

<table>
<tr><th colspan="4">PHTHISIS PULMONALIS.</th></tr>
<tr><th colspan="2">EARLY STAGE.</th><th colspan="2">ADVANCED STAGE.</th></tr>
<tr><th>Vital Capacity. Diseased.</th><th>Vital Capacity. Healthy.</th><th>Vital Capacity. Diseased.</th><th>Vital Capacity. Healthy.</th></tr>
<tr><th>Cubic inches.</th><th>Cubic inches.</th><th>Cubic inches.</th><th>Cubic inches.</th></tr>
<tr><td>113</td><td>220</td><td>59</td><td>135</td></tr>
<tr><td>115</td><td>173</td><td>89</td><td>224</td></tr>
<tr><td>105</td><td>173</td><td>108</td><td>254</td></tr>
<tr><td>130</td><td>204</td><td>72</td><td>135</td></tr>
<tr><td>128</td><td>220</td><td>80</td><td>229</td></tr>
<tr><td>120</td><td>229</td><td>75</td><td>254</td></tr>
<tr><td>100</td><td>193</td><td>34</td><td>246</td></tr>
<tr><td>140</td><td>246</td><td>171</td><td>270</td></tr>
<tr><td>100</td><td>204</td><td>60</td><td>237</td></tr>
<tr><td>110</td><td>220</td><td></td><td></td></tr>
<tr><td>136</td><td>229</td><td></td><td></td></tr>
<tr><td>135</td><td>204</td><td></td><td></td></tr>
<tr><td>192</td><td>230</td><td></td><td></td></tr>
<tr><td>225</td><td>300</td><td></td><td></td></tr>
<tr><td>145</td><td>220</td><td></td><td></td></tr>
<tr><td>200</td><td>240</td><td></td><td></td></tr>
<tr><td>185</td><td>230</td><td></td><td></td></tr>
<tr><td>218</td><td>240</td><td></td><td></td></tr>
<tr><td>129</td><td>220</td><td></td><td></td></tr>
<tr><td>344</td><td>434</td><td></td><td></td></tr>
<tr><td>220</td><td>260</td><td></td><td></td></tr>
<tr><td>196</td><td>254</td><td></td><td></td></tr>
</table>

165.—These cases were not from my own diagnosis, but individuals sent to me by others, well skilled in auscultation.

41:5

The division of the thoracic movements.

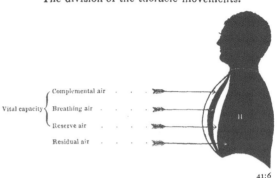

	Complemental air . . . ➤
Vital capacity {	Breathing air . . . . ➤
	Reserve air . . . . ➤
	Residual air . . . . ➤

41:6

Hutchinson defines the components of a tidal breath in relation to the thoracic movement during breathing. He then examines a large number of healthy subjects (top table) and establishes the normal value of the vital capacity of the lung. Based on this data, he is able to show (left table) how spirometry can be used to distinguish patients with phthisis, the fibrotic complication of tuberculosis.

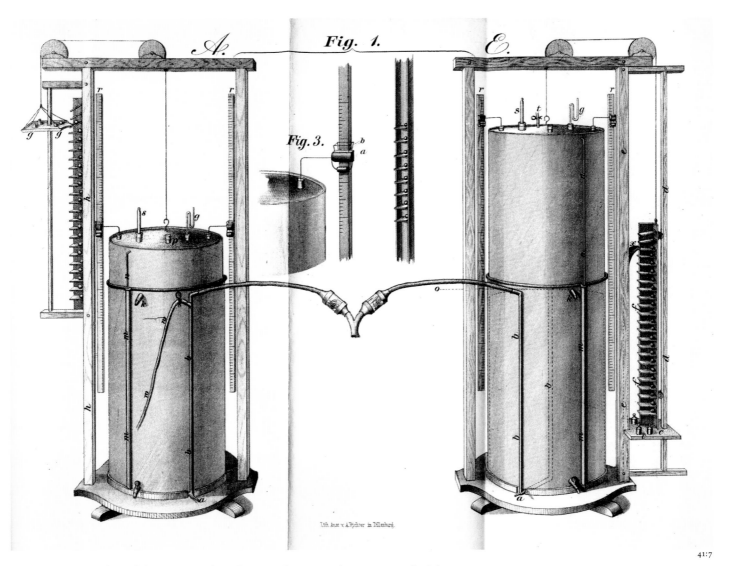

Carl Speck (1828–1916) describes a much improved spirometer, which he uses in 1871 to measure respiratory gas exchange at rest and also during exercise, making him a pioneer of sport medicine.

41:7

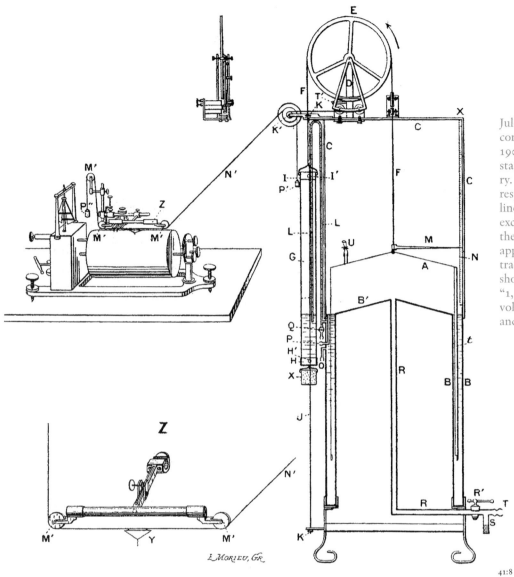

Jules Tissot (1864–1918) constructs a spirometer in 1904 that remains the "gold standard" for half a century. It is designed to give low respiratory resistance and a linear relation between the excursion of the bell and the volume change. The apparatus and a typical tracing obtained from it are shown. The spikes marked "1, 2, 3" represent known volumes of 1 litre, 0.5 litres and 0.25 litres.

L. MORIEU, GR.

41:8

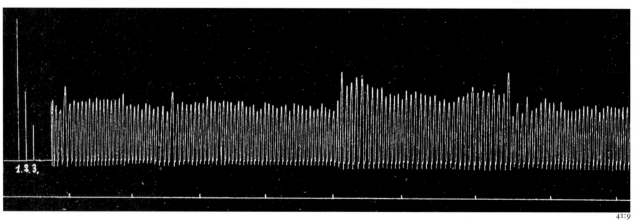

41:9

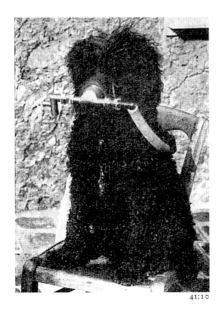

41:10

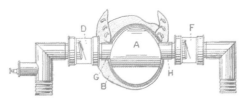

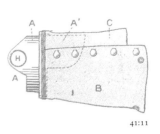

41:11

Tissot also develops novel devices, with low resistance to breathing, to provide a tight connection between man or animal and his spirometer. In many clinical applications maintaining the integrity of the connection between apparatus and patient remains a challenge even today.

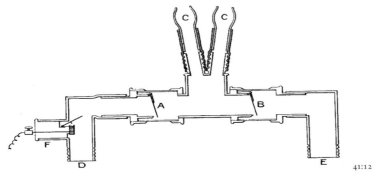

41:12

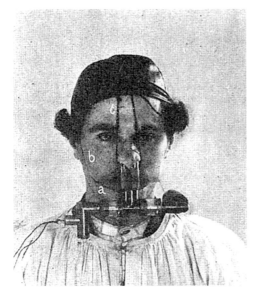

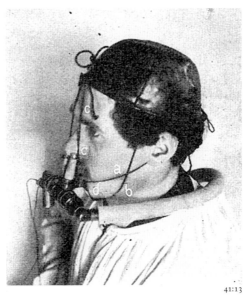

41:13

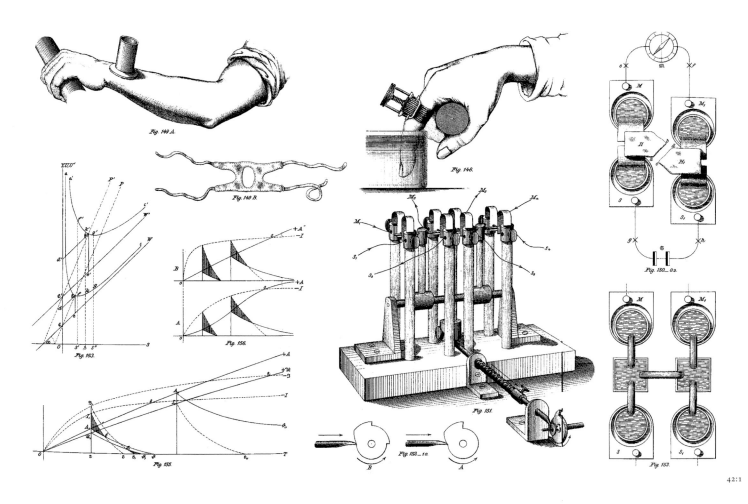

On the right Emil Du Bois-Reymond's (1818–1896) "Willkurversuch", where he demonstrates the direction of the current generated by voluntary muscular contraction. Above some of the devices and experiments of his pioneering neurophysiological investigations.

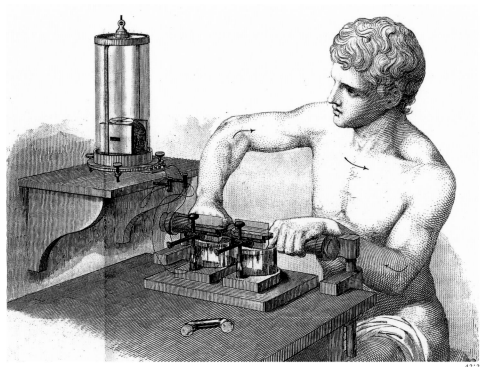

Du Bois-Reymond was born in Berlin in 1818. He attended French high school and later at the University of Berlin he studied a wide variety of subjects from theology, philosophy, psychology and literature to botany, geology, natural sciences, logic and mathematics. Eventually, he settled on medicine and soon took the study of the electrical phenomenon in animals (42.1)(42.2) as a lifelong task. Thanks to Humboldt's interest in this topic (42.3), he was elected to the Prussian Academy of Sciences in 1851. On the death of his teacher Johannes Müller in 1858, he succeeded him as professor of physiology in Berlin. Du Bois-Reymond had a great gift for language and a sharp pen, blending French eloquence with German thoroughness. He considered the history of science the most important but most neglected part of cultural history. His speeches on scientific and cultural matters set a standard that few, if any, could rival in his own time or later (42.4).

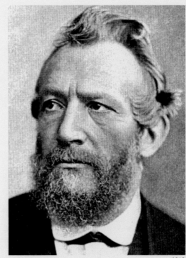

Emil Du Bois-Reymond

42:3

Untersuchungen über thierische Elektricität.

Band 1, Band 2 (2 Abteilungen) Berlin: Reimer G; 1848–1884.

In these collected electrophysiological works, Du Bois-Reymond describes many new phenomena related to nerve activity and muscle contraction, including the existence of the "injury current" in the muscle and the nerve and also the phenomenon of "negative oscillations" in the muscle. He studies extensively the polarisation that occurs when a current flows through the nerve (electrotonus) and the polarisation that arises at the interface between different electrolytes. He obtains these experimental results by careful avoidance of many sources of measuring error and by developing new instruments such as highly sensitive coils for detecting weak currents, non-polarisable electrodes and special switching devices.

IN PERSPECTIVE:
Du Bois-Reymond continued the work initiated by Jallabert (42.5), Galvani (42.6) and particularly Humboldt (42.3), but his interest arose as a direct result of the book published by Matteucci in 1840 on animal electricity (42.1). Apart from his discoveries in electrophysiology Du Bois-Reymond, together with his friends Helmholtz (42.7), Ludwig and Brucke (42.8), introduced the broad use of physical methods and instrumentation to break new ground in physiology. In a famous prologue to the first volume of the work cited above, Du Bois-Reymond once and for all settled the dispute with the adherents of the theory of vital force (Lebenskraft)(42.9). One of his prominent disciples, Pflugger, continued his electrophysiological studies and also made other important contributions, particularly in respiration physiology and in the study of blood gases (42.10).

42.1 Matteucci C. *Essai sur la phénomènes électrique des animaux.* Paris; 1840.
42.2 Du Bois-Reymond E. Ueber den sogennanten Froschstrom. *Ann Phys* 1843; 58:1.
42.3 See ref. 19.9.
42.4 Du Bois-Reymond E. *Reden*, 2 vols. Leipzig (1912).
42.5 See #19 Jallabert page 110.
42.6 See ref. 19.4 and ref. 19.7.
42.7 See #43 Helmholtz page 228 and #45. Helmholtz page 236.
42.8 See ref. 35.5 and ref. 45.8.
42.9 See ref. 4.7.
42.10 See ref. 37.4.

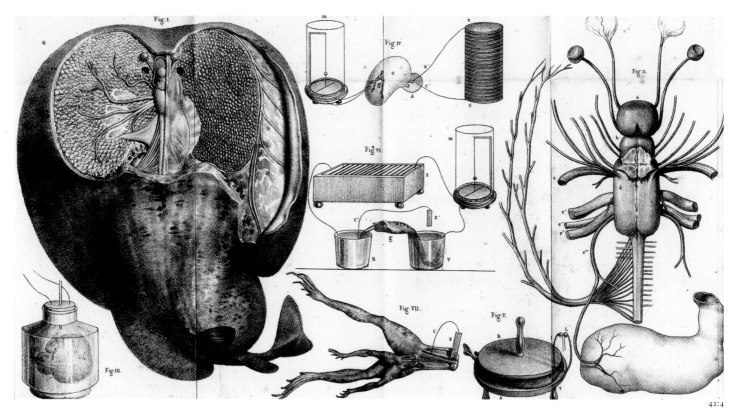

42:4

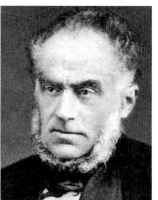

42:6

Carlo Matteucci's (1811–1868) investigations in 1840 of the electricity generated in the torpedo and in the frog nerve (illustrated above) are the starting point of Du Bois-Reymond's work.

Johannes Müller (1801–1858) (see also picture 25:12) directs Du Bois-Reymond's interest to electrophysiology. On Müller's death, Du Bois-Reymond succeeds him in the Chair of Physiology in Berlin.

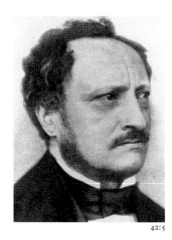

42:5

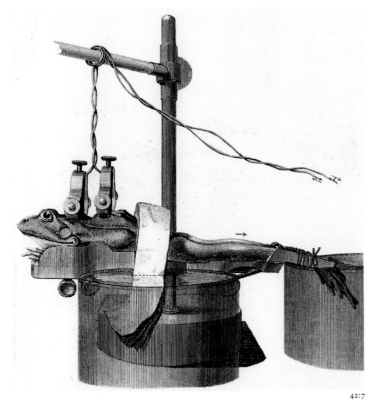

42:7

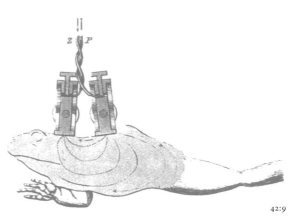

42:9

By developing sensitive instruments and with a careful experimental design, Du Bois-Reymond discovers new neurophysiological phenomena of fundamental importance such as the resting nerve current, the "injury current" in the muscle and the nerve and the "negative oscillations" in the muscle.

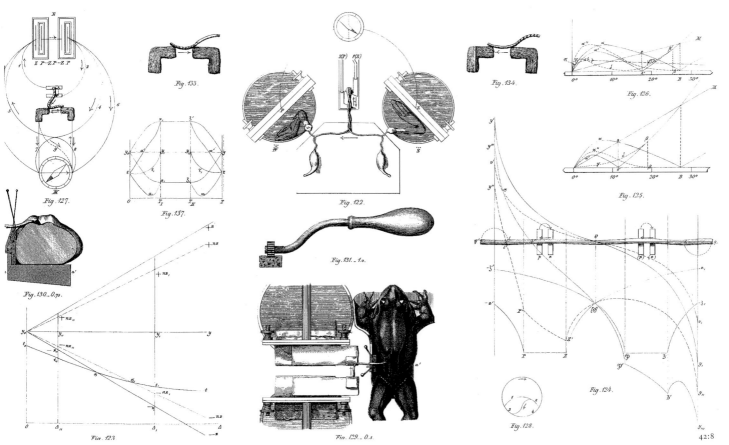

42:8

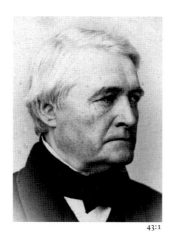

In 1844 Claude Pouillet (1790–1868) introduces the concept of the ballistic galvanometer. By generating a current at the firing of a projectile and allowing the projectile to interrupt the current at various distances from the firing point, he is able to measure the time of very short flight intervals despite the use of rather slowly responding instrumentation.

43:1

Hermann von Helmholtz's (1821–1894) illustration of his ballistic galvanometer, which he designs to measure the propagation velocity of nerve impulses.

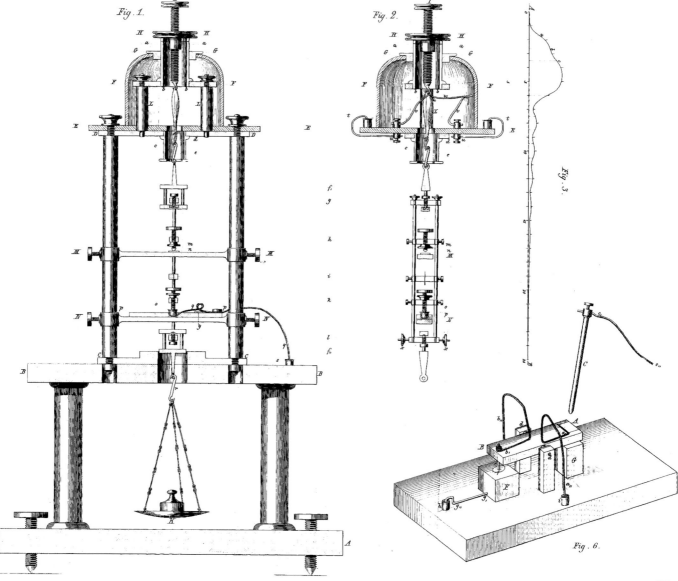

43:2

HELMHOLTZ was born in 1821, the oldest of four children of a Potsdam college teacher. Helmoltz was drawn to physics early on, but the family could only afford a medical education, for which state scholarships were available. After taking his degree in 1842, Helmholtz started his eight-year duty as an army surgeon, a commitment he made to receive a stipend. In 1847 he presented his classic paper on the fundamental law of the conservation of energy (43.1). On Humboldt's (43.2) request, Helmholtz was soon released from his obligations as a surgeon and was appointed professor of physiology in Königsberg. For more than two decades he held similar positions in Bonn and in Heidelberg, doing research primarily on sensory physiology (43.3). In 1871, he succeeded Magnus (43.4) in Berlin as professor of physics and devoted himself particularly to problems in thermodynamics and in electrodynamic action. He also wrote extensively on philosophical issues particularly concerning scientific methodology (43.5).

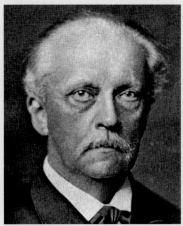

Hermann von Helmholtz ⁴³:³

Messungen über den zeitlichen Verlauf der Zuckung animalischer Muskeln und die Fortpflanzungsgeschwindigkeit der Reizung in den Nerven.

ARCH ANAT PHYSIOL BERLIN: VEIT; 1850. P276.

HELMHOLTZ DESCRIBES an ingenious arrangement to determine the velocity of a nerve impulse. He generates inductively a current that makes the muscle contract and thereby interrupt the flow of the current. The slowly reacting galvanometer produces a deflection in proportion to the duration of the current impulse. By allowing the impulse to travel different lengths along the nerve he calculates the velocity to be around 30 m/s.

IN PERSPECTIVE:
Helmholtz's method (which he completed with a graphical technique two years later (43.6)) may be traced back to the earliest efforts by Hooke to determine the velocity of a projectile (43.7)(43.8). The basic idea of Hooke's ballistic experiment was that if the projectile hit and fused with a large enough body at rest the resulting motion of this body, as governed by the law of conservation of momentum, would be slow enough to be measured. In analogy, Pouillet introduced the ballistic galvanometer technique by generating a current at the firing of a projectile and allowing the projectile to interrupt the current at various distances from the firing point (43.9). The deflection of the galvanometer was then proportional to the duration of the impulse. As stated in ref. (43.8) "a primary attribute of inventiveness, if not genius itself, is the ability to recognise the broader applicability of concepts developed by other sciences and to adapt them as tools for new purposes". Helmholtz, who was probably the last scholar fully embracing most of the sciences, philosophy and the fine arts, was able to do just that.

43.1　von Helmholtz H. *Über die Erhaltung der Kraft, eine physikalische Abhandlung vorgetragen in der Sitzung der physikalisches Gesellschaft zu Berlin am 23sten juli 1847.* Berlin; 1847.

43.2　For Humboldt's influence see #36 Dumas page 192, #39 Liebig page 208 and #42 Du Bois-Reymond page 224 and also ref. 19.9.

43.3　See ref. 5.13 and also #45 Helmholtz page 236 and ref. 19.3.

43.4　See #37 Magnus page 196.

43.5　von Helmholtz H. *Die Thatsachen in der Wahrnehmung.* Berlin; 1879 and also ref. 4.9.

43.6　von Helmholtz H. Messungen über Fort pfanzungsgeschwindigkeit der Reizung in den Nerven. *Arch Ant Physiol Berlin*; 1852. p199.

43.7　Günther RT. *Early science in Oxford* Vol.VI The life and work of Robert Hooke (Part I) Oxford; 1930. See also #11 Hooke page 72.

43.8　Hoff HE, Geddes LA. Ballistics and the Instrumentation of Physiology: The Velocity of the Projectile and of the Nerve Impulse. *J Hist Med* 1960; 15:133.

43.9　Pouillet CS. Note sur un moyen de mésurer des intervalles de temps extrémement courts, ... *C R Acad Sci* 1844; 19:1384.

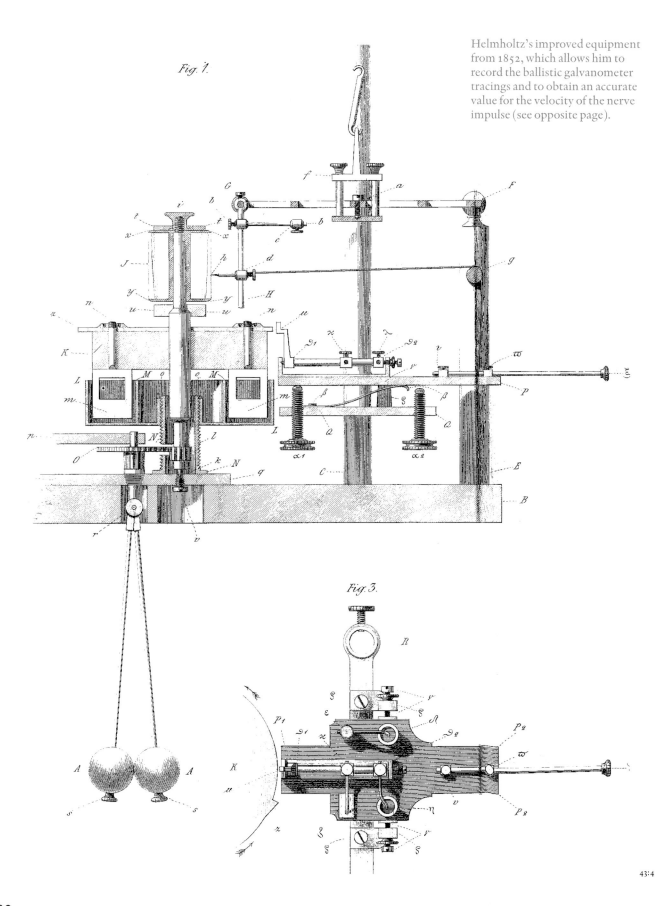

Fig. 1.

Helmholtz's improved equipment from 1852, which allows him to record the ballistic galvanometer tracings and to obtain an accurate value for the velocity of the nerve impulse (see opposite page).

Fig. 3.

43:4

Reihe X.

Am 29sten Decb. mit den Muskeln eines seit vier Monaten aufbewahrten Frosches angestellt. Durch die entferntere Nervenstelle wird ein stärkerer Strom geleitet, der durch die sich berührenden Spiralen erzeugt wird, durch die nähere ein schwächerer bei 2½ Ctm. Abstand der Spiralen· Nach je zwei Beobachtungen wird der Muskel neu eingestellt.

A. Rechter Muskel. Nervenstrecke 40 mm. Ablenkung vorher 116,09, nachher 112,45, im Mittel 114,27.

No.	Ueberlastung.	Erhebungshöhe.	Differenz der Ausschläge bei Reizung der entfernteren	näheren Nervenstrecke.
1	20 gr.	1,19	100,69	
2	—	1,22	96,15	
3	—	1,22		93,92
4	—	1,15		97,19
5	—	1,10	97,70	
6	—	1,10	104,33	
7	—	1,17		93,87
8	—	1,12		92,27
9	—	1,15	106,43	
10	—	1,15	101,74	
11	—	1,12		98,00
12	—	1,17		98,60
13	—	1,12	96,81	
14	—	1,10	103,99	

Mittel			100,98	95,64
Wahrscheinl. Fehler des Mittels			± 0,86	± 0,66
Derselbe der einzelnen Beobachtung			± 2,42	± 1,61
Zeitdauer in Secunden von der Reizung bis zur Erhebung			0,02437	0,02307
Wahrscheinl. Fehler derselben .			± 0,00020	± 0,00016

Zeitunterschied wegen der Fortpflanzung: 0,00130 ± 0,00027

Fortpflanzungsgeschwindigkeit: 30,8 ± 6,4 Mt.

43:5

The result of one of Helmholtz's experiments for measuring the velocity of the nerve impulse. An electric stimulation starts the nerve impulse current, which is then interrupted when the muscle contracts. The propagation lengths differ by 40 mm and the corresponding time difference is determined to be 0.0013 seconds, which gives a velocity of 30.8 m/seconds.

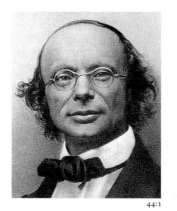

Wilhelm Weber (1804–1891) works in the 1820s, together with his elder brother Ernst Heinrich, on the experimental aspects of fluid dynamics in the circulatory system.

Ernst Heinrich Weber (1795–1878) determines the arterial pulse velocity to about 9 m/second and shows that the elasticity and resistance of the blood vessels transform the pulsatile movement of the blood in the aorta into a continuous flow through the arterioles and the capillaries.

44:1

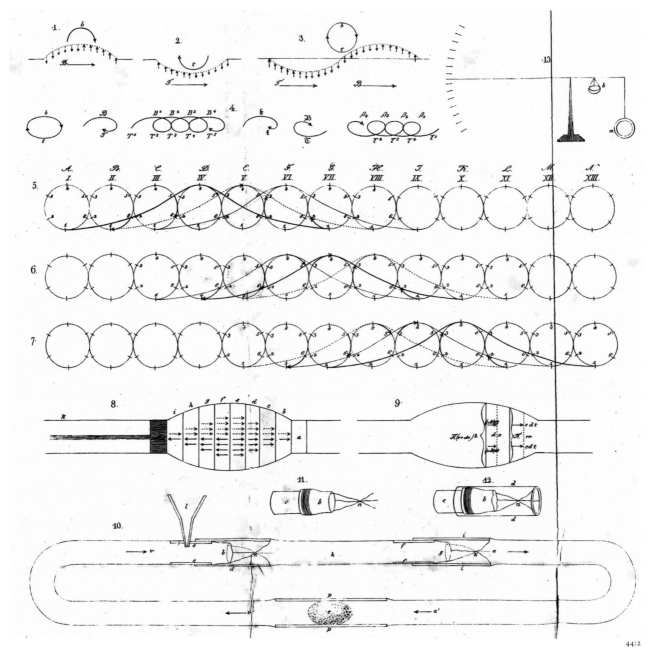

44:2

WEBER was born in 1795 in Wittenberg, where his father was professor of theology. As a boy he met Chladni (44.1) and became interested in physics. He started to study medicine in Wittenberg and received his degree in Leipzig in 1817. Four years later he was appointed professor of comparative anatomy, a position that he held for fifty years, till his retirement. From 1840 to 1866, when he was succeeded by Ludwig (44.2), he also held the chair of physiology. Weber made many important contributions to anatomy. Some of the structures that he discovered still bear his name. In physiology, working with his youngest brother Eduard, he made the famous demonstration of the inhibitory effect of the vagus nerve on the heart (44.3). He also pioneered sensory physiology, particularly concerning tactile sensations related to skin and muscle (44.4), making him one of the founders of psychophysics (the study of stimulus versus sensation).

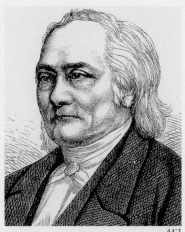

Ernst Heinrich Weber   44:3

Ueber die Anwendung der Wellenlehre auf die Lehre vom Kreislaufe des Blutes und insbesondere auf die Pulslehre.

ARCH ANAT PHYSIOL BERLIN: VEIT; 1851. P497.

WEBER SUMS up a decade of research starting in 1825 (44.5) on the movement of fluids in elastic tubes as applied to the circulation of the blood (44.6). Using tubes of rubber or small intestines as models, Weber studies flow and pressure in open and closed circuits of flow. He explores the elastic nature of the arterial wall and its effect on pulse wave propagation and the resistance to and the attenuation of this wave by the capillary bed. He also discovers that the diameter of the blood vessels is under muscular and nervous control.

IN PERSPECTIVE:

The science of hydrodynamics started with the work of Bernoulli (44.7).Young studied the blood circulation and the function of the heart from a hydrodynamic standpoint in 1809 (44.8). Poiseuille established the laws of fluid flow in capillary tubes with rigid walls in the 1840s (44.9). Weber was the first to investigate fluid flow in elastic tubes in 1825, working together with a younger brother, Wilhelm (who is most well-known for his work on earth magnetism, the unit of magnetic flux being named after him) (44.5)(44.6). The paper cited above summarises his results, which remain valid despite many thorough subsequent investigations. They are still one of the cornerstones of modern concepts in haemodynamics. The three Weber brothers, Ernst, Wilhelm and Eduard, were forerunners of the "physico-mathematical" approach to physiology that was fully adopted by Du Bois-Reymond, Helmholtz and Ludwig (44.10) and their disciples (44.11) during the late 19th century.

44.1   See ref. 13.5.
44.2   See ref. 35.5 and ref. 37.5.
44.3   Weber E, Weber EH. Experimenta, quibus probaturnervos vagos ... *Ann Univ Med.* (Milano) 3ser. 1845; 20:227.
44.4   Weber EH. Der Tastsinn und das Gemeingefühl. R. Wagner *Handwörterbuch Physiol* III part 2 1850. p481.
44.5   See ref. 18.9.
44.6   Weber EH. Programma, Pulsum arteriarum non in omnibus arteriis simul, ... *Annot anat physiol.* 1 Leipzig; 1827.
44.7   See #18 Bernoulli page 104.
44.8   Young T. On the function of the heart and arteries. *Phil.Trans.* 1809; I:12.
44.9   See #35 Poiseuille page 188 and ref. 35.10.
44.10 See #42 Du Bois-Reymond page 224, #43 Helmholtz page 228, and ref. 35.5 and ref. 37.5.
44.11 Rothschuh C. *History of Physiology.* New York: R.E.Krieger; 1978.

PHILOSOPHICAL

TRANSACTIONS.

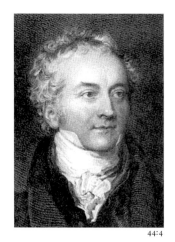

I. *The Croonian Lecture.   On the Functions of the Heart and Arteries.   By* Thomas Young, *M. D. For. Sec. R. S.*

Read November 10, 1808.

44:4

44:5

In examining the functions of the heart and arteries, I shall inquire, in the first place, upon the grounds of the hydraulic investigations which I have already submitted to the Royal Society, what would be the nature of the circulation of the blood, if the whole of the veins and arteries were invariable in their dimensions, like tubes of glass or of bone ; in the second place, in what manner the pulse would be transmitted from the heart through the arteries, if they were merely elastic tubes ; and in the third place, what actions we can with propriety attribute to the muscular coats of the arteries themselves.   I shall lastly add some observations on the disturbances of these motions, which may be supposed to occur in different kinds of inflammations and of fevers.

44:6

Thomas Young (1773–1829) makes many important contributions both in physics and in physiology (see #5). In this lecture from 1808 he discusses the properties of the circulatory system from a remarkably modern standpoint. His work exerts significant influence on the subsequent studies of the Weber brothers.

When we consider the blood vessels as tubes of invariable dimensions, we may suppose, in order to determine the velocity of the blood in their different parts, and the resistances opposed to its motion, that this motion is nearly uniform, since the alternations, arising from the pulsation of the heart, do not materially affect the calculation, especially as they are much less sensible in the smaller vessels than in the larger ones, and the principal part of the resistance arises from these small vessels. We are to consider the blood in the arteries as subjected to a certain pressure, by means of which it is forced into the veins, where the tension is much less considerable; and this pressure, originating from the contractions of the heart, and continued by the tension of the arteries, is almost entirely employed in overcoming the friction of the vessels: for the force required to overcome the inertia of the blood is so inconsiderable, that it may, without impropriety, be wholly neglected. We must therefore inquire, what the magnitude of this pressure is, and what degree of resistance we can suppose to arise from the friction of the internal surface of the blood vessels, or from any other causes of retardation. The magnitude of the pressure has been ascertained by Hales's most interesting experiments on a variety of animals, and may thence be estimated with sufficient accuracy for the human body; and for determining the magnitude of the resistance, I shall employ the theorems which I have deduced from my own experiments on very minute tubes, compared with those which had been made by former observers under different circumstances; together with some comparative experiments on the motion of water and of other fluids in the same tubes.

B 2

44:7

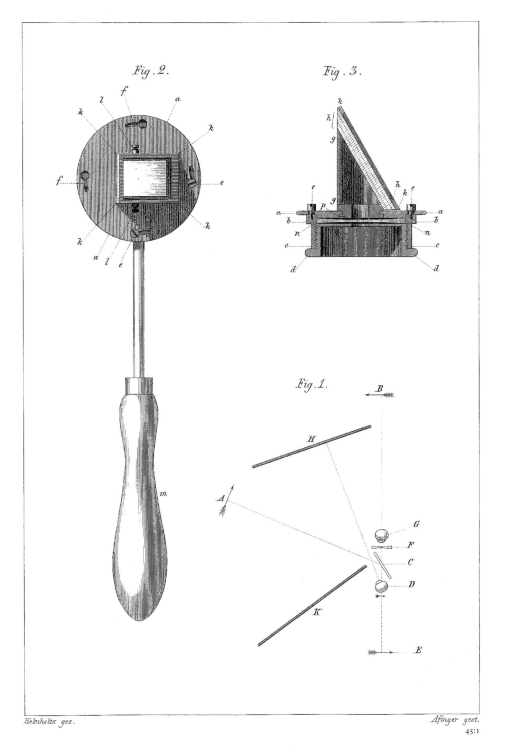

In 1850 Hermann von Helmholtz (1821–1894) announces the invention of the ophthalmoscope. His illustration of the device is shown on the right. After eight days of work Helmholtz has a prototype instrument ready and reports "I had the great pleasure to be the first to observe the retina in a living human being." He examined the eye of his wife Olga.

Although the great ophthalmologist Alfred von Graefe (1828–1870) declares "Helmholtz has unfolded to us a new world", others are less enthusiastic. Helmholtz reminisced "As regards the ophthalmoscope, a highly regarded surgical colleague told me that he would never use the instrument, that it was too dangerous to allow its harsh light to impinge upon a diseased eye; another declared that the ophthalmoscope might be of use to doctors with bad eyes, but that he had very good eyes and had no call for it."

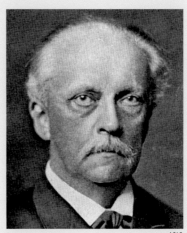

ELMHOLTZ was born in 1821, the oldest of four children of a Potsdam collage teacher with strong aesthetically and philosophical interests. He was drawn to physics early on, but the family could only afford a medical education, for which state scholarships were available. After taking his degree in 1842, Helmholtz started his eight-year duty as an army surgeon, a commitment he made to receive a stipend. In 1847 he presented his classic paper on the conservation of energy (45.1). On Humboldt's (45.2) request, Helmholtz was soon released from his obligations as a surgeon and was appointed professor of physiology in Königsberg. For more than two decades he held similar positions in Bonn and in Heidelberg, doing research primarily on sensory physiology (45.3). In 1871 he succeeded Magnus (45.4) in Berlin as professor of physics and devoted himself primarily to problems in thermodynamics and in electrodynamic action. He also wrote extensively on philosophical issues particularly concerning problems of scientific methodology (45.5)

Beschreibung eines Augen-Spiegels zur Untersuchung der Netzhaut im lebenden Auge.

BERLIN: FÖRSTNER'SCHE VERLAGSBUCHHANDLUNG; 1851.

HELMHOLTZ FIRST recounts how the work of Ernst Brücke led him to the invention of the ophthalmoscope. He then explains his line of thinking when solving the practical problems of observing the retina from outside and then gives a description of the instrument. He also derives a formula for the amount of light reflected from the retina that reaches the eye of the observer.

IN PERSPECTIVE:

Scheiner in 1619 was the first to locate the seat of vision as the retina (45.6). Cumming and Brücke independently noted that the human eye could be made luminous and Cumming considered its diagnostic potential (45.7)(45.8)(45.9). Stimulated by Brücke's research, Helmholtz developed the ophthalmoscope in eight days. He first used it to look into the eyes of his wife Olga and dedicated a copy of his book to her with the words "in remembrance that her eye was the first whose interior revealed itself to the searching eye". Helmholtz said on the early reception of his invention (45.10): "one of my very famous surgical colleagues told me that he would never use such an instrument, since in his opinion it was far too dangerous to allow the entrance of such bright light into the eye". The electric ophthalmoscope, with its built-in light source, was introduced in 1896. During the following years many practical improvements were made (45.9) and in particular the co-operation between Gullstrand and the Carl Zeiss company led to significant advances in design (45.11) and also to many other new ophthalmologic instruments.

45.1 See ref. 43.1.
45.2 On Humboldts influence see #36 Dumas page 192, #39 Liebig page 208 and #42 Du Bois-Reymond page 224 and also ref. 19.9.
45.3 See ref. 43.3.
45.4 See #37 Magnus page 196.
45.5 See ref 43.5.
45.6 See ref. 5.7 and also #5 Kepler page 42.
45.7 Cumming W. On a luminous appearance of the human eye, and its application to the detection of disease of the retina and psoterior part of the eye. *Med.-Chir Trans Med Chir Soc* London. 1846; 29:283.
45.8 Brücke E. Über das Leuchten der menschlichen Augen. *Anat Phys wis Med* 1847. p225.
45.9 Friedenwald H. *The History of the Invention and of the Development of the Ophthalmoscope.* JAMA 1902; 38(9):549.
45.10 See ref. 4.9 p.20.
45.11 Gullstrand A. Die reflexlose Ophtalmoskopie. *Arch Augenheilkunde* 1911; 68:101. See also #64 Abbe page 328.

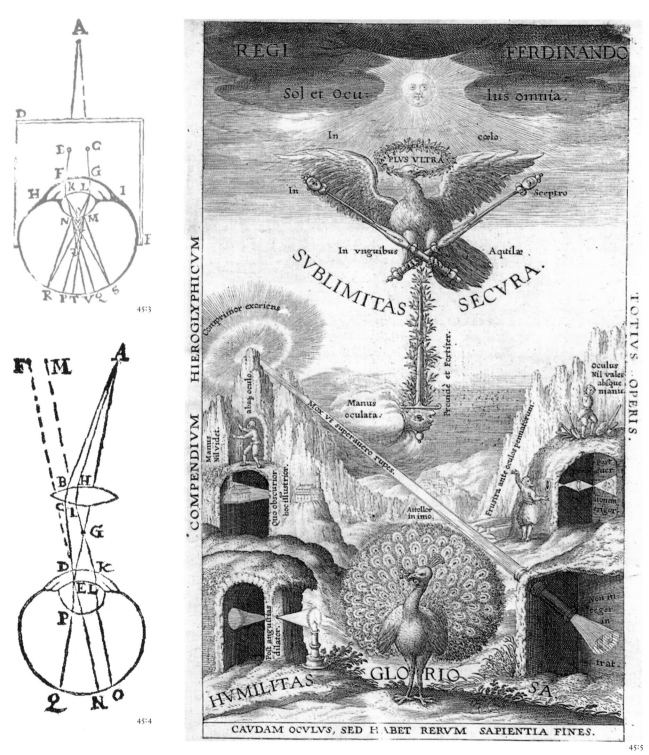

45:3

45:4

REGI FERDINANDO

Sol et Ocu: lus omnia.

In cœlo

PLVS VLTRA

In Sceptro

In vnguibus Aquilæ

SVBLIMITAS SECVRA.

COMPENDIVM HIEROGLYPHICVM

TOTIVS OPERIS.

Compressior exoriens

Oculus Nil valet absque manu

absq; oculo.

Manus Nil videt.

Quo obscurior hoc illustrior.

Manus oculata.

Mox vt superauero rupes.

Prcunde et Fortiter.

Frustra ante oculos pennatorum.

Post euer.

tionem erigor.

Attollor in imo.

Post angustias dilator.

Nen in teger in trat.

HVMILITAS GLO RIO SA

CAVDAM OCVLVS, SED HABET RERVM SAPIENTIA FINES.

45:5

Christoph Scheiner (1573–1650) is the first to show that the retina is the seat of vision. He demonstrates that accommodation is an active process and makes accurate diagrams of the eye. The illustrations on the left are taken from his investigations.

The famous frontispiece of Scheiner's book "Oculus hoc est fundamentum opticum" from 1619, which shows six small scenes (three on the right and three on the left) symbolising his studies of vision and the image formation in the eye.

ON A
LUMINOUS APPEARANCE
OF
THE HUMAN EYE,
AND ITS APPLICATION TO THE DETECTION OF DISEASE OF THE RETINA AND POSTERIOR PART OF THE EYE.

By WILLIAM CUMMING,
LATE HOUSE-SURGEON TO THE LONDON HOSPITAL.

COMMUNICATED BY T. B. CURLING,
ASSISTANT-SURGEON TO THE LONDON HOSPITAL.

Received June 1st—Read June 23rd, 1846.

THE luminous appearance of the eyes of cats, dogs, rabbits, oxen, sheep, and other animals, has been long known, and referred to the reflection of light by the tapetum; as also the reflection from the eye of the Albino, the reflection produced by morbid deposits in, and other changes of, the retina; and from the deficiency of pigment in persons not Albinoes.

Müller, (page 93, by Baly,) in a paragraph on the development of light in the higher animals, says, "The luminous appearance of the eyes of some animals arises from the reflection of the light from a brilliant tapetum which is devoid of black pigment; for which reason the eye of the white rabbit is especially brilliant, and the eyes of the Albino Sachs are said to have been luminous. Prevost was the first to explain the phenomenon: he showed that it could never be seen in complete darkness, and is dependent neither on the will, nor on the passions, but is the effect of the reflection of light which enters the eye from without."

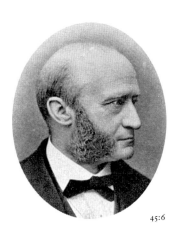

Ernst Brücke (1819–1892) observes the reflected light from the eyes of rabbits, cats and man, but fails to make the invention of the ophthalmoscope because, as Helmholtz put it, "he did not ask himself how an optical image is formed by the light returning from the eye."

45:6

45:7

Already in 1846 William Cumming (1812–1886) establishes that every healthy human eye can be made luminous. He is also the first to suggest the use of this phenomenon for the examination of the retina and the porterior portion of the eyeball.

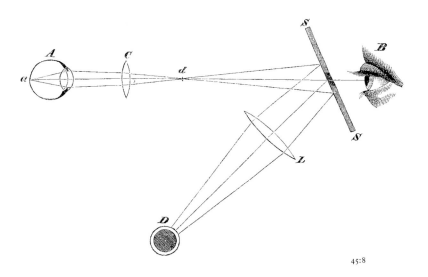

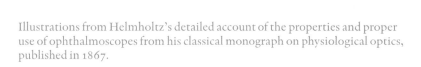

45:8

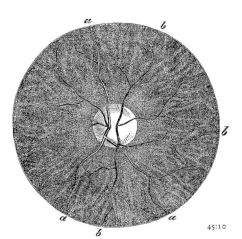

45:10

Illustrations from Helmholtz's detailed account of the properties and proper use of ophthalmoscopes from his classical monograph on physiological optics, published in 1867.

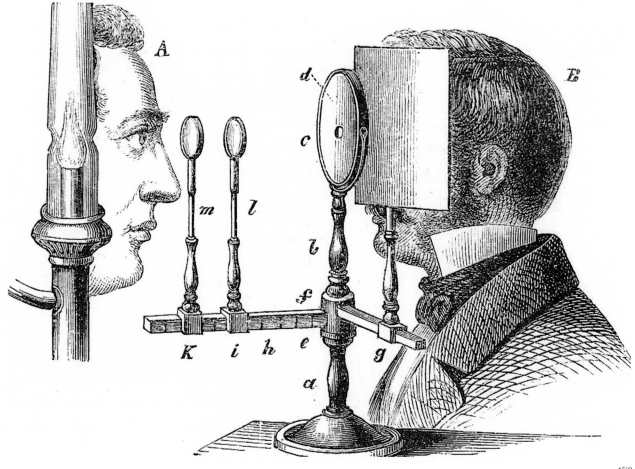

45:9

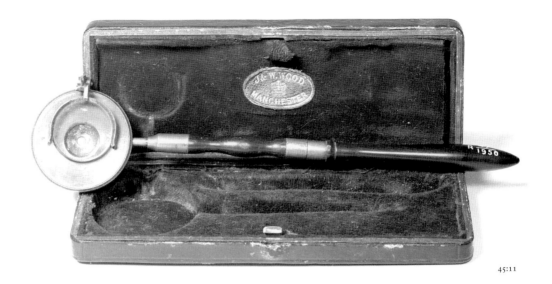

45:11

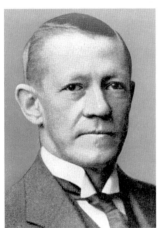

45:12

Alvar Gullstrand (1862–1930) presents a detailed mathematical analysis of the accommodation mechanism of the eye and, in collaboration with the company Carl Zeiss, constructs a superior ophthalmoscope in 1911 (right).

Top picture shows ophthalmoscope designed ca. 1860 by Richard Liebreich (1830–1917), who publishes an Atlas of Ophthalmoscopy in 1863. It is the first iconography of the fundus oculi.

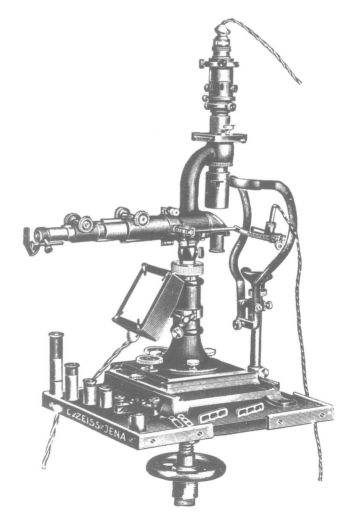

45:13

46:1

Adolf Fick (1829–1901) gives, in "Die medicinische Physik", the first comprehensive overview of the various applications of physics in medicine.

Fick sets up the diffusion equation and establishes the definition of the diffusion coefficient "k". He points out the analogy to Fourier's theory of heat flow (see #32).

nicht streng richtig ist) übertragen hat. Man darf nur in dem Fourier'schen Gesetz das Wort Wärmequantität mit dem Worte Quantität des gelösten Körpers, und das Wort Temperatur mit Lösungsdichtigkeit vertauschen. Der Leitungsfähigkeit entspricht in unserem Falle eine von der Verwandtschaft der beiden Körper abhängige Constante.

Das Gesetz kann nun in Bezug auf die Verbreitung eines in Wasser löslichen Salzes, dessen spezifisches Gewicht das des Wassers übertrifft, in diesem letzteren so ausgedrückt werden (wobei auf die kleine Verdichtung bei der Mischung ungleich concentrirter Lösungen keine Rücksicht genommen wird). In einer Masse von Salzlösung sei in jeder horizontalen Elementarschicht die Concentration constant und $= y$ einer Function der Höhe x dieser Schicht über irgend einer als Anfang angenommenen Horizontalebene, wobei noch die Einschränkung zu machen ist, dass die Function y mit wachsendem x abnehmen müsse, d. h. dass jede höhere Schicht weniger concentrirt (also leichter) als alle darunter liegenden sein müsse, weil nur in diesem Falle die Diffusion nicht durch die Schwere gestört wird; dann wird aus der Elementarschicht zwischen den Horizontalebenen bei x und $x + dx$ (in welcher die Concentration y ist) während des Zeitdifferentials dt in die nächst höher liegende, von den Horizontalebenen bei $x + dx$ und $x + 2dx$ begrenzte, in welcher die Concentration $y + \frac{dy}{dx} dx$ herrscht, eine Salzmenge übertreten $= - Q . k . \frac{dy}{dx} dt$, wo Q die Oberfläche der Schicht und k eine von der Natur der Substanzen abhängige Constante bedeutet. Gleichzeitig tritt natürlich eine an Volum jener Salzmenge gleiche Wassermenge aus der oberen Schicht in die untere.

Genau nach dem Muster der Fourier'schen Entwicklung für den Wärmestrom leitet man aus diesem Grundgesetze für den Diffusionsstrom die Differentialgleichung her

$$\frac{\delta y}{\delta t} = - k \left(\frac{\delta^2 y}{\delta x^2} + \frac{1}{Q} \frac{dQ}{dx} . \frac{\delta y}{\delta x} \right) \quad . . . . . \quad (1)$$

wenn der Querschnitt Q des Gefässes, in welchem der Strom statthat, eine Funktion seiner Höhe über dem Boden ist. Ist der Querschnitt constant (d. h. das Gefäss cylindrisch oder prismatisch), so vereinfacht sich die Differentialgleichung zu

$$\frac{\delta y}{\delta t} = - k \frac{\delta^2 y}{\delta x^2} \quad . . . . \quad (2).$$

46:2

FICK was born in 1829 in Kassel, where his father was municipal architect. The youngest of nine children, he started to study mathematics and physics in Marburg, where one of his brothers was professor of anatomy. He soon turned to medicine and was guided not only by his brother but also by Carl Ludwig (46.1). In Berlin Fick met and made friends with Du Bois-Reymond and Helmholtz (46.2). In 1851 Fick obtained his doctorate and left for Zürich to work as prosector in anatomy with Ludwig and later as professor of anatomy and physiology. He moved to the chair of physiology in Würzburg in 1868 and remained there till his retirement in 1899. Fick was a modest man with strong convictions that he always stood by without hesitation. Apart from his remarkably diverse scientific interests, he also wrote on social issues. In particular he strongly opposed the abuse of alcohol (46.3).

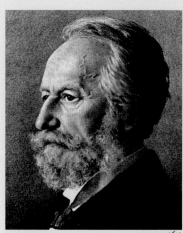

Adolf Fick   46:3

Die medicinische Physik.

BRAUNSCHWEIG: VIERWEG F UND SOHN; 1856.

IN EIGHT chapters Fick gives a concise account of science and technology as applied to medicine and physiology. The following topics are covered: Molecular physics (diffusion of gases and liquids), Mechanics (statics and dynamics of muscular action), Hydrodynamics (fluid flow in blood vessels, blood pressure), Sound (propagation and auscultation), Heat (chemical processes of heat generation, conservation of energy), Optics (geometrical optics and its application to the eye, ophthalmoscopy and colour vision), Electricity (currents and their role in nerve and muscle and electrotherapy) and finally Useful instrumentation (sphygmograph, microscope, ophthalmoscope, electric induction equipment, galvanometer).

IN PERSPECTIVE:
Fick mastered all advances in mathematics, physics and chemistry and was able to apply them to problems in medicine and physiology (46.4). Thus he was the first to approach muscular contraction from the principle of the conservation of energy (46.5) and to design a test of the chemical theory of the energy production in the muscle, proposed by Liebig (46.6). Fick set up the diffusion equation and introduced the collodion membrane in the study of diffusion through porous media (46.7)(46.8). His contributions to haemodynamics include the introduction of the principle of plethysmography (46.9) and the method of cardiac output determination that is named after him (46.10). He also developed the first practical device for intraocular pressure measurements (46.11). Fick and his generation of 19th century German physiologists (46.1)(46.2) worked with the simplest possible arrangements, under constant or controlled conditions, making observations with scientific methods and measuring devices often of their own construction or modified to suit the particular purpose of the experiment.

46.1 See ref. 35.5 and ref. 37.5 also #42 Du Bois-Reymond page 224 and #44 Weber page 232.

46.2 See #42 Du Bois-Reymond page 224 and #43 Helmholtz page 228, #45 Helmholtz page 238.

46.3 Fick A. *Die Alkoholfrage*. (Vortrag Würzburg am 16 März 1892) Würzburg; 1892.

46.4 Fick A. *Gesammelte Schriften*. Band I–IV Würzburg; 1903–1905.

46.5 Fick A. *Experimenteller Beitrag zur Lehre von der Erhaltung der Kraft bei der Muskelzusammenziehung*. Untersuchungen aus dem physiologischen Laboratorium der Züricher Hochschule. Wien; 1869.

46.6 Fick A, Wislicenus J. Ueber die Entstehung der Muskelkraft. *Vierteljahresschrift Zurch Natur Gesell* Vol. X 1865. See also #39 Liebig page 208.

46.7 Fick A. Ueber Diffusion. *Ann Phys Chem* 1855; 94:59. See also Tyrell HJ. The Origin and Present Status of Fick's Diffusion Law. *J Chem Ed*. 1964; 41(7):397.

46.8 Fick A. Ueber Endosmose. *Wiener med Wochenschrift* 1857; 45:809/810.

46.9 Fick A. *Die Geschwindigkeitskurve in der Arterie des lebenden Menschen*. Untersuchungen aus dem physiologischen Laboratorium der Züricher Hochschule Wien; 1869.

46.10 See #56 Fick page 290.

46.11 Fick A. Ueber Messung des Druckes im Auge. *Pfluger's Arch ges Physiol* 1888; 42:86.

VII. THE BAKERIAN LECTURE.—*On Osmotic Force.*
By THOMAS GRAHAM, *F.R.S.* &c.

Received June 15,—Read June 15, 1854.

THE expression " Osmotic Force " (from ὠσμὸς, *impulsio*) has reference to the endosmose and exosmose of DUTROCHET.

We may succeed in covering a solution of salt occupying the lower part of a glass jar by a stratum of pure water without much intermixture of the two liquids. A force, however, is thereby brought into action which carries up the salt in a gradual manner, dispersing it and ultimately producing a uniform mixture of the salt with the whole volume of water. The molecules of salt have the liquid condition when in solution as well as those of water itself, and we have in the experiment the contact of two different liquids, which must of necessity diffuse through each other, the molecules of a liquid being self-repellent, or subject to a force the same in kind but less in degree as that which gives to gases their elasticity and diffusibility.

The force of liquid diffusibility will still act if we interpose between the two liquids a porous sheet of animal membrane or of unglazed earthenware; for the pores of such a septum are occupied by water, and we continue to have an uninterrupted liquid communication between the water on one side of the septum and the saline solution on the other side.

46:5

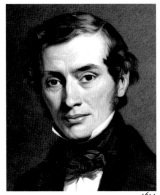

46:4

Thomas Graham (1805–1869) studies diffusion in gases and solutions and discovers and names the phenomenon now known as the osmotic force. He finds that certain substances (i.e. glue) pass more slowly through membranes than others (i.e. common salt). He calls the former colloids and the latter crystalloids and introduces the notion of dialysis to describe these observations. The beginning of his famous lecture "On osmotic force" with illustrations of his equipment is shown on the right.

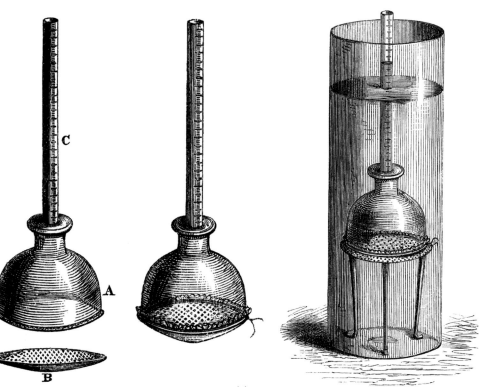

46:6

46:7

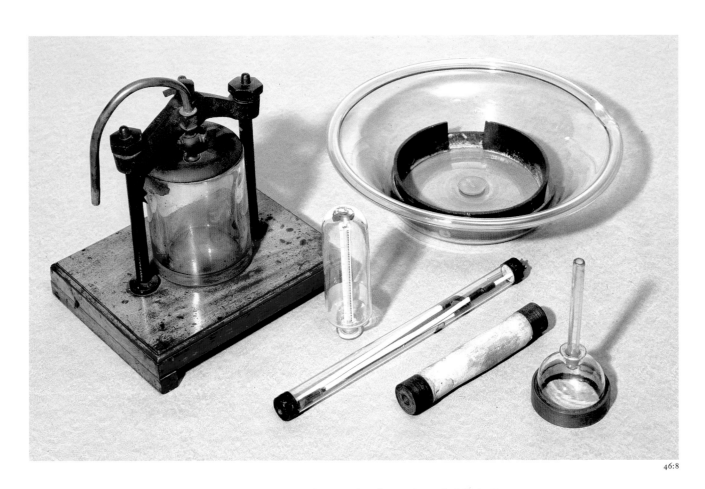

46:8

Graham's osmometer, where a semi-permeable membrane is fitted over the end of the bell jar.
Compare with drawings from his publication from 1854 on the opposite page.

Sonnabend den 7. November.   № **45.**   Siebenter Jahrgang 1857.

Bureau: Stadt, Herrengasse Nr. 252.   Jeden Sonnabend erscheint eine Nummer.

Wiener Medizinische Wochenschrift.

Man pränumeriert in Wien im Bureau der „Wiener mediz. Wochenschrift" und in Seidel's Buchhandlung, Graben §122. Ausser Wien in den Buchhandlungen und Postämtern. Geldsendungen müssen frankirt werden.

Preis dieser Wochenschrift für Wien und im Buchhandel ganzjährig 8 fl., halbjährig 4 fl., mit Postzusendung ganzjährig 10 fl., halbjährig 5 fl. C.-Mze. Inserate werden mit 8 kr. pr. zweispaltige Petitzeile berechnet.

Ueber Endosmose.

Von **Professor A. Fick** in Zürich.

Die unsicheren und widerspruchsvollen Resultate der meisten endosmotischen Versuche mit thierischen Häuten hatten schon lange in mir die Vermuthung rege gemacht, dass zwei ganz verschiedene Prozesse des Durchganges flüssiger Körper durch permeable Scheidewände unter dem Begriffe der Endosmose zusammengeworfen würden, und dass diese beiden Vorgänge bei thierischen Membranen in den meisten Fällen gleichzeitig auftreten und so der eine das gesetzmässige Erscheinen des andern verdeckt. Die Bestätigung dieser Vermuthung sehe ich als das wichtigste Resultat einer umfassenderen Experimentaluntersuchung an, die ich der Naturforscher-Versammlung in Bonn vorzulegen die Ehre hatte, und die demnächst ausführlich in ihrem ganzen Umfange in der physiologischen Zeitschrift des Hrn. Moleschott erscheinen wird. *)

Es hat sich nämlich ganz wie ich vermuthete herausgestellt, dass der Austausch heterogener aber mischbarer Flüssigkeiten durch Struktur- also porenlose Scheidewände, — der demnach durch die eigentlichen Molekularinterstitien vor sich gehen muss, — nach ganz anderen Gesetzen geschieht als der Austausch solcher Flüssigkeiten durch eine Scheidewand mit wirklichen Poren oder Löchern. Zur Untersuchung des erstbezeichneten Vorganges dienten mir Beutelchen von Kollodium, zur Untersuchung des andern Thonscheidewände; als heterogene Flüssigkeiten habe ich bis jetzt auf der einen Seite immer Wasser, auf der andern Lösungen verschiedener Salze, namentlich von Chlornatrium angewandt. Ich kann in dieser kurzen Ankündigung nicht näher auf die Methode meiner Versuche eingehen. Nur eine Bemerkung kann ich nicht unterdrücken. Es hat mir trotz wiederholter ernsthafter Bemühungen nie gelingen wollen, eine Kollodiummembran horizontal auszuspannen, so dass sie zu einer ausgedehnteren Versuchsreihe brauchbar gewesen wäre, und ich habe mich desshalb mit den erwähnten Beutelchen begnügen müssen, was mancherlei Missstände und Fehler herbeiführte, die eine sonst überflüssige Vervielfältigung der Versuche nothwendig machte.

Die Gesetze der wahren Endosmose durch eine aus quellungsfähiger Substanz gebildete aber strukturlose Scheidewand — wie meine Kollodiummembranen — scheinen sehr einfach, so weit sie sich auf die Abhängigkeit des Vorganges von der Konzentration der angewandten Salzlösung beziehen. Auf diesen Punkt hatte ich zunächst allein mein Augenmerk gerichtet. Befindet sich in einem Kollodiumbeutelchen eine Salzlösung, und wird dasselbe gleichzeitig umspült von reinem Wasser, so wird die Substanz des Beutels, wie Jedermann bekannt, von zwei entgegengesetzt gerichteten endosmotischen Strömen durchsetzt. Es geht ein Wasserstrom von aussen nach innen und ein Salzstrom von innen nach aussen. Es ist ferner allgemein bekannt, dass der Wasserstrom viel stärker ist als der Salzstrom, es ging beiläufig gesagt in den meisten meiner Versuche mehr als hundertmal so viel Wasser in der Zeiteinheit nach innen als Salz nach aussen. Das Verhältniss dieser beiden Stromstärken bezeichnet man gemeiniglich als das endosmotische Aequivalent, doch dürfte diese

*) Der geehrte Verfasser hat auf unser ausdrückliches Ersuchen obigen Artikel uns freundlichst überlassen.   D. Red.

Grösse zunächst kaum von dem hohen Interesse sein, das man ihr vielfach beigelegt hat.

Ich habe an meinen Kollodiumhäuten vor Allem eine höchst merkwürdige und vielleicht für eine dereinstige Theorie lehrreiche Veränderlichkeit mit der Zeit beobachtet. Sie hat mich theils im Allgemeinen sehr überrascht, da ich gewiss mit Allen in Uebereinstimmung von dem Vortheil ausging, eine Kollodiumhaut sei ein ganz konstantes Ding; theils noch ganz im Besonderen, weil sie nur eine relative ist. In Beziehung auf den endosmotischen Wasserstrom verhält sich nämlich die Membran in der That ganz konstant, d. h. sie lässt unter sonst gleichen Bedingungen — bei gleicher Temperatur, gleicher Konzentration etc. — immer gleich viel Wasser durchtreten, mag sie zum erstenmal mit Flüssigkeiten in Berührung kommen oder schon wochenlang damit in Berührung gewesen sein. Die Durchgängigkeit der Membran für Salz ist dagegen, abgesehen von allen andern Umständen, abhängig von der Zeit, während welcher die Membran bereits mit Lösungen in Berührung war. Die Durchgängigkeit für Salz ist im Anfang Null und wächst mit der Zeit, und zwar langsamer als die Zeit, so dass vermuthlich nach einer gewissen Zeit ein stationärer Zustand eintritt, den ich aber leider nie habe beobachten können, weil mir die Membranen — sehr zerbrechlich wie sie sind — immer vor Erreichung desselben zu Grunde gingen. Beispielsweise ging durch eine gewisse Membran bei einer Konzentration von etwa 0,084 während 5 Minuten 8 Tage nach Beginn der Versuchsreihe 0,025 Mgr. Salz, einige Tage später 0,029 Mgr., noch später 0,08 Mgr. — Am besten springt die Gesetzmässigkeit dieser Veränderung der Membran in die Augen, wenn man ihre Durchgängigkeit für Salz als Funktion der Zeit graphisch darstellt durch die Ordinaten einer Kurve. Diese kehrt alsdann ihre konkave Seite gegen die Abscissenaxe, auf welcher die Zeiten gemessen werden, und geht durch den Ursprung der Koordinaten.

Die Abhängigkeit der endosmotischen Stromstärken von der Dichtheit der Lösungen im Innern der Membran ist folgende: Die Wasserstromstärke wächst durchweg und stetig mit zunehmender Lösungsdichtheit, jedoch in den meisten Fällen etwas langsamer als diese, so dass zu einer doppelt so dichten Lösung ein nicht ganz doppelt so starker Wasserstrom geht. Als Maass der Dichtheit ist dabei der Quotient des gelösten Salzes dividirt durch das Gewicht der Lösung anzusehen. In Versuchsreihen, wo die Wasserstromstärke überall nicht bedeutend war, ist die der soeben bezeichneten Grösse nahezu proportional, nicht aber der Grösse, durch welche Jolly die Konzentration misst und welcher er die Wasserstromstärke proportional setzt — nämlich dem Quotienten des gelösten Salzes dividirt durch das lösende Wasser. Die Abhängigkeit der Salzstromstärke von der Konzentration lässt sich aus meinen Versuchsreihen wegen der vorhin erwähnten Veränderung der Membran nur mittelbar folgern. Ceteris paribus scheint die Salzstromstärke mit zunehmender Konzentration noch langsamer zu wachsen als die Wasserstromstärke, so dass also das Verhältniss beider Ströme — das sogenannte endosmotische Aequivalent — mit zunehmender Konzentration selbst zunimmt.

Was das Verhalten verschiedener Salze bei dem fraglichen Vorgange betrifft, so habe ich bis jetzt erst wenig Material zur Vergleichung, jedoch sind zwei Beispiele, die ich vorführen kann, gerade

46:9

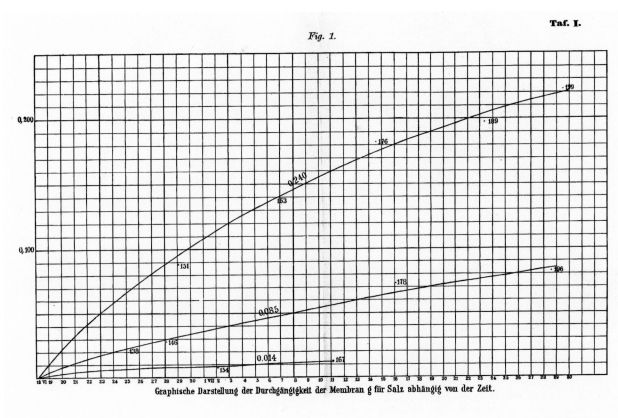

Fig. 1.

0,200

0,240

153

0,100

151

· 199

· 189

· 176

· 196

· 178

0,085

146

139

0,014

154

· 167

Graphische Darstellung der Durchgängigkeit der Membran g für Salz abhängig von der Zeit.

Versuche über Endosmose.

46:10

The graphs above show results from Fick's experiment with diffusion of a salt through a semipermeable collodion membrane.

In 1846 Christian Schönbein (1799–1868) discovers how to make pyroxylin ("guncotton"), a substance that soon finds important applications (see #38), including in medicine (see #77). A solution of pyroxylin in alcohol or ether produces collodion. Fick describes his experiment with a collodion membrane, in this way " … the exchange of heterogeneous, miscible fluid though a structure—here the non-porous septa—which must take place via the actual intermolecular interstices—occurs in accordance with quite different laws from the exchange of such fluids through a septum with actual pores or holes. In order to investigate the first mentioned process, I availed myself of phials of collodion and in order to investigate the second, septa from tuna; as heterogeneous fluids, I have hitherto used water on one side and on the other solutions of various salts, in particular chloride of soda."

sequently, whilst there is no impediment to the free passage of air through the apparatus, no ether escapes till it has been breathed by the patient. The mouth-piece I have adopted is furnished with the cushion and India-rubber described by Mr. Tracy in a recent number of the MED. GAZETTE. I use,

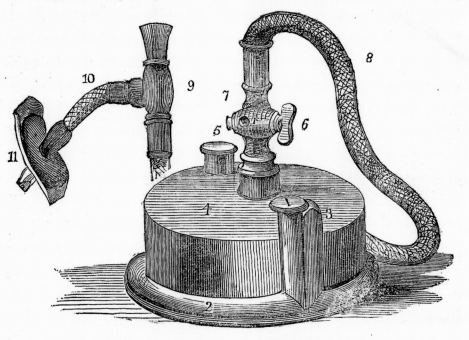

The first description given by John Snow (1813–1858) of his ether inhaler in the London Medical Gazette 1847.

1, Cap which unscrews to admit the air to
2, Metal pipe.
3, Entrance of ditto into
4, Spiral chamber.
5, Star closing aperture for putting in or pouring out ether.
6, Two-way tap.

7, External opening of ditto.
8, Flexible tube.
9, Ebony tube, containing ball valves of cedar wood.
10, Portion of flexible tube to admit of change of position of
11, Mouth-piece, with soft cushion, &c.

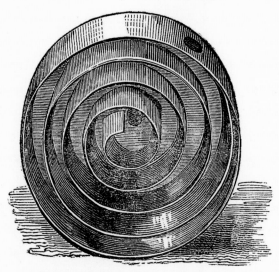

Interior of spiral chamber, the bottom being removed.
N.B.—The spiral tin plate is soldered to the top, and reaches nearly to the bottom.

47:1

248

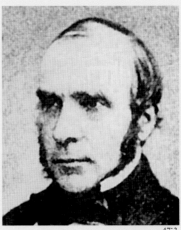

John Snow   47:2

J OHN Snow was born in 1813 in York and became a general practitioner in London in 1838. Having taken an interest in respiration physiology and the design of equipment for re-suscitation, he was soon able to improve on the methods of administering the new inhalation anaesthetic agents, (sulphuric) ether and chloroform, that were introduced in 1846–47. Snow, was the first full-time specialist in anaesthesia. Renowned for his insights and skills, he was invited to administer chloroform to Queen Victoria at the births of two of her children. The Queen's satisfaction greatly contributed to the acceptance of chloroform as anaesthetics in midwifery. Richardson, a prominent anaesthesiologist himself and a good friend of Snow, later wrote in a memoir of Snow (from the book cited below): "the naked truth, for its own sake, was what he sought and loved. No consideration of honour or profit seemed to have power to bias his opinions on any subject".

On Chloroform and Other Anaesthetics: Their Action and Administration.

LONDON; J. CHURCHILL 1858.

IN THIS last and major work of Snow, he reports experimental animal research on the physiology of the anaesthetic state and describes the first use of endotracheal anaesthesia. Snow investigates the physical and chemical properties of the anaesthetic agents and their concentrations in air and blood. The physiological effects of these concentrations are also elucidated. Fatal outcomes of chloroform anaesthesia are discussed and new improved inhalers for ether and chloroform are described.

IN PERSPECTIVE:
Paracelsus at the end of 16th century already recognised the anaesthetic effect of ether and Turner recommended it against headaches in 1761 (47.1). The clinical usefulness of ether inhalation was established by Long in 1842 (47.2), but widely accepted only after Morton's demonstration of pain relief during surgery (47.3). The first users of ether and chloroform were practical men with little scientific training (47.4)(47.5), unused to handling more elaborate equipment. Therefore, inhalation anaesthesia, particularly with chloroform, soon led to many fatal outcomes raising justified concerns (47.6). While Snow put the administration of anaesthetics on a firm scientific footing, prominent physiologists Longet and Bernard investigated the mechanism of anaesthetic action (47.7)(47.8). Subsequently, new agents, improved equipment and advances in respiration physiology have gradually improved the safety and efficacy of clinical anaesthesia. The evaporation method used in Snow's vaporisers is still the standard in modern equipment (47.9), although other systems have also been developed using direct pneumatic (47.10) and electronic (47.11) injection of the anaesthetic liquid into the breathing circuit.

47.1 See ref. 3.2 and ref. 3.6.
47.2 See ref. 3.7.
47.3 See ref. 3.9.
47.4 See ref 3.7, 3.9 and ref. 36.11.
47.5 Weiger J. Über Ether und Chloroform. Wien; 1850.
47.6 Report of the committee, appointed to inquire into the uses and the physiological, therapeutical and toxical effects of chloroform. *Medico-Chirurgical Trans The Roy.* Med Chir Soc London; 1864. See also ref. 23.10, and 23.11.
47.7 Longet F-A. *Expériences relatives aux effects de l'inhalation de l'éther sulphurique sur le système nerveux.* Paris; 1847.
47.8 Bernard C. *Leçons sur les anesthésiques et sur l'asphyxie.* Paris; 1875.
47.9 Dorsch JA, Dorsch SE. *Understanding Anesthesia Equipment.* Baltimore: Williams & Wilkins; 1994.
47.10 Gedeon A, Olsson SG. A new type of anæsthetic vaporizer. In: *30-th Ann Conf Eng Med Biol* 1977; 19: 203. See also ref. 47.9 p103.
47.11 Cooper JB et al. A new anesthesia delivery system. *Anesthesiology* 1978; 49:310.

Experiment 28. A young rabbit, rather more than half-grown, was made insensible by breathing air charged with four per cent. of vapour of chloroform in a large jar. The trachea was then opened, and a tube was introduced and tied. The lungs and heart were then exposed, by making an incision and removing the lower half of the sternum, with the adjoining part of the cartilages of the ribs on each side. The front of the pericardium was also cut away, to expose the heart. Whilst these operations were performed, artificial respiration was kept up by means of a bladder of air attached to the tube in the trachea. The heart contracted vigorously and quickly, and the lungs were of a light red colour. The rabbit was beginning to show signs of returning sensibility, when the bladder of air was changed for one containing ten per cent. of vapour of chloroform. The bladder contained 125 cubic inches, and twelve minims of chloroform were put in before it was filled with the bellows. Three or four inflations of the lungs only were made, when I perceived that the heart was beginning to be affected, and I changed the chloroform for a bladder containing only air. These three or four inflations of the lungs with chloroform, had the effect of causing the right cavities of the heart to become distended with blood, and its pulsations to become much slower. In two or three minutes, however, the action of the heart was quite reestablished by the artificial respiration, the pulsations being vigorous and

47:3

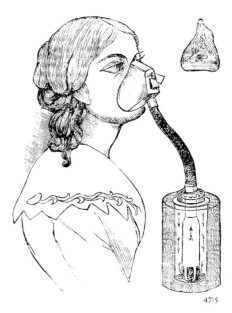

47:5

Snow's chloroform inhaler.

Left, description of the first intratracheal anaesthesia that Snow performs on a young rabbit, from 1858.

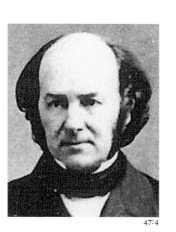

47:4

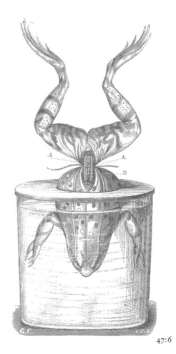

47:6

The mechanism of anaesthetic action is first explored in extensive animal experimentation by François Longet (1811–1871) (left). Later Claude Bernard (1813–1878) studies the effects of chloroform on the central nervous system using the frog preparation shown above.

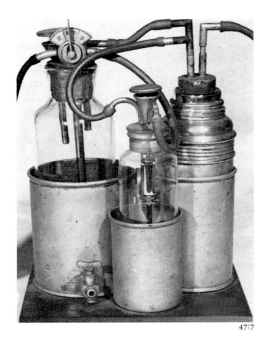

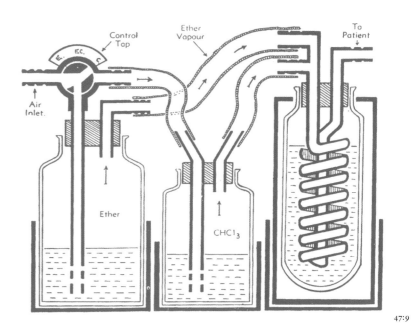

47:7

47:9

The principle and the realisation of a warm ether/chloroform vaporiser from 1916.

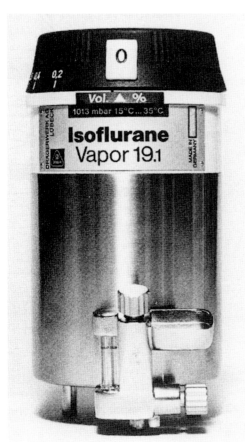

47:8

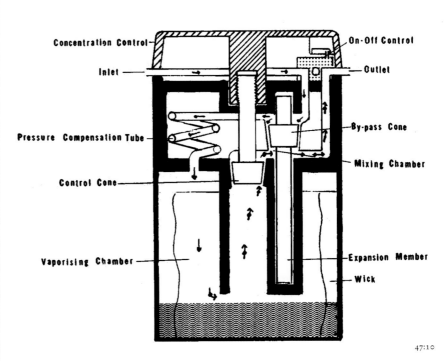

47:10

The principle and the realisation of a modern vaporiser for isoflurane. Basically the devices shown on this page are developments and refinements of the draw-over type of vaporiser that goes back to the original design of Snow illustrated in 47:1.

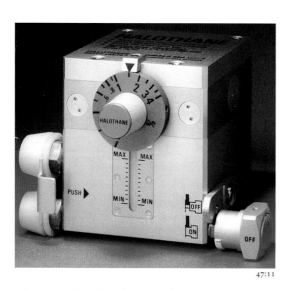

47:11

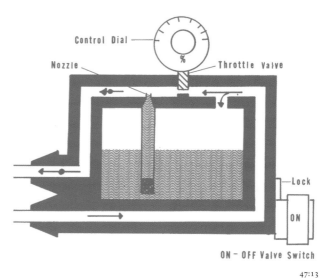

Control Dial

Nozzle   Throttle Valve

Lock

ON

ON − OFF Valve Switch

47:13

The principle and realisation of a vaporiser employing an injector of the anaesthetic liquid which is driven by the carrier gas flow.

An electronic anaesthetic liquid injection system with the vaporising coil (left). Also shown when mounted into the first electronic anaesthesia delivery unit from 1978.

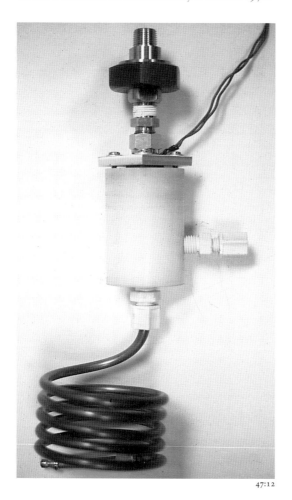

47:12

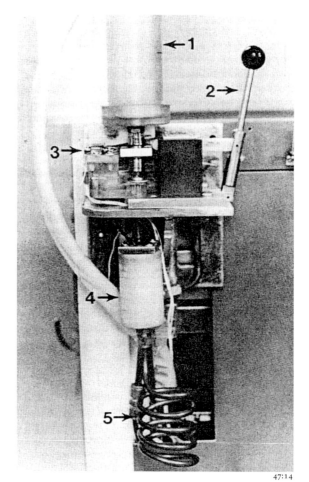

47:14

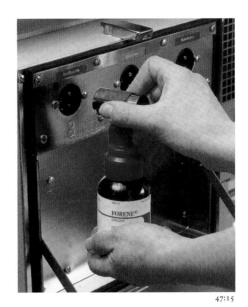

The vaporiser system of the first commercially available electronic anaesthesia machine from the late 1980s. The liquid anaesthetic is introduced through a keyed connector at the back of the unit. The liquid is vaporised in a temperature control chamber (below left) and the concentrated anaesthetic gas obtained in this way is electronically injected into the fresh gas flow.

47:15

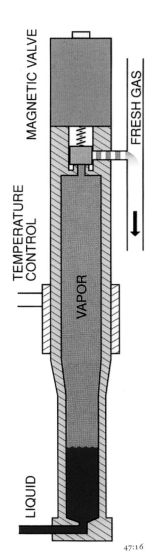

MAGNETIC VALVE

FRESH GAS

TEMPERATURE CONTROL

VAPOR

LIQUID

47:16

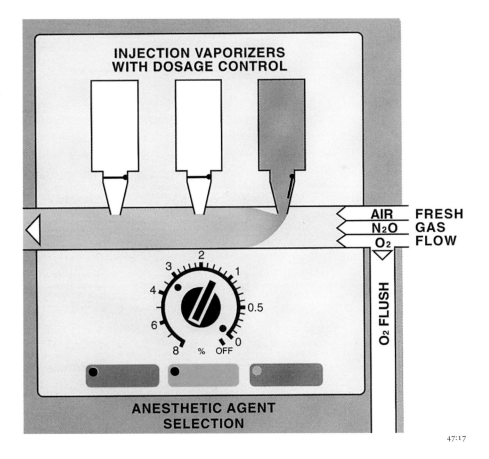

INJECTION VAPORIZERS WITH DOSAGE CONTROL

AIR
N₂O
O₂

FRESH GAS FLOW

O₂ FLUSH

ANESTHETIC AGENT SELECTION

47:17

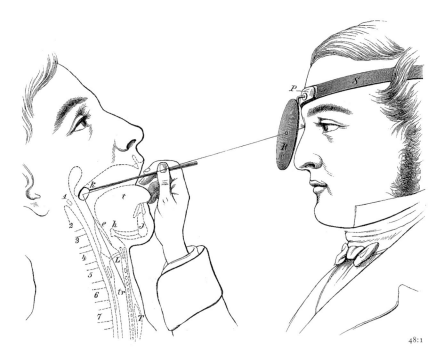

48:1

Johann Czermak (1828–1873) develops laryngoscopy into a practical method of examination. He substitutes artificial light for sunlight, develops special mirrors and lectures extensively to promote the clinical use of the technique.

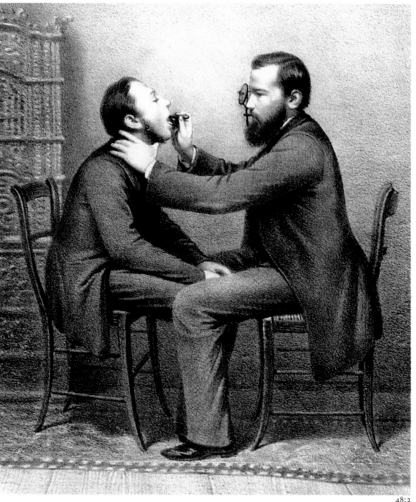

48:2

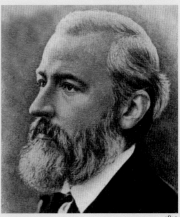

Johann Czermak

48:3

CZERMAK was born in 1828 in Prague. His father, grandfather and uncle were all physicians. As a boy he played the piano and showed both practical and theoretical talents. After the death of his father in 1843, he studied medicine, first in Vienna and later in Breslau where Purkinje, a friend of the family, became his life long mentor (48.1). In 1850 he concluded his studies in Würzburg and became assistant to Purkinje at the newly founded Physiological Institute in Prague. He was appointed professor of physiology in 1858 in Budapest, where his interest in the mechanism of speech lead him to laryngoscopic investigations. Two years later, unable to comply with the requirement to teach in Hungarian introduced by a new nationalistic government, he resigned. During his last years he worked in Prague, Jena and Leipzig and died at the age of only forty-five from the effects of diabetes.

Physiologische Untersuchungen mit Garcia's Kehlkopfspiegel.

SITZUNGSBERICHTE D K K AKADEMIE DER WISSENSCHAFTEN. WIEN; 1858; 29:557.

THIS IS the first detailed account published by Czermak of his improvements to the mirror arrangement of Garcia for the investigation of the larynx. Czermak introduces the use of a large perforated concave mirror to reflect light onto the laryngoscopic mirror and the use of artificial illumination to make the procedure easy to perform.

IN PERSPECTIVE:
Fothergill gave a classic description of malignant sore throats in 1748 (48.2). In the early 19th century the time was ripe to try to differentiate the various kinds of ulceration of the larynx (48.3). To this end Bozzini (1807), Babington (1829), Liston (1837) and others developed more or less impractical instruments for the investigation of the larynx (48.3). However, in 1855 Garcia, a singing teacher in London interested in the movements of his vocal cords when singing, described a mirror arrangement that, with the sun as the light source, could be used for such an investigation (48.4). Two years later, independently, Turk tried a similar mirror arrangement on his patients (48.5), but soon abandoned it as impractical for clinical work. Czermak borrowed Turk's mirrors and improved both the mirrors and the entire method. In the ensuing controversy with Turk over priority, Czermak justly argued that without his efforts "laryngoscopy would have been a dead-born child". Subsequently, both Turk and Czermak wrote and lectured extensively on laryngoscopy, helping to promote its rapid dissemination (48.6)(48.7)(48.8)(48.9). Mackenzie's epoch-making work established the technique as a useful clinical tool (48.10).

48.1 Kruta V. J. *E. Purkyne (1787–1869) Physiologist. A Short Account of His Contributions to the Progress of Physiology With a Bibliography of His Works*. Prag; 1969.

48.2 Foothergill J. *An Account of the Sore Throat*. London; 1748. See also ref. 23.3.

48.3 Stevenson RC, Guthrie G. *A History of Oto-Laryngology*. Edinburgh; 1949.

48.4 Garcia M. Observations on the Human Voice. *Phil Mag* 1855; 10:218.

48.5 Turk L. Der Kehlkopfrachenspiegel und die Methode seines Gebrauchs. *Zeit k k Ges Aertzte zu Wien* 1858; 1:401.

48.6 Czermak J. *Der Kehlkopfspiegel und seine Verwerthung für Physiologie und Medicin*. Leipzig; 1860.

48.7 Turk L. *Praktische Anleitung zur Laryngoskopie*. Wien; 1860.

48.8 Czermak J. *Gesammelte Schriften*. Bd. I, II Leipzig; 1879.

48.9 Czermak J. Populäre physiologische Vorträge III *Gesammelte Schriften* Bd II, Leipzig; 1879. p60.

48.10 Mackenzie M. *Essays on Growths in the Larynx*. London; 1871.

"Observations on the Human Voice." By Manuel Garcia, Esq.
The pages which follow are intended to describe some observations made on the interior of the larynx during the act of singing. The method which I have adopted is very simple. It consists in placing a little mirror, fixed on a long handle suitably bent, in the throat of the person experimented on against the soft palate and uvula. The party ought to turn himself towards the sun, so that the luminous rays falling on the little mirror, may be reflected on the larynx. If the observer experiment on himself, he ought, by means of a second mirror, to receive the rays of the sun, and direct them on the mirror, which is placed against the uvula. We shall now add our own deductions from the observations which the image reflected by the mirror has afforded us.

48:4

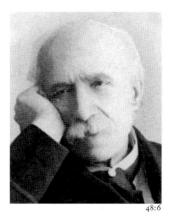

48:6

Manuel Garcia (1805–1906), a singing teacher interested in seeing the movements of his vocal cords while singing, describes a mirror arrangement that with the sun as the light source can be used for such a purpose.

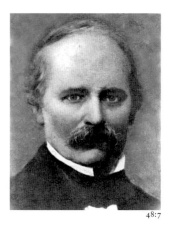

48:7

Ludwig Turck (1810–1868) attempts to use Garcia's technique clinically, but finds it impractical since he is dependent on sunlight, as illustrated in his book from 1866 (left). Later a bitter dispute develops between him and Czermak about the priority to have introduced clinical laryngoscopy.

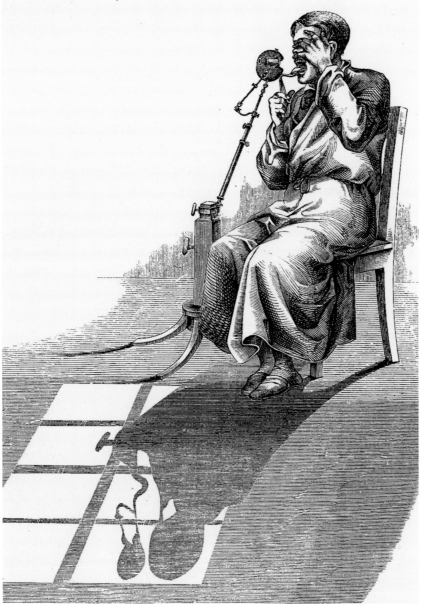

48:5

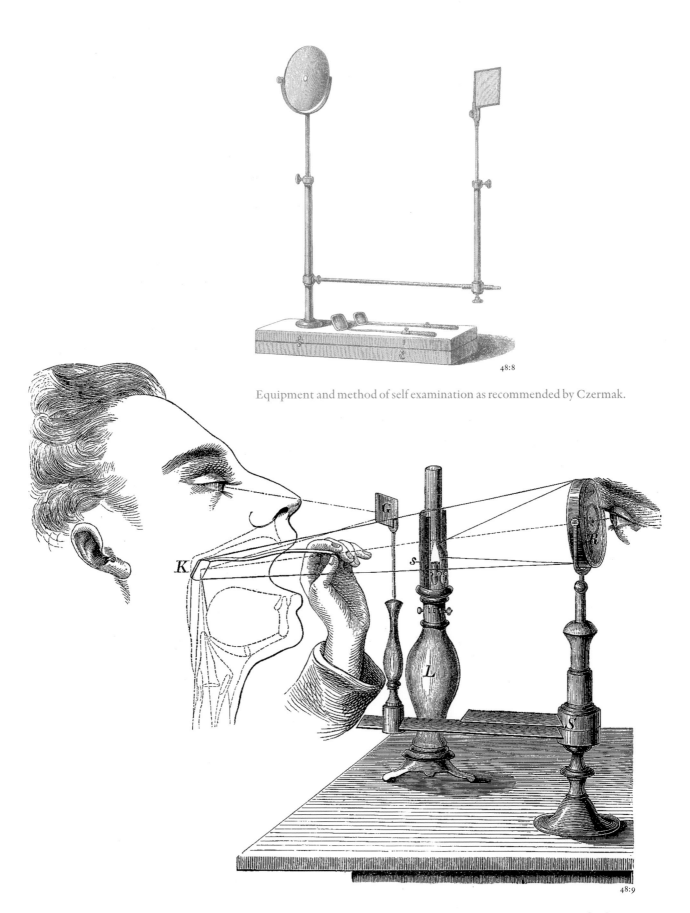

48:8

Equipment and method of self examination as recommended by Czermak.

48:9

Untersuchungen über das Sonnenspectrum und die Spectren der chemischen Elemente.

Von
Hⁿ· G. KIRCHHOFF.

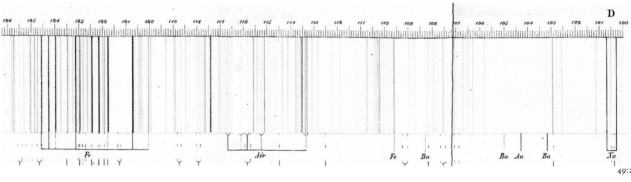

[Vorgetragen in der Akademie der Wissenschaften am 11. Juli 1861 von Hrn. Magnus.]

Das Sonnenspectrum.

Entwirft man durch ein Prisma ein Sonnenspectrum, das so rein als möglich ist, und betrachtet dasselbe durch ein Fernrohr von geringer Vergröfserung, so erblickt man zwischen den Linien, die Fraunhofer durch Buchstaben bezeichnet hat, ein Gewirre von feinen Linien und nebeligen Streifen, das dem Auge nur wenigen Anhalt darbietet. Wendet man mehr Prismen und eine stärkere Vergröfserung an, so treten, wenn die Apparate die nöthige Vollkommenheit besitzen, aus demselben mehr und mehr Liniengruppen hervor, die so characteristisch sind, dafs sie leicht aufgefafst und leicht wieder erkannt werden, Liniengruppen, die füglich verglichen werden können mit den Sterngruppen, die einzelne Sternbilder so leicht auffinden lassen. Von diesen Liniengruppen sind in der Fraunhoferschen Zeichnung des Sonnenspectrums (¹) nur sehr wenige kenntlich, und dasselbe gilt von der in gröfserem Maafstabe ausgeführten Zeichnung, die in neuester Zeit von Brewster und Gladstone (²) veröffentlicht ist. Ich habe dieselben für den hellsten Theil des Sonnenspectrums so vollständig und treu, als möglich, abzubilden gesucht; die Tafeln I und II sind lithographische Copieen der Zeichnung, die ich ausgeführt habe (³).

(¹) Denkschriften der Münchner Akademie für 1814 und 1815.

(²) *Phil. Trans. of the royal soc. of London for* 1860.

(³) Meine Zeichnung umfafst das Stück des Spectrums von *A* bis *G*; ich mufs mich darauf beschränken, jetzt nur einen Theil derselben zu veröffentlichen, da das Übrige noch Revisionen erfordert, die ich in nächster Zeit vorzunehmen aufser Stande bin, weil meine Augen durch die anhaltenden Beobachtungen des Spectrums zu sehr angegriffen sind.

49:1

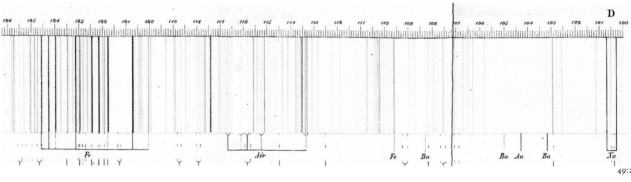

49:2

Gustav Kirchhoff

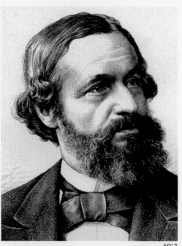

Gustav Kirchhoff   49:3

BORN in 1824 in Königsberg, Kirchhoff had a rather un-
eventful life. His father was a law counsellor and taught
Kirchhoff loyalty to the Prussian state but otherwise to
hold rather liberal values. Kirchhoff studied at the University of Königsberg and graduated in 1847. In 1851 he was
named professor of physics in Breslau, where he met and made
friends with Bunsen. In 1854, on Bunsen's initiative, Kirchhoff
moved to Heidelberg, where they worked together on the development of spectral analysis. Kirchhoff was an excellent teacher
and his lecture notes on theoretical physics set a standard at German universities. He was of a somewhat reserved but cheerful
character, which he maintained even during a long illness at the
end of his life. When his failing health prevented experimental
work, he accepted the chair of theoretical physics in Berlin, a post
that he held till his death in 1887.

Untersuchungen über das Sonnen-spectrum und die Spectren der chemischen Elemente.

ABHANDLUNGEN D K AKADEMIE D WISS ZU BERLIN JAHRE 1861.
BERLIN; 1862. P63.

IT WAS an unexplained fact that the dark bands in the light of the
sun, as first reported by Fraunhofer (49.1), coincided with the
bright lines emitted by sodium vapour in a "Bunsen burner".
Kirchhoff describes here his and Bunsen's remarkable discovery
(49.2)(49.3) that these dark bands get even darker if the sunlight is
allowed to pass through the sodium vapour. This observation
leads them to the conclusion that emission and absorption spectra
uniquely identify an element such as sodium.

IN PERSPECTIVE:
The impetus to this work came from Bunsen's desire to identify salts from their
colour in the flames of a "Bunsen burner", a device that had very high temperature
but low luminosity (49.4). Beginning with coloured pieces of glass, on Kirchhoff's
suggestion he turned to spectrographic recordings. These studies soon led to the
discovery of several new elements such as caesium and rubidium (49.2)(49.3) and
eventually to Kirchhoff's law of the spectral distribution of radiation from a
"black body". Although the colour of urine has been an important diagnostic indicator for many centuries (49.5), the scientific techniques introduced by spectroscopy were first used in medicine by Hoppe-Seyler to determine the properties
of his newly isolated "Blutfarbstoffe" (haemoglobin) (49.6). In 1873 Vierordt developed a double slit spectrometer to allow for quantitative spectroscopy (49.7)
and he used this instrument for measuring the spectra of blood, bile and urine
(49.8). Fluorescence spectroscopy for tissue characterisation, photodynamic therapy of malignant tissue and novel biosensors are but a few of today's many applications of optical spectroscopy in medicine (49.9)(49.10).

49.1 See ref. 9.8.
49.2 Kirchhoff G, Bunsen R. Chemische
     Analyse durch Spectralbeobachtungen.
     Ann Phys Chem 1860; 60:161.
49.3 Kirchhoff G, Bunsen R. Analyse chimique
     fondée sur les observations du spectre. *Ann
     Chim Phys* 1862; 64:257.
49.4 Bunsen R. *Gesammelte Abhandlungen*. Bd.
     1–3 Leipzig; 1904.
49.5 Pinder U. *Epiphanie Medicorum*. Nuren-
     berg; 1506.
49.6 See # 51 Hoppe-Seyler page 268.
49.7 Vierordt K. *Die anwendung des Spectralappa-
     rates zur Photometrie der Absortionsspectren
     und zur quantitativen chemischen Analyse.*
     Tubingen; 1873.
49.8 Vierordt K. *Die Quantitative Spectralanalyse
     in ihrer Anwendung auf Physiologie, Physik,
     Chemie und Technologie.* Tubingen; 1876.
49.9 Svanberg S. Time-Resolved spectroscopic
     Techniques in Laser Medicine. In: *Ultrafast
     Spectroscopy* G. Mourou et al. Editors.
     Springer; 1994.
49.10 Sevick-Muraca E, Benaron D, editors. Bio-
     medical Optical Spectroscopy & Diagnos-
     tics (*Trends in Optics & Photonics* Vol. 3) Op
     tical Society of America; 1996.

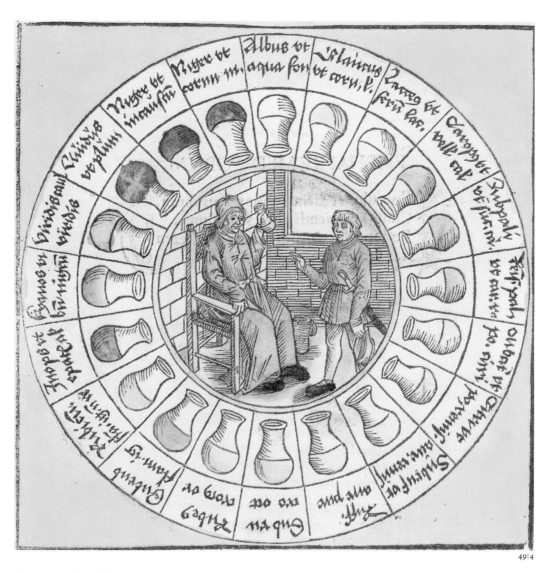

49:4

The diagnostic use of the colour of body fluids, particularly urine, has ancient traditions. Here a physician is shown demonstrating uroscopic analysis to a student in 1506. The twenty different colours of urine correspond to different diagnostics of the movement of the heart and the pulse as well as fevers caused by disease or emotional states.

A colorimeter with samples from the Bausch & Lomb Optical Co. from the early 1920s.

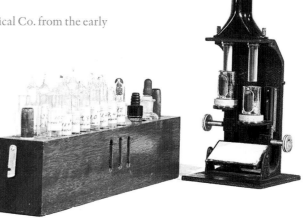

49:5

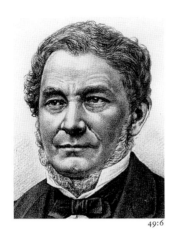

49:6

Bunsen's desire to identify salts from their colour in the flame of his "Bunsen burner" led to the invention of the spectrometer. Kirchhoff and Bunsen soon used it to discover new chemical elements, sodium, rubidium and caesium being among the first, as shown below.

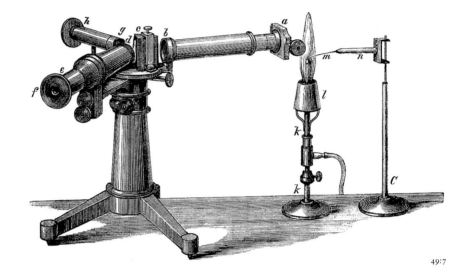

49:7

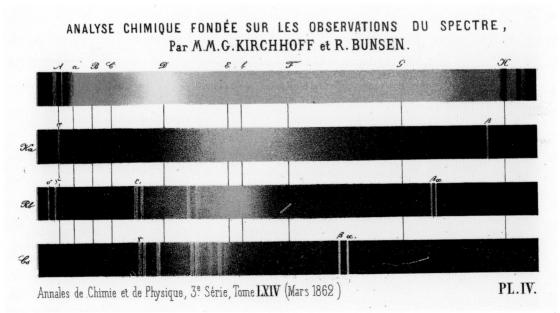

ANALYSE CHIMIQUE FONDÉE SUR LES OBSERVATIONS DU SPECTRE, Par M.M.G. KIRCHHOFF et R. BUNSEN.

Annales de Chimie et de Physique, 3e Série, Tome LXIV (Mars 1862)

PL. IV.

49:8

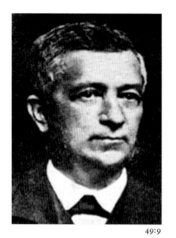

Karl Vierordt (1818–1884) invents new devices and techniques often useful in addressing medical problems (see #35). In 1873 his double slit spectrometer allows quantitative spectroscopy for the first time (right). Three years later he uses this technique to determine the spectra of blood (see table), bile and urine.

49:9

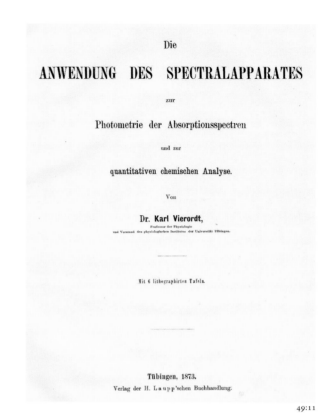

Die

ANWENDUNG DES SPECTRALAPPARATES

zur

Photometrie der Absorptionsspectren

und zur

quantitativen chemischen Analyse.

Von

Dr. Karl Vierordt,
Professor der Physiologie
und Vorstand des physiologischen Institutes der Universität Tübingen.

Mit 6 lithographirten Tafeln.

Tübingen, 1873.
Verlag der H. Laupp'schen Buchhandlung.

49:11

Die meisten der in Tabelle 42 enthaltenen Messungen wurden im Januar und Februar 1875 angestellt. Der erforderliche Blutstropfen wurde durch Anstechen eines Fingers gewonnen.

Tabelle 42.

Hämoglobulingehalt des Menschenblutes ausgedrückt in den Werthen des Exstinctionscoëfficienten für die Region des zweiten Absorptionsbandes des 100fach verdünnten Blutes.

		Mein Blut		
Studirender (sehr blass)	0,924	1. Jan. 7ʰ 40'	1,3936	Vor dem Frühstück.
Studirender	1,566	» » 9ʰ 45'	1,2879	8ʰ 15, eine Tasse Kaffe u. 1 Weck.
35j. Mann	1,364	» » 11ʰ	1,2396	
42j. Mann	1,433	» » 12ʰ 20'	1,3034	
34j. Frau. Caries des Kniegelenkes (mittlerer Ernährungsstand), kein Fieber	1,086	» » 2ʰ 15'	1,2918	12ʰ 30' bis 1 Uhr Mittagessen; sammt ³/₄ Lit. Wein.
29j. Mann. Caries des Kniegelenkes	1,213	» » 4ʰ 15'	1,2432	2ʰ 30' bis 3ʰ 15' Spaziergang.
30j. Frau. Blass. Scrofulöse Geschwüre	1,115	» » 6ʰ	1,2653	4ʰ 20' bis 4ʰ 50' eine Flasche Bier getrunken.
49j. Mann. Sehr mager. Kein Fieber. Gonarthritis fungosa seit 1½ Jahren	0,838	» » 7ʰ 50'	1,2396	
Mein Blut 6. Jan.	1,232			
» » 31. Dec.		» » 10ʰ Abends.	1,2322	8ʰ 15'—8ʰ 30' Abendessen.
Stich im 5. Finger.	1,1249	2. Jan. 4ᵏ 15' Morg.	1,2690	Von 11ʰ bis 4ʰ 15' geschlafen.
» » Stich im 4. Finger.	1,1157	» » 8ʰ Morgens.	1,3112	Von 5ʰ bis 7ʰ wieder geschlafen. Vor dem Frühstück.

also 1/122 Differenz.

49:10

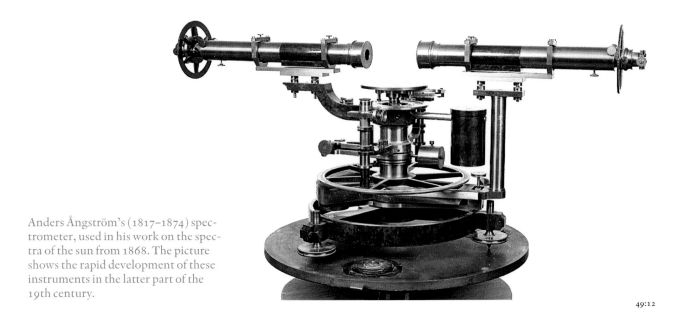

Anders Ångström's (1817–1874) spectrometer, used in his work on the spectra of the sun from 1868. The picture shows the rapid development of these instruments in the latter part of the 19th century.

49:12

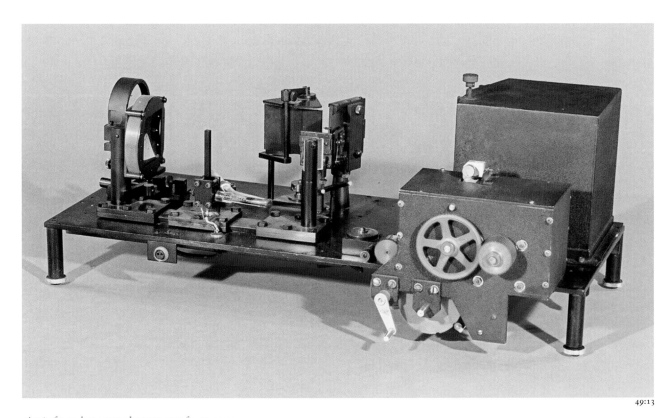

49:13

An infrared spectrophotometer from 1905.

Louis Pasteur's (1822–1895) simple but ingenious experimental apparatus for proving conclusively that spontaneous generation did not occur or in his own words that "there is no circumstance known in which it can be affirmed that microscopic beings came into the world without germs, without parents similar to themselves." The flasks with long, narrow, "swan-like" necks kept the fermentable liquid in the flask sterile even when open to the ambient air, as long as the liquid did not come into contact with the sides of the neck.

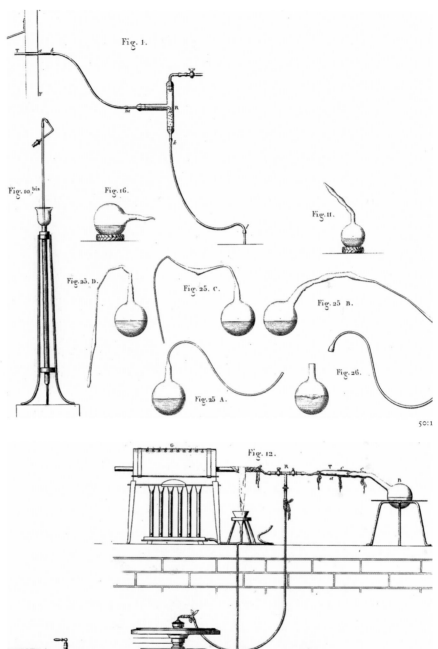

50:1

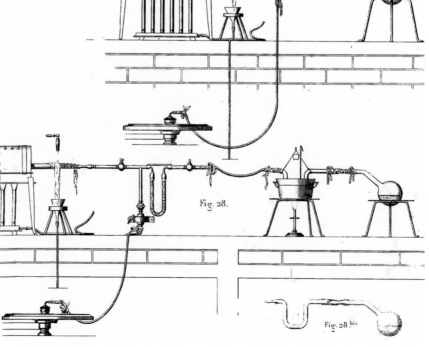

50:2

264

PASTEUR was born in Dole as the only son of a tanner. In elementary school he was a mediocre student and considered a career as an artist. His awakening interest in chemistry and science made him prepare for and, in 1843, enter the École Normale Supérieure in Paris. After receiving his doctorate in 1848, he was professor of chemistry in Strasbourg and Lille before he returned to the École Normale in 1857 as director of scientific studies and later director of the laboratory for physiological chemistry. Pasteur was ambitious, self-assured and opportunistic and argued in scientific debates with devastating efficiency. Although an excellent teacher, his authoritarian views strained his relations with students. Pasteur had little interest in social, political, philosophical or religious issues. He believed that his work resulted inevitably from the underlying scientific truths, a view reflected in his sayings that "experiment imposed the view on me" and "chance favours a prepared mind". He led the Institut Pasteur from 1888 to 1895, when a stroke ended his life. Many of his projects were extensively supported by the French government, which also granted him a generous life annuity and, on his death, a state funeral.

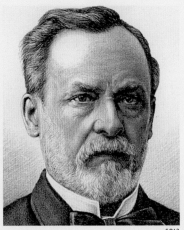

Louis Pasteur   50:3

Mémoire sur les corpuscules organisés qui exist dans l'atmosphère, examen de la doctrine de générations spontanées.

ANN CHIM PHYS 1862; 64:5.

PASTEUR GIVES a historic review of the controversy of spontaneous generation, that is the belief that living organisms can arise without any immediate living parent from inorganic or organic material. He then presents in eight chapters ingenious experiments leading to convincing evidence that this concept is incorrect and that the growth of microbial life in previously sterile liquids such as milk and urine is exclusively due to contamination by micro-organisms carried by airborne particles.

IN PERSPECTIVE:

Redi, a member of Accademia del Cimento (50.1), showed in 1668 that no maggots arose spontaneously in rotting meat if flies were prevented from reaching the meat (50.2). Spallanzani reported in 1765 (50.3) that if chicken broth was boiled after evacuating the air from the bottle, no growth of organisms took place. However, none of these studies were entirely conclusive and the idea of spontaneous generation could not be dismissed until Pasteur published his results. Although Pasteur's work on immunology and vaccination had direct and spectacular medical applications (50.4)(50.5), his studies on fermentation (50.6)(50.7) and his experiments for disproving spontaneous generation founded the science of microbiology (50.8) and the germ theory of disease (50.9), which in turn led to the development of aseptic surgery (50.10).

50.1 See ref. 7.3.
50.2 Redi F. *Esperienze intorno alla generazione degl'insetti.* Firenze; 1668. See also ref. 7.3.
50.3 Spallanzani L. *Saggio di osservazioni microscopiche concernenti il sistema della generazione. In Dissertazioni due . . .* Modena; 1765.
50.4 Pasteur L, Joubert JF. Charbon et septicémie. *C R Acad Sci* 1877; 85:101.
50.5 Pasteur L, et al. Sur la rage. *C R Acad Sci* 1881; 92:1259.
50.6 Pasteur L. Mémoire sur la fermentation appelée lactique. *C R Acad Sci* 1857; 45:913.
50.7 Pasteur L. Recherches sur la putréfaction. *C R Acad Sci.* 1863; 56:1189.
50.8 See #61 Koch page 316.
50.9 Pasteur L, Joubert JF, Chamberland CE. La théorie des germes et ses applications à la médecine et la chirurgie. *C R Acad Sci* 1878; 86:1037.
50.10 See #54 Lister page 282.

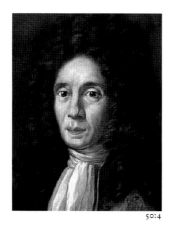

50:4

Almost two centuries before Pasteur, Francesco Redi (1626–1697) publishes a book with compelling observations that disprove the concept of spontaneous generation. He declares "I know that from the flesh of a goat, fed twenty days only on leaves of mulberry, nothing but worms were born, which transformed into flies; and from the flesh of the same goat, kept in a closed jar, nothing at all was born."

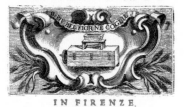

ESPERIENZE
INTORNO ALLA GENERAZIONE
DEGL' INSETTI
FATTE
DA FRANCESCO REDI
ACCADEMICO DELLA CRVSCA,
E DA LVI SCRITTE IN VNA LETTERA
ALL' ILLVSTRISSIMO SIGNOR
CARLO DATI·

IN FIRENZE.
All' Insegna della STELLA. MDCLXVIII.
Con licenza de' Superiori.

50:5

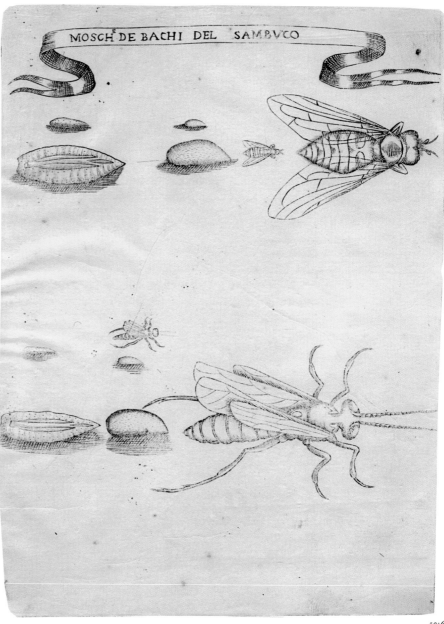

MOSCH DE BACHI DEL SAMBVCO

50:6

50:7

In 1765, about a century after Redi and a century before Pasteur, Lazzaro Spallanzani (1727–1799) studies the various life forms that develop in different infusions (i.e. from pumpkin seeds fig 2, urine fig 6, and white beans fig 9) and takes a major step in finally disproving the theory of spontaneous generation of life by showing that all infusions remain free from micro-organisms when they are boiled for an hour and hermetically sealed in a flask.

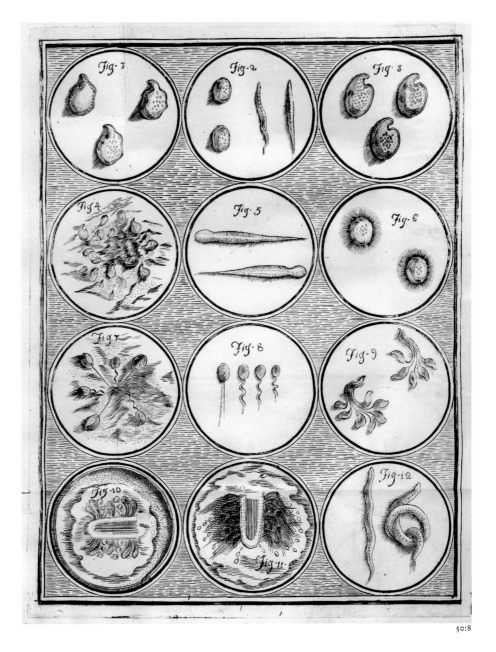

50:8

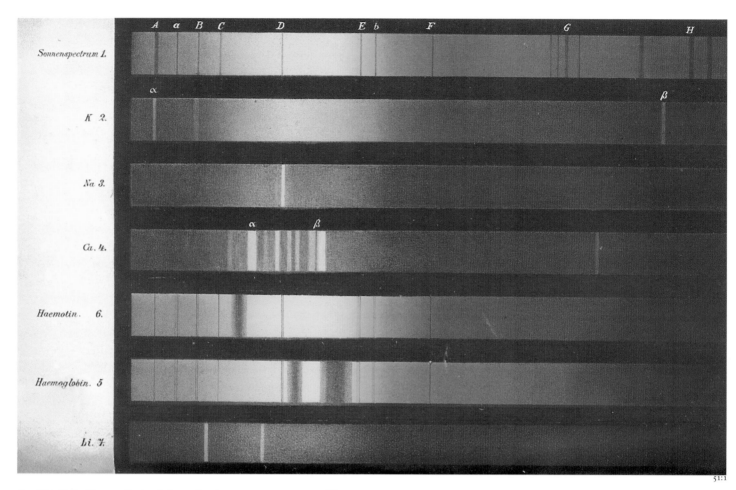

In 1862 Felix Hoppe-Seyler (1825–1895) prepares a pure crystalline form of the pigment of blood, which he calls haemoglobin. The illustration shows his registration of the spectra of haemoglobin together with those of the sun and several other common elements.

HOPPE was born in Freiburg in 1825 as the tenth child of a minister. From the age of six, as both his parents had died, a brother-in-law Dr Seyler raised him and also formally adopted him in 1864. As a result Hoppe changed his name to Hoppe-Seyler. He entered medical school in Halle in 1846, but a chance meeting with the Weber brothers (51.1) convinced him to continue his studies in Leipzig. He received his M.D. in 1851 in Berlin and worked for a short time as a practitioner before he accepted a post as prosector in anatomy at the pathological institute. In 1861 he was appointed professor of chemistry at the Medical Faculty of Tubingen. From 1872 till his death in 1895 he was professor in physiological chemistry in Strasbourg. He founded the "Zeitschrift fur Physiologische Chemie" and together with prominent disciples promoted biochemistry as a separate science. Hoppe-Seyler was a kind and engaging man with frugal habits, an expert mountaineer who enjoyed sailing and other outdoor activities.

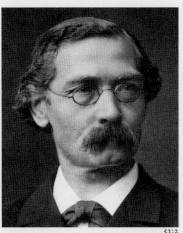

Felix Hoppe-Seyler   51:2

Ueber das Verhalten des Blutfarbstoffe im Spectrum des Sonnenlichtes.

ARCH PATH ANAT PHYSIOL BERLIN: G. REIMER; 1862; 23:446.

HOPPE-SEYLER DESCRIBES how he prepares a pure form of the pigment of the blood by inducing it to crystallise. He also subjects this substance, which he calls haemoglobin, to the novel method of spectral analysis developed by Kirchoff and Bunsen (51.2) and presents the absorption spectra of haemoglobin.

IN PERSPECTIVE:
During the 18th century Menghini had shown that red blood cells contained iron (51.3). Berzelius (51.4) and later LeCanu (51.5) demonstrated that the iron was localised to the coloured pigment of the blood that LeCanu called "hematosine" and that this carried more oxygen than the remaining part of the blood, called "globulin" (serum). After preparing pure "blutfarbstoffe" (haemoglobin), Hoppe-Seyler showed spectroscopically (51.6) that oxygen was loosely bound to it and that it could be easily replaced by carbon monoxide and even more so by nitric oxide (51.7)(51.8). Following Vierordt's studies of the spectrum of blood (51.9), in 1894 Hufner determined the correct value of the oxygen binding capacity of haemoglobin (51.10). Hoppe-Seyler's studies extended to many branches of what is today called biochemistry and his disciples Miescher and Kossel started the chemical exploration of the structure of the cell-nucleus. Miescher was the first to suggest the existence of the genetic code (51.11). The full molecular structure of haemoglobin and its related forms were revealed first in the 1950s by the work of Perutz and Kendrew (51.12).

51.1   See #44 Weber page 232.
51.2   See #49 Kirchhoff page 258.
51.3   Menghini V. De ferrearum particularum sede in sanguine. Bonon. *Sci Art Inst Acad Comment* 1746; 2(2):244.
51.4   See ref. 14.4.
51.5   LeCanu LR. De l'Hematosine, au Matière Colorante du Sang. *Ann Chim Phys* 1830; 45:5.
51.6   Hoppe-Seyler EF. Ueber den chemischen und optischen Eigenschaften des Blutfarbstoffs. *Virchows Arch Pathol Anat* 1864; 29:233 and p597.
51.7   Herman L. Ueber die Wirkungen des Stickstoffoxydgases auf das Blut. *Arch Anat Physiol wiss Med* 1865. p469.
51.8   Hoppe-Seyler F. *Handbuch der physiologisch- und pathologisch-Chemischen Analyse für Ärtzte und Studirenden*. Berlin; 1865. p201.
51.9   See ref. 49.8.
51.10 Hufner CG. Neue Versuche zur Bestimmung der Sauerstoffkapazität des Blutfarbstoffs. *Arch Pat Anat. Physiol* 1894. p130.
51.11 Olby R, Posner E. An early reference to genetic coding. *Nature* 1967;215:556.
51.12 Perutz MF. *X-ray Analysis of Haemoglobin*. Nobel Lecture. Stockholm; 1962.

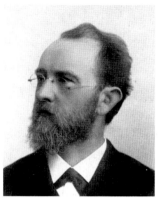

Carl Hufner (1840–1908) and the
equipment used by him to determine the oxygen carrying capacity
of haemoglobin. He finds that 1.34
ml oxygen (at 0°C and 760 mm
Hg) is bound to one gram of
haemoglobin, a value still accepted
today.

51:3

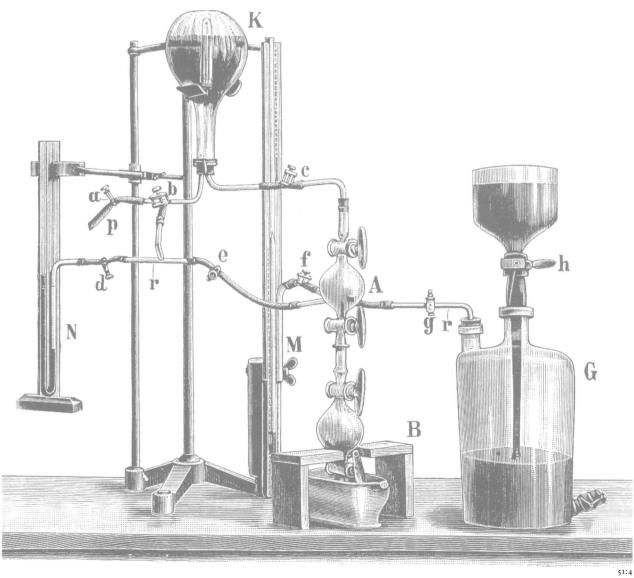

51:4

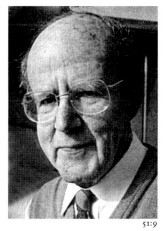

51:5

51:8

Max Perutz (1914–2002) shares the 1962 Nobel Prize in Chemistry for his work on the structure of globular proteins such as haemoglobin. The illustrations show the structure of the haemoglobin molecule and the chemical make up of the part called the haem group, which contains the iron atom. The basic tool used to determine the structure is Fourier analysis of X-ray diffraction data, now for the first time making full use of the improving electronic digital computers (see #32 and #85).

51:9

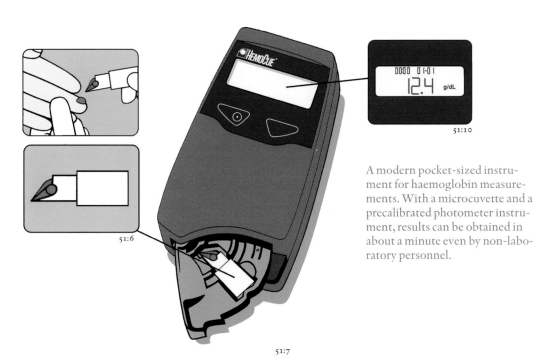

51:10

51:6

51:7

A modern pocket-sized instrument for haemoglobin measurements. With a microcuvette and a precalibrated photometer instrument, results can be obtained in about a minute even by non-laboratory personnel.

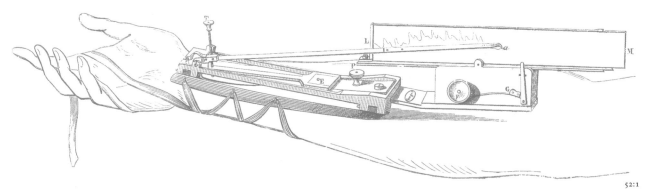

52:1

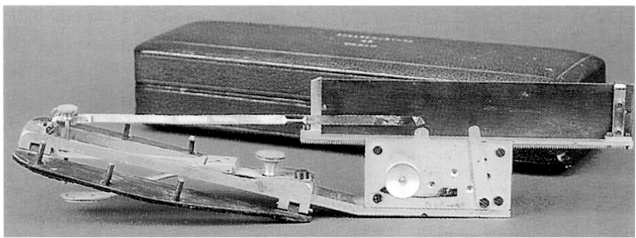

52:2

Étienne-Jules Marey's (1830–1904) greatly improved sphygmograph. This is the first design robust enough to lend itself to practical work. A drawing from his book and a photo of a contemporary device show the construction and the way it was intended to be used.

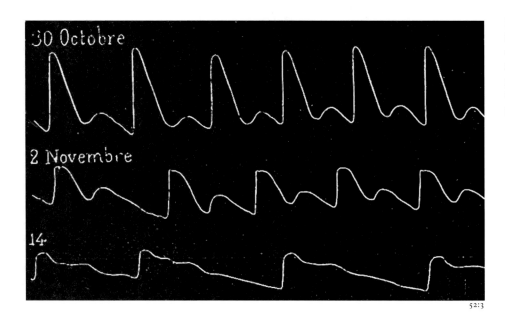

52:3

30 Octobre

2 Novembre

14

Marey studies the pulse shape for a variety of pathological cardio-vascular conditions but also in other diseases. The graphs show the progressive effect of typhoid fever on the pulse.

M AREY was born in Beaune in 1830. After his dissertation in 1857, he set up a private laboratory for experimental physiology in Paris. For a decade his studies concerned the function of the heart and the circulatory system, where he developed new instrumentation for graphical recording of the physiological parameters (52.1). In 1868 he succeeded Flourens (52.2) as professor of natural history at the Collège de France and turned his attention to the mechanics of locomotion. From 1881 these studies were extended to animal motion outdoors, an area where he broke new ground by improving the techniques of cinematography (52.3)(52.4)(52.5). In 1878 he was elected to the Académie des Sciences and became president there in 1895. A few years before his death in 1904, Marey founded an institute, named after him, for the standardisation and improvement of graphical recording devices.

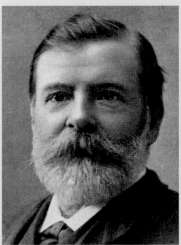
Étienne-Jules Marey   52:4

Physiologie médicale de la circulation du sang basée sur l'étude graphique des mouvements du coer et du puls artériel.

PARIS: A. DELAHAYE; 1863.

IN THE first part of this book Marey describes his new sphygmograph (52.6), cardiograph (52.7) and probes for cardiac catheterisation. Using this equipment he makes the first recordings of "cardiac sound" and detailed observations on pressure changes in the heart and the arteries. He studies the effect of respiration on the arterial pulse and establishes the relationship between blood pressure and heart rate. Marey also describes a hydro-mechanical model of the circulatory system that he builds in order to simulate the physiological observations and to test and improve his equipment. The second part of the book gives many examples of graphical recordings illustrating various pathological conditions of the heart and the vessels.

IN PERSPECTIVE:
Constantly striving for accuracy, Marey nevertheless always kept the ease of use of equipment in mind. His sphygmograph was a dramatic improvement both in performance and in clinical applicability over the previous work of Ludwig and Vierordt (52.8). Another important innovation was the "Marey's tambour", a device for pressure transmission that allowed rather free movement during a recording and was still in use during the 1950s. Following Fick's pioneering work (52.9), Marey also developed the technique of volume plethysmography and applied it to the arm for measuring blood pressure (52.1). These studies can be considered a forerunner to the modern method of blood pressure measurement introduced by Riva-Rocci in 1896 (52.10).

52.1 Marey E-J. *La méthod graphique dans les sciences expérimentales et particulièrement en physiologie et en médecine.* Paris; 1878.
52.2 See ref. 36.9.
52.3 Marey E-J. *Le Vol des Oiseaux.* (Physiologie du Mouvement) Paris; 1890.
52.4 See ref. 12.11.
52.5 See ref. 38.4 chapter 34.
52.6 Marey E-J. *Recherches sur le pouls au moyen d'un nouvel appareil enregistreur le spyghmographe.* Paris; 1860.
52.7 Chauveau JB, Marey E-J. Appareils et expériences cardiographiques. *Mém Acad imp de Méd* 1863; 26:268.
52.8 See #35 Poiseuille page 188 ref. 35.5 and ref. 35.7.
52.9 See #46 Fick page 242 and ref. 46.9.
52.10 See #68 Riva-Rocci page 350.

Marey introduces an improved plethysmographic technique for the registration of blood pressure in the arm. The volumetric change of the arm is detected and a counter pressure is applied through a cuff surrounding the arm.

In another important advance, Marey constructs a sensitive pressure sensor dome, that he calls "tambour", for on-site measurements or for transmitting pressure variations to other instrumentation. The device is used in a variety of experimental arrangements in his cardio-vascular studies but also as shown below, with the "pneumograph", a device for registering respiratory movements.

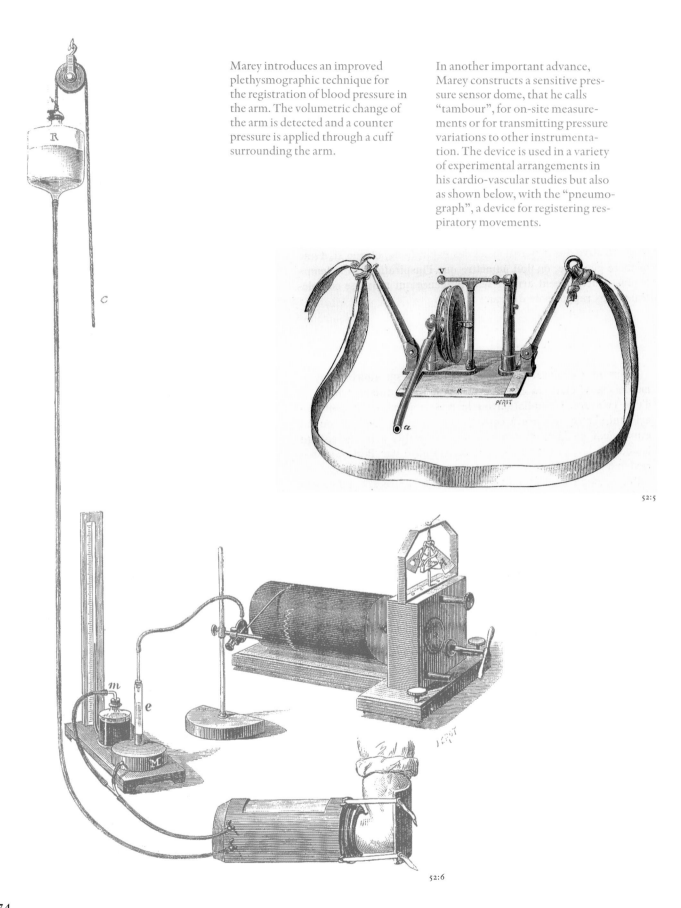

52:5

52:6

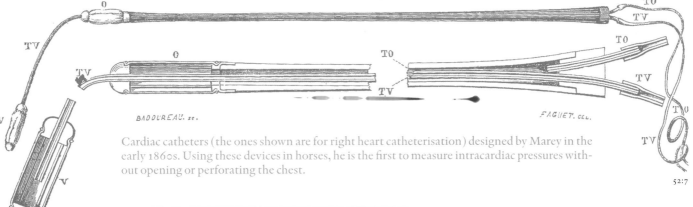

BADOUREAU. sc.   FAGUET. del.

Cardiac catheters (the ones shown are for right heart catheterisation) designed by Marey in the early 1860s. Using these devices in horses, he is the first to measure intracardiac pressures without opening or perforating the chest.

52:7

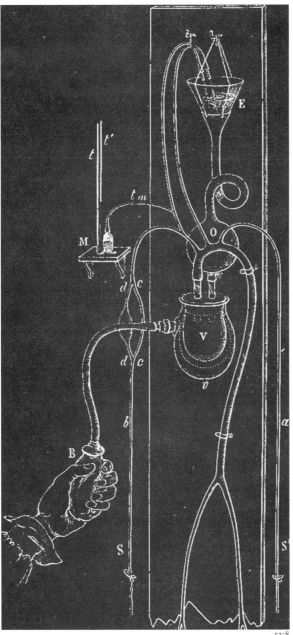

52:8

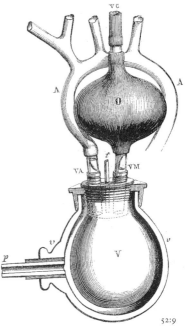

52:9

Well aware of the work of the Weber brothers (see #44), Marey builds a rather sophisticated model of the circulatory system. He uses the model for testing new apparatus and to simulate and verify experimental results, including the effect of an arterial aneurysm on the arterial pulse.

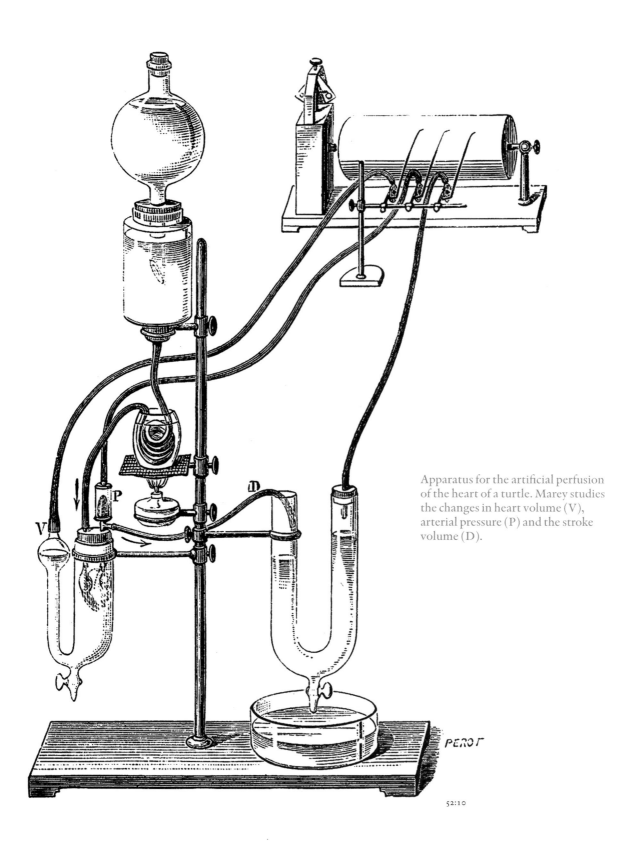

Apparatus for the artificial perfusion
of the heart of a turtle. Marey studies
the changes in heart volume (V),
arterial pressure (P) and the stroke
volume (D).

PEROT

52:10

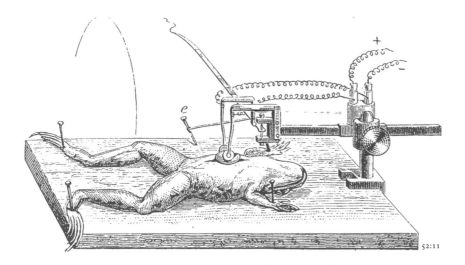

52:11

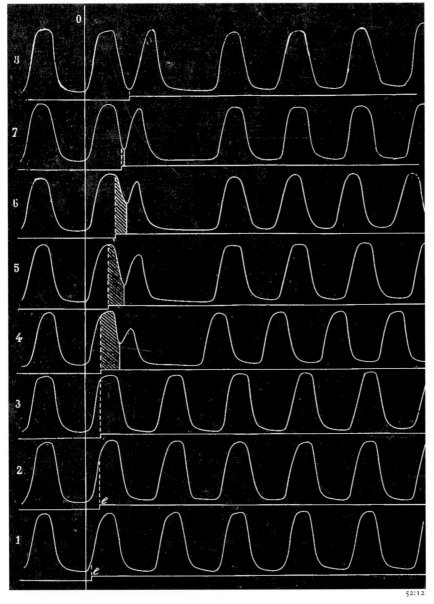

Marey investigates the effect of electric stimulation on the frog heart. He demonstrates the changing susceptibility of the heart to weak electric excitation (applied at the time of the offset shown in the baseline) at different times during the cardiac cycle.

52:12

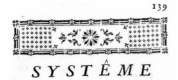

SYSTÊME DE LA NATURE.

ESSAI

SUR LA FORMATION DES CORPS ORGANISÉS.

I.

Uelques Philofophes ont cru qu'avec la *matiere* & le *mouvement* ils pouvoient expliquer toute la Nature : & pour rendre la chofe plus fimple encore, ils ont averti que par la matiere ils n'entendoient que l'*étendue*. D'autres fentant l'infuffifance de cette fimplicité, ont cru qu'il falloit

53:1

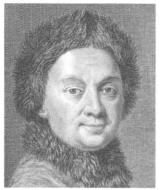

53:3

Already in the mid-18th century Pierre Maupertius (1698–1759) (see portrait above) publishes important observations that foreshadow Mendel's laws of heredity. He studies the dominant trait of polydactyly (more than five digits) in a family and postulates that separate hereditary components come from the male and the female parent and that the trait could be inherited from either parent.

Gregor Mendel (1822–1884) announces the result of his extensive study on plant hybridisation. Mendel's experiments aim at finding a generally applicable law governing the formation of hybrids. He is convinced that such a law exists "since unity in the plan of development of organic life is beyond doubt." His work is all but ignored for over three decades.

Below right William Bateson's (1861–1926) English translation from 1909, which quickly makes Mendel's results more generally available and accepted.

Versuche über Pflanzen-Hybriden.

Von

Gregor Mendel.

(Vorgelegt in den Sitzungen vom 8. Februar und 8. März 1865.)

Einleitende Bemerkungen.

Künstliche Befruchtungen, welche an Zierpflanzen desshalb vorgenommen wurden, um neue Farben-Varianten zu erzielen, waren die Veranlassung zu den Versuchen, die her besprochen werden sollen. Die auffallende Regelmässigkeit, mit welcher dieselben Hybridformen immer wiederkehrten, so oft die Befruchtung zwischen gleichen Arten geschah, gab die Anregung zu weiteren Experimenten, deren Aufgabe es war, die Entwicklung der Hybriden in ihren Nachkommen zu verfolgen.

Dieser Aufgabe haben sorgfältige Beobachter, wie Kölreuter, Gärtner, Herbert, Lecocq, Wichura u. a. einen Theil ihres Lebens mit unermüdlicher Ausdauer geopfert. Namentlich hat Gärtner in seinem Werke „die Bastarderzeugung im Pflanzenreiche" sehr schätzbare Beobachtungen niedergelegt, und in neuester Zeit wurden von Wichura gründliche Untersuchungen über die Bastarde der Weiden veröffentlicht. Wenn es noch nicht gelungen ist, ein allgemein giltiges Gesetz für die Bildung und Entwicklung der Hybriden aufzustellen, so kann das Niemanden Wunder nehmen, der den Umfang der Aufgabe kennt und die Schwierigkeiten zu würdigen weiss, mit denen Versuche dieser Art zu kämpfen haben. Eine endgiltige Entscheidung kann erst dann erfolgen, bis Detail-Versuche aus den verschiedensten Pflanzen-Familien vorliegen. Wer die Ar-

1*

53:2

EXPERIMENTS IN PLANT-HYBRIDISATION*.

By Gregor Mendel.

(*Read at the Meetings of the 8th February and 8th March*, 1865.)

Introductory Remarks.

Experience of artificial fertilisation, such as is effected with ornamental plants in order to obtain new variations in colour, has led to the experiments which will here be discussed. The striking regularity with which the same hybrid forms always reappeared whenever fertilisation took place between the same species induced further experiments to be undertaken, the object of which was to follow up the developments of the hybrids in their progeny.

To this object numerous careful observers, such as Kölreuter, Gärtner, Herbert, Lecoq, Wichura and others, have devoted a part of their lives with inexhaustible perseverance. Gärtner especially, in his work "Die Bastarderzeugung im Pflanzenreiche" (The Production of Hybrids in the Vegetable Kingdom), has recorded very valuable observations ; and quite recently Wichura published the results of some profound investigations into the hybrids of the Willow. That, so far, no generally applicable law governing the formation and development of hybrids has been successfully formulated can hardly be wondered at by anyone who is acquainted with the extent of the task, and can appreciate the difficulties with which experiments of

* [This translation was made by the Royal Horticultural Society, and is reprinted with modifications and corrections, by permission. The original paper was published in the *Verh. naturf. Ver. in Brünn, Abhandlungen,* IV. 1865, which appeared in 1866.]

53:4

ENDEL was born in 1822 in Heinzendorf, Austrian Silesia. His father was a peasant and in his mother's family many were professional gardeners. He attended church school and later the Philosophical Institute of Olmutz. In 1843 he entered the Augustinian Monastery in old Brno. After studies in theology, agriculture, pomology and viticulture, he was ordained a priest in 1847. From 1856, when Mendel was in charge of the gardens at the monastery, he experimented with pea plants, which led him in 1864 to the rules of heredity, now named after him. In 1868 he was elected abbot of the monastery, a post that prevented him from further scientific work. Mendel was a friendly person and an enthusiastic teacher. He had a weak mental constitution and the political controversies that he got involved with embittered the last ten years of his life.

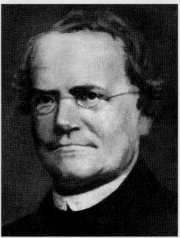

Gregor Mendel   53:5

Versuche über Pflanzen-Hybriden.

VERHANDLUNGEN DES NATURFORSCHENDEN VEREINES IN BRÜNN 1865; 4:3.
BRÜNN: G. GASTL; 1866.

MENDEL REPORTS the results of his observations on more than 28,000 pea plants cultivated over an eight-year period. He analyses seven pairs of seed and plant characteristics and observes the $128 (= 2^7)$ constant associations of these seven alternative and mutually exclusive traits. Using the concept of "dominant" and "recessive" characteristics, he explains "the evolutionary history of organic forms" and claims that his rules are general as "no basic difference could exist in important matters, since unity in the plan of development of organic life is beyond doubt".

IN PERSPECTIVE:
Maupertuis studied the laws of heredity of a dominant trait (polydactyly or extra digits) a century before Mendel (53.1). He postulated that separate hereditary components came from the male and the female parent and that they would fuse due to chemical attraction. He demonstrated that the trait was inherited from either parent by recording a complete family history in three successive generations and showing that the outcome could not occur by chance. Based on observations on large populations, Galton, a contemporary of Mendel, studied inherited traits between different generations (53.2). Mendel's work went unnoticed until 1900 when, independently, Correns (53.3), de Vries (53.4) and Tschermak (53.5) rediscovered it. Bateson introduced Mendel's ideas to a wide audience (53.6) and coined the word "genetics". The concept of natural selection (53.7) operates on the variability in populations that occur according to Mendel's law and due to the existence of mutations (53.8). While Mendel knew and approved of Darwin's theory (53.9), Darwin was unaware of Mendel's work. In 1932 Haldane (53.10) presented a synthesis of the two.

53.1 Maupertuis P. *Oeuvres.* Vol.1–4 Lyon; 1756. particularly Vol.2 p139 Systeme de la Nature.

53.2 See ref. 30.8.

53.3 Correns C. G Mendel's Regel über das Verhalten der Nachkommenschaft der Rassen bastarde. *Ber dtsch bot Ges* 1900; 18:158.

53.4 deVries H. Das Spaltungsgesetz der Bastarde. *Ber dtsch bot Ges* 1900; 18:83.

53.5 von Tschermak-Seysenegg E. Über künstliche Kreuzung von Pisum sativum. *Z landwirtsch Versuchsw in Österreich* 1900; 3:465.

53.6 Bateson W. *Mendel's principles of Heredity.* Cambridge; 1909.

53.7 Darwin C, Wallace AR. On the Tendency of Species to form Varieties; and on the Perpetuation of Varieties and Species by Natural Means of Selection. *J Proc Linnean Soc* 1858; 3(9):45.

53.8 deVries H. *Die Muthationstheorie.* Vol. 1,2 Leipzig; 1901–1903.

53.9 Darwin C. *On the Origin of Species by Means of Natural Selection.* London; 1859.

53.10 Haldane JB. *The causes of evolution.* London; 1932.

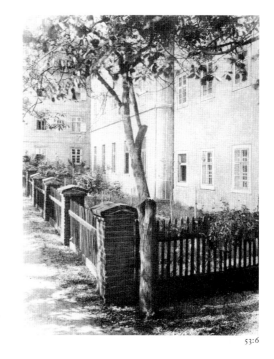

The Monastery Garden at the end of the 19th century (below) where Mendel performed his experiments in a special experimental garden. This garden, about 35×7 m in size, is shown right as it appeared in the beginning of the 20th century.

53:6

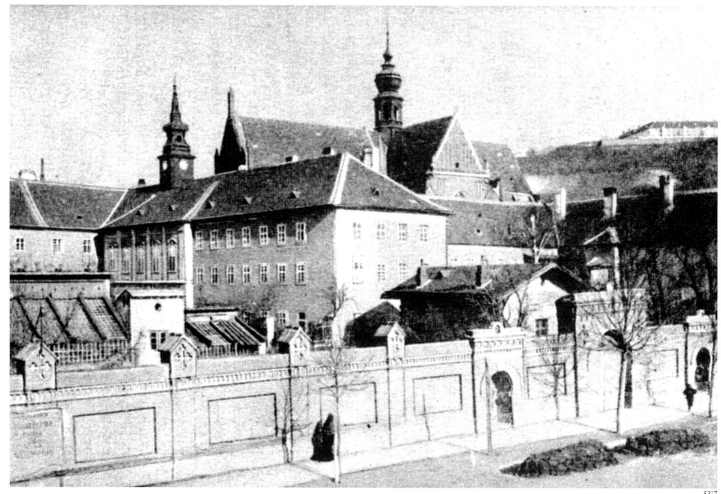

53:7

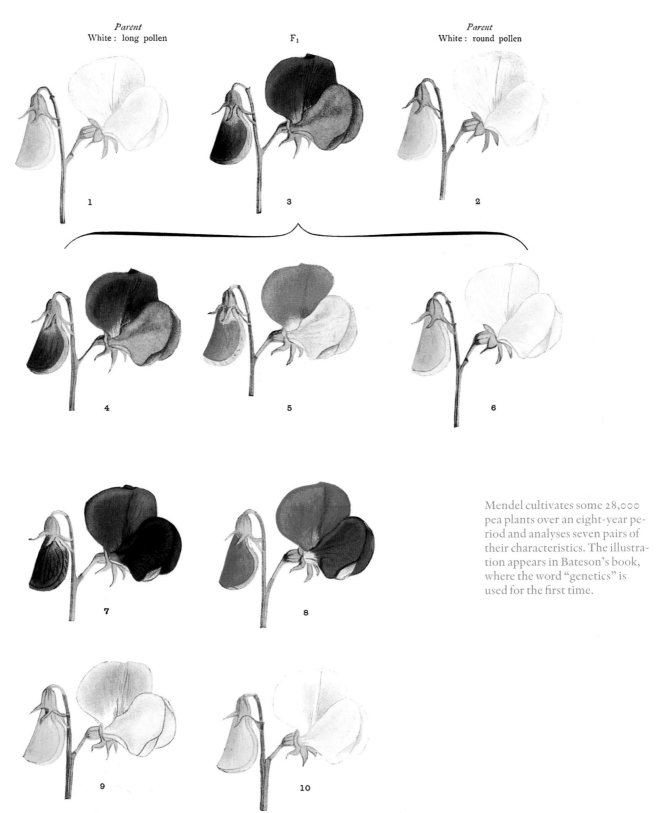

Mendel cultivates some 28,000 pea plants over an eight-year period and analyses seven pairs of their characteristics. The illustration appears in Bateson's book, where the word "genetics" is used for the first time.

1 and 2. Emily Henderson, white.   3. F₁ Purple Invincible.   4—10. The various F₂ types obtained by self-fertilising F₁.   4. Purple Invincible.   5. Painted Lady.   6. White.   7. Purple with purple wings.   8. Miss Hunt.   9. Purple Picotee.   10. Pink Picotee, or Tinged White.   In the red class 5, 8 and 10 correspond respectively to 4, 7 and 9 in the purple classes.

53:8

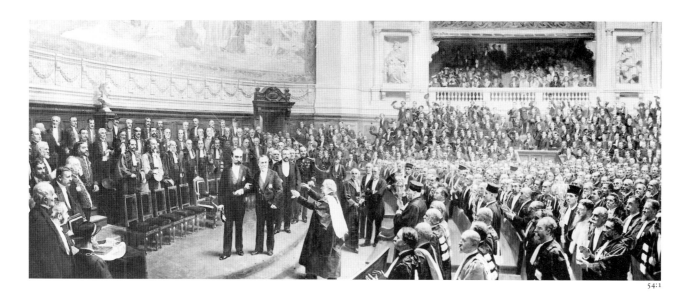

54:1

Lister acclaims Louis Pasteur (1822–1895) at Pasteur's Jubilee in Paris 1892.

Joseph Lister's (1827–1912) account of the background to his idea of a system for aseptic surgery. The importance of Pasteur's germ theory of disease obviously plays an important role in this major advance in surgery.

Turning now to the question how the atmosphere produces decomposition of organic substances, we find that a flood of light has been thrown upon this most important subject by the philosophic researches of M. Pasteur, who has demonstrated by thoroughly convincing evidence that it is not to its oxygen or to any of its gaseous constituents that the air owes this property, but to minute particles suspended in it, which are the germs of various low forms of life, long since revealed by the microscope, and regarded as merely accidental concomitants of putrescence, but now shown by Pasteur to be its essential cause, resolving the complex organic compounds into substances of simpler chemical constitution, just as the yeast plant converts sugar into alcohol and carbonic acid.

A beautiful illustration of this doctrine seems to me to be presented in surgery by pneumothorax with emphysema, resulting from puncture of the lung by a fractured rib. Here, though atmospheric air is perpetually introduced into the pleura in great abundance, no inflammatory disturbance supervenes; whereas an external wound penetrating the chest, if it remains open, infallibly causes dangerous suppurative pleurisy. In the latter case the blood and serum poured out into the pleural cavity, as an immediate consequence of the injury, are decomposed by the germs that enter with the air, and then operate as a powerful irritant upon the serous membrane. But in case of puncture of the lung without external wound, the atmospheric gases are filtered of the causes of decomposition before they enter the pleura, by passing through the bronchial tubes, which, by their small size, their tortuous course, their mucous secretion, and ciliated epithelial lining, seem to be specially designed to arrest all solid particles in the air inhaled. Consequently the effused fluids retain their original characters unimpaired, and are speedily absorbed by the unirritated pleura.

54:2

LISTER was born in Upton in 1827 into a Quaker family. His father was a well-known physicist (54.1). After a broad education in private schools, he entered University College London and received his medical degree in 1852. After seven years as assistant surgeon in Edinburgh Lister's reputation as an original investigator and excellent clinician landed him the professorship of surgery in Glasgow. He introduced the antiseptic method in surgery during 1865–1867. In 1877 the position as Head of Clinical Surgery at Kings College in London gave him a better platform from which to promote his ideas and he soon received worldwide recognition and many honours. As a man Lister was deeply religious, charming but reserved, and with an honest, unassuming character. A stroke in 1903 led to declining health and eventually to his death in 1912.

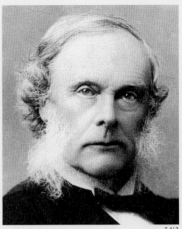

Joseph Lister

54:3

On a New Method of Treating Compound Fracture, Abscess, etc. with Observations on the Conditions of Suppuration.

LANCET 1867; 1: 326, 357, 387, 507 AND LANCET 1867; 2:95.

BASED ON Pasteur's proof (54.2) that airborne germs cause putrefaction and having heard that treating sewage with carbolic acid (phenol) removed any odour, Lister decides to use this compound for wound treatment. He reports eleven cases of compound fractures (which normally carried a mortality of about 40%), all cleansed with a solution of carbolic acid and covered with a dressing soaked with the acid and with a tin plate to diminish evaporation. Nine of his patients survive. He also reports that if abscesses are opened antiseptically, recovery is better than if they are not opened at all.

IN PERSPECTIVE:
According to Liebig, oxygen was the main agent required for organic putrefaction (54.3)(54.4). Pasteur on the other hand had shown (54.2) that this process was initiated by airborne micro-organisms. The dramatic improvement in the outcomes with Lister's antiseptic method (54.5)(54.6) soon led to extensive carbolic spraying of the entire operating area. However by 1890, realising that most of the airborne microbes were neither pathogenic nor killed by the spray, Lister withdrew his support for this procedure (54.7). Koch's development of steam sterilisation techniques (54.8)(54.9) and the risk of interfering with the natural healing process when using chemical antiseptics led to a controversy between proponents of aseptic procedures and those stressing the importance of antisepsis in wound treatment. Lister, always conciliatory, invited both Koch and Pasteur to a meeting in London in 1881. Eventually, the conflict was set aside by the adaptation of both points of view, as advocated by Lister.

54.1 See ref. 9.5.
54.2 See #50 Pasteur page 264.
54.3 See #39 Liebig page 208.
54.4 von Liebig J. Ueber die Erscheinungen der Gährung, Fäulniss und Verwesung und ihre Ursache. *Ann d. Pharm* 1839; 30(31):38.
54.5 Lister J. On the Effects of the Antiseptic System of Treatment upon the Salubrity of a Surgical Hospital. *Lancet* 1870; I p4. and p40.
54.6 *The Collected Papers of Joseph, Baron Lister*. Vol. 1,2 Oxford; 1909. Vol.2 part III The antiseptic system.
54.7 Lister J. An Address on the present Position of Antiseptic Surgery, delivered before the International Medical Congress Berlin; 1890. In: *Brit Med J* 1890; II:377.
54.8 See #61 Koch page 316.
54.9 Koch R. Ueber Desinfection. *Mittheil kais Gesundheitsamt* 1881; 1:234.

Applying these principles to the treatment of compound fracture, bearing in mind that it is from the vitality of the atmospheric particles that all the mischief arises, it appears that all that is requisite is to dress the wound with some material capable of killing these septic germs, provided that any substance can be found reliable for this purpose, yet not too potent as a caustic.

In the course of the year 1864 I was much struck with an account of the remarkable effects produced by carbolic acid upon the sewage of the town of Carlisle, the admixture of a very small proportion not only preventing all odour from the lands irrigated with the refuse material, but, as it was stated, destroying the entozoa which usually infest cattle fed upon such pastures.

My attention having for several years been much directed to the subject of suppuration, more especially in its relation to decomposition, I saw that such a powerful antiseptic was peculiarly adapted for experiments with a view to elucidating that subject, and while I was engaged in the investigation the applicability of carbolic acid for the treatment of compound fracture naturally occurred to me.

My first attempt of this kind was made in the Glasgow Royal Infirmary in March 1865, in a case of compound fracture of the leg. It proved unsuccessful, in consequence, as I now believe, of improper management; but subsequent trials have more than realized my most sanguine anticipations.

Carbolic acid [1] proved in various ways well adapted for the purpose.

[1] Carbolic acid is found in the shops in two forms—the glacial or crystalline, solid at ordinary temperatures of the atmosphere; and the fluid, which sometimes passes under the name of German creosote. The fluid variety is sold in various degrees of purity. The crude forms are objectionable from their offensive odour; but the properly rectified product is almost fragrant. Different samples, however, differ much in energy of action, and hence, though I have hitherto employed the liquid

54:4

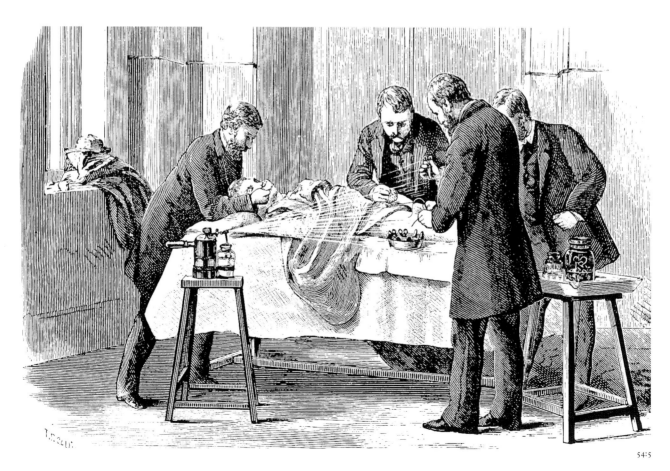

54:5

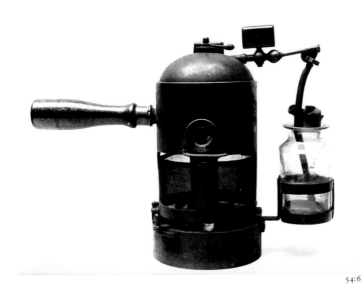

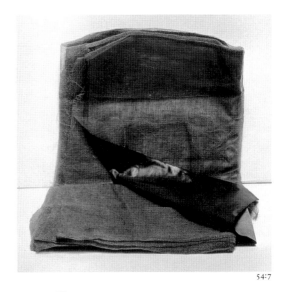

54:6

54:7

The carbolic steam spray, the carbolised gauze and their proper arrangement as used by Lister in major operations.

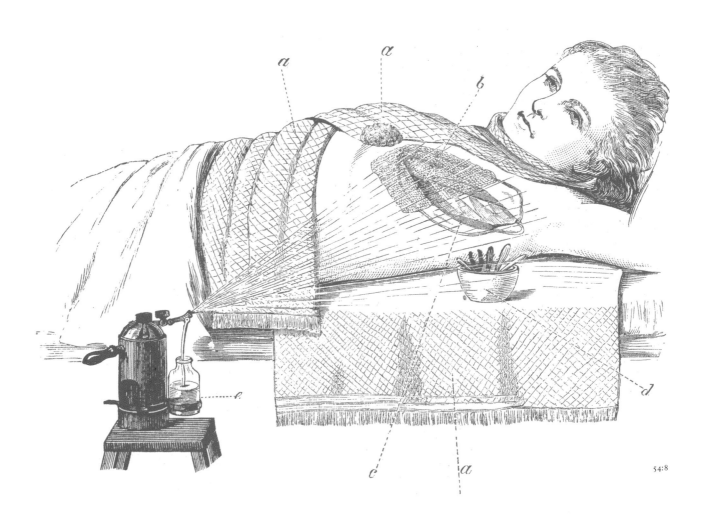

54:8

XXXIV. *On Governors.*

A GOVERNOR is a part of a machine by means of which the velocity of the machine is kept nearly uniform, notwithstanding variations in the driving-power or the resistance.

Most governors depend on the centrifugal force of a piece connected with a shaft of the machine. When the velocity increases, this force increases, and either increases the pressure of the piece against a surface or moves the piece, and so acts on a break or a valve.

In one class of regulators of machinery, which we may call *moderators*[*], the resistance is increased by a quantity depending on the velocity. Thus in some pieces of clockwork the moderator consists of a conical pendulum revolving within a circular case. When the velocity increases, the ball of the pendulum presses against the inside of the case, and the friction checks the increase of velocity.

In Watt's governor for steam-engines the arms open outwards, and so contract the aperture of the steam-valve.

In a water-break invented by Professor J. Thomson, when the velocity is increased, water is centrifugally pumped up, and overflows with a great velocity, and the work is spent in lifting and communicating this velocity to the water.

In all these contrivances an increase of driving-power produces an increase of velocity, though a much smaller increase than would be produced without the moderator.

But if the part acted on by centrifugal force, instead of acting directly on the machine, sets in motion a contrivance which continually increases the resistance as long as the velocity is above its normal value, and reverses its action when the velocity is below that value, the governor will bring the velocity to the same normal value whatever variation (within the working limits of the machine) be made in the driving-power or the resistance.

I propose at present, without entering into any details of mechanism, to direct the attention of engineers and mathematicians to the dynamical theory of such governors.

It will be seen that the motion of a machine with its governor consists in general of a uniform motion, combined with a disturbance which may be expressed as the sum of several component motions. These components may be of four different kinds :—

1. The disturbance may continually increase.
2. It may continually diminish.
3. It may be an oscillation of continually increasing amplitude.
4. It may be an oscillation of continually decreasing amplitude.

The first and third cases are evidently inconsistent with the stability of the motion ; and the second and fourth alone are admissible in a good governor. This condition is mathematically equivalent to the condition that all the possible roots, and all the possible parts of the impossible roots, of a certain equation shall be negative.

I have not been able completely to determine these conditions for equations of a higher degree than the third ; but I hope that the subject will obtain the attention of mathematicians.

[*] See Mr C. W. Siemens "On Uniform Rotation," *Phil. Trans.* 1866, p. 657.

In 1868 James Clerk Maxwell (1831–1879) lays the foundation for control theory. At about the same time Claude Bernard (1813–1878) introduces the notion that a regulatory mechanism controls all vital functions of an organism and maintains stability (homeostasis) in health. Almost a century later the Greek word for Maxwell's "governor" gives the name "cybernetics" to this scientific field.

MAXWELL, the son of a prominent Scottish family, was born in Edinburgh in 1831. He studied at the Edinburgh Academy and published his first paper at the age of fourteen. After studies at Edinburgh University, he went to Cambridge in 1850. From 1855, when he became a fellow of Trinity, he held several professorships before he retired from regular academic life in 1865. However, in 1871 he was appointed professor of experimental physics at Cambridge, where he planned, developed and even gave economic support to the Cavendish Laboratory. Maxwell was a religious man with a bent for mysticism. Maxwell is most well known for his landmark theory of the electromagnetic field (55.1) and his contributions to the kinetic theory of gases (55.2). He died of cancer at the age of only forty-eight.

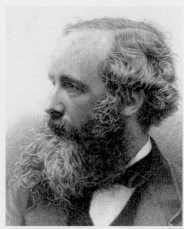

James Clerk Maxwell   55:2

On Governors.

PROCEEDINGS OF THE ROYAL SOCIETY OF LONDON 1868; 16:270.

WITH THIS paper Maxwell establishes the foundations of control theory. Introducing his analyses, he starts by saying: "A Governor is a part of a machine by means of which the velocity of the machine is kept nearly uniform, notwithstanding variations in the driving-power or the resistance" He continues: "I propose at present, without entering into any details of the mechanism, to direct the attention of engineers and mathematicians to the dynamic theory of such governors."

IN PERSPECTIVE:

Theories of control and communication are closely linked, since adequate control requires the exchange of proper information between the system and its "governor". Nyquist and Black made important advances in both these areas in the 1930s (55.3)(55.4)(55.5). More recently, Wiener introduced the word "cybernetics" (derived from the Greek for governor or steersman) and discussed bio-medical applications of control systems (55.6). A decade before Maxwell's paper Bernard, studying the vasomotor nerves, discovered that a physiological equilibrium was created by the simultaneous workings of two antagonistic (the vasoconstrictor and the vasodilator) innervations (55.7). From these observations evolved Bernard's general notion that a regulatory mechanism controlled all vital functions of an organism and maintained stability of the "milieu intérieur" (55.8) and that disease states represented deviations from this homeostasis. The modern theory of communication is based on the statistical concept of entropy (55.9), which was originally introduced by Boltzman, who in extending Maxwell's kinetic theory of gases (55.2) wanted to define a measure for the orderliness of a gaseous state (55.10). In one recent medical signal processing application, the entropy concept is shown to be useful for analysing the EEG signal to assess the depth of clinical anaesthetic sedation (55.11).

55.1 Maxwell JC. *Treatise on Electricity and Magnetism*. Vol. 1,2 Oxford; 1873.

55.2 Niven WD editor. *The Scientific Papers of James Clerk Maxwell*. Vol. 1,2 Cambridge; 1890. Vol.1 p377 Illustrations of the Dynamic theory of Gases. 1860. Vol.2 p26 On the dynamic Theory of Gases. 1866.

55.3 Nyquist H. Thermal agitation of electric charge in conductors. *Phys Rev* 1928; 32:110.

55.4 Nyquist H. Regeneration theory. *Bell Syst Tech J* 1932; 11:126.

55.5 Black HS. Stabilized feedback amplifiers. *Bell Syst Tech J* 1934; 13:1.

55.6 Wiener N. *Cybernetics or control and communication in the Animal and the Machine*. MIT Press; 1961.

55.7 Bernard C. *Leçons sur la physiologie et la pathologie du système nerveux*. Paris; 1858.

55.8 See ref. 4.8.

55.9 Shanon C, Weaver W. *The Mathematical Theory of Communication*. Urbana; 1949.

55.10 Boltzmann L. Über die Beziehung zwischen dem zweiten Hauptsatze, . . . *Sitzung d Kaiserl Akad Wiss* LXXVI, Oktober 1877 Wien; 1878.

55.11 Viertiö-Olja HE, et al. Entropy of EEG signal is a robust index for depth of hypnosis. *Anesthesiology* 2000; 93:1369.

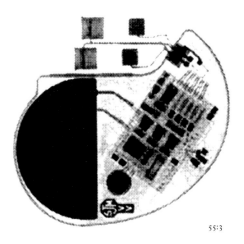

55:3

Rate Hysteresis

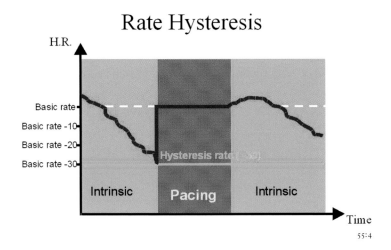

55:4

Ventricular Sensing / Inhibition

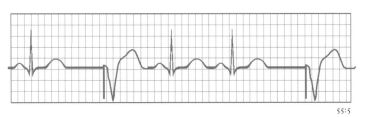

55:5

An X-ray image of a modern cardiac pacemaker, the operation of which is an example of a complex control system that, as illustrated by the graphs on the right, adapts to different physiological parameters that continuously reflect the status and the needs of the patient.

Modern infusion apparatus for pain relief. Physiological parameters can be set to control the dosage level but, using the handset shown in the foreground, patient controlled analgesia (PCA) can also be implemented. In this mode the patient becomes a part of the control loop.

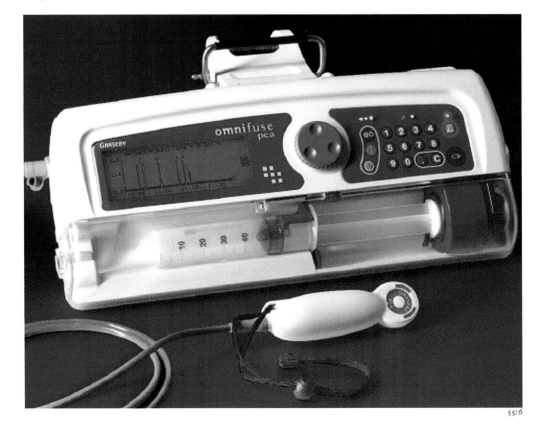

55:6

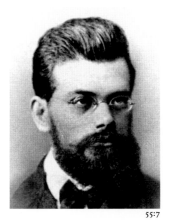

55:7

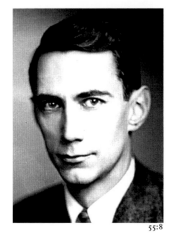

55:8

Control and communication are closely linked areas, since adequate control requires exchange of proper information between the system and its "governor". Modern communication theory dates back to 1948 and the work of Claude Shannon (1916–2001) (shown above). The key concept of his theory, that of "entropy", was introduced by Ludwig Boltzmann (1844–1906) (top portrait) seventy years before as a measure of the orderliness of the gaseous state. The page on the right shows Shannon's explanation of the entropy concept for the simplest of information systems, that having only two possible outcomes with probability p, and 1-p. The least ordered state (largest entropy) is when both outcomes are equally possible, each with a probability of 0.5.

Quantities of the form $H = -\Sigma\, p_i \log p_i$ (the constant K merely amounts to a choice of a unit of measure) play a central role in information theory as measures of information, choice and uncertainty. The form of H will be recognized as that of entropy as defined in certain formulations of statistical mechanics[8] where p_i is the probability of a system being in cell i of its phase space. H is then, for example, the H in Boltzmann's famous H theorem. We shall call $H = -\Sigma\, p_i \log p_i$ the entropy of the set of probabilities $p_1, \cdots, p_n$. If x is a chance variable we will write $H(x)$ for its entropy; thus x is not an argument of a function but a label for a number, to differentiate it from $H(y)$ say, the entropy of the chance variable y.

The entropy in the case of two possibilities with probabilities p and $q = 1 - p$, namely

$$H = -(p \log p + q \log q)$$

is plotted in Fig. 7 as a function of p.

The quantity H has a number of interesting properties which further substantiate it as a reasonable measure of choice or information.

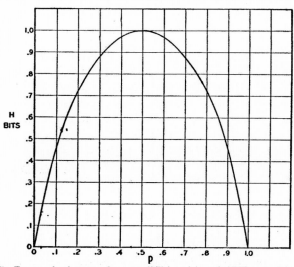

Fig. 7—Entropy in the case of two possibilities with probabilities p and $(1-p)$.

[8]See, for example, R. C. Tolman, *Principles of Statistical Mechanics*, Oxford, Clarendon, 1938.

55:9

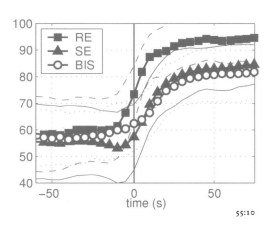

55:10

A modern clinical application of the information entropy concept is the assessment of the state of consciousness of a patient through an analysis of the electric variations in the brain activity as presented by an EEG signal. The picture illustrates how the rising consciousness of patients emerging from anaesthesia (at time zero) is revealed in the increasing entropy (RE and SE) and spectral index (BIS) of the EEG.

XIV. Sitzung am 9. Juli 1870.

Inhalt: **Fick**: Ueber die Messung des Blutquantums in den Herzventrikeln. — **Rinecker**: Ueber Rötheln und Masern.

1) Das Protokoll der letzten Sitzung wurde verlesen und genehmigt.

2) Neu eingelaufene Bücher werden in Vorlage gebracht.

3) Hr. Dr. phil. **Röntgen** wird als Mitglied angemeldet.

4) Hr. **Fick** hält einen Vortrag über die Messung des Blutquantums, das in jeder Systole durch die Herzventrikel ausgeworfen wird, eine Grösse, deren Kenntniss ohne Zweifel von grösster Wichtigkeit ist. Gleichwohl sind darüber die abweichendsten Ansichten aufgestellt. Während Th. **Young** die in Rede stehende Grösse auf etwa 45^{ccm} anschlägt, cursiren in den neueren Lehrbüchern der Physiologie meist sehr viel höhere Angaben, welche, gestützt auf die Schätzungen von **Volkmann** und **Vierordt**, sich bis auf 180^{ccm} belaufen. Bei dieser Sachlage ist es seltsam, dass man noch nicht auf folgenden naheliegenden Weg gekommen ist, auf dem diese wichtige Grösse wenigstens an Thieren direkter Bestimmung zugänglich ist. Man bestimme, wie viel Sauerstoff ein Thier während einer gewissen Zeit aus der Luft aufnimmt und wie viel Kohlensäure es abgibt. Man nehme ferner dem Thiere während der Versuchszeit eine Probe arteriellen und eine Probe venösen Blutes. In beiden ist der Sauerstoffgehalt und der Kohlensäuregehalt zu ermitteln. Die Differenz des Sauerstoffgehaltes ergibt, wie viel Sauerstoff jedes Cubiccentimeter Blut beim Durchgang durch die Lungen aufnimmt, und da man weiss, wie viel Sauerstoff im Ganzen während einer bestimmten Zeit aufgenommen wurde, so kann man berechnen, wie viel Cubiccentimeter Blut während dieser Zeit die Lungen passirten, oder wenn man durch die Anzahl der Herzschläge in dieser Zeit dividirt, wie viel Cubiccentimeter Blut mit jeder Systole des Herzens ausgeworfen wurden. Die entsprechende Rechnung mit den Kohlensäuremengen gibt eine Bestimmung desselben Werthes, welche die erstere controllirt.

Da zur Ausführung dieser Methode 2 Gaspumpen gehören, so ist der Vortragende leider nicht in der Lage, experimentelle Bestimmungen mitzutheilen. Er will daher nur noch nach dem Schema der angegebenen Methode eine Berechnung der Blutstromstärke des Menschen geben, gegründet auf mehr oder weniger willkürliche Data. Nach den von **Scheffer** in Ludwig's Laboratorium ausgeführten Versuchen enthält 1^{ccm} arterielles Hundeblut 0,146^{ccm} Sauerstoff (gemessen bei 0^0 Temperatur und 1^m Quecksilber Druck), 1^{ccm} venöses Hundeblut enthält 0,0905^{ccm} Sauerstoff. Jedes Cubiccentimeter Blut nimmt also beim Durchgang durch die Lungen 0,0555^{ccm} Sauerstoff auf. Nehme man an, das wäre beim Menschen gerade so. Nehme man ferner an, ein Mensch absorbirte in 24^h 833^{gr} Sauerstoff aus der Luft. Sie nehmen bei 0^0 und 1^m Druck 433200^{ccm} Raum ein. Demnach würden in den Lungen des Menschen jede Secunde 5^{ccm} Sauerstoff absorbirt. Um diese Absorption zu bewerkstelligen, müssten aber der obigen Annahme gemäss $\frac{5}{0,0555}$^{ccm} Blut die Lungen durchströmen, d. h 90^{ccm}. Angenommen endlich, dass 7 Systolen in 6 Secunden erfolgten, würden mit jeder Systole des Ventrikels 77^{ccm} Blut ausgeworfen.

56:1

The report from the annual meeting for the year 1870 of the Society for Physics and Medicine in Würzburg. Adolf Fick (1829–1901) gives a lecture where he introduces his method for calculating cardiac output from the oxygen uptake and the difference in the arterio-venous oxygen content of blood (Fick's principle). Using values reported by others and relying on blood gas data from dogs, he nevertheless estimates the stroke volume in man to be 77 ml, an entirely reasonable estimate even by modern standards. Just preceding the lecture of Fick, the 25 year-old Dr Wilhelm Röntgen is elected member of the Society.

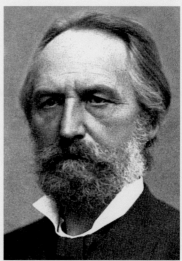

FICK was born in 1829 in Kassel, where his father was municipal architect. The youngest of nine children, he started to study mathematics and physics in Marburg, where one of his brothers was professor of anatomy. He soon turned to medicine and was guided not only by his brother but also by Ludwig (56.1). In Berlin, Fick met and made friends with Du Bois-Reymond and Helmholtz (56.1). In 1851 Fick obtained his doctorate and left for Zürich to work as prosector in anatomy with Ludwig and later as professor of anatomy and physiology. He moved to the chair of physiology in Würzburg in 1868 and remained there till his retirement in 1899. Fick was a modest man with strong convictions that he always stood by without hesitation. Apart from his remarkably diverse scientific interests, he also wrote on social issues. In particular he strongly opposed the abuse of alcohol (56.2).

Ueber die Messung des Blutquantums in den Hertzventrikeln.

SITZUNGSBER D PHYSIKAL-MED GES ZU WÜRZBURG. GESELLSCHAFTS-JAHR 1870. STAHEL'SCHEN BUCH U KUNSTHANDLUNG; 1872. P16.

IN THESE minutes from the meeting of the Medico-Physical Society in Würzburg, two entries are notable, Dr.phil. Röntgen is accepted as a new member of the Society and Fick gives a lecture on the measurement of the amount of blood passing the ventricles of the heart. With no access to gas pumps, Fick regrets that he cannot report experimental results but, using data on blood gases from the laboratory of Ludwig (56.3), he shows how to calculate cardiac output in man assuming that man and dog have the same difference in the arterio-venous oxygen content. The result he arrives at is 5.4 litres/minute.

IN PERSPECTIVE:
Gréhant and Quinquaud measured the pulmonary perfusion of dogs in 1886 using Fick's principle but applied to the carbon dioxide balance over the lungs (56.4). A decade later Zuntz and Hagemann determined the cardiac output of horses from the oxygen balance to be 75 ml/min/kg (56.5), a value that has stood the test of time (56.6). The first measurements in man were made by Löwy and v. Schrötter in 1905, utilising the oxygen balance (56.7) and soon many improvements to their methodology followed (56.8). The dye dilution method for measuring cardiac output was introduced in the 1940s (56.9) and, more recently, the thermodilution technique (56.10) has gained wide acceptance. Among the many techniques now available for estimating cardiac output clinically (56.11), Fick's method is the only one that is based on first principles. Formulated in differential form it also allows entirely non-invasive measurements of the pulmonary blood flow (56.12).

56.1 See ref. 46.1 and ref. 46.2.
56.2 See ref. 46.3.
56.3 See ref. 37.5.
56.4 Gréhant N, Quinquaud CE. Recherches expérimentales sur la mesure du volume de sang qui traverse les poumons en un temps donné. *C R Séance et Mém d Soc biol* 1886; 38:159.
56.5 Zuntz N, Hagemann O. *Untersuchungen über den Stoffwechsel des Pferdes bei Ruhe und Arbeit.* Berlin; 1898.
56.6 Fischer EW, Dalton RG. Cardiac Output in Horses. *Nature* 1959; 184:2020.
56.7 Löwy A, von Schrötter H. Untersuchungen über die Blutcirculation beim Menschen. *Zeit f exp Pathol u Therapie* 1905; 1:197.
56.8 Kisch F, Schwarz H. Das Herzschlagvolumen und die Methodik seiner Bestimmung. *Erg Inner Med u Kinderh* 1925; 27:169.
56.9 Hamilton WF, et al. Comparison of the Fick and dye injection methods of measuring the cardiac output in man. *Am J Physiol* 1948; 153:309.
56.10 Ganz W, et al. A new technique for measurement of cardiac output by thermodilution in man. *Am J Cardiol* 1971; 17:392.
56.11 Robertson JI, Birkenhäger WH. Editors. *Cardiac Output Measurement* London: Saunders; 1991.
56.12 Gedeon A, et al. A new method for noninvasive bedside determination of pulmonary blood flow. *Med. & Bio Eng & Comp* 1980; 18:411.

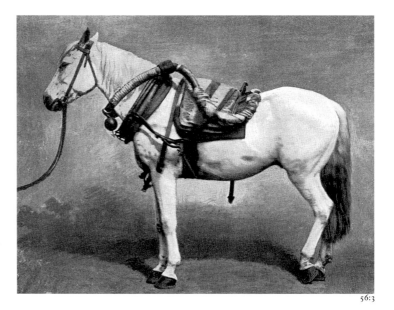

The apparatus developed by Nathan Zuntz (1847–1920) to measure the cardiac output of horses using Fick's principle (see #37). He obtains the value of 75 ml/min/kg, the accuracy of which is confirmed more than half a century later.

56:3

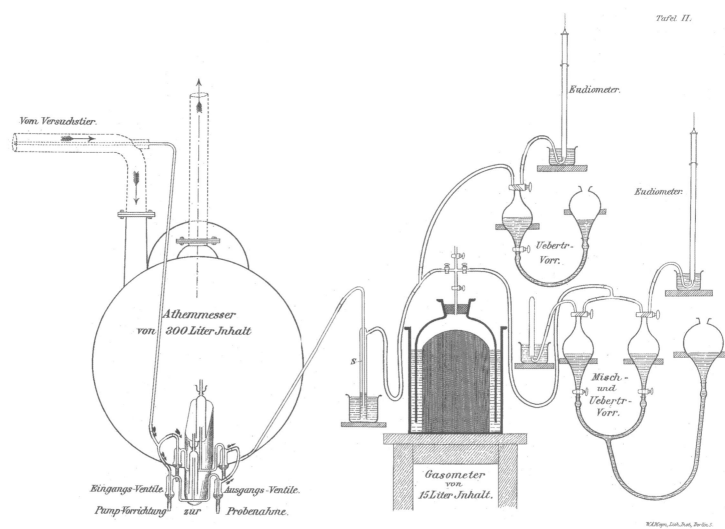

Tafel II.

Vom Versuchstier.

Eudiometer.

Eudiometer.

Uebertr-Vorr.

Athemmesser von 300 Liter Jnhalt

S.

Misch- und Uebertr- Vorr.

Eingangs-Ventile. *Ausgangs-Ventile.*

Pump-Vorrichtung *zur* *Probenahme.*

Gasometer von 15 Liter Jnhalt.

W.A.Meyn, Lith.Inst., Berlin.S.

56:4

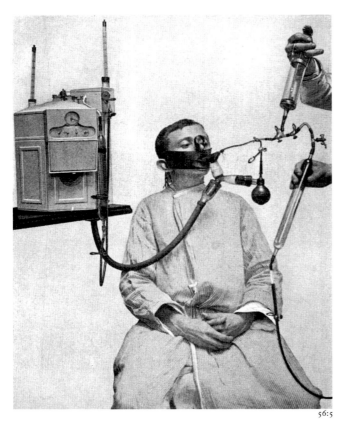

56:5

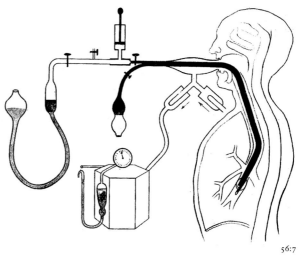

56:7

Adolf Löwy (1862–1937) in Berlin and Hermann von Schrötter (1870–1928) in Vienna collaborate in 1905 to make the first non-invasive determination of cardiac output using Fick's principle. As shown by their schematic diagram (above), venous blood gas samples are obtained through a catheter placed in a closed off section of the lung. They report a reasonable average cardiac output value of 3.85 litre/min, but with very large variations in the individual measurement.

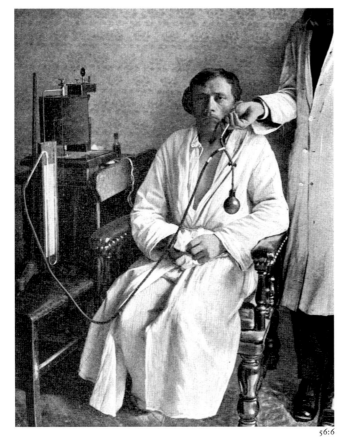

56:6

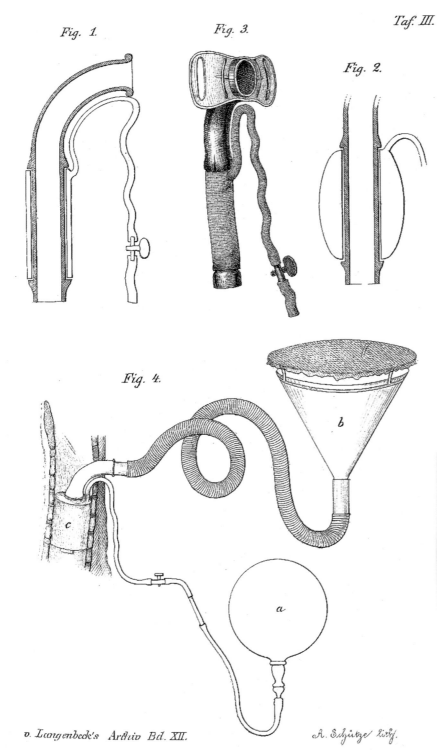

Fig. 1. Fig. 3. Taf. III. Fig. 2. Fig. 4. v. Langenbeck's Archiv Bd. XII. A. Schütze lith.

In 1871 Friedrich Trendelenburg (1844–1924) introduces a cuffed canule that prevents aspiration. As shown in his illustration, a funnel-shaped attachment can be connected to it through the tracheostomy for convenient administration of inhalation anaesthetics.

Below, a set of tracheotomy instruments from the end of the 19th century.

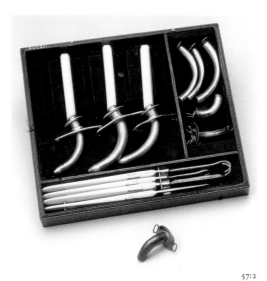

57:2

57:1

TRENDELENBURG was born in Berlin in 1844, the son of the famous German philosopher Friedrich Adolf Trendelenburg. For his early studies in medicine he went to Glasgow and Edinburgh, but returned to Berlin and received his medical doctorate in 1866 with a dissertation on ancient surgery in India. During the years 1868 to 1874, Trendelenburg worked as an assistant surgeon and developed the tampon cannula to be described below. He was a founder of the German Surgical Society in 1872. Trendelenburg left Berlin for Rostock, where he was appointed professor of surgery in 1875. He stayed here for seven years, but then moved to Bonn and in 1885 to a position as surgeon-in-chief at the university clinic in Leipzig. He retired in 1911 and died thirteen years later.

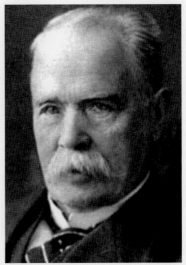

57:3

Friedrich Trendelenburg

Beiträge zu den Operationen an den Luftwegen.

ARCH KLIN CHIR 1871; 12:112. BERLIN: A. HIRSCHWALD; 1871.

TRENDELENBURG CITES his own experience in a recent case and also the experience of others showing the problems of aspiration in connection with major surgery of the larynx. He then describes a procedure based on tracheotomy and a newly designed piece of equipment (Tampon-Canule) that is intended to prevent aspiration and the associated complications. He lists six different operations where his technique could be indicated and closes by reporting his first case, performed in December 1869, which fully confirmed the advantage of his method. His paper also shows illustrations of his device and its use with inhalation anaesthesia.

IN PERSPECTIVE:
Both Roman (Galen) and Arabic (Rahzes, Avicenna) surgeons knew about tracheotomy (57.1). Casseri gave a magnificent illustration of it in 1600 (57.2), while Santorio described the procedure from his own experience (57.3) using a trocar and a cannula that he left in the wound for three days. Heister suggested the name tracheotomy (57.4) and Martine (57.5) in 1730 was the first to use double tubes, the inner being removable to keep the tracheostomy tube free from mucus. Operations on the larynx started with Desault around 1810 (57.6)(57.1). Trendelenburg had to adapt his device to the funnel used at the time in Berlin to deliver chloroform anaesthesia. In 1900 Kuhn started experimenting with oral and nasal intubation (57.7) and by 1905 he had developed a technique that allowed anaesthesia to be delivered using positive pressure ventilation (57.8). The first such procedure in man was reported by Barthélemy and Dufour in 1907 (57.9). Subsequently Elsberg, following the work of Meltzer, developed the apparatus needed for the clinical use of positive pressure ventilation (57.10)(57.11).

57.1 See ref. 48.3.
57.2 See ref. 25.3.
57.3 See p363 in the main work cited in #7 Santorio page 54.
57.4 Heister L. *Chirurgie in welcher alles was zur Wund-Artzney gehöret, nach der neuesten und besten Art.* Nurnberg; 1718.
57.5 See ref. 7.4 for another of Martine's contributions to medicine.
57.6 Desault PJ. *Oevres chirurgicales.* 3 vols. Paris; 1798–1803.
57.7 Kuhn F. Die perorale Intubation. *Zbl Chir* 28/52 Leipzig; 1901.
57.8 Kuhn F. Perorale Tubagen mit und ohne Druck. *Dtsch Z Chir* 1905; 76:148.
57.9 Barthélemy M, Dufour L. L'anesthésie dans la chirugie de la face. *La Presse Médicale* 27 Juillet 1907. p475.
57.10 Elsberg CA. Zur Narkose beim Menschen mittelst der kontinuerlichen intratracheal Insufflation von Meltzer. *Berl klin Wschr* 1910; 47(21):957.
57.11 Gwathmey JT. *Anesthesia.* Chapter X. NewYork: D.Appleton and Co; 1914.

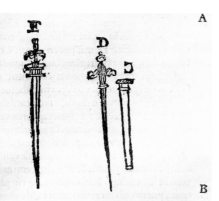

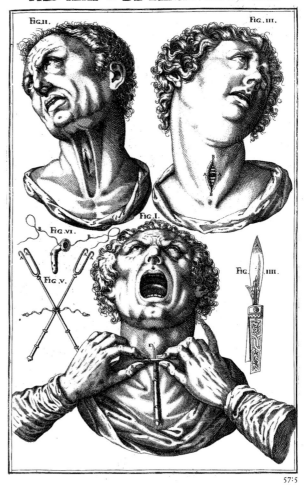

57:5

Julius Casserius (1561–1616) gives an accurate illustration of tracheotomy in 1600.

Sed pro infantibus & adultis, qui suffocantur, si nullum aliud remedium iuuet, nostra perforatio facta infra laryngem cum instrumento E à subita morte ad subitam salutem tutò patientem reuocat : dummodo materia suffocans sit à larynge supra, vel supra perforationem, quia si infra, vel in ipso pulmone existat vana redditur perforatio. Instrumentum C est fistula argentea perforata. Instrumentum D est acus mucronata, quæ intromittitur in instrumentũ C quo tamen acus longior est, & intromissa fit instrumentum E, quod cum illo fit ita vnitum, vt tactui nulla occurrat asperitas : imo instrumentum E vnum continuum, & non duo esse videntur. Dum igitur volumus dicto instrumento perforare, prius curamus, vt patientes inclinent caput retrorsum, hoc fine, vt aspera arteria distendatur : deinde sub larynge post duos, vel tres circulos, circuli intermedium perforamus : hac lege seruata quod dum incipit instrumentum ingredi cauitatem tracheæ statim retrahatur, & auferatur ab ipsa fistula acus interna, ne pungat partem oppositam tracheæ : quo peracto fistula tutò intimius impellitur : inde per fistulam perforatam acu ablata, libera fit inspiratio, & expiratio, omninoque prohibetur suffocatio non solum in angina suffocante, sed in quocumque simili affectu : imo si illa vti liceret in laqueo interimendis, ipsos quoque à suffocatione præseruaret. Tamdiu in trachea detinetur fistula, donec superetur suffocationis causa, qua solum superata, fistula aufertur. Sanabitur verò perexiguum vulnus eodem die ne dicam hora, si foramini pauxillum chollirij nostri, quod fit ex iulapio, & lithargyro, applicetur.

Notanda est differentia inter respiratione crebram & velocem, de qua in tex. mentionem facit Auicennas :
crebritas enim respicit terminum : velocitas
verò respicit
motum,
seu
spacium per quod
fit motus.

∴

In 1625 Santorio Santorio (1561–1636) describes tracheotomy from his own experience in this way: "But our perforation, done under the larynx with instrument E, safely restores children and adults, who are choking, from sudden death to sudden salvation, if no other cure helps, provided that the suffocating matter is located over the larynx or over the perforation, because if it is located under it or in the lung itself, the perforation is done in vain.

Instrument C is a perforated silver pipe. Instrument D is a pointed needle, which is placed in instrument C. The needle is longer than instrument C. This should introduce instrument E, because they should make a unity together, so that no difficulty arises when it comes to the operation;" "When we have made sure that the instrument is starting to enter the cavity of the trachea, it is pulled back immediately and the inner needle removed from the pipe, so that it does not sting the opposite side of the trachea. When this has been accomplished, the pipe is safely pushed further in. Thereafter the inhalation and exhalation should be free through the pipe, deprived of the needle. On the whole, suffocation is prevented not only when it comes to choking in the throat, but in all similar cases."

57:4

In 1900 Franz Kuhn (1866–1929) starts to experiment with oral and nasal intubation and by 1905 he has developed a technique that allows anaesthesia to be delivered using positive pressure ventilation.

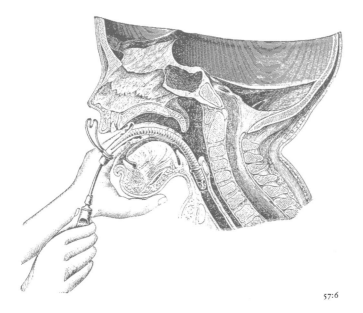

57:6

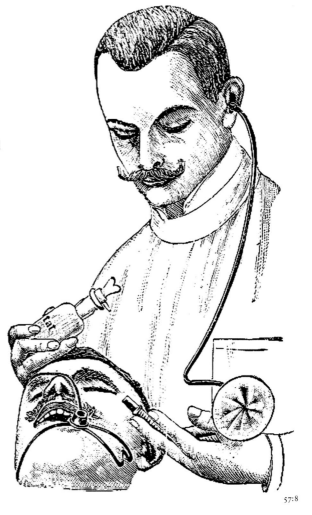

57:8

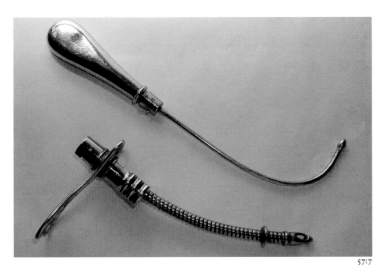

57:7

Kuhn's tracheal intubation set.

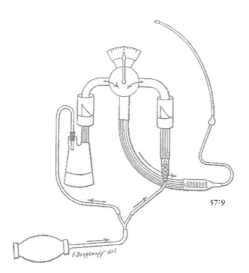

57:9

In 1907 Marc Barthélemy and Léon Dufour report the first clinical insufflation endotracheal anaesthesia in man using chloroform during a facial operation. The equipment (see figure above) and the method are described in this way: "a hand-operated bellows is connected to a tube in the flask of chloroform, the other end of which is attached to one of the inhalation valves. In addition, the same bellows controls the other inhalation valve directly, which will thus pass only pure air. The proportion of pure air to chloroform-bearing air is governed by the pointer on the central disk at which the two streams end up; they meet in the medial tube, which ends in a No. 18 Gelly's urethal catheter. Introduced into the larynx, the catheter does not block off the glottis and the patient can breathe freely alongside it. In this way, one remains in absolute control of the mixture, which is absorbed in its entirety every time the bellows is operated, and when one ceases to operate it, the patient breathes pure air." "In order to spare the patient the disagreeable sensation of having the catheter introduced, and particularly to avoid reflexes that could be dangerous, this apparatus must be used only for the maintenance of anaesthesia induced by the normal procedures. It also allows pure air to be injected at any given time as needed—that is to say provision of artificial respiration: it is sufficient to set the pointer to 0."

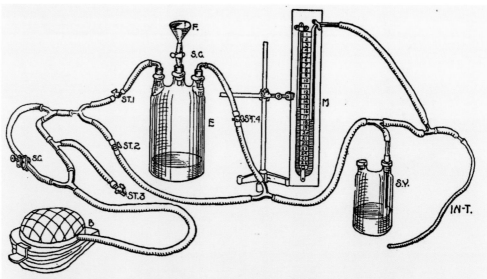

MELTZER'S SIMPLE APPARATUS FOR INTRATRACHEAL INSUFFLATION. B, foot-bellows; S. T, stopcocks; E, ether bottle with S. C, stopcock and F, funnel; M, manometer; S. V, mercury safety valve; IN-T, intratracheal tube.

57:10

Samuel Meltzer's (1851–1920) improved intratracheal insufflation apparatus. Meltzer notes that a continuous flow of air can keep dogs alive for hours, an observation made already more than two centuries before by Hooke (see #11).

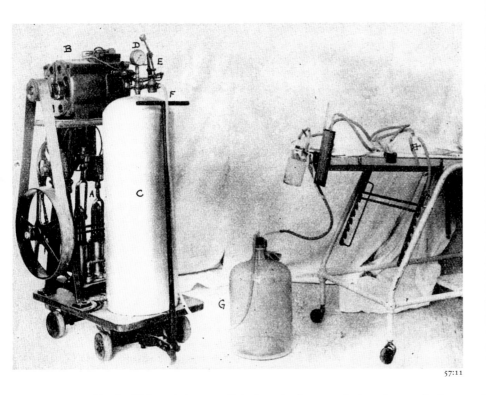

57:11

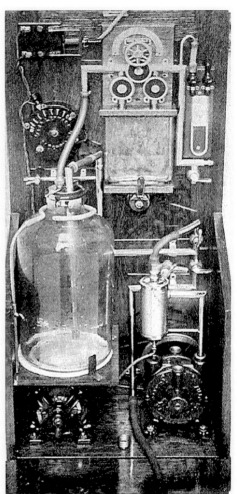

ELSBERG'S APPARATUS, FOR HOSPITAL USE.

57:12

Charles Elsberg (1871–1948) designs the first practical equipment for intratracheal insufflation, which marks the beginning of modern endotracheal anaesthesia. Illustrations show his prototype unit (left) and his apparatus for hospital use (right).

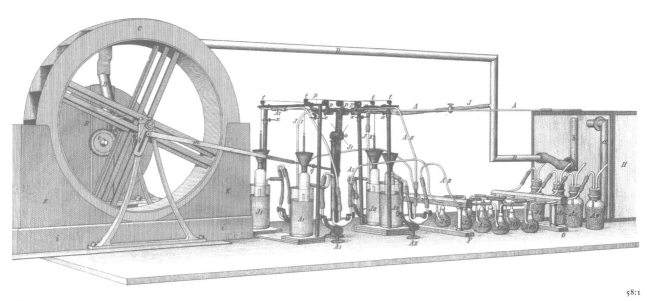

58:1

Illustration of the respiration apparatus of Carl Voit (1831–1908). It is a small but much improved version of Max Pettenkofer's (1818–1901) huge machine (see next pages). It allows the accurate determination of the gas exchange in animals and is used in Voit's important studies on substrate utilisation in the metabolic process.

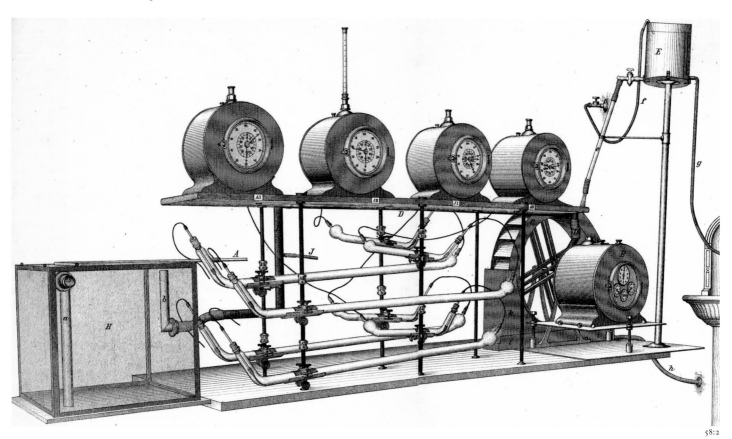

58:2

VOIT, the son of an architect, was born in Amberg in 1831. At seventeen years of age he began studying medicine in Munich. He then received training in analytical chemistry in Göttingen and also in Munich, where he attended the lectures of Liebig (58.1). In 1856 he became assistant to Bischoff at the Physiological Institute of Munich and four years later joined the laboratory of Pettenkofer, who became his lifelong friend. In 1863 Voit was appointed professor of physiology and for the next three decades he carried out an ambitious programme of metabolic research. Later he devoted most of his time to official duties at the university. All his life he enjoyed lecturing and continued to do so till 1907, the year before his death.

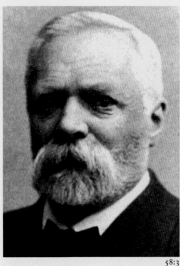

Carl von Voit   58:3

Beschreibung eines Apparates zur Untersuchung der gasförmigen Ausscheidungen des Thierkörpers.

ABH D K AKAD D WISS MÜNCHEN; 1876; 12(1):219.

VOIT GIVES a detailed description of his apparatus for the measurement of gas exchange in animals. The technique is based on an open-circuit approach, where air is allowed to flow through an enclosure where the experimental animal is confined. Accurate methods of gas analysis and ingenious absolute calibration techniques are combined to improve on the performance of a similar but much larger installation built by Pettenkofer in 1861 (58.2).

IN PERSPECTIVE:
In 1849 Regnault and Reiset presented the first quantitative study of gas exchange in animals (58.3). Measuring the changes in gas concentration in a closed space (closed circuit method), they demonstrated the general effect of nutrition on oxygen uptake and carbon dioxide elimination. The closed circuit method was subsequently perfected by Krogh (58.4). In 1860 Bischoff and Voit showed that all of the nitrous intake of a meat diet could be accounted for by collection of the excretions of the animal and by taking the body weight changes into account (58.5). To measure rather than just estimate the amount of carbon and oxygen exhaled as a result of the metabolic process of the other substrates, Pettenkofer built a huge apparatus for determining the carbon dioxide elimination in man (58.2). It was basically a ventilated room where the gas flow and concentrations of carbon dioxide were carefully measured, not unlike the hood technique used clinically in modern times (58.6). The resting energy expenditure in healthy man was determined in 1919 (58.7) and Weir showed that it could be calculated from gas exchange measurements (58.8). Modern metabolic carts can be used to monitor and tailor therapy in severe disease states, both acute and chronic (58.9)(58.10)(58.11).

58.1   See #39 Liebig page 208.
58.2   Pettenkofer M. Ueber einen neuen Respirations-Apparat. *Abh d k b Akad d Wiss* 1861. p231.
58.3   Regnault HV, Reiset J. Recherches Chimique sur la Respiration des Animaux des Diverses Classes. *Ann chim phys* 1849; 26:299.
58.4   Krogh A. *The respiratory exchange of animals and man.* London:Longmans Green & Co; 1916. Chapter 2. See also ref. 37.7.
58.5   See ref. 39.9.
58.6   Askanazi J, et al. Nutrition for the patient with respiratory failure: glucose vs fat. *Anesth* 1981; 54:373.
58.7   Harris JA, Benedict FG. *A Biometric Study of Basal Metabolism in Man.* Publ.279 Washington DC: Carnegie Institute of Washington; 1919.
58.8   de Weir JB. New methods to calculating metabolic rate with special reference to protein metabolism. *J Physiol* 1949; 109:1.
58.9   AARC Clinical Guideline 949: Metabolic Measurement using Indirect Calorimetry during Mechnical Ventilation. *Resp Care* 1994; 39(12):1170.
58.10   Bursztein S. editor. *Energy Metabolism, Indirect Calorimetry and Nutrition.* Baltimore: Williams and Wilkins; 1989.
58.11   Nixon DW, et al. Resting energy expenditure in lung and colon cancer. *Metabolism* 1988; 37:1059.

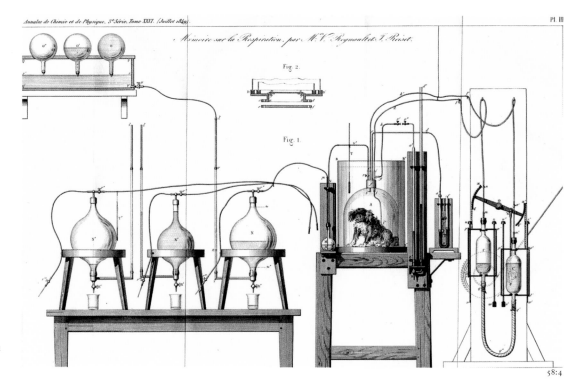

The experimental arrangement of Victor Regnault (1810–1878) and Jules Reiset (1818–1896). Their study in 1849 is the first to demonstrate the effect of nutrition on oxygen uptake and carbon dioxide elimination.

58:4

Supported by funds from King Maximilian of Bavaria, Max Pettenkofer (1818–1901) builds an apparatus where the experimental chamber has the size of an ordinary room. The amount of carbon dioxide exhaled by the subject in the room is calculated from concentrations of the air entering and exiting the room.

58:5

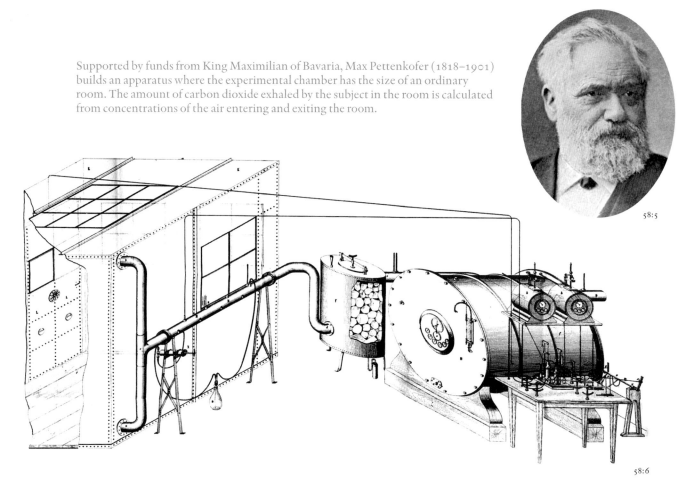

58:6

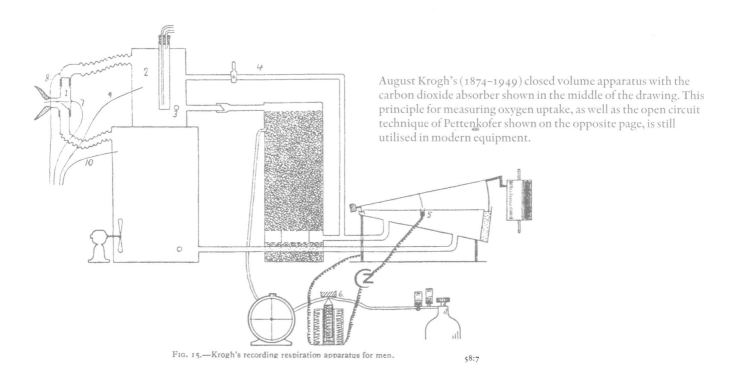

August Krogh's (1874–1949) closed volume apparatus with the carbon dioxide absorber shown in the middle of the drawing. This principle for measuring oxygen uptake, as well as the open circuit technique of Pettenkofer shown on the opposite page, is still utilised in modern equipment.

FIG. 15.—Krogh's recording respiration apparatus for men.

58:7

The apparatus used by Francis Benedict (1870–1957) in 1919 to establish the basal metabolic rate in healthy human volunteers.

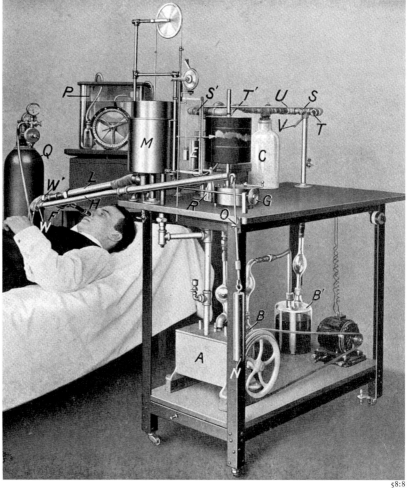

58:8

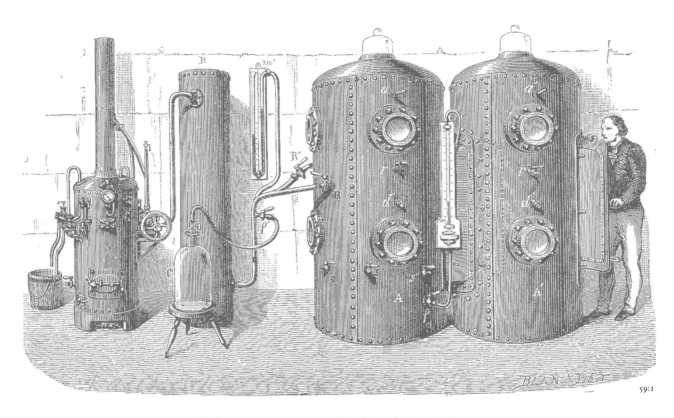

The low pressure apparatus of Paul Bert (1833–1886)
used to determine the oxygen content of blood at
subatmospheric pressures. Graphs are shown in a live
animal (C), and in vitro, blood at body temperature
(B) and at room temperature (A).

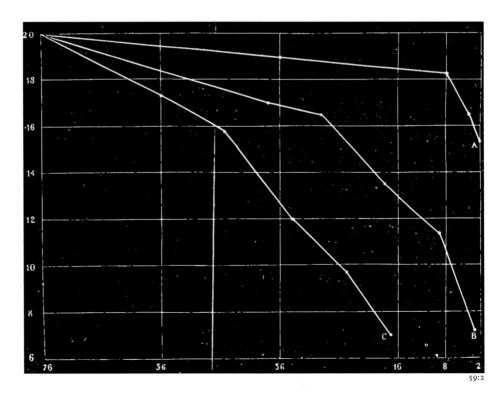

59:2

ERT was born in Auxerre in 1833. He studied medicine in Paris, receiving his M.D. degree in 1863. After three years as assistant to Bernard (59.1), he was appointed professor in zoology and physiology in Bordeaux, but returned in 1869 to Paris to succeed Bernard in the chair of physiology at the Sorbonne. In the following year he entered politics with a programme to reform elementary education in France. His proposals to incorporate elements of science in order to sharpen the intellect and stimulate causal thinking were enacted in 1880. When in 1885 a revolt erupted in Indochina against the French colonial regime, Bert was appointed the first civil governor there. His ambitious activities to improve relations with the local population were cut short by his death in Hanoi in 1886.

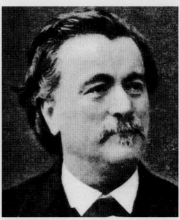

Paul Bert

59:3

La pression barométrique. Recherches de physiologie expérimentale.

PARIS: G. MASSON; 1878.

IN THIS monumental work of more than 1,150 pages and 89 illustrations Bert examines the effect of pressure on an organism, using elaborate newly designed apparatus. He establishes for the first time the dissociation curve of oxygen and carbon dioxide in blood and shows that it is the partial pressure of the gases and not the barometric pressure that is of physiological significance. He explains the mechanism of decompression sickness and high altitude sickness and observes the toxic effect of pure oxygen at high pressures. He also shows that carbon dioxide can act as an anaesthetic. At the end, Bert discusses the physiological background to the fatal outcome of the ascent of the balloon "Zénith" to 8,600 m, where only one out of the three scientists on board escaped with his life.

IN PERSPECTIVE:
Bert's work was based on previous knowledge about blood gases (59.2), the properties of haemoglobin (59.3) and the anaesthetic effects of nitrous oxide (59.4) at normal atmospheric pressures. His work clarified many outstanding physiological issues. Thus, in 1824 Hickman discovered that carbon dioxide could be used as a stupefying agent (59.5) but his method, which he called suspended animation, was met everywhere with disinterest or distrust (59.6). Bert, vindicating Hickman's assertions concluded, "Anaesthesia produced by carbon dioxide deserves a new the attention of surgeons"(59.7). Bert used mixtures of oxygen and nitrous oxide (in the ratio 1/6) and produced adequate anaesthesia by elevating the total pressure by about 20% (59.8). His pioneering measurements of the oxygen dissociation relationship of blood was subsequently improved on by Hufner (59.9) and later extensively studied by Barcroft (59.10), Douglas and Haldane (59.11).

59.1 See ref. 55.7, ref. 47.8 and ref. 4.8.
59.2 See #37 Magnus page 196.
59.3 See #51 Hoppe-Seyler page 268.
59.4 See #28 Davy page 156 and ref. 28.11.
59.5 Hickman H. *A letter on suspended animation, containing experiments showing that it may be safely employed during operations on animals,* ... Ironbridge; 1824.
59.6 Sykes WS. *Essays on the first hundred years of anaesthesia.* Vol. I Chap. 7 Churchill Livingstone; 1982.
59.7 Main work cited above p1018.
59.8 Bert P. Sur la possibilité d'obtenir, à l'aide du protoxyde d'azote, une insensibilité du long durée et sur l'innocuité de cet anesthésieque. *C R Acad Sci* 1878; 87:728. See also ref. 28.8 p318–323.
59.9 See ref. 51.10.
59.10 Barcroft J. *The respiratory function of the blood.* Cambridge University Press; 1913.
59.11 Haldane JC. *Respiration.* New Haven: Yale University Press; 1922.

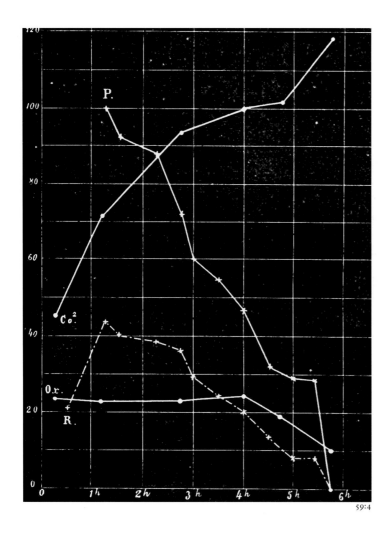

59:4

In 1823 Henry Hickman (1800–1830) argues in vain that carbon dioxide can be used as a stupefying agent. Half a century later Bert's work vindicates Hickman's assertions. The diagram left shows the effect of the rising carbon dioxide tension in blood (Co) on blood pressure (P), oxygen tension (Ox) and respiration (R).

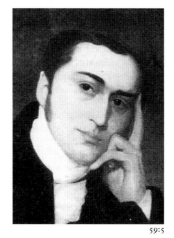

59:5

The pneumatic chamber constructed by Bert for oxygen and nitrous oxide anaesthesia is first used in 1879. Delivering a 15/85 oxygen/nitrous oxide mixture at 15% above the atmospheric pressure, it is reported to produce satisfactory anaesthesia in a short operation on a toe-nail.

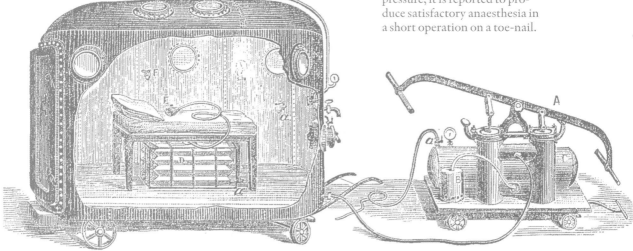

59:6

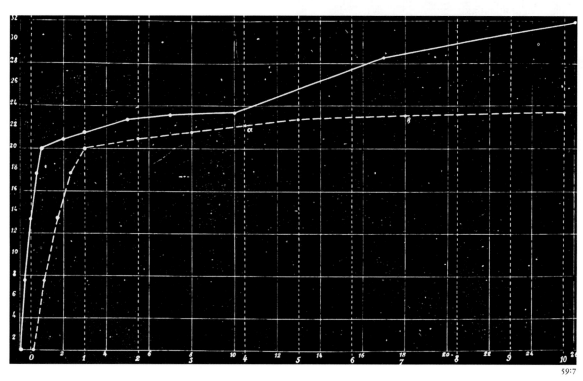

59:7

Bert determines the increase in the oxygen content of blood with increasing pressure (dashed line 0–10 atmospheres, full line 0–26
atmospheres) and discusses the application of his results to diving.
He also demonstrates the toxic effects of hyperbaric oxygen.

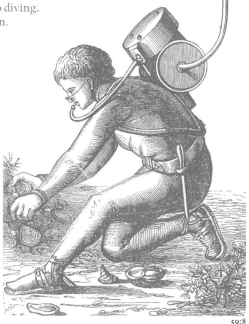

59:8

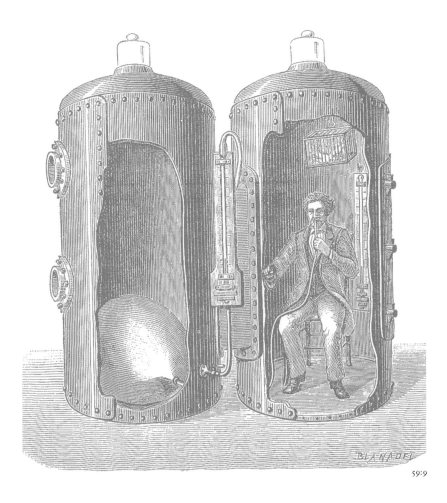

59:9

Bert's apparatus for studying the effect of impaired oxygenation when oxygen is diluted by a pressure reduction. Also shown is the relation that he obtains between oxygen content and oxygen tension of blood. This measurement is the first determination of the "oxygen dissociation curve", a relation of major physiological importance.

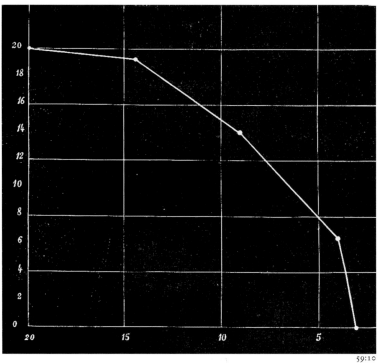

59:10

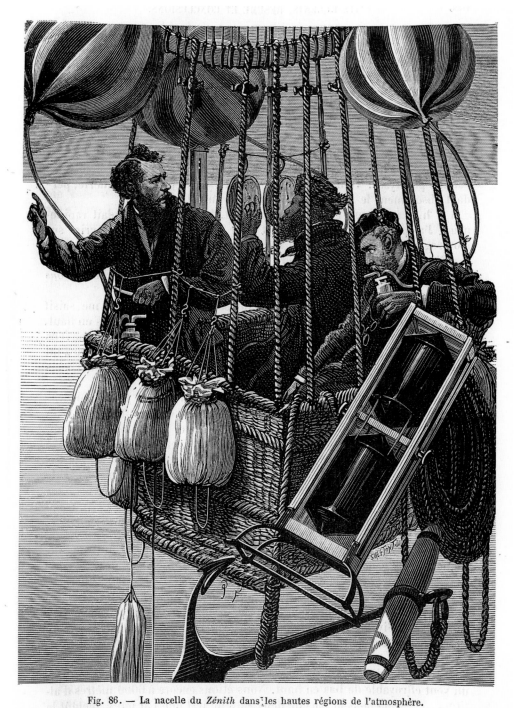

Fig. 86. — La nacelle du *Zénith* dans les hautes régions de l'atmosphère.

SIVEL	G. TISSANDIER	CROCÉ-SPINELLI
coupe les cordelettes qui retiennent à la nacelle les sacs de lest remplis de sable.	observe les baromètres.	après avoir fait les observations spectroscopiques, va respirer l'oxygène.

59:11

The famous picture of the three scientists conducting physical experiments while their balloon, the Zénith, ascends to 8,600 metres. Only one of them, Tissandier, survives the trip and Bert is able to explain the cause of the tragedy as inadvertently spending too long at the highest altitudes with inadequate levels of oxygen.

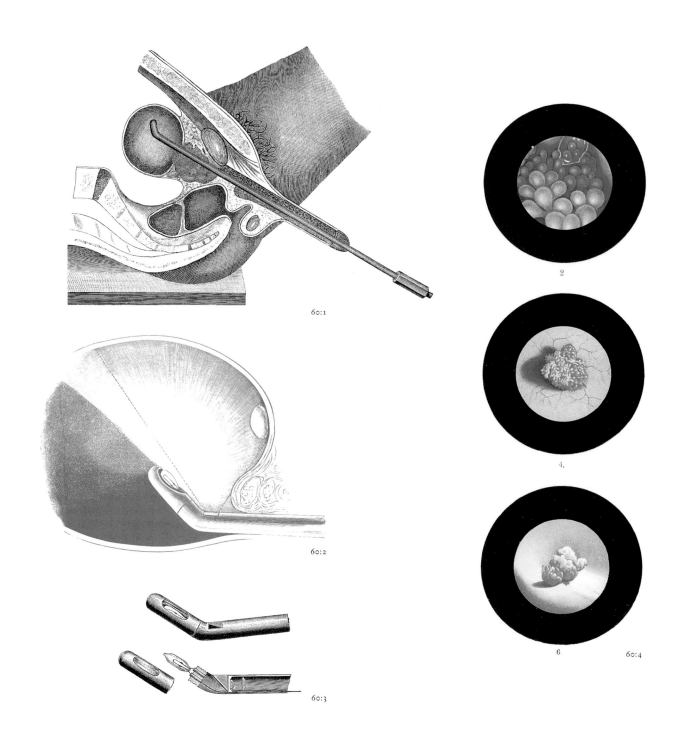

60:1

60:2

60:3

2

4.

6

60:4

In 1879 Max Nitze (1848–1906) introduces a newly designed cystoscope for the examination of the urinary bladder. This instrument uses a platinum wire as a light source and
needs to be water-cooled. However, the same year Thomas Edison (1847–1931) invents
the incandescent electric lamp, which by 1886 is sufficiently small to allow Nitze to incorporate it into his instrument. The resulting superior device, shown here, gains rapid
acceptance and the technique also finds many new applications.

Images from the cystoscope of
Nitze showing malignancies of
the urinary bladder.

N ITZE was born in 1848 in Berlin. He studied medicine in Heidelberg, Würzburg and Leipzig and started his career in 1874 as assistant surgeon at the City Hospital of Dresden. Three years later he moved to Vienna, where he established collaboration with Josef Leiter, a highly talented designer and manufacturer of medical apparatus and supplies. In 1879 Nitze was able to demonstrate for the first time his newly developed cystoscope. In 1890 he was appointed extraordinary professor of urology in Berlin. On his death in 1906 he had just completed the second edition of his textbook on cystoscopy (60.1), which summarises his life work.

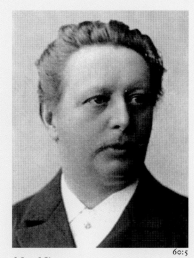

Max Nitze   60:5

Eine neue Beobachtungs- und Untersuchungsmethode für Harnröhre, Harnblase und Rectum.

WIEN MED WSCHR WIEN; 1879; 29:649, AND P688, 713, 776, 806.

IN THESE reports Nitze describes the first version of his cystoscope and its proper use. The major advance compared to previous efforts is the platina wire that he places at the tip of the device as a light source for the illumination of the urinary bladder. The instrument needs to be fitted with water cooling to remove the excess heat produced by the light source but, together with an optical arrangement for wide angle viewing of the interior of the bladder, it is far superior to earlier devices (60.2).

IN PERSPECTIVE:
In 1865 Desormeaux made the first clinical investigation using an "endoscope" that introduced light into the urinary bladder by reflection (60.2). This instrument was modified by Pantaleoni to accomplish the first hysteroscopy in 1869. Nitze's first design cited above was greatly improved when in 1886 he was able to replace the platina wire light source with the new invention of Edison, the incandescent light bulb (60.3). Subsequently Nitze developed special versions of the cystoscope for irrigation, photography and surgery (60.1)(60.4). Leiter also developed modified versions of the instrument for other purposes, including his "hysteroskop" "endoskop", "stomatoskop", "laryngoskop" (60.5), "otoskop" and "gastroskop" (60.6).Very soon Mikulicz-Radecki reported the successful clinical use of Leiter's gastroscope (60.7) and in 1898 Killian described the first direct broncoscopy using Leiter's equipment (60.8). Following the ideas of Kelling (60.9), Jacobaeus introduced clinical laparoscopy and thoracoscopy in 1910 (60.10). In the early 1960s Hopkins improved the imaging systems considerably by employing rods rather than conventional lenses. Image transmission by optical fibre bundles was conceived in 1954 by Hopkins and Kapany and independently by Heel, and this technology plays a key role today in endoscopic instrumentation (60.11)(60.12).

60.1 Nitze M. *Lehrbuch der Kystoskopie ihre Technik und klinische Bedeutung*. Wiesbaden; 1907.

60.2 Desormeaux AJ. *De l'endoscope et de ses applications au diagnostic et au traitment des affections de l'urèthre et de la vessie*. Paris; 1865.

60.3 Edison TA. *Electric-Lamp*. U.S. Patent 223,898 January 27 1880.

60.4 Nitze M. *Kystophotographischer Atlas*. Wiesbaden; 1894.

60.5 See # 48 Czermak page 254.

60.6 Leiter J. *Instrumente und Apparate zur direkten Beleuchtung Menschlicher Körperhöhlen durch Elektrischen Glühlicht*. Wien; 1880.

60.7 von Mikulicz-Radecki J. *Ueber Gastroscopie und Oesophagoskopie*. Wien med Presse 1881; 22:1405. p1437, p1473, p1505, p1537, p1573 and p1629.

60.8 Killian G. Ueber directe Bronchoskopie. *Munch med Wschr* 1898; 45:844.

60.9 Kelling G. Über die Besichtigung der Speiseröhre und des Magens mit biegsamen Instrumente. *Verh Gesell Dtsch Naturf u Ärzte* 1901; 73:117.

60.10 Jacobaeus HC. Ueber die Möglichkeit die Zystoscopie bei Untersuchungen seröser Höhlungen anzuwenden. *Münch med Wschr* 1910; 57:2090.

60.11 Kapany NS, et al. *Fiber Optics*. Part I–IV. J.O.S.A 1957; 47:413. p423, p594 and p1109.

60.12 Sircus W, Flisk E, Craigs B. Milestones in the evolution of endoscopy: A short history. *J Roy Coll Physicians Edinb* 2003; 33:124.

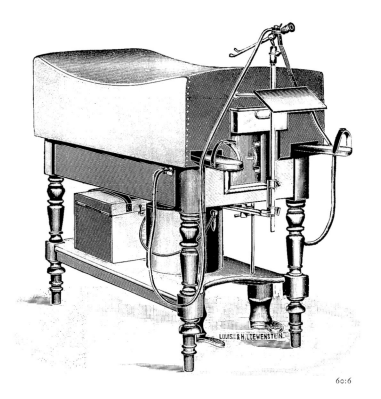

60:6

The first special examination table for cystoscopy.

Devices developed for formalin sterilisation (below left) and steam sterilisation of cystoscopes.

The irrigation cystoscope shown right has an extra channel which, in other versions of the instrument, is used to introduce a loop of platinum wire that allows cauterisation of malignancies.

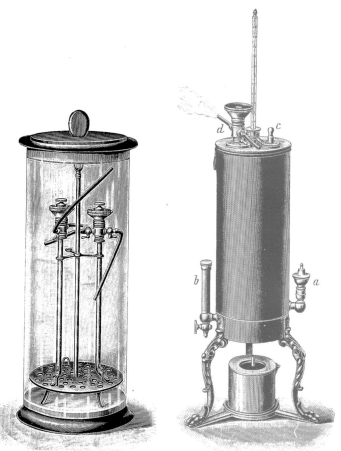

60:7

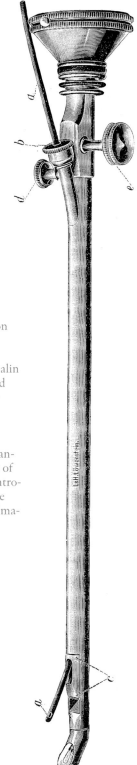

60:8

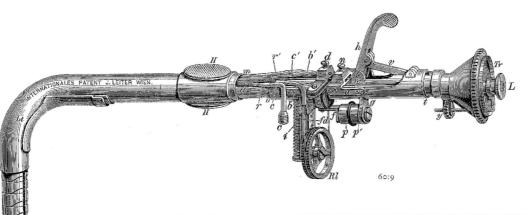

60:9

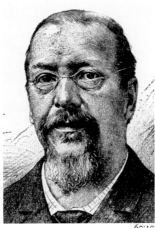

60:10

Josef Leiter (1830–1892) is a highly competent manufacturer of medical equipment and supplies in Vienna. In collaboration with prominent physicians, he develops a series of improved endoscopic instruments, including the new gastroscope shown here.

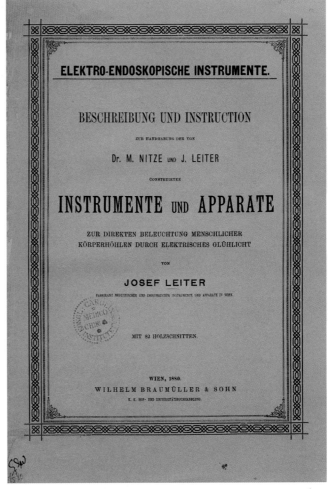

ELEKTRO-ENDOSKOPISCHE INSTRUMENTE.

BESCHREIBUNG UND INSTRUCTION

ZUR HANDHABUNG DER VON

Dr. M. NITZE UND J. LEITER

CONSTRUIRTEN

INSTRUMENTE UND APPARATE

ZUR DIREKTEN BELEUCHTUNG MENSCHLICHER
KÖRPERHÖHLEN DURCH ELEKTRISCHES GLÜHLICHT

VON

JOSEF LEITER

FABRIKANT MEDICINISCHER UND CHIRURGISCHER INSTRUMENTE UND APPARATE IN WIEN.

MIT 82 HOLZSCHNITTEN.

WIEN, 1880.
WILHELM BRAUMÜLLER & SOHN
K. K. HOF- UND UNIVERSITÄTSBUCHHANDLUNG.

60:11

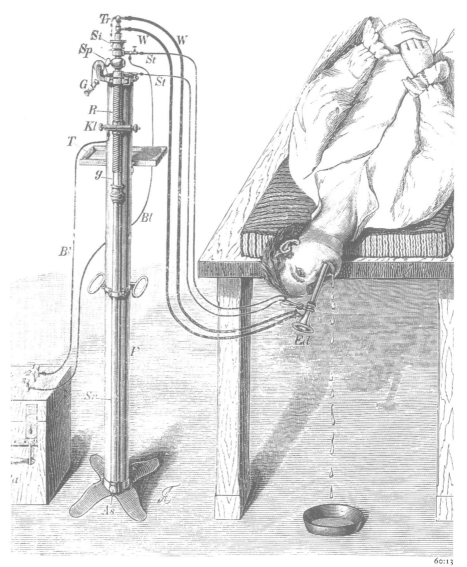

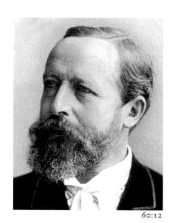

Leiter's gastroscope is conceived and first used clinically in 1881 by Johann Mikulicz-Radecki (1850–1905). The illustration shows him and his equipment connected to a patient.

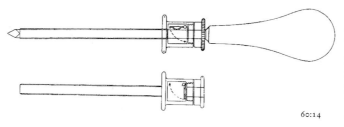

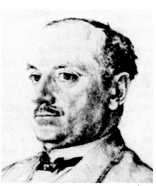

Hans Christian Jacobaeus (1879–1937) introduces thoracoscopy and, following the work of Georg Kelling (1866–1945), also laparoscopy as a clinical method of examination. The illustration shows his first equipment from 1910.

On the right, Gustav Killian (1860–1921) and assistants perform bronchoscopic examination of a patient in sitting and in supine position.

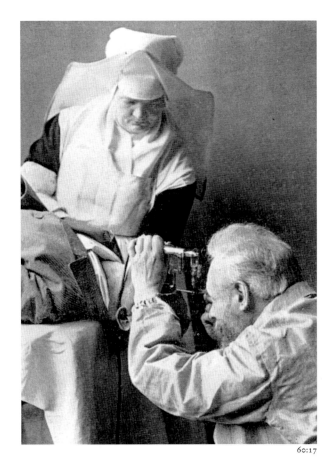

60:17

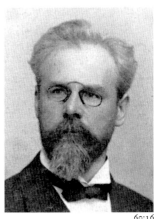

60:16

Killian demonstrates the new technique of bronchoscopy in 1897. That same year he reports the first endoscopic removal of a foreign body from the lungs, a small piece of bone accidentally swallowed by the patient while eating vegetable soup.

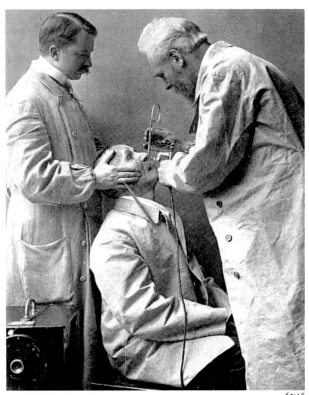

60:18

A microscope from Carl Zeiss Jena that was used by Robert Koch (1843–1910) in his studies of micro-organisms. In 1882 he makes the famed discovery of the tubercle bacillus using such an instrument.

Koch illustrates his microscopic techniques with eighty-four images. Six of these showing micro-organisms from a dermal streptococcal infection (erysipelas) are reproduced here.

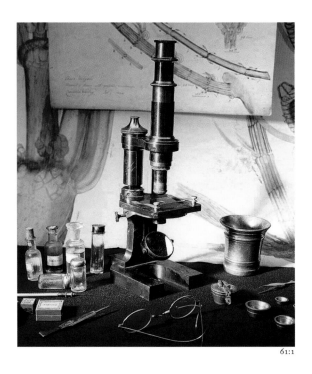

61:1

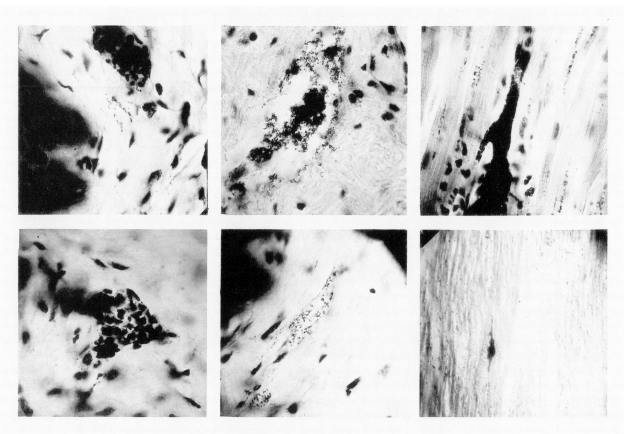

61:2

Robert Koch

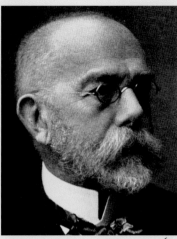

Robert Koch

61:3

KOCH was born in Claustal in 1843 into a family with thirteen children. After mediocre results in elementary school he considered emigrating to America, but settled on studies in medicine at the University of Göttingen. In 1866 he left with a degree of distinction, got married and then struggled for six years to find a position that could support his family. In 1880 he was appointed to a research position at the new Imperial Department of Health in Berlin. Later as professor of hygiene and advisor to the government, he travelled to Africa and India to study cholera, bubonic plague, malaria and other diseases and at home he helped fight epidemics of cholera and typhoid fever. Koch's motto was never to be idle and never give up. He could be arrogant but, while reserved with strangers, he was kind and entertaining with friends. He received the Nobel Prize in Medicine in 1905, five years before his death.

Zur Untersuchung von pathogenen Organismen.

MITTHEIL D KAIS GESUNDHEITSAMTE 1881;1:1. BERLIN: DRUCK U VERLAG DER NORDDEUTSCHEN BUCHDRUCKEREI; 1881.

KOCH DESCRIBES his methods of producing and studying bacterial cultures. He uses gelatine solutions, differential staining with aniline and a heat treatment to produce films of bacteria for microscopic investigation and photography. He discusses the pathogenic properties and mechanism of spread of micro-organisms, and how to take samples from air, dust, water and soil. He also touches on effective new methods of disinfection (61.1)(61.2). Eighty-four microphotographs of various micro-organisms illustrate the presentation.

IN PERSPECTIVE:
Koch's famed discoveries, including that of the tubercle bacillus (61.3), were made possible by a decade of methodological developments (61.4) and his use of the advanced microscopes just made available from Zeiss and Abbe (61.5). His study of the bacterial inhibitory action of different substances showed that Lister's carboxyl acid (61.6) was inferior to mercuric chloride (61.1). Koch also took issue with Pasteur's research on anthrax (61.7) and a long heated debate ensued. In an important contribution, Koch and his assistants demonstrated the effectiveness of steam sterilisation as compared to dry heat treatment (61.2). The technique was first put to clinical use in 1882 by Trendelenburg (61.8) and the first central sterilisation unit was installed in Berlin in 1890. Tyndall, studying the germs carried by atmospheric dust, discovered a less aggressive method of sterilisation based on repeated cycles of heating and cooling (Tyndallisation) (61.9). Gas sterilisation and irradiation sterilisation, both common today, were developed as alternative technologies in the late 1950s (61.10)(61.11).

61.1 See ref. 54.9.
61.2 Koch R, Gaffky G,Loeffler F. Versuche über die Verwerthbarkeit heisser Wasserdämpfe zu Desinfectionszwecke. *Mitthei d Kais Gesundheitsamte* 1881; 1:322.
61.3 Koch R. Die Aetilogie der Tuberkulose. *Berl Klin Wschr* 1882; 19:221.
61.4 Koch R. Verfahren zur Untersuchung, zum Conservieren und Photografieren der Bakterien. *Beitr Biol. Pflanz* 1876. p399.
61.5 See #64 Abbe page 328.
61.6 See #54 Lister page 282.
61.7 Koch R. Zur Aetiologie des Milzbrandes. *Mitthei d Kais Gesundheitsamte* 1881; 1:49. See also #50 Pasteur page 264.
61.8 See #57 Trendelenburg page 294.
61.9 Tyndall J. *Essays on the floating-matter of the air in relation to putrefaction and infection.* London: Longmans, Green and Co; 1881. p210.
61.10 Skeehan Jr RA, King Jr JH, Kaye S. Ethylene oxide sterilization in opthalmology. *Am J Opthalmol.* 1956; 42:424.
61.11 Woolston J. Irradiation Sterilization of Medical Devices. *Medical Device Technology* 1990; 1(4):25.

		Dauer des Versuches	Temperatur			Wirkung auf Sporen
			im Apparat	in der Rolle am Ende des Versuches		
				in der Mitte	in der halben Dicke	
Im Des-infectionsapparat des Baracken-lazarethes	Flanellrolle	4 Stunden	140—150° C.	83,0° C.	92,0° C.	Weder Milzbrandsporen noch die in der Erde ent-haltenen waren getödtet.
	Tuchrolle	4 Stunden	140—150° C.	81,0° C.		
Im Dampfkochtopf	Flanellrolle	1½ Stunden	120° C.	117° C.		Sporen von Milzbrand und in Erde getödtet.
		1 Stunde	110° C.	96,5° C.	100° C.	Milzbrandsporen getödtet, Sporen in der Erde nicht sämmtlich entwickelungs-unfähig.
	Tuchrolle	½ Stunde	120—126° C.	118° C.		

61:4

Koch makes comparative evaluations of various methods of sterilisation and discovers (see table above) the
superior effect obtained with steam sterilisation.

An early high pressure autoclave developed by F & M.
Lautenschläger and installed at the Charité Hospital
in Berlin, where the first central sterilisation unit is
established in 1890.

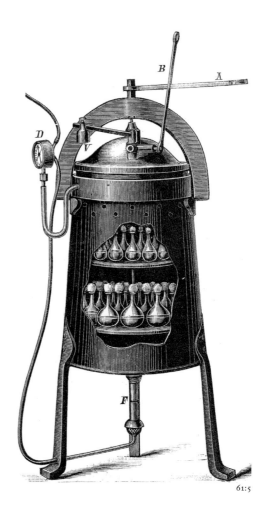

61:5

This, then, is my mode of proceeding:—Before the latent period of any of the germs has been completed (say a few hours after the preparation of the infusion), I subject it for a brief interval to a temperature which may be under that of boiling water. Such softened and vivified germs as are on the point of passing into active life are thereby killed; others not yet softened remain intact. I repeat this process well within the interval necessary for the most advanced of those others to finish their period of latency. The number of undestroyed germs is further diminished by this second heating. After a number of repetitions, which varies with the character of the germs, the infusion, however obstinate, is completely sterilized.

61:6

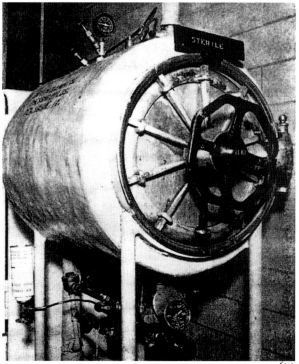

61:8

In 1877 John Tyndall (1820–1893) conceives a new method for sterilisation ("Tyndallisation" or fractional sterilisation) that uses "discontinuous heating" at relatively low temperatures. The citation above is from his first description of the procedure. The simple apparatus shown below left is constructed by Dr. Robert Muencke in Berlin after the instructions of Koch and is well suited for Tyndallisation.

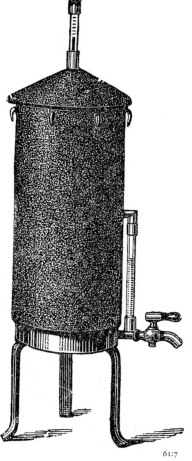

The modified autoclave from 1959, shown on the right, is the first experimental device developed for ethylene oxide sterilisation.

61:7

61:9

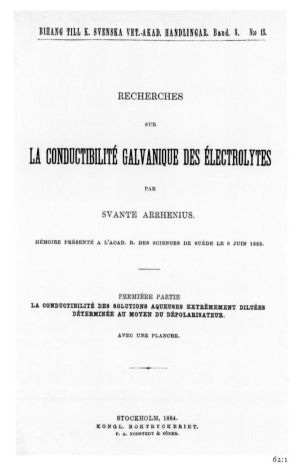

The dissertation of Svante Arrhenius (1859–1927) where, using the experimental setup shown, he measures the conductivity of dilute solutions of salts, acids and bases and explains the results by postulating an "active" electrolytic part expressed as a fraction of the total quantity of electrolyte.

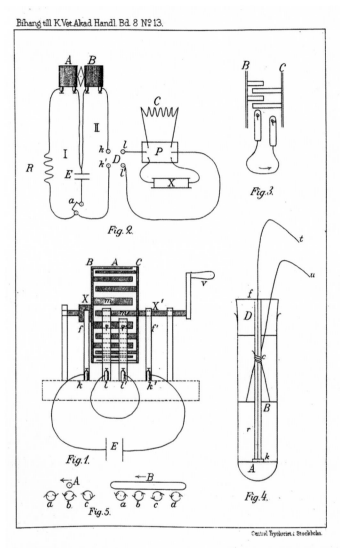

ARRHENIUS was born near Uppsala in Sweden in 1859. He entered the University of Uppsala in 1876 to study mathematics, physics and chemistry. His dissertation (cited below) received only mediocre grades, but it was appreciated abroad. In 1895 despite other attractive offers, he accepted the post as professor of physics at Stockholms Högskola. In 1903 he received the Nobel Prize in Chemistry and two years later he was made director of the physical chemistry department of the Nobel Institute. Arrhenius was a simple and good-natured person not without humour. He believed in the importance of sharing scientific knowledge with the public and published popular scientific treatises on a variety of topics from immunochemistry to earth sciences and cosmology (62.1)(62.2)(62.3). These books were widely acclaimed and read in many languages long after his death in 1927.

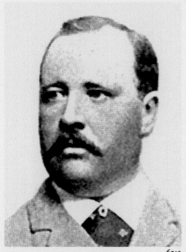

Svante Arrhenius

62:3

Recherches sur la conductibilité galvanique des électrolytes 1, 2.

BIHANG K SV VET.-AKAD HANDL.
STOCKHOLM: NORDSTEDT PA & SÖNER; 1884; 8(13) AND 1884; 8(14).

ARRHENIUS' DISSERTATION deals with the conductivity of dilute solutions of salts, acids and bases at different temperatures and degrees of dilution. The first part presents experimental results and the second part a theoretical discussion. Arrhenius believes the solution consists of the solvent and in addition an "active" electrolytic and a "passive" non-electrolytic part. He introduces the concept of a coefficient of activity of the electrolyte and at the end summarises his fifty-six separate conclusions by stating that at a given temperature and dilution the active part conducts electricity and can always be expressed as a fraction of the total quantity of the electrolyte.

IN PERSPECTIVE:
Although Kohlrausch and Lenz had made measurements similar to Arrhenius' before (62.4)(62.5), their studies were less extensive and they did not attempt to explain the results obtained. By 1887 Arrhenius had revised and extended his theory, introducing explicitly the concept of electrolytic dissociation (62.6). He also incorporated the new discovery of van't Hoff about the equivalence between the laws of osmotic pressure in the liquid state and the laws of the gaseous state (62.7). He did this by relating his activity coefficient to the constant of proportion introduced by van't Hoff between absolute temperature and the product of the pressure and volume of a gas (62.7). The importance of Arrhenius' work in medicine was first demonstrated by Hamburger who in 1902, while studying cell permeability for ions and haemolysis, discovered that bicarbonate and chloride ions could be exchanged across cell membranes (62.8). Based on these advances, Henderson explored the acid base regulation in blood (62.9).

62.1 Arrhenius S. *Immunochemistry*. New York; 1907.
62.2 Arrhenius S. *Ueber den Einfluss des Atmosphärischen Kohlensäuregehalts auf die Temperatur der Erdoberfläche*. Bihang K Sv Vet-Akad Handl 22, Avd. I No. 1 Stockholm; 1896.
62.3 Arrhenius S. *The Life of the Universe, as conceived by Man from the Earliest Ages to the Present time*. London: Harper; 1909.
62.4 Kohlrausch F. Das elektrische Leitungsvermögen der wässerigen Lösungen von den Hydraten und Salzen der leichte Metallen ... *Ann Phys Chem* 1879; 6:167. p1. and p145.
62.5 Lenz HF. Ueber das galvanische Leitungsvermögen alcoholischer Lösungen. *Mém l'Acad Imp Sci* St. Petersbourg VIII:e Sér. 1882; 30(9).
62.6 Arrhenius S. Über die Dissociation der in Wasser gelösten Stoffe. *Zeit Phys Chem* 1887; 1:631.
62.7 See #63 van't Hoff page 324.
62.8 Hamburger HJ. *Osmotische Druck und Ionenlehre in den Medicinischen Wissenschaften*. 3 Bde Wiesbaden; 1902–1904.
62.9 Henderson LJ. Das Gleichgewicht zwischen Basen und Säuren im tierischen Organismus. *Ergebn Physiol* 1909; 8:254.

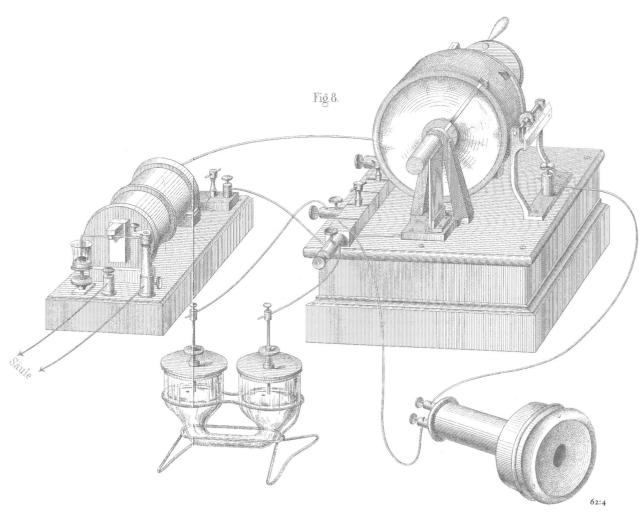

Fig 8.

Säule

62:4

In 1879 Friedrich Kohlrausch (1840–1910) develops a sensitive instrument for conductivity measurements using a battery, an induction coil and an electric bridge, the balance of which is detected by a telephone. He measures the resistance of wires and electrolytes. Although predating Arrhenius's experiments, Kohlrausch makes no attempt to explain the observed phenomena.

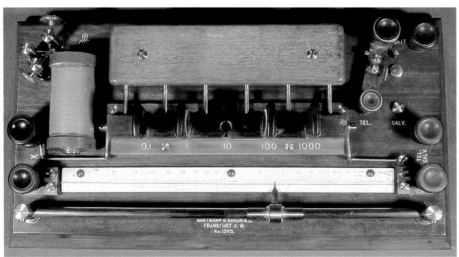

62:5

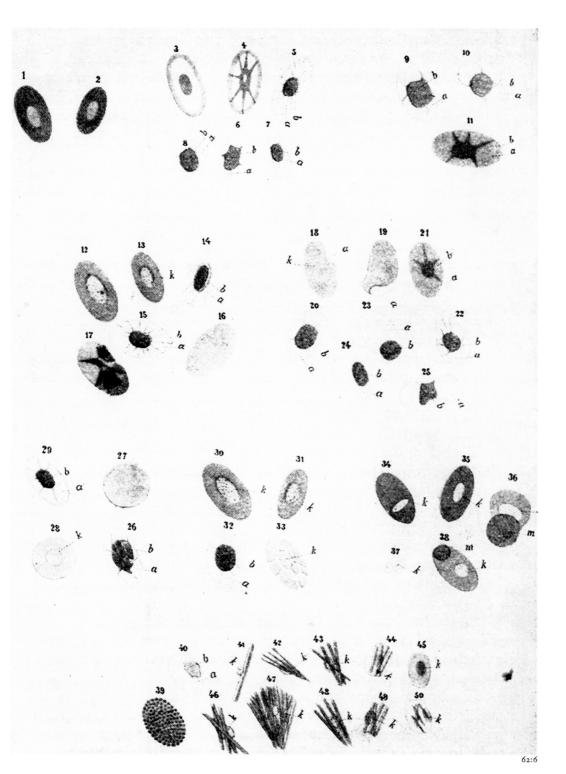

62:6

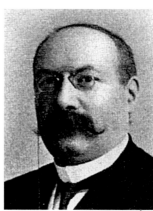

62:7

In the first years of the 20th century Hartog Hamburger (1859–1924) demonstrates the importance of Arrhenius's discoveries for medicine. He studies cell permeability and hemolysis and discovers that bicarbonate and chloride ions can be exchanged across cell membranes. The illustration shows blood cells of a frog (and those marked 39–50 from a fish) after 48–72 hours in sodium chloride and cane sugar solutions of varying concentrations.

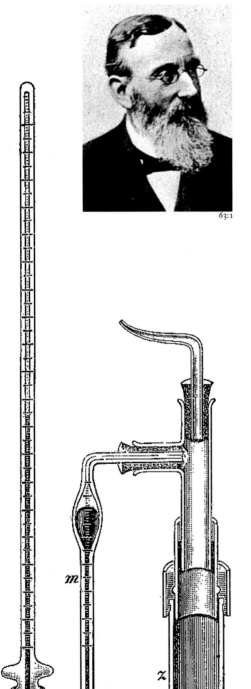

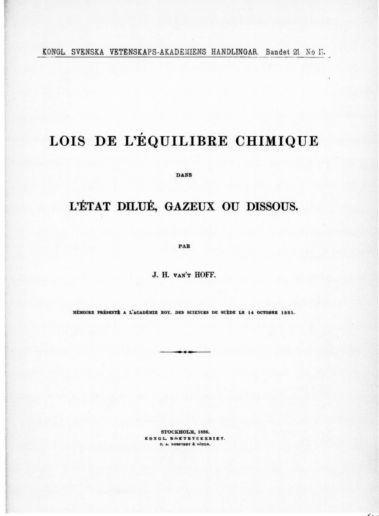

In 1877 Wilhelm Pfeffer (1845–1920) makes the first quantitative measurements of osmotic pressure using cane sugar solutions. His study is made possible by an invention of Moritz Traube (1826-1894), a decade before, that allows the preparation of mechanically strong semi-permeable membranes. The illustrations show Pfeffer and his equipment.

63:1

63:2

63:3

The title page of Jacobus van't Hoff's (1852–1911) famous theoretical investigation of the laws of chemical equilibrium for dilute solutions. He uses the experimental results of Pfeffer in support of the theory.

BORN in 1852 in Rotterdam, van't Hoff was the third of the seven children of a physician. After elementary school he studied technology and mathematics for three years in Delft. In 1871 he entered the University of Leiden. After three years of study, including short periods in Bonn and in Paris, he obtained a Ph.D. in chemistry from the University of Utrecht. In 1878 he became a lecturer at the University of Amsterdam and later professor and head of the department of chemistry. In 1887 van't Hoff turned down an invitation to Leipzig but, despite being given excellent facilities, he accepted a position in Berlin two years later. After his move he changed from a somewhat reserved to a more happy, extrovert character. During the last decade of his life he received many honours, including the first Nobel Prize in Chemistry in 1901, awarded for his work on chemical dynamics and on osmotic pressure in solutions.

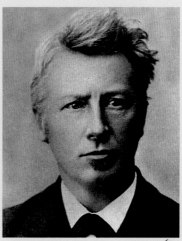

Jacobus van't Hoff 63:4

Lois de l'équilibre chimique dans l'état dilué, gazeux ou dissous.

KUNGL SV VET AKAD HANDL
STOCKHOLM: NORDSTEDT PA & SÖNER; 1886; 21(17):1.

FROM THERMODYNAMIC principles applied to diffusion through a semi-permeable membrane, van't Hoff derives the laws of chemical equilibrium for dilute solutions. He obtains the relationship between osmotic pressure, the concentration of a solute, the volume of the solution and the temperature and compares his calculations with experimental results for a number of specific chemical reactions. In a paper (63.1) immediately following this main treatise, van't Hoff expands on the striking similarity between the laws governing osmotic pressure and the ideal gas laws as established by Boyle, Gay-Lussac and Avogadro (63.2).

IN PERSPECTIVE:

Dutrochet observed in 1828 that membranes of organic material could allow the passage of water, while stopping the passage of a substance dissolved in it (63.3). In 1854 Graham presented his extensive experimental work on the "osmotic force" in solutions (63.4). He introduced the concept of a "dialyzer", noting that some substances "dialyzed" slowly, while others did so much faster through a membrane. At about the same time Fick developed the diffusion equation and introduced the collodion semi-permeable membrane (63.5). Van't Hoff referred primarily to the experimental observations of the biologist Pfeffer (63.6) in support of his theory. However, further tests were provided by measurements on the lowering of the freezing point of a solution (63.7). Also, the studies on red blood cells reported by Hamburger (63.8) produced isotonic coefficients in agreement with van't Hoff's theory and Arrhenius showed that his results based on the electrolytic dissociation concept also lent support to van't Hoff's work (63.9).

63.1 van't Hoff J. Une propriété générale de la matière diluée. *Kungl Sv Vet Akad Handl* Stockholm; 1886; 21 (17):42.
63.2 See ref. 8.6, ref. 7.2, ref.18.4 and ref. 18.5.
63.3 Dutrochet RJ. Nouvelles Recherches sur l'Endosmose et l'Endosmose. *Ann Chim Phys* 1828; 37:191.
63.4 Graham T. The Bakerian Lecture: On Osmotic Force. *Phil Trans Roy Soc* 1854; 144:177.
63.5 See # 46 Fick page 242 and ref 46.8.
63.6 Pfeffer W. *Osmotische Untersuchungen.* Leipzig; 1877.
63.7 Raoult F-M. Loi de congélation des solutions acqueuses des matières organiques. *C R l'Acad Sci* 1882; 94:1517.
63.8 See ref. 62.8.
63.9 See #62 Arrhenius page 320.

3. *Détermination de i à l'aide de la pression isotonique. La valeur de i est égale à la moitié du coëfficient isotonique.*

Comme la valeur de i répond à l'expression:

$$i = \frac{PV}{RT},$$

et comme R a été trouvé égal à 845, on a:

$$i = \frac{PV}{845\,T}$$

où P indique la pression osmotique en K^0 par Mr $\underline{2}$, V le volume en Mr $\underline{3}$ dans lequel se trouve la quantité moléculaire en K^0.

Or le sucre de cannes étant un des corps dont la pression citée est le mieux connue, ou calculera pour lui la valeur de i d'après les données de M. PFEFFER[1]) obtenues avec une solution contenant 1 partie de sucre sur 100 parties d'eau, ce qui conduit à:

$$V = \frac{342 \times 101}{1000} = 34{,}54 \quad (342 = C_{12}H_{22}O_{11}).$$

Comme M. PFEFFER indique la pression en millimètres de mercure (p) et la température en degrés Celsius (t) on a:

$$P = \frac{p}{760}\,10333 = 13{,}6\ p \quad \text{et} \quad T = t + 273$$

par conséquent:

$$i = \frac{34{,}54}{845(t + 273)}\,13{,}6\ p = \frac{0{,}556\ p}{t + 273}.$$

C'est ainsi qu'on a calculé i d'après les données suivantes:

t	p	$i = \dfrac{0{,}556\,p}{t + 273}$
6,8	505	1 —
13,7	525	1,01
14,2	510	0,99
15,5	520	1 —
22	548	1,03
32	544	0,99
36	567	1,02

Il en résulte que pour le sucre de cannes la valeur de i est égale à l'unité.

63:5

Left, Van't Hoff defines the ratio "i" (a constant that equals 1 for an ideal gas) and using the data of Pfeffer he finds that it has a value of 1 for cane sugar solutions. In this way he demonstrates the similarity between the laws governing osmotic pressure and those known to apply to ideal gases.

Francois-Marie Raoult (1830–1901) and his experimental apparatus for measuring the lowering of the freezing point of dilute solutions. This phenomenon and the lowering of the vapour pressure of a solution gives quantitative support to the theories of van't Hoff and Arrhenius (see #62).

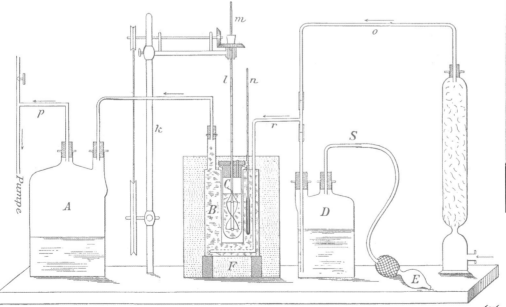

63:6

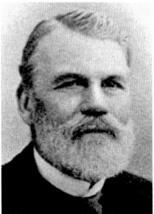

63:7

Substanz	Formel	α	$i = \dfrac{\Delta}{1,85}$ (aus der Gefrierpunkts- erniedrigung)	$i = 1 + (k - 1)\,\alpha$ (aus dem elektrischen Leitvermögen)
Aethylalkohol . .	$C_2H_5(OH)$	0,00	0,94	1,00
Glycerin	$C_3H_5(OH)_3$	0,00	0,92	1,00
Mannit	$C_6H_8(OH)_6$	0,00	0,97	1,00
Rohrzucker . . .	$C_{12}H_{22}O_{11}$	0,00	1,00	1,00
Baryumhydroxyd .	$Ba(OH)_2$	0,84	2,69	2,67
Lithiumhydroxyd .	$LiOH$	0,83	2,02	1,83
Natriumhydroxyd .	$NaOH$	0,88	1,96	1,88
Ammoniak . . .	NH_3	0,01	1,03	1,01
Anilin	$C_6H_5 \cdot NH_2$	0,00	0,83	1,00
Chlorwasserstoff .	HCl	0,90	1,98	1,90
Jodwasserstoff . .	HJ	0,96	2,03	1,96
Schwefelsäure . .	H_2SO_4	0,60	2,06	2,19
Borsäure	H_3BO_3	0,00	1,11	1,00
Milchsäure . . .	$C_3H_6O_3$	0,03	1,01	1,03
Chlorkalium . . .	KCl	0,86	1,82	1,86
Chlornatrium . . .	$NaCl$	0,82	1,90	1,82
Chlorammonium . .	$(NH)_4Cl$	0,84	1,88	1,84
Jodkalium	KJ	0,92	1,90	1,92
Kaliumnitrat . . .	KNO_3	0,81	1,67	1,81
Kaliumcarbonat . .	K_2CO_3	0,69	2,26	2,38
Natriumcarbonat .	Na_2CO_3	0,61	2,18	2,22
Kaliumsulfat . . .	K_2SO_4	0,67	2,11	2,33
Natriumsulfat . .	Na_2SO_4	0,62	1,91	2,24
Calciumnitrat .	$Ca(NO_3)_2$	0,67	2,02	2,33
Magnesiumsulfat .	$MgSO_4$	0,40	1,04	1,40

63:8

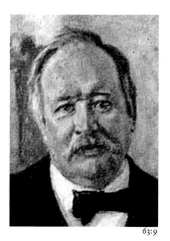

Svante Arrhenius (1859–1927) is able to show that both his electrolytic "activity" coefficient alpha, and the phenomenon of the lowering of the freezing point of a solution are in general agreement with van't Hoff's theory for a wide range of substances (compare the last two columns in the table above).

63:9

da u' hier nach der früheren Festsetzung negativ ist. Nun ist:

$$\frac{L\,l}{L'\,l'} = \frac{y}{-y'} = -\frac{1}{\beta},$$

also wird schließlich:

$$\frac{sin\,u'}{sin\,u} = \frac{n}{n'}\,\frac{1}{\beta} \quad \cdot \cdot \cdot \cdot \cdot \cdot \cdot \cdot \quad (10)$$

Rein dioptrisch ist diese Sinusbedingung identisch damit, daß die verschiedenen Zonen des Systems vom Objekt ein im

Fig. 10.

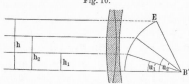

gleichen Verhältnis β vergrößertes Bild am gleichen Orte (Vereinigungspunkt der Nullzone) entwerfen.

Eine sehr einfache Gestalt nimmt die Sinusbedingung an, wenn entweder der Objekt- oder der Bildpunkt im Unendlichen liegt. Dann geht die Sinusbedingung (vgl. Fig. 10)

$$\frac{sin\,u_1}{sin\,u_1'} = \frac{sin\,u_2}{sin\,u_2'} = const$$

über in:

$$\frac{h_1}{sin\,u_1'} = \frac{h_2}{sin\,u_2'} = const,$$

da sich bei unbegrenzt wachsendem Objektabstand der Quotient $\frac{sin\,u_1}{sin\,u_2}$ unbegrenzt dem Wert h_1/h_2 nähert. Es gilt also:

$$\frac{h}{sin\,u'} = const;$$

da für sehr kleine Werte von u' gilt:

$$\frac{h}{sin\,u'} = \frac{h}{tg\,u'} = F',$$

so lautet also die Sinusbedingung in diesem speziellen Falle:

$$\frac{h}{sin\,u'} = F' \quad \cdot \cdot \cdot \cdot \cdot \cdot \cdot \cdot \quad (11\,\text{a})$$

bzw. wenn das Bild im Unendlichen liegt:

$$\frac{h'}{sin\,u} = F \quad \cdot \cdot \cdot \cdot \cdot \cdot \cdot \cdot \quad (11\,\text{b})$$

64:1

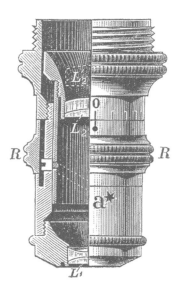

64:2

Ernst Abbe's (1840–1905) derivation of the sine law for lens design, as published after notes taken during his lectures in 1887.

The figure, top right, shows Abbe's drawing of an optical system and his calculations of its properties.

Abbe's renowned apocromatic lens system. The rotation of the ring "R" can reposition the lenses "L2".

64:3

ABBE was born in 1840 in Eisenach, where his father worked long hours as a spinning-mill worker. Young Abbe's distaste for oppression and dedication to social justice arose from experiences during the revolution in 1848. With a scholarship from his father's employer, he studied physics under Wilhelm Weber (64.1) and received his degree in Göttingen in 1861. Two years later he was appointed lecturer in mathematics, physics and astronomy at Jena University. In 1866 Zeiss, a mechanic at the university who had a small company that manufactured microscopes, feared competition from abroad and wanted to improve his products but did not know how (64.2). He approached Abbe, who was soon able to help and in 1875 Zeiss offered him a partnership in his firm. In 1888, when Zeiss died, Abbe alone controlled the company, but the following year he chartered the Carl Zeiss Foundation, turning over his shares but remaining as "one of the management" till his death in 1905.

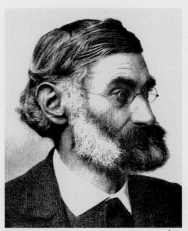

Ernst Abbe   64:4

Über Verbesserungen des Mikroskops mit hilfe neuer Arten optischen Glases.

SITZ D MED-NATURW GESELLSCHAFT ZU JENA. 9 JULI 1886.

ABBE REPORTS here his final improvements on the reduction of chromatic aberrations of optical systems. The advances, he says, are made possible by the development of new glass materials containing phosphorus and boron, which exhibit desirable dispersion characteristics, including at higher values of the refractive index. He describes the resulting apochromatic objective and the ocular adapted to it and draws attention to the potential usefulness of the arrangement in microphotography (64.3)

IN PERSPECTIVE:
Fraunhofer's ambition to improve the material and production methods of optical glass and to better understand optical imaging strongly influenced Zeiss (64.2)(64.4). In Schott, a small glassworks owner, he found an ideal partner who was able to develop the first two areas, while Abbe provided the theoretical insights and performed the mathematical calculations (64.2)(64.5). Abbe's "sine law" of lens design reduced image distortions, and his diffraction analysis of the resolving power of an objective as determined by its numerical aperture and his success in reducing chromatic aberrations all contributed to the superiority of Zeiss' new microscopes (64.6). These instruments helped Koch's discover the tubercle bacillus (64.7). Abbe's theory of image formation is fundamental to all optical instrumentation design (64.8) and it played also an important role in the understanding of electron microscopy (64.9)(64.10). The Carl Zeiss Foundation was chartered to promote studies in science and mathematics, but its statutes also called for far-reaching social benefits (even by modern standards) for all of its employees. Today the Foundation still controls a large commercial enterprise.

64.1 See # 44 Weber page 232.
64.2 Volkmann H. *Carl Zeiss und Ernst Abbe ihr Leben und ihr Werk*. Deutsches Museum 34 Heft 2 1966.
64.3 See # 61 Koch page 316 and also ref. 38.6.
64.4 See ref. 9.8, ref. 9.7.
64.5 Lummer O, Reiche F. editors. E Abbe. *Die Lehre von der Bildentstehung im Mikroskop*. Brauschweig; 1910.
64.6 *Gesammelte Abhandlungen von Ernst Abbe*. 5vols. Jena; 1904–1940.
64.7 See # 61 Koch page 316 and ref. 61.3.
64.8 See ref. 9.7, ref. 9.10, ref. 9.11.
64.9 Bruche E, Johansson H. Elektronenoptik und Elektronenmikroskop. *Die Naturwissen*. 1932; 20(21):353.
64.10 See # 83 Ruska page 428.

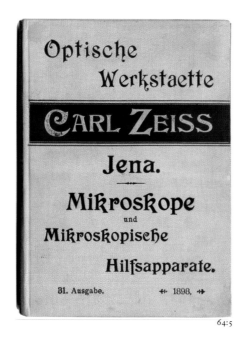

A catalogue from the company Carl Zeiss Jena in 1898.

Abbe's condenser unit and an objective lens mounted to allow precise centre alignment.

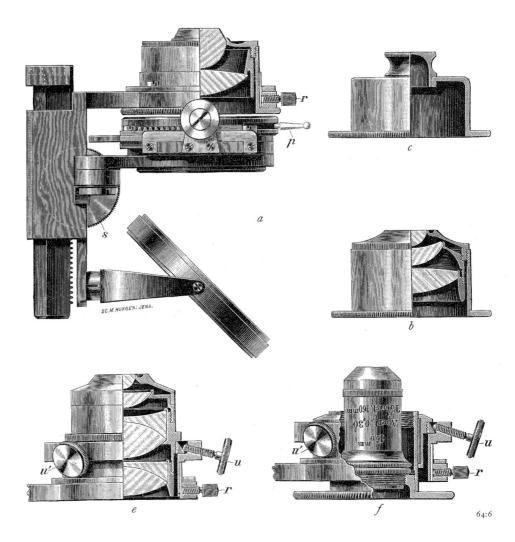

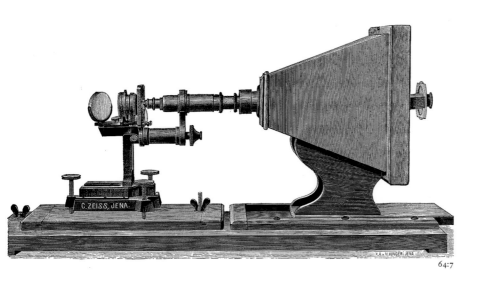

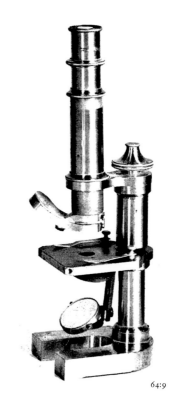
64:7

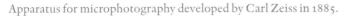

Apparatus for microphotography developed by Carl Zeiss in 1885.

Microtome for microscopic sample preparation from 1885 (below left).

A Zeiss microscope from 1860 before Abbe introduced his new design methods (top right) and the first instrument, built in 1875, incorporating the improvements invented by him.

64:9

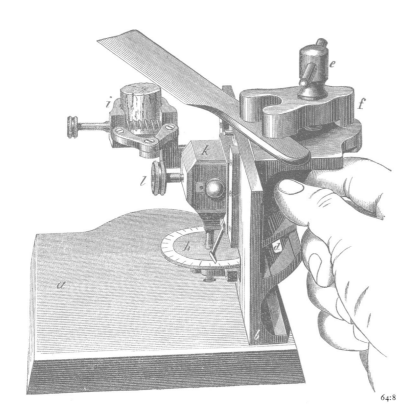
64:8

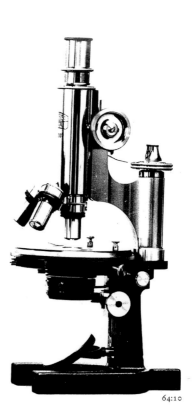
64:10

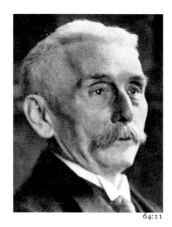

Otto Schott (1851–1935), the owner of the small glassworks shown below as it appeared around 1884. Schott, Abbe and Carl Zeiss (1816–1888) formed a successful partnership in 1879. Their combined talents enabled them to design and produce optical systems of superior quality.

Neue

Mikroskop-

Objective und Oculare

aus

Special-Gläsern

des

Glastechnischen Laboratoriums
(Schott & Gen.)

hergestellt

von

Carl Zeiss
Optische Werkstätte
JENA.
1886.

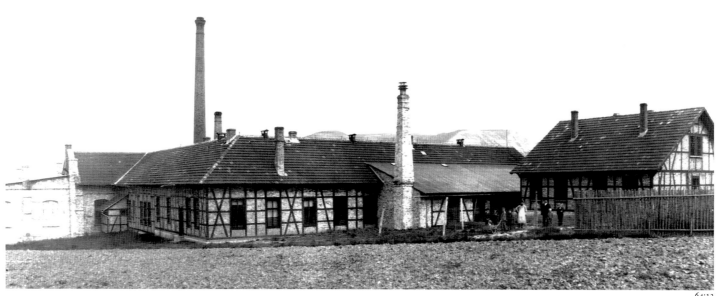

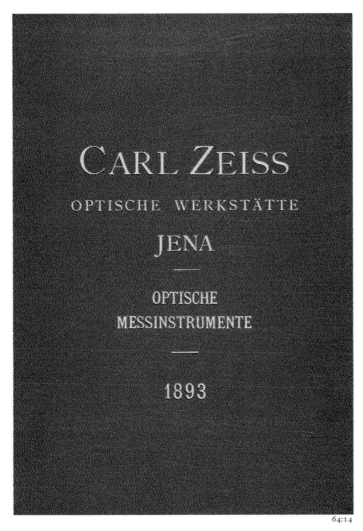

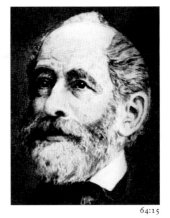

Top right, Carl Zeiss two years before his death. A Carl Zeiss catalogue of optical measuring instruments from 1893 that introduces Abbe's large crystal refractometer (right).

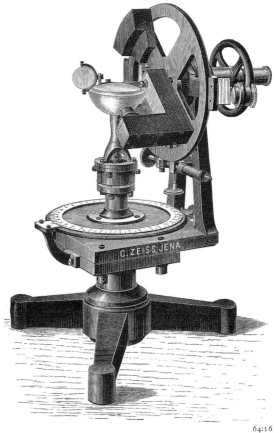

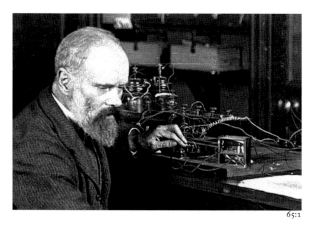
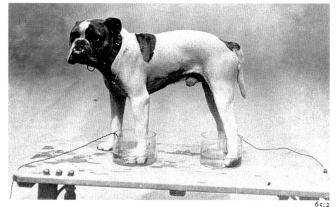

Augustus Waller (1856–1922) in his laboratory, making electric registrations on his bulldog "Jimmy".

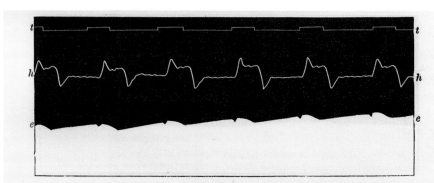

FIG. 1. Man. Heart led off to electrometer from front and back of chest (front to Hg; back to H_2SO_4).

65:3

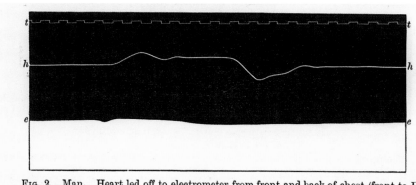

FIG. 2. Man. Heart led off to electrometer from front and back of chest (front to Hg; back to H_2SO_4).

e.e. electrometer.   *h.h.* cardiograph.   *t.t.* time in $\frac{1}{5}$th sec.

65:4

In 1887 Waller makes a dramatic public demonstration showing that electric signals related to the heart beat can be registered from the surface of the body.

WALLER was born in Paris in 1856, the son of the prominent physiologist A.V. Waller. Throughout his life Waller strived to follow in his father's footsteps. After receiving his M.D. in 1881, Waller joined the department of physiology at University College London. He was then appointed lecturer at St. Mary's Hospital in Paddington, where he held the first public demonstration of electrocardiography. In 1892, at the same age as his father, Waller was elected to the Royal Society. Subsequently he was the Director of the Physiological Laboratory of the University of London and also held corresponding posts in Paris, Moscow and Rome. Waller, a humorous extrovert person, enjoyed giving public lectures and demonstrations, often drawing on his wife and his dog for help in experiments.

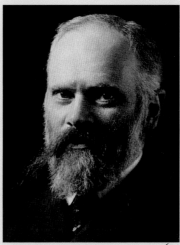

Augustus Désiré Waller   65:5

A Demonstration on Man of Electromotive changes accompanying the Heart Beat.

J PHYSIOL LONDON; 1887; 8:29.

WALLER DESCRIBES electrocardiographic recordings made on one of his assistants in the laboratory, using Lippmann's mercury capillary electrometer (65.1). Waller connects the electrodes to various parts of the body, for instance the front and back of the chest, and displays the movement of the mercury by optical projection. He notes that the electric signal always precedes the arterial pulse and that the appearance of the signal depends on the location of the electrodes.

IN PERSPECTIVE:

In 1842 Matteucci observed in a frog that a current is generated with every beat of the heart (65.2). He used the contraction of a muscle in a frog's leg as an indicator. Kölliker and Müller made proper measurements of the potential at different locations on the heart in 1856 (65.3). The time course of these electric signals were able to be studied when the highly sensitive capillary electrometer of Lippmann (65.1) was combined with the registration technique of Marey (65.4)(65.5)(65.6). Thus Burdon Sanderson and Page investigated the potential signal of uninjured and injured hearts and defined the two intervals later to be called QRS and T (65.7). Since the body was known to conduct electricity, Waller suspected that similar information could also be obtained from external parts of the body. He made the celebrated demonstration of this on himself and on his bulldog Jimmy (65.8). Subsequent improvements in instrumentation allowed Einthoven to register the ECG signal as we know it today (65.9)(65.10). Initially Waller did not believe in the clinical usefulness of his technique, but by 1917 he had made 2,000 recordings and was ready to change his mind.

65.1 Lippmann G. Relation entre les phénomènes électriques et capillaires. *C R Acad Sci* 1873. p1407.

65.2 Matteucci C.: Sur un phenomene physiologique produit par les muscles en contraction. *Ann Chim Phys* 1842; 6:339. See also # 42 Du Bois-Reymond page 224 and ref. 42.1.

65.3 Kölliker Rv, Müller H. Nachweis der negativer Schwankung des Muskelstroms am naturlich sich contrahirenden Muskel. *Verh phys-med Ges Würzburg* 1856; 6:528.

65.4 See #52 Marey page 272.

65.5 Marey E-T. Inscription photographique des indications de l'électromètre de Lippmann. *C R Acad Sci* 1876. p278.

65.6 Ref. 52.1 p525.

65.7 Burdon Sanderson J, Page FJ. Experimental Results relating to the Rythmical and Excitatory Motions of the Ventricle of the Heart of the Frog, and of the Electrical Phenomena which accompany them. *Proc Roy Soc* 1878; 27:410.

65.8 Waller AD. Introductory Address on The Electromotive Properties of the Human Heart. *Brit Med J* 1888; 2: 751.

65.9 See #71 Einthoven page 366.

65.10 Waller AD. *The signs of life from their electrical aspekt*. New York: E.P.Dutton & Co; 1903.

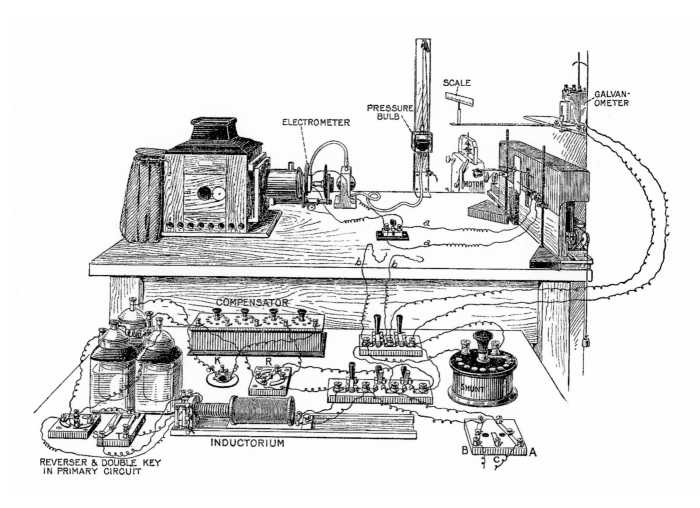

ELECTROMETER

SCALE

PRESSURE BULB

GALVAN- OMETER

MOTOR

COMPENSATOR

K

R

SHUNT

INDUCTORIUM

REVERSER & DOUBLE KEY
IN PRIMARY CIRCUIT

B C A

65:6

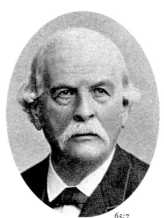

Rudolf von Köllicker (1817–1905) (left) makes the first measurements of potentials at different locations on a beating heart. Two decades later John Burdon-Sanderson (1828–1905) studies the potential signal from injured and uninjured frog hearts and defines two intervals, later to be called QRS and T.

65:7

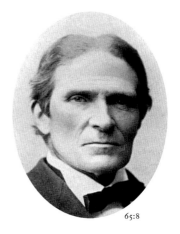

65:8

ELECTRICAL ACTION OF HUMAN HEART

First Demonstration.—The disc of light upon the transparent screen in front of you is from the field of a microscope illuminated from behind. The vertical shadow is that of a fine capillary tube filled half with mercury, half with sulphuric acid—

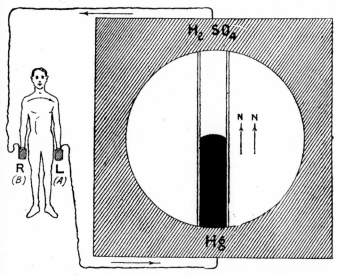

FIG. I.—On suddenly throwing an electrical current into the apparatus there is a movement of the mercury column in the direction of such current. When the two hands are connected with the two poles of the apparatus as shown in the figure, the mercury column is seen to move upwards in the field as indicated by the arrow N ; this "positive" movement indicates current in the body from right to left. If the hands are transposed, or if the pole connections are reversed, the column pulsates downwards in the field, indicating as before current in the body from right to left.

65:9

The illustration on the opposite page shows a capillary galvanometer set up. In 1873 Gabriel Lippman (1845–1921) invents the capillary galvanometer, a highly sensitive instrument where a potential change sets a mercury column in a capillary tube in motion. This motion is projected with a microscope onto a display or fed into a registration device.

The figure on the left explains the principle of Waller's demonstration of the electric action of the human heart using the capillary galvanometer.

Willem Einthoven (1860–1927) introduces mathematical techniques to compensate for the inadequate response time of the capillary galvanometer. In 1894 he obtains more truthful ECG traces, as shown in the illustration by the dashed line, which is to be compared to the graph traced out by the moving dark shadow of the capillary galvanometer.

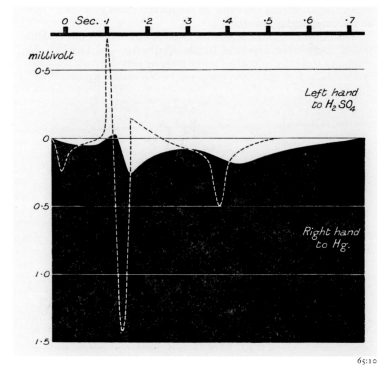

65:10

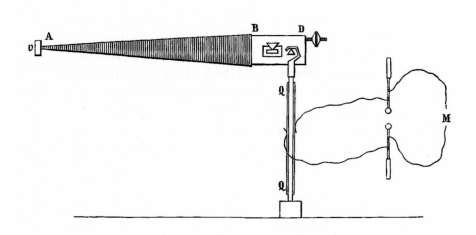

66:1

Pierre Curie (1859–1906) explores the piezoelectric effect in quartz. Using a microscope and a lever, he measures the expansion of the crystal when a voltage is applied (top) and studies the voltage generated when the crystal is compressed (bottom). The arrangement in the middle illustration shows a double beam of quartz glued together that bends on the application of a voltage (one beam contracts while the other expands).

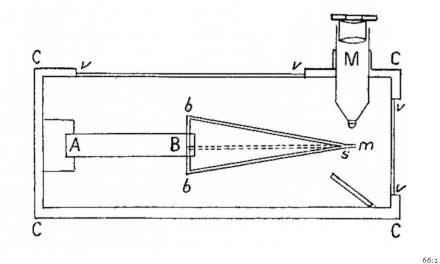

66:2

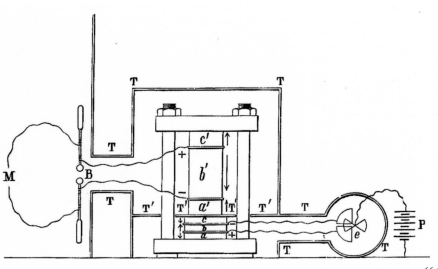

66:3

CURIE was born in 1859 in Paris, the son of a physician. He never went to elementary school, but studied on his own and with his mother and father. Curie enrolled in the Faculty of Sciences in Paris in 1875 and started working with his elder brother Jacques, who was an assistant at the mineralogy laboratory of the Sorbonne. Their collaboration, which resulted in the discovery of piezoelectricity (66.1), ended in 1883 when Curie was appointed director of the laboratory at École de Physique et Chimie. Here in 1895 he met and married a student, Maria Sklodowska (66.1). In 1903, they shared the Nobel Prize in Physics with Becquerel for his work on radioactivity. Curie was a serious, reserved man with a gentle and kind disposition. His work was cut short by his sudden death in 1906, when struck by a cart while crossing a street in Paris.

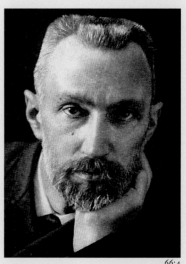

66:4

Pierre Curie

Dilatation électrique du Quartz.

J DE PHYS 2SER. PARIS; 1889; 8:149.

THIS PAPER, written together with his brother Jacques, first analyses the electrical output of a quartz crystal for different directions of compression. Then experimental results are presented from a piezoelectric manometer gauge built for large pressures. Next Curie employs a lever as a mechanical amplifier and observes with a microscope the dilation of a crystal caused by an applied electrical field. Finally, an arrangement is described which has two beams of quartz glued together and flexes when electrically driven.

IN PERSPECTIVE:
Curie later developed piezoelectric instrumentation that played a major role in his and his wife's successful research on radioactivity (66.1). In 1916 Curie's pupil Langevin invented the technique of generating ultrasonic waves with piezoelectric transducers (66.2). His aim was to locate underwater objects, an urgently needed capability at the time because of the First World War. Spallanzani had noticed ultrasonic waves already in 1794, as he understood that bats navigated not by sight but by using inaudible sound (66.3). Langevin noted the destructive power of ultrasonic waves and early medical use was mostly confined to applications in physiotherapy (66.4) and to attempts at cancer treatment and wound healing. The first diagnostic methods appeared at the end of the 1940s (66.5), but the major advance came when the pulse echo technique was developed for non-destructive testing in industry (66.6). In 1959 Sauerbrey showed that quartz crystals could be used as highly sensitive microbalances (66.7). This led to the development of clinical instruments for anaesthetic gas monitoring (66.8) and to a variety of liquid phase biomedical sensors for research purposes (66.9)(66.10).

66.1 *Oevres de Pierre Curie.* Société Francaise de Physique. Paris: Gauthier-Villars; 1908 and #70 Marie Curie page 362.

66.2 Chilowsky C, Langevin P. *Procédés et appareils pour la production de signaux sous-marins dirigés et pour la localisation à distance d'obstacles sous-marins.* Brevet d'invention No 502.913 1920. Application 1916.

66.3 Spallanzani L. *Lettere sopra il sospetto di un nuovo senso nei pipistrelli.* Torino; 1794 and Galambos R. *The Avoidance of Obstacles by flying Bats: Spallanzani's Ideas (1794) and Later Theories.* Isis 1942; 34:132.

66.4 Pohlman R, Richter R, Parow E. Über die Ausbreitung und Absorption des Ultraschalls im menschlichen Gewebe und seine therapeutische Wirkung in Ischias und Plexusneuralgie. *Dtsch Med Wschr* 1939; 52(7):251.

66.5 Dussik KTh, Dussik F, Wyt L. Auf dem Wege zur Hyperphonographie des Gehirnes. *Wiener Med Wsch* 1947; 38/39:425.

66.6 Firestone FA. The Supersonic Reflectoscope, an Instrument for Inspecting the Interior of Solid Parts by Means of Sound Waves. *J Acoust Soc Am* 1946; 17(3):287. See also #90 Edler-Hertz page 466.

66.7 Sauerbrey G. Verwendung von Schwingquartzen zur Wägung dünner Schichten und zur Mikrowägung. *Z Phys* 1959; 155:206.

66.8 Gedeon A. Anesthetic Agent Analysis Using Piezoelectric Microbalance. *Biom Instr Tech* Nov/Dec 1989.

66.9 Kanazawa KK, Gordon III JG. Frequency of quartz microbalance in contact with liquid. *Anal.Chem.* 1985; 57:1770.

66.10 Höök F, et al. Structural changes in hemoglobin during adsorption to solid surfaces: Effects of pH, ionic strength and ligand Binding. *Proc Natl Acad Sci* 1998; 95:12271.

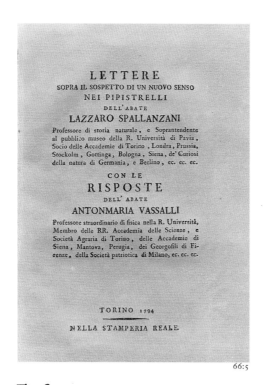

In this letter from 1794 Lazzaro Spallanzani (1729–1799) describes his experiments with blinded bats. He finds that they can navigate without recourse to sight and reluctantly draws the conclusion that they must have an unknown sense that guides them. This is the discovery of the phenomenon of ultrasound. It takes another hundred and fifty years before the navigation of bats is understood in some detail.

Paul Langevin (1872–1946) builds the first piezoelectric transducers suitable for efficient generation of ultrasound. The illustration shows his patent application from 1916, which was aimed at detecting underwater objects, a capability badly needed during the First World War.

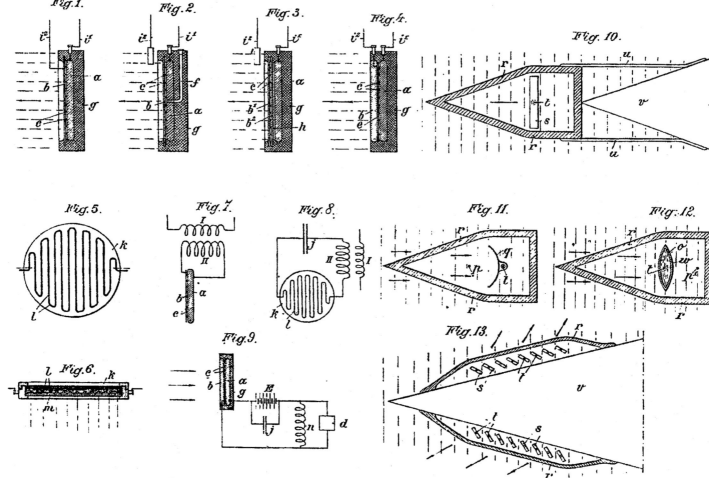

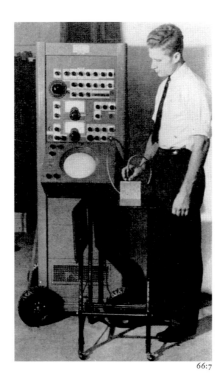

The Supersonic Reflectoscope is developed in the mid-1940s for examining the interior of bodies in industrial applications. Typical tracings obtained from the device are shown and explained below.

66:7

FIG. 9. Wall thickness measurement. We sometimes wish to know the wall thickness of a cored casting or of a pipe carrying corrosive material, where the inside surface is inaccessible. The crystal is placed against the wall and a series of successive reflections is obtained; the average distance between them is read off of the inch mark scale and is the thickness of the wall. Above is the series of reflections through a wall one inch thick; note that a reflection follows each one inch mark. The accuracy of this method is of the order of five percent; it depends on the smoothness, flatness, and parallelism of the wall faces.

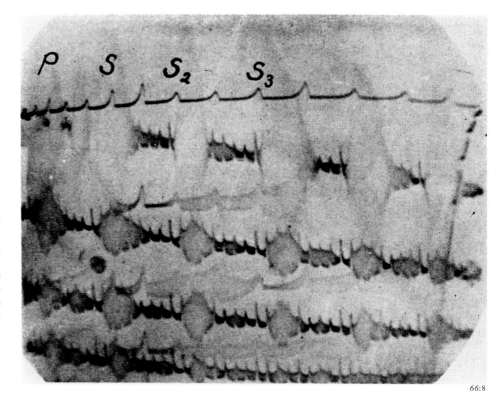

66:8

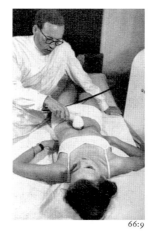

66:9

Until the 1940s medical use of ultrasound is primarily confined to physiotherapy. The picture shows equipment from that time being used in this application.

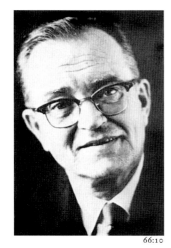

66:10

Karl Dussik (1908–1968) pioneers the use of ultrasound for medical diagnostic purposes. In 1947 he describes his equipment (in the picture he stands next to the device that he calls a "Hyperphonograph") and publishes the image of the brain shown below.

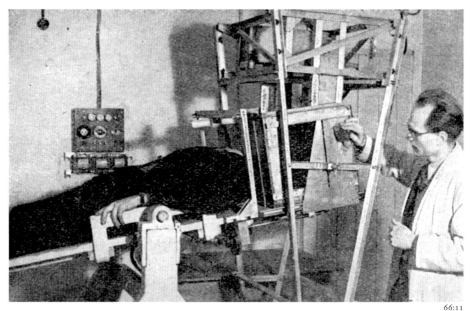

66:11

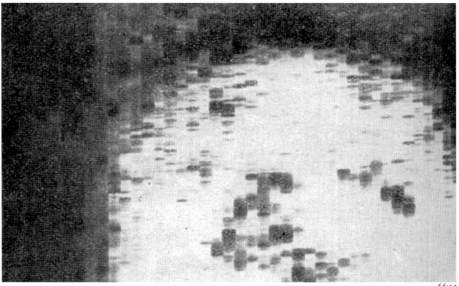

66:12

COATED CRYSTAL RESONATOR

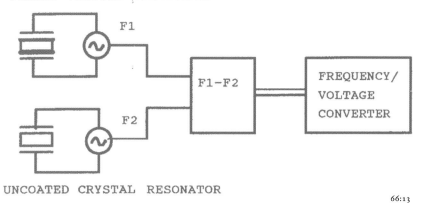

F1

F2

F1−F2

FREQUENCY/
VOLTAGE
CONVERTER

UNCOATED CRYSTAL RESONATOR

66:13

The principle and a photograph of a piezo-electric quartz crystal sensor used to detect anaesthetic gases. Both crystals have gold electrodes and resonate at about 10 MHz. However, one of them is also coated with a substance to which the gas can adsorb. The frequency of this crystal is decreased in proportion to the gas concentration, which can therefore be determined using the differential frequency arrangement shown.

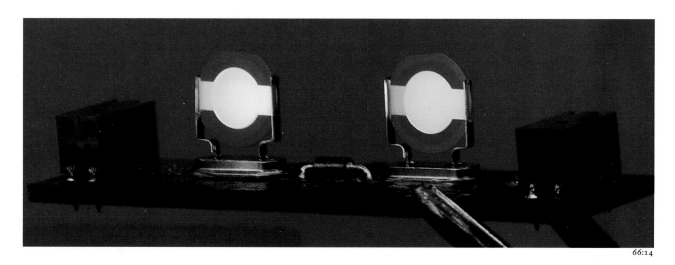

66:14

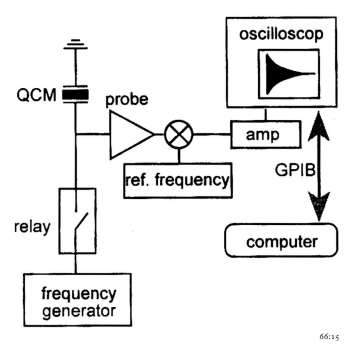

QCM

probe

oscilloscop

amp

ref. frequency

GPIB

relay

computer

frequency
generator

66:15

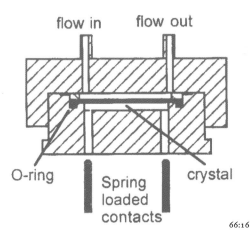

flow in   flow out

O-ring   Spring
loaded
contacts   crystal

66:16

The quartz crystal microbalance (QCM) technique used for measuring surface loading effects in liquid phase biomedical sensors. The figure shows the cuvette with a crystal and the electronics that drive the crystal and register the exponentially decaying amplitude that reflects the molecular load on the crystal surface.

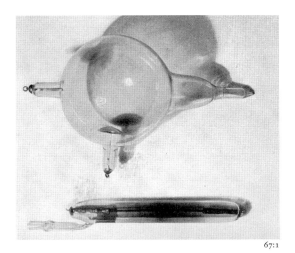

67:1

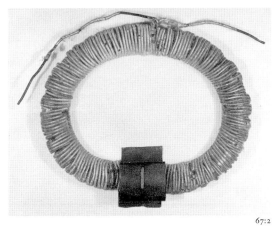

67:2

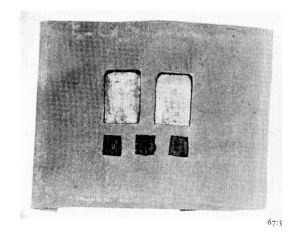

67:3

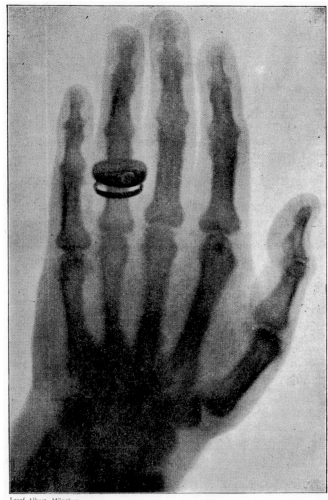

Josef Albert, München, repr.

Hand des Anatomen Geheimrath von Kölliker.

Im Physikal. Institut der Universität Würzburg
mit X-Strahlen aufgenommen
von **Professor Dr. W. C. Röntgen.**

67:4

The famous X-ray picture of the hand of Albert von Köllicker (see #65), from the first publication of Röntgen's discovery.

The equipment used by Wilhelm Röntgen (1845–1923) in his very first experiments with X-rays. Vacuum tubes, an electromagnetic coil employed in his attempts to deflect the X-rays and a plate of lead with apertures for studying the absorption of different materials.

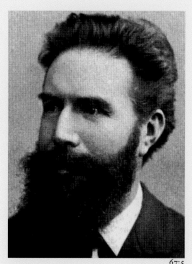

Wilhelm Conrad Röntgen 67:5

ORN in Lennep in 1845, Röntgen was the only child of a cloth manufacturer. He was first educated at the Utrecht Technical School and later entered the Polytechnic at Zürich, where he received his diploma and doctorate in mechanical engineering in 1868. He was appointed to the chair of physics at the University of Giessen in 1879 and became director of the Physical Institute at the University of Würzburg and, after his epochal discovery of X-rays in 1895, he was also made honorary doctor of medicine. In 1900 Röntgen moved to Munich and the following year he received the first Nobel Prize in Physics. Of a retiring nature, Röntgen shunned public engagements, even declining to deliver the Nobel lecture. He retired in 1920 and died after a short illness three years later.

Ueber eine neue Art von Strahlen.

SITZUNGB D WÜRZBURGER PHYSIK-MED GES JAHRG 1895. P132.
WÜRZBURG: VERLAG DER STAHEL'SCHEN BUCHHANDLUNG; 1896

RÖNTGEN ANNOUNCES his discovery of an unknown radiation "X-Strahlen" emanating from a cathode ray tube covered with black paper. He finds that the ray penetrates easily many materials, including aluminium, but not a 1.5-mm thick lead plate. He is unable to reflect, refract or diffract the radiation, nor can he produce interference phenomena or deflection with electrical fields. He notes that X-rays always emanate at the glass wall where the tube is struck by the cathode ray. Finally, he observes that the radiation blackens photographic plates and uses this to document his experiments and to produce "shadows of handbones".

IN PERSPECTIVE:
At the end of the 19th century cathode ray tubes were extensively used in investigations of electrical discharge phenomena in gases (67.1)(67.2)(67.3). These studies culminated in the discovery of the electron by Thomson in 1897 (67.4). Following Röntgen's announcement, Carl Müller (later "Röntgenmüller") promptly started commercial production of X-ray tubes, and developed a much improved water-cooled model in 1899. The modern tungsten filament X-ray tube was invented by Coolidge at the General Electric Research Laboratory in 1913 (67.5). The medical community immediately recognised and continuously developed the extraordinary potential of X-rays for diagnostic purposes, the CAT scanner being among the latest developments in this field (67.6). Sjögren reported the first successful use of X-rays for cancer treatment in 1899 (67.7). Also many new diagnostic techniques were able to be developed under X-ray image control (67.8). In a major advance, Laue discovered the X-ray diffraction method in 1913 (67.9) that has ever since been the cornerstone of structural determinations of complex molecules in general (67.10) and those of biomedical interest in particular (67.11).

67.1 Plücker J. Über die Einwirkung des Magneten auf die elektrischen Entladungen in verdünnten Gasen. *Ann Phys Chem* 1858; 103:88. p151, p113.
67.2 Hittorf W. Über die Elektricitätsleitumg der Gase. Erste Mitteilungen. *Ann Phys Chem* 1869; 136:1.
67.3 Crooks W. Contributions to molecular physics in high vacua. *Phil Trans Roy Soc* 1879; 170:641.
67.4 See #69 Thomson page 356.
67.5 Coolidge WD. *Improved x-ray tube.* US Patent 1,203,495 1916.
67.6 See #95 Hounsfield page 492.
67.7 Sjögren TA. *Fall af epiteliom behandladt med Röntgenstrålar.* Förh Sv Läkare-Sällsk Sammank Stockholm; 1899. p208.
67.8 Seldinger SI. Catheter replacement of the needle in percutaneous angiography. A new technique. *Acta radiol* 1953; 39:368. See also ref. 56.10.
67.9 See #76 Laue page 390.
67.10 See ref. 78.6.
67.11 See #76 Laue page 390 and #88 Watson-Crick page 456.

William Coolidge (1873–1975) with his newly developed X-ray tube, which was first used in a clinical setting in 1913. A major advance in X-ray technology, it has a high-vacuum tube with heated tungsten filament as cathode and a tungsten disc as an anode.

Vacuum tubes designed by William Crookes (1832–1919) (at the back of the image) and by Coolidge (in the middle) and by Carl Müller (1845–1912) (front). Crookes builds vacuum tubes in the last decades of the 19th century as part of his investigations of the properties of rarefied gases. Müller starts commercial manufacture of X-ray tubes only months after Röntgen's discovery.

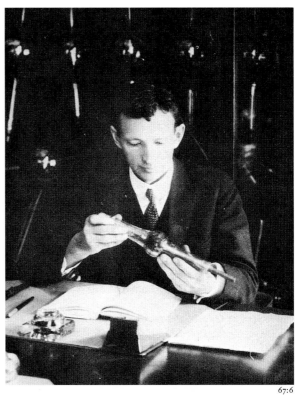

67:6

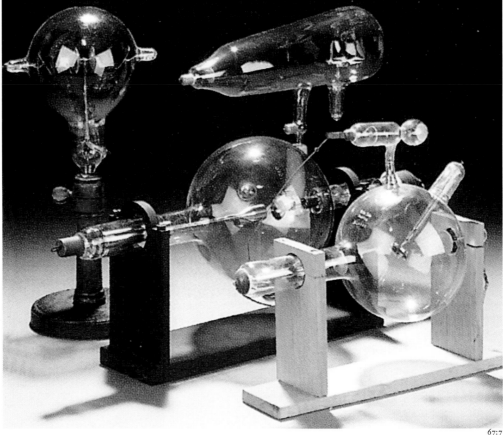

67:7

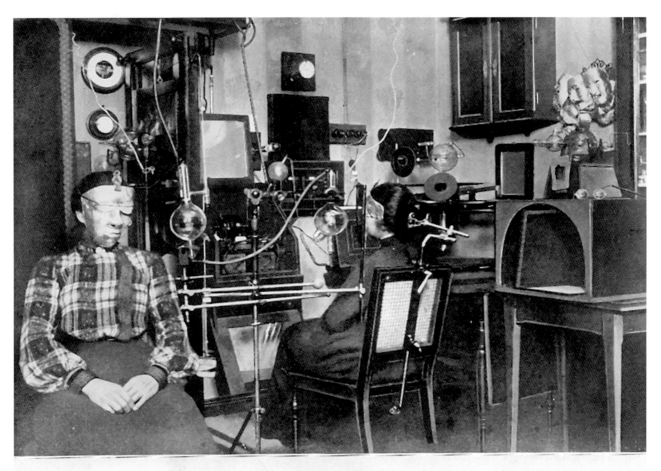

Röntgenbestrahlung im ärztlichen Sprechzimmer, *1900.*

X-ray treatment in the doctor's office in 1900.

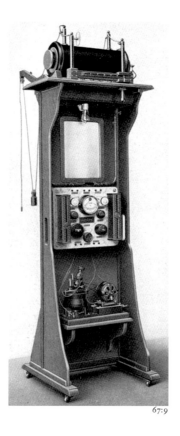

67:9

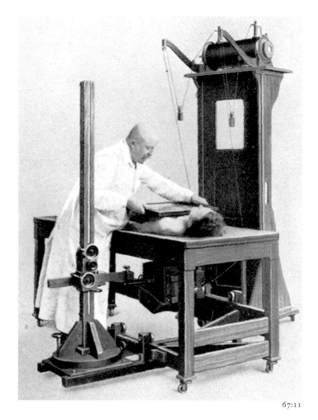

67:11

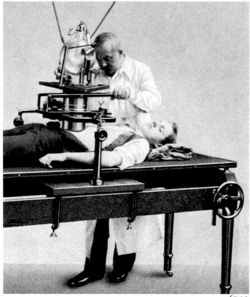

67:10

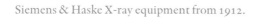

Siemens & Haske X-ray equipment from 1912.

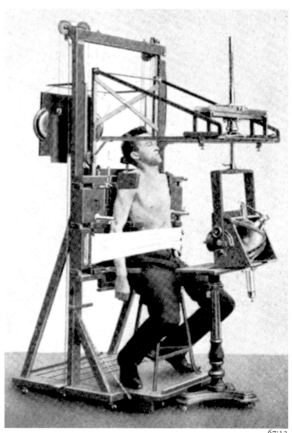

67:12

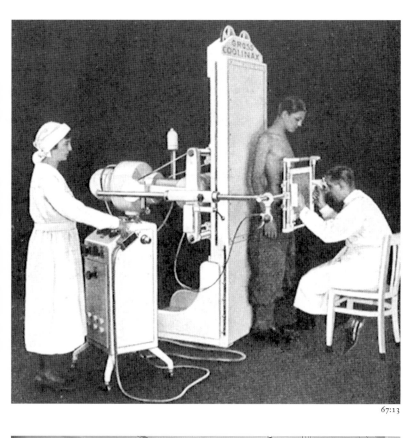

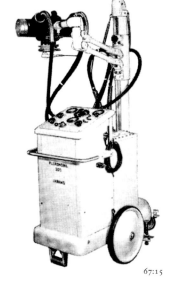

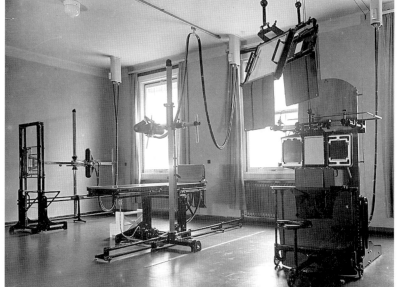

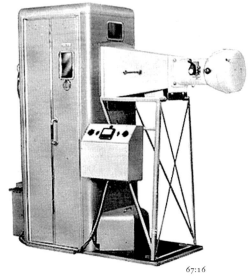

X-ray equipment "Grosscoolinax" from 1933 (at the top).

X-ray room in Caecilien-Krankenhaus Berlin 1935.

X-ray equipment for mass radiography and a
mobile X-ray unit ("Pleromobil") for operating
rooms, both from 1952.

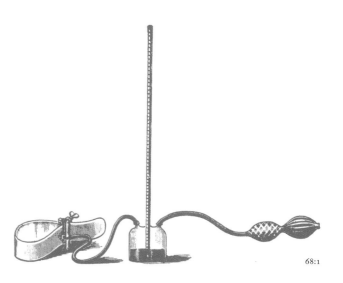

68:1

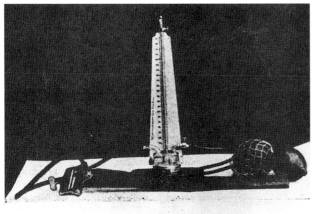

68:2

Scipione Riva-Rocci (1863–1937) invents the first clinically practical sphygmomanometer in 1896. The illustration above shows his drawing of the device and the instrument (left) is used by Nicolai Korotkoff (1874–1920), as explained on the following pages.

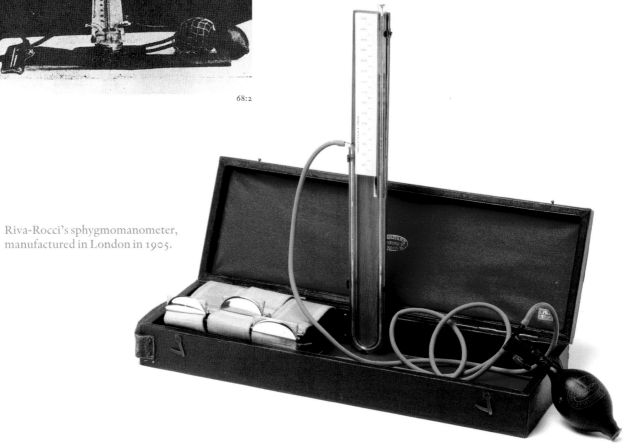

Riva-Rocci's sphygmomanometer, manufactured in London in 1905.

68:3

R IVA-ROCCI was born in Almese in 1863. He obtained his doctorate in medicine and surgery from the University of Torino in 1888and remained there as assistant lecturer for ten years. At the end of this period he invented the sphygmomanometer that brought him fame. From 1894 he was a qualified pathologist and in 1907 he also became a certified paediatrician. Starting in 1900 and for almost three decades he was the head physician at the Ospedale civico di Varese and most of this time he held an additional appointment as lecturer at the paediatric clinic of the University of Pavia. He died in Rapallo at the age of seventy-four.

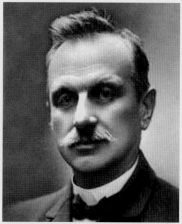

Scipione Riva-Rocci   68:4

Un Sfigmomanometro nuovo.

GAZ MED TORINO TORINO; 1896; 47:981 AND P1001.

RIVA-ROCCI ANNOUNCES his invention of a simple blood pressure measuring device. Inflating a rubber hose from a bicycle that is wrapped around the upper arm and measuring the pressure in the hose with a mercury manometer, he determines the blood pressure in the brachial artery by feeling the pulse disappearing or reappearing as the hose is inflated or deflated.

IN PERSPECTIVE:

In 1881 Basch invented the first clinically useful sphygmomanometer (68.1). Pressing a water-filled bulb attached to a vertical mercury column against the radial artery, he was able to determine the systolic pressure by noting when the pulsations disappeared. Riva-Rocci's method described in the cited paper was much more practical. Its function was based on a combination of the counter-pressure technique introduced by Vierordt (68.2), the volume plethysmographic method invented by Fick (68.3) and developed by Marey (68.4) and the ancient Chinese art of feeling the pulse (68.5). In 1897 Hill and Barnard made Riva-Rocci's device even more convenient to use by replacing the mercury manometer with a pressure gauge (68.6) and von Recklinghausen increased the width of the cuff for greater accuracy in 1901 (68.7). Korotkoff, serving as a surgeon in the Russo-Japanese war of 1904, used auscultation to study the formation of collateral vessels in aortic aneurysms (68.8). In the course of this work he discovered, while using Riva-Rocci's device, that auscultation offered an attractive alternative to palpating the arterial pulse (68.9). Korotkoff used a binaural stethoscope developed from the original concept of Laennec (68.10) in 1856 (68.11). By 1920 these non-invasive methods of measuring blood pressure were in general use both in hospitals and by general practitioners. Since 1970 automatic blood pressure devices have been available that allow reliable measurements to be made without the assistance of medical personnel (68.12).

68.1 Basch SS. Ueber die Messung des Blutdrucks am Menschen. *Z Klin Med* 1881; 2:79.

68.2 See ref. 35.7.

68.3 See # 46 Fick page 242 and ref. 46.9.

68.4 See # 52 Marey page 272 and ref 52.1.

68.5 Cleyer A. *Specimen Medicinae Sinicac, sive Opuscula Medica ad Mentem Sinensium, . . .* Frankfurt am Main; 1682.

68.6 Hill L, Barnard H. A simple and accurate form of sphygmomanometer or arterial pressure gauge contrived for clinical use. *Brit med J* 1897; 2:904.

68.7 von Recklinghausen H. Ueber Blutdruckmessung beim Menschen. *Arch exp Path Pharm.* 1901; 46:78.

68.8 Segall HN. Nicolai S Korotkoff. *Experiments for determining the efficiency of arterial collaterals (translation of thesis 1910) with preface and biographical notes.* Montreal; 1980.

68.9 Korotkoff NC. To the question of methods of determining the blood pressure. *Reports Imp mil med Acad* 1905; 11:365 being Appendix l in ref. 68.8.

68.10 See # 31 Laennec page 172.

68.11 Leared A. On the self-adjusting double stethoscope. *Lancet* 1856; 2:138. and p202.

68.12 Geddes LA. *Handbook of Blood Pressure Measurements.* Clifton NJ: Humana Press; 1991.

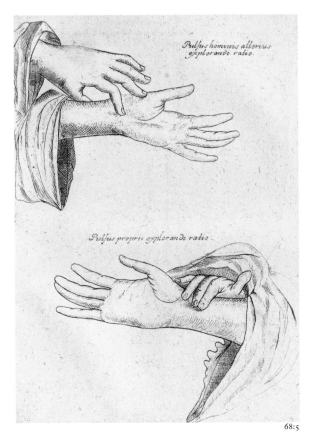

Chinese teachings according to Wang Shu-Ho (300 AD) on the examination of the pulse as translated and brought to Europe in 1682 by Andreas Cleyer (1634–1698).

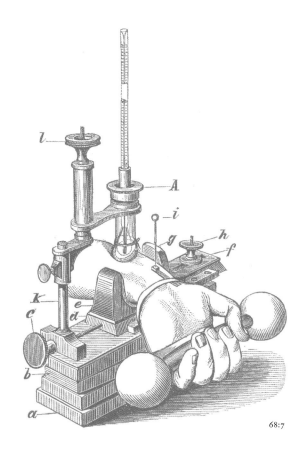

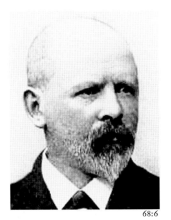

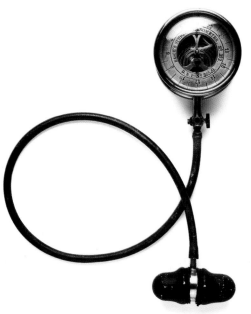

Samuel von Basch (1837–1905) employs a water and mercury filled rubber bulb that presses against the artery and obliterates the pulse, thereby indicating the arterial pressure on a mercury manometer. The pictures show his original drawing from 1880 and a later model of his device, where a pressure gauge has replaced the manometer tube.

A SIMPLE AND ACCURATE FORM OF SPHYGMOMETER OR ARTERIAL PRESSURE GAUGE CONTRIVED FOR CLINICAL USE.

BY

LEONARD HILL, M.B., and HAROLD BARNARD,
Lecturer on Physiology,   M.S., F.R.C.S., Surgical Registrar,
London Hospital.   London Hospital.

THIS instrument consists of: (1) A broad armlet, which is strapped round the upper arm. The armlet is formed of a flexible steel band, on the inside of which there is fastened a bag of thin indiarubber. The rubber bag is connected by a Y-tube with (2) a small compressing air pump fitted with a valve and (3) a pressure gauge.

The pressure gauge is of special construction. Roughly, it consists of a metal tambour, the expansion of which is

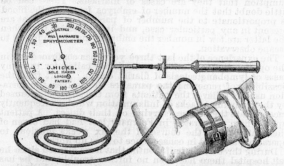

exhibited in a highly magnified form by means of an index or pointer which travels round a dial. This dial is graduated in millimetres of mercury. The armlet, pump, and pressure gauge when not in use fit conveniently into a leather case. The instrument is used thus: (1) The armlet is strapped round the upper arm so that it fits closely to the skin. (2) By means of the pump the pressure is raised within the rubber bag until the pulsation indicated by the index of the pressure gauge becomes of maximal excursion. (3) At this point the pressure indicated by the gauge is read, and this pressure is the mean arterial pressure.

The armlet can be applied to the arm of any individual with the greatest ease, for the flexible steel band adapts itself to any shape or size. In children the armlet can be fitted equally well to the thigh, and the pressure is then taken in the femoral artery. The armlet is bound closely round the arm so that the rubber bag may be but slightly distended when the pressure is raised within up to the arterial tension. If the bag were greatly distended the elasticity of the bag would come into play, and from this an error in the readings would arise. To avoid this error the rubber bag is made thin and flaccid. By raising the pressure within the bag the venous outlets are blocked. This, if continued for long, produces great congestion of the arm and discomfort. For this reason the readings must be taken rapidly. The pressure is never to be maintained on the arm for more than a minute or so. The following is a convenient plan of work:

(1) Force up the pressure rapidly till pulsation appears. (2) Continue to force up the pressure till pulsation disappears or obviously becomes lessened. (3) Slightly open the valve and allow slow leakage. As the pressure falls, note where the pulsation becomes maximal. (4) Let the air out entirely, and empty the arm of venous blood either by elevation of the limb or friction. (5) Repeat the operation and take another reading.

By following this plan no pain or discomfort will arise.

In studying the effect of exercise, posture, drugs, etc., successive readings must be taken in the above manner, first during the normal, and then during the experimental condition.

Owing to the effect of position on the circulation, the readings must be taken uniformly, with the arm placed by the side and on the same level as the heart. The muscles of the arm must be relaxed during the observations. The arterial tension is constantly varying slightly, owing to changes in the force of the heart beat and the respiratory oscillations of pressure. Thus the maximal pulsation may be found now at one place and now at another, a few millimetres higher or lower. The mean of the different readings must be taken just as is done when the mercurial manometer is used in physiological experiments on animals. In conditions of quiet respiration these variations are often not great, and the pressure may be read at each observation within 2 or 3 millimetres. Variations of pressure by 5 to 10 mms. Hg. are of frequent occurrence, are physiological, and of no importance.

When the rubber bag presses upon the outside of the arterial wall, with a pressure equal to that mean pressure exerted from within, the wall is able to oscillate with the greatest freedom. In systole the artery is fully expanded, while in diastole it is collapsed by the pressure of the bag.

The accuracy of this index has been proved by repeated experiment. Thus the armlet was strapped round the neck of a dog (excluding the trachea). A cannula was inserted into the femoral artery, and connected with a mercurial manometer. Simultaneous readings were then taken of the pressure in the femoral artery, as indicated by the mercurial manometer, and the pressure in the carotid arteries as indicated by the sphygmometer. The maximal pulsation of the index of the sphygmometer was thus found to occur always at a pressure which exactly corresponded with the mean pressure in the femoral artery.

It is well known that the carotid and femoral mean pressures are practically the same in the dog when the animal is lying in the horizontal position. To show in yet another way the accuracy of this instrument the following experiment was performed. Whilst one arm was passively elevated above the head and the other remained dependent by the side, simultaneous readings were taken from either brachial artery by means of two sphygmometers. From the dependent arm the higher reading was obtained. The difference was equivalent in mercury to the height of the vertical column of blood which separated the two points of observation.

The facility with which the instrument can be used for clinical purposes is illustrated by a series of observations which we have made upon patients placed under the influence of anæsthetics. Before and during administration a series of readings were taken at intervals of time, and from the figures thus obtained curves were plotted out. In 8 cases of anæsthesia with gas and oxygen (sitting posture) the arterial pressure either rose a few millimetres of mercury or remained constant. In 4 cases of anæsthesia with ether the arterial pressure remained constant or fell a very few millimetres of mercury. In 6 cases of anæsthesia with chloroform the sphygmometer indicated an extensive and rapid fall of arterial pressure. This fall equalled 20 to 40 mm. of mercury. The normal arterial pressure in most healthy young men appears to be 110 to 130 mm. Hg. in the sitting posture.

We shall shortly be in a position to publish a series of preliminary observations on arterial pressure in different pathological states. By means of this instrument, which is made for us by Mr. J. Hicks, of 8, Hatton Garden, E.C., we believe that the arterial pressure can be taken in man as rapidly, simply, and accurately as the temperature can be taken with the clinical thermometer.

68:9

Independent of Riva-Rocci's work, Leonard Hill (1866–1952) and Harold Barnard (1868–1908) introduce a convenient armlet method of blood pressure measurement using an aneroid manometer in 1897. They also note that the maximal pulsation occurs at the "mean arterial pressure".

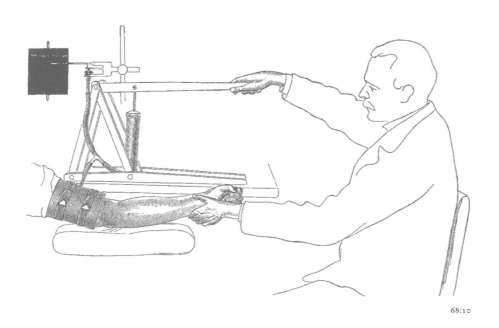

68:10

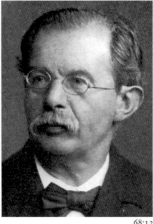

68:12

In 1901 Heinrich von Recklinghausen (1867–1943) studies how the cuff parameters affect the accuracy of blood pressure measurements. He demonstrates the benefit of wider cuffs (11–13 cm) and constructs an all-metal manometer. The illustration shows his experimental arrangement and a registration of the oscillations of the pressure in the cuff at different cuff pressures.

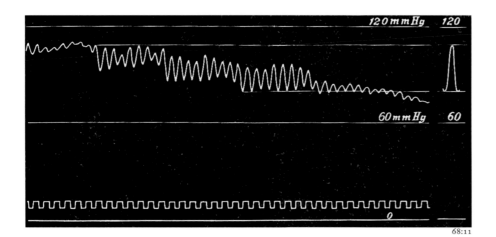

68:11

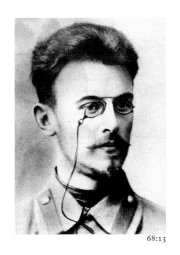

68:13

Korotkoff presents his new auscultation technique, which allows the determination of both the systolic and the diastolic blood pressure. He develops the method while working as a surgeon during the Russo-Japanese war (1904–1905) studying aneurysms and the effect of arterial compression. The graph shows a typical registration from these studies. He soon realises the advantage of auscultation as compared to feeling the pulsation in the artery.

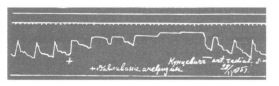

KUNTSEVICH: 28 Jan. 1905
left radial artery
compression of aneurysm at +
compression discontinued at −

68:14

N.C. Korotkoff: To the question of methods of determining the blood pressure (from the clinic of Professor C.P. Federoff). Reports of the Imperial Military Medical Academy, 11:365-367, 8 Nov. 1905.

On the basis of his observations the reporter has come to this conclusion: that the completely compressed artery under normal circumstances does not produce any sounds. Utilizing this phenomenon he proposes the auditory method of determining the blood pressure in man. The cuff of Riva-Rocci is placed on the middle thrid of the upper arm, the pressure within the cuff is quickly raised up to complete cessation of circulation below the cuff. Then, letting the mercury of the manometer fall, one listens to the artery just below the cuff with a children's stethoscope. At first, no sounds are heard. With the falling of the mercury in the manometer, down to a certain height, the first short tones appear; their appearance indicates the passage of part of the pulse wave under the cuff. It follows that the manometric figure at which the first tone appears corresponds to the maximal pressure. With the further fall of the mercury in the manometer one hears the systolic compression murmurs, which pass again into tones (second). Finally, all sounds disappear. The time of the cessation of sounds indicates the free passage of the pulse wave; in other words, at the moment of the disappearance of the sounds the minimal blood pressure within the artery preponderates over the pressure in the cuff. It follows that the manometric figures at this time correspond to the minimal blood pressure. Experiments on animals gave confirmative results. The first sound-tones appear (10 to 12 mm.) earlier than the pulse, for the palpation of which (e.g. in the radial artery) the inrush of the greater part of the pulse wave is required.

68:15

$$\theta = \frac{Fe}{m}\frac{l}{v^2}.$$

If, instead of the electric intensity, the rays are acted on by a magnetic force H at right angles to the rays, and extending across the distance l, the velocity at right angles to the original path of the rays is

$$\frac{Hev}{m}\frac{l}{v},$$

so that ϕ, the angle through which the rays are deflected when they leave the magnetic field, is given by the equation

$$\phi = \frac{He}{m}\frac{l}{v}.$$

From these equations we get

$$v = \frac{\phi}{\theta}\frac{F}{H}$$

and

$$\frac{m}{e} = \frac{H^2\theta \cdot l}{F\phi^2}.$$

In the actual experiments H was adjusted so that $\phi = \theta$; in this case the equations become

$$v = \frac{F}{H},$$

$$\frac{m}{e} = \frac{H^2 l}{F\theta}.$$

The apparatus used to measure v and m/e by this means is that represented in fig. 2. The electric field was produced by connecting the two aluminium plates to the terminals of a battery of storage-cells. The phosphorescent patch at the end of the tube was deflected, and the deflexion measured by a scale pasted to the end of the tube. As it was necessary to darken the room to see the phosphorescent patch, a needle coated with luminous paint was placed so that by a screw it could be moved up and down the scale; this needle could be seen when the room was darkened, and it was moved until it coincided with the phosphorescent patch. Thus, when light was admitted, the deflexion of the phosphorescent patch could be measured.

The magnetic field was produced by placing outside the tube two coils whose diameter was equal to the length of the plates; the coils were placed so that they covered the space

occupied by the plates, the distance between the coils was equal to the radius of either. The mean value of the magnetic force over the length l was determined in the following way: a narrow coil C whose length was l, connected with a ballistic galvanometer, was placed between the coils; the plane of the windings of C was parallel to the planes of the coils; the cross section of the coil was a rectangle 5 cm. by 1 cm. A given current was sent through the outer coils and the kick a of the galvanometer observed when this current was reversed. The coil C was then placed at the centre of two very large coils, so as to be in a field of uniform magnetic force: the current through the large coils was reversed and the kick β of the galvanometer again observed; by comparing a and β we can get the mean value of the magnetic force over a length l; this was found to be

$$60 \times \iota,$$

where ι is the current flowing through the coils.

A series of experiments was made to see if the electrostatic deflexion was proportional to the electric intensity between the plates; this was found to be the case. In the following experiments the current through the coils was adjusted so that the electrostatic deflexion was the same as the magnetic:—

Gas.	θ.	H.	F.	l.	m/e.	v.
Air	8/110	5·5	$1\cdot5\times10^{10}$	5	$1\cdot3\times10^{-7}$	$2\cdot8\times10^9$
Air	9·5/110	5·4	$1\cdot5\times10^{10}$	5	$1\cdot1\times10^{-7}$	$2\cdot8\times10^9$
Air	13/110	6·6	$1\cdot5\times10^{10}$	5	$1\cdot2\times10^{-7}$	$2\cdot3\times10^9$
Hydrogen	9/110	6·3	$1\cdot5\times10^{10}$	5	$1\cdot5\times10^{-7}$	$2\cdot5\times10^9$
Carbonic acid	11/110	6·9	$1\cdot5\times10^{10}$	5	$1\cdot5\times10^{-7}$	$2\cdot2\times10^9$
Air	6/110	5	$1\cdot8\times10^{10}$	5	$1\cdot3\times10^{-7}$	$3\cdot6\times10^9$
Air	7/110	3·6	1×10^{10}	5	$1\cdot1\times10^{-7}$	$2\cdot8\times10^9$

The cathode in the first five experiments was aluminium, in the last two experiments it was made of platinum; in the last experiment Sir William Crookes's method of getting rid of the mercury vapour by inserting tubes of pounded sulphur, sulphur iodide, and copper filings between the bulb and the pump was adopted. In the calculation of m/e and v no allowance has been made for the magnetic force due to the coil in

69:1

Joseph Thomson (1856–1940) discovers the electron. By balancing electrostatic and magnetic deflection of the charged "corpuscle" (electron) (see his illustrations of the equipment used), he can determine the velocity, which then allows him to measure the charge to mass ratio by deflection in a magnetic field. He finds this ratio to be about 1,000 times larger than that for a hydrogen ion (see his calculations and the table above summarising his results).

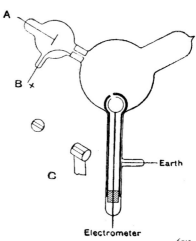

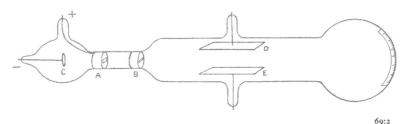

69:2

THOMSON was born near Manchester in 1856, the son of a bookseller. He planned a career in engineering, but in 1876 he won a minor scholarship that allowed him to enter Trinity College in Cambridge. He remained there for the rest of his life. In 1884, following Maxwell and Rayleigh (69.1), Thomson was appointed Cavendish Professor of Experimental Physics. He trained seven Nobel Prize winners during his tenure, winning the Nobel Prize in Physics himself in 1906. Thomson was an enthusiastic, imaginative and resourceful person capable of delegating less important matters, all of which made him an excellent director of research. He was a good teacher and an outstanding lecturer and took pedagogy seriously, writing textbooks for all levels of scientific study. He resigned his professorship in favour of Rutherford in 1919 and died in 1940.

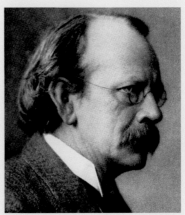

Joseph John Thomson

69:4

Cathode Rays.

PHILOSOPHICAL MAGAZINE
LONDON: TAYLOR AND FRANCIS; 1897; 44:293.

THOMSON REPORTS on his successful attempt to elucidate the nature of cathode rays. Improving the vacuum of the cathode ray tube, he discovers that electrostatic forces can deflect the rays. Next he balances the forces of electrostatic deflection against the forces of magnetic deflection and so determines the velocity of the "corpuscle" (electron). From the known kinetic energy and from the deflection produced by a homogenous magnetic field, he determines the charge/mass ratio and finds it to be about 1,000 times larger than that of a hydrogen ion. He proves this to be true in the presence of different gases and for different cathode materials.

IN PERSPECTIVE:

The controversy surrounding the nature of cathode rays (69.2)(69.3) was the driving force behind both Thomson's and Röntgen's (69.4) investigations and landmark discoveries. While the existence of the electron opened up an entirely new view on the structure of matter, Thomson turned his attention to "positive rays" (ion beams). By 1913 his newly designed equipment was able to separate isotopes of the stable element of neon (69.5), work that led his student Aston to develop the analytic technique of mass spectrometry (69.6). In 1928 Dirac predicted the existence of a positively charged electron (positron) from pure theoretical considerations (69.7). Today PET imaging in medicine is based on the detection of gamma rays emitted when such a positron is annihilated with an electron (69.8). In 1946 Wilson suggested the radiological use of protons (69.9) and five years later Leksell described the use of proton beams for stereotactic brain surgery (69.10). During the last decade ion beams have gained increasing importance in cancer therapy (69.11) and electron beams are nowadays widely used as a preferred method of sterilising certain medical products (69.12).

69.1 See #55 Maxwell page 286 and ref. 13.10.
69.2 Darrigol O. *Electrodynamics from Ampere to Einstein.* Oxford University Press; 2000. Chapt. 7. See also ref. 67.1, ref. 67.2 and ref. 67.3
69.3 Lenard P. Über die Absoption der Kathodenstrahlen. *Ann phys Chem* 1895; 56:255.
69.4 See #67 Röntgen page 344.
69.5 Thomson JJ. Rays of positive electricity. *Proc Roy Soc A* 1913; 89:I.
69.6 See #79 Aston page 406.
69.7 Dirac P. The Quantum Theory of the Electron. *Proc Roy Soc A* 1928; 117:610.
69.8 See #99 Phelps page 514.
69.9 Wilson RR. Radiological use of fast protons. *Radiology* 1946;47:487.
69.10 Leksell L. The stereotaxic method and radiosurgery of the brain. *Acta Chir Scand* 1951;102:316.
69.11 Alonso JR. Review of ion beam therapy: present and future. *Proc EPAC* 2000. p235.
69.12 See ref. 61.11.

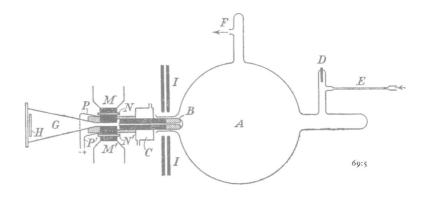

PLATE I.

69:5

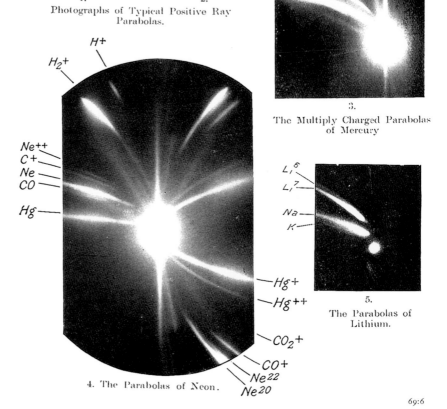

1. — 2.
Photographs of Typical Positive Ray Parabolas.

3.
The Multiply Charged Parabolas of Mercury

4. The Parabolas of Neon.

5.
The Parabolas of Lithium.

By 1913 Thomson's positive ion beam apparatus (top diagram) is sensitive enough to separate many ions and also the isotopes of neon. The photographs show some results from his experiments. This work initiated the development of the modern mass spectrometer instrumentation (see #79).

69:6

The general interpretation of non-relativity quantum mechanics is based on the transformation theory, and is made possible by the wave equation being of the form

$$(\mathbf{H} - \mathbf{W})\,\psi = 0, \tag{2}$$

i.e., being linear in W or $\partial/\partial t$, so that the wave function at any time determines the wave function at any later time. The wave equation of the relativity theory must also be linear in W if the general interpretation is to be possible.

The second difficulty in Gordon's interpretation arises from the fact that if one takes the conjugate imaginary of equation (1), one gets

$$\left[\left(-\frac{\mathbf{W}}{c} + \frac{e}{c}\,\mathbf{A_0}\right)^2 + \left(-\mathbf{p} + \frac{e}{c}\,\mathbf{A}\right)^2 + m^2 c^2\right]\psi = 0,$$

which is the same as one would get if one put $-e$ for e. The wave equation (1) thus refers equally well to an electron with charge e as to one with charge $-e$. If one considers for definiteness the limiting case of large quantum numbers one would find that some of the solutions of the wave equation are wave packets moving in the way a particle of charge $-e$ would move on the classical theory, while others are wave packets moving in the way a particle of charge e would move classically. For this second class of solutions W has a negative value. One gets over the difficulty on the classical theory by arbitrarily excluding those solutions that have a negative W. One cannot do this on the quantum theory, since in general a perturbation will cause transitions from states with W positive to states with W negative. Such a transition would appear experimentally as the electron suddenly changing its charge from $-e$ to e, a phenomenon which has not been observed. The true relativity wave equation should thus be such that its solutions split up into two non-combining sets, referring respectively to the charge $-e$ and the charge e.

69:8

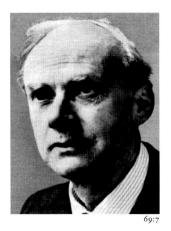

Paul Dirac (1902–1984) deduces the existence of positively charged electrons (positrons) from purely theoretical considerations in 1928.

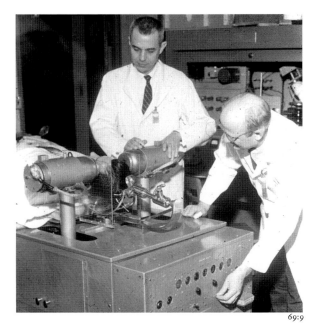

Gordon Brownell (left) with the first clinical positron imaging device, built in 1952 specifically for brain imaging (see #99).

69:9

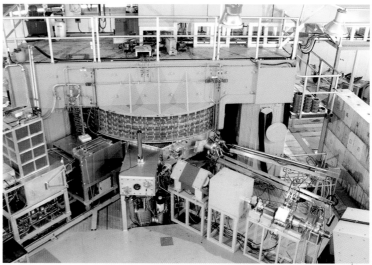

69:10

The proton cyclotron of the Svedberg Laboratory in Uppsala (top) and patients being treated at the facility with a narrow beam of protons to the head (right) and to the prostate. Today an estimated total of 30,000 patients have received proton irradiation therapy for various forms of malignancies worldwide.

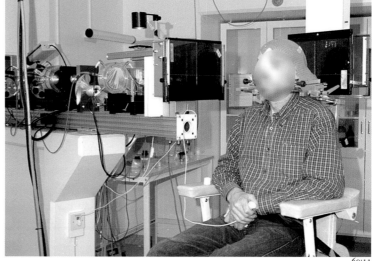

69:11

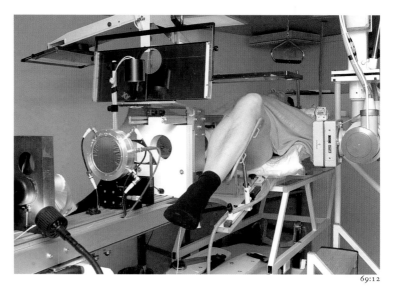

69:12

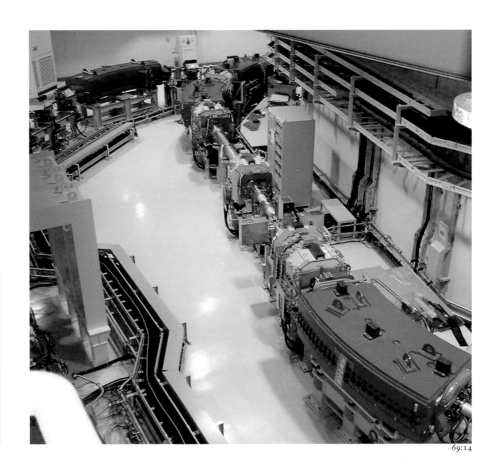

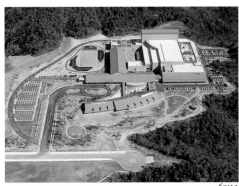

The image above shows an aerial view of the Hyogo Ion Beam Medical Center in Japan, its main accelerator (top) and a treatment room. The facility is designed also to produce synchrotron radiation about 100 million times more powerful than conventional X-rays. It opened in 2001 for the treatment of primary tumours with both proton and carbon ion beams.

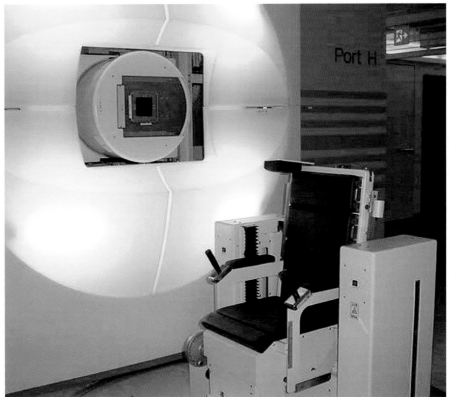

The laboratory of Marie Curie (1867–1934) for measuring radioactivity. The key apparatus, the electrometer balance, is seen on the table in the middle of the picture. An exploded view of the instrument that was originally developed by Pierre and Jacques Curie (see #66) is displayed below right.

Left below, to measure the radioactivity (R), the substance is placed on a lead plate (A) and 100 V is applied to an electrode plate (M) that is connected to a bridge including the highly sensitive piezoelectric balance. The zero of the bridge is adjusted by minute increments of the weight loading the electrometer ("To Weight"). The principle of the measurement is illustrated by the diagram.

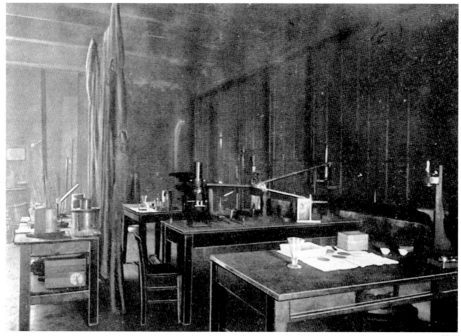

70:1

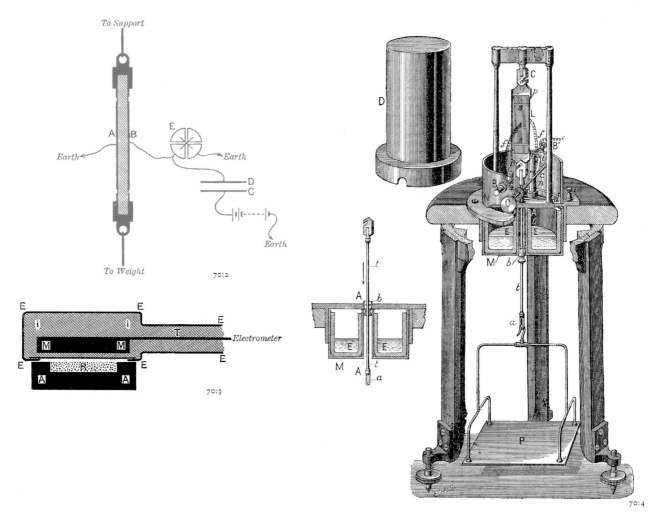

70:2

70:3

70:4

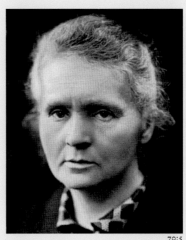

Maria Sklodowska Curie

70:5

KLODOWSKA was born in Warsaw in 1867. A brilliant
student, she worked as a private tutor and governess to
support herself and a sister who studied in France. In
1891, on the invitation her sister, she moved to Paris.
Sklodowska obtained her degrees in mathematics and physics
with the highest distinction and was invited to work in Lippmann's laboratory (70.1). She married Pierre Curie in 1895 and
both were soon caught up in the excitement created by Röntgen's
X-ray discovery and Becquerel's report of the rays emanating from
uranium (70.2). For her work on radioactivity she shared the 1903
Nobel Prize in Physics with her husband and with Becquerel, but
she also received her own Nobel Prize in Chemistry in 1911 for her
discoveries of the elements radium and polonium. Assisted by her
daughter Irène, she continued her work until her death in 1934,
which was partly caused by damages from the huge amount of radioactive material that she had handled.

Rayon émis par les composés de l'uranium et du thorium.

COMPTES RENDUS PARIS: GAUTHIER-VILLARS ET FILS; 1898; 126:1101.

IN HER first paper on radioactivity Sklodowska Curie describes
the measuring technique she was to employ in all her future work.
The substance to be studied, in this case compounds of uranium
and thorium, is placed between two condensor plates that are kept
at 100 volts. The current drawn from the condensor is taken as a
measure of the activity of the material. To detect the very weak
currents (typically $< 10^{-11}$ A) she uses a zero balance technique involving the condensor and a highly sensitive piezoelectric quartz
electrometer previously designed by the brothers Pierre and
Jacque Curie (70.3).

IN PERSPECTIVE:
On hearing about Röntgen's discovery, Becquerel started investigating fluorescent materials, believing in error that X-rays would be emitted from them. Within a month he found that potassium uranyl phosphate blackened photographic
plates wrapped in black paper (70.2). The subsequent pioneering investigations of
the Curie couple (70.3) were soon overshadowed by the experimental and theoretical work of Rutherford (70.4). He explained the laws of radioactive decay and
made collision experiments that led to the first hypothesis about the structure of
the atom (70.5) and the first demonstration of artificial transmutation (70.6). Radioactive techniques were introduced in chemistry and biology by Hevesy (70.7).
In 1959 Yalow and Berson conceived the radioimmunoassay technique (RIA)
(70.8), which revolutionised the chemical analysis of blood and tissue. Radioactive methods are also common in perfusion diagnostics (70.9), in many cases of
cancer treatment (70.10) and for medical sterilisation purposes (70.11).

70.1 See ref. 65.1.
70.2 Becquerel H. Émission de radiation nou-
       velles par l'uranium métallique. *C R Acad
       Sci* 1896; 122:1086.
70.3 See ref 66.1 p 335–516.
70.4 Rutherford E. *Radio-Activity*. Cambridge
       At the University Press; 1904.
70.5 Rutherford E. The Scattering of alfa and
       beta Particles by Matter and the Structure
       of the Atom. *Phil Mag* 6ser. 1911; 21:669.
70.6 Rutherford E. Collision of alfa Particles
       with Light Atoms IV. An Anomalous Ef-
       fect in Nitrogen. *Phil Mag* 6ser. 1919;
       37:581.
70.7 Hevesy G. Applications of isotopes in biol-
       ogy. *J Chem Soc* 1939; 39(2):1213.
70.8 Berson SA, Yalow RS. *Isotopic tracers in the
       study of diabetes.* In: Adv Biol Med Phys To-
       bias CA, Lawrence JH. Editors. Vol.VI
       New York:Academic Press; 1958. p349. See
       also ref. 81.9.
70.9 Kety SS. Measurement of regional circula-
       tion by the local clearance of radioactive
       sodium. *Am Heart J* 1949; 38:321.
70.10 Washington CM, Leaver D. Editors. *Princi-
       ples and Practice of Radiation Therapy*. Mos-
       by; 2003.
70.11 See ref. 61.11.

Ernst Rutherford's (1871–1937) theoretical and experimental work explains the laws of radioactive decay, leading to the first hypothesis of the structure of the atom and the first demonstration of artificial transmutation. The text is reproduced from his classic book "Radioactivity", published in 1904.

CHAPTER IV.

NATURE OF THE RADIATIONS.

PART I.

COMPARISON OF THE RADIATIONS.

65. **The Three Types of Radiation.** All the radio-active substances possess in common the power of acting on a photographic plate and of ionizing the gas in their immediate neighbourhood. The intensity of the radiations may be compared by means of their photographic or electrical action; and, in the case of the strongly radio-active substances, by the power they possess of lighting up a phosphorescent screen. Such comparisons, however, do not throw any light on the question whether the radiations are of the same or of different kinds, for it is well known that such different types of radiations as the short waves of ultra-violet light, Röntgen and cathode rays, all possess the property of producing ions throughout the volume of a gas, lighting up a fluorescent screen, and acting on a photographic plate. Neither can the ordinary optical methods be employed to examine the radiations under consideration, as they show no trace of regular reflection, refraction, or polarization.

Two general methods can be used to distinguish the types of the radiations given out by the same body, and also to compare the radiations from the different active substances. These methods are as follows:

(1) By observing whether the rays are appreciably deflected in a magnetic field.

(2) By comparing the relative absorption of the rays by solids and gases.

Examined in these ways, it has been found that there are three different types of radiation emitted from radio-active bodies, which for brevity and convenience have been termed the α, β, and γ rays.

(i) The α rays are very readily absorbed by thin metal foil and by a few centimetres of air. They have been shown to consist of positively charged bodies projected with a velocity of about 1/10 the velocity of light. They are deflected by intense magnetic and electric fields, but the amount of deviation is minute in comparison with the deviation, under the same conditions, of the cathode rays produced in a vacuum tube.

(ii) The β rays are far more penetrating in character than the α rays, and consist of negatively charged bodies projected with velocities of the same order as the velocity of light. They are far more readily deflected than the α rays and are in fact identical with the cathode rays produced in a vacuum tube.

(iii) The γ rays are extremely penetrating, and non-deviable by a magnetic field. Their true nature is not yet known, but they are analogous in some respects to very penetrating Röntgen rays.

The three best known radio-active substances, uranium, thorium, and radium, all give out these three types of rays, each in an amount approximately proportional to its relative activity. Polonium stands alone in giving only the α or easily absorbed rays[1].

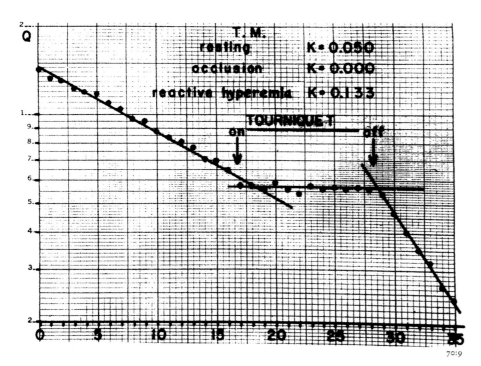

T. M.
resting   K = 0.050
occlusion   K = 0.000
reactive hyperemia   K = 0.133

TOURNIQUET
on   off

70:9

Seymour Kety (1915–2000) introduces the isotope clearance method for perfusion measurements in 1949. The clearance (shown by the slope of the lines) of the sodium isotope $Na^{24}Cl$ from the human gastrocnemius (calf) reflects the perfusion variations when applying and releasing a tourniquet about the thigh.

Lars Leksell (1907–1986) shown next to his first apparatus for gamma radiation surgery. The unit has more than 200 separate radioactive (cobalt) sources that irradiate a selected area of the brain. The first installation for clinical use is made in Stockholm in 1968.

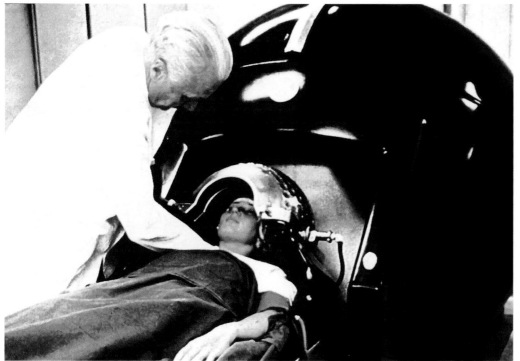

70:10

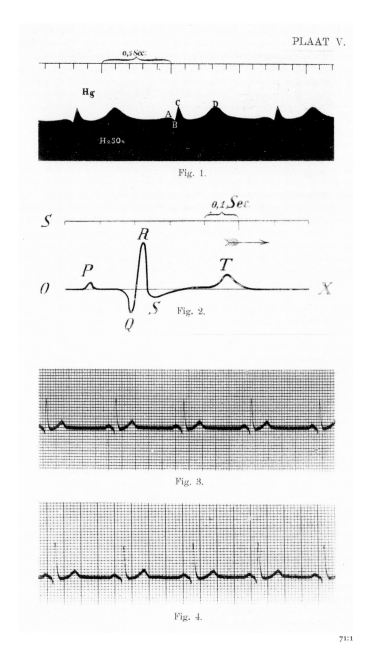

PLAAT V.

Fig. 1.

Fig. 2.

Fig. 3.

Fig. 4.

71:1

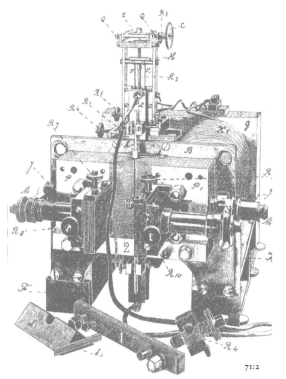

71:2

In a short publication from 1902 Willem Einthoven (1860–1927) includes the first modern ECG registration (the graph marked O-X), which is obtained with his newly developed string galvanometer. A drawing and a photograph of the original device are shown right. The key sensing element of the apparatus is a thin silver-coated quartz string that is placed in a strong magnetic field.

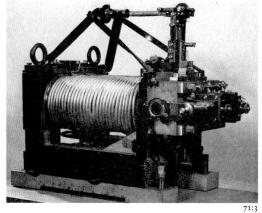

71:3

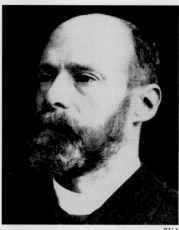

EINTHOVEN was born in Semarang, Java, in 1860. When he was six years of age his father, a physician, died and the family moved to Utrecht. There Einthoven entered medical school in 1879 and received his degree in medicine with distinction six years later. He was appointed professor of physiology in Leiden in 1886. Stimulated by the work of Waller (71.1), he started to improve on the techniques for recording the electrical signals of a heartbeat. His work not only improved previous methods but eventually also led to the development of a new instrument, the string galvanometer, for which he received the Nobel Prize in Medicine in 1924 (71.2). Einthoven was married to a cousin and had four children. He died in 1927.

Galvanometrische registratie van het menschelijk electrocardiogram.

IN: HERINNERINGSBUNDEL PROF S S ROSENSTEIN.
LEIDEN: E.IJDO; 1902. P101.

EINTHOVEN DEMONSTRATES the improved results obtained with his new equipment for registering the electrical activity of the heart. He shows the superior performance of the string galvanometer (71.3) by comparing the original technique of Waller (71.1), employing Lippmann's capillary galvanometer (71.4), and the results of his own improvement of this method (71.5) with the tracings obtained with the new device. His report is illustrated with the first modern ECG recording and with the customary P,Q,R,S,T notation.

IN PERSPECTIVE:
In 1842 Matteucci observed electrical phenomena when contacting the muscle of a beating heart directly (71.6), but it was Waller who showed that the signal could also be obtained from contact with the body surface (71.1). However, Waller's instrument had a rather slow response and so Einthoven first applied mathematical corrections to improve its frequency characteristics (71.5). Abandoning these efforts and starting with the compensatory principle of the mirror galvanometer of D'Arsonval and Deprez (71.7), he constructed a new device using a thin string of silver-coated quartz placed in a magnetic field as the sensing element. He subsequently developed many versions of this instrument (71.2) and used it to register various physiological signals such as the ECG, heart sounds and action currents of sympathetic nerves. Connecting patients in the hospital to the equipment in his laboratory Einthoven made "telecardiograms" at a distance of 1.6 km. Until about 1950 the string galvanometer remained the standard of reference (71.8), but was then overtaken by the faster direct-writing ink-jet devices invented by Elmquist (71.9). In 1947 Holter designed the first "radioelectrocardiography" unit and a decade later the original 80-pound backpack system had been reduced sufficiently in size to make clinical applications possible (71.10)(71.11).

71.1 See #65 Waller page 334.
71.2 Einthoven W. *The string galvanometer and the measurement of the action current of the heart.* The Nobel Lecture Stockholm; 1925.
71.3 Einthoven W. Un nouveau galvanomètre. *Arch N Sc Ex Nat* 1901; 6:625.
71.4 See ref. 65.1.
71.5 Einthoven W. Lippmann's Capillar-Electrometer zur Messung schnell wechselnder Potentialunterschiede *Pfluger's Arch ges Physiol* 1894; 56:528.
71.6 See ref. 65.2.
71.7 D'Arsonval JA, Deprez M. Galvanomètre apériodique. *C R Acad Sci* 1882; 94:1347. See also ref. 2.7.
71.8 Barron SL. *The development of the electrocardiograph.* Cambridge Monogr. 5 London; 1952.
71.9 *Swedish Special Apparatus for heart clinics. Electrocardiograph-Elmquist system.* AB Elema-Järnhs 1952. See also #91 Elmquist-Senning page 470.
71.10 Holter NJ. Radioelectrocardiography: A New Technique for Cardiovascular Studies. *Ann N Y Acad Sci* 1957; 65:913.
71.11 MacInnis HF. The Clinical Application of Radioelectrocardiography. *Can Med Assoc J* 1954; 70:574.

In March 1905 Einthoven makes the first ECG registration at a distance, in a laboratory about 1.6 km from the hospital. The picture shows the patient and the "telecardiogram" obtained on this particular occasion.

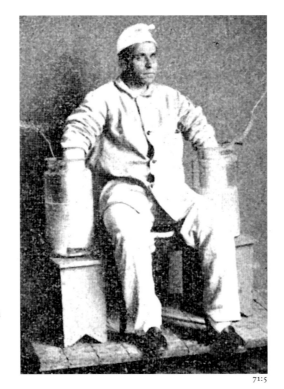

71:5

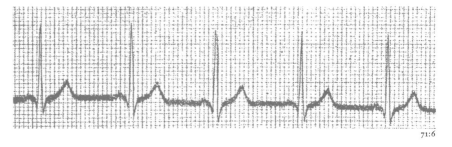

71:6

Little more than half a century after the first "telecardiogram" of Einthoven, Norman Holter (1914-1983) designs the first ambulatory apparatus for radio transmission of an ECG signal. The device weighs 80 kg and is carried on the back, as shown in the photograph below.

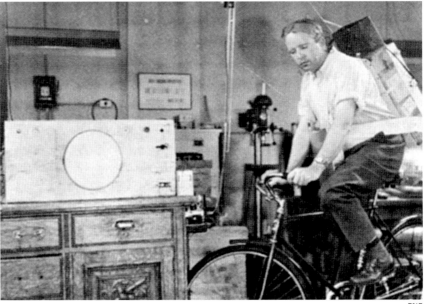

71:7

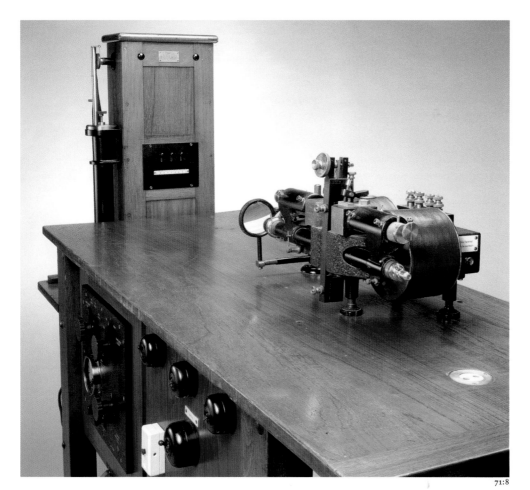

An electrocardiograph manufactured by Cambridge Instrument Company in England in 1930 and, below, a French Boulitte electrocardiograph in use on an ambulatory patient at S:t Eriks Hospital in Stockholm in 1930.

71:8

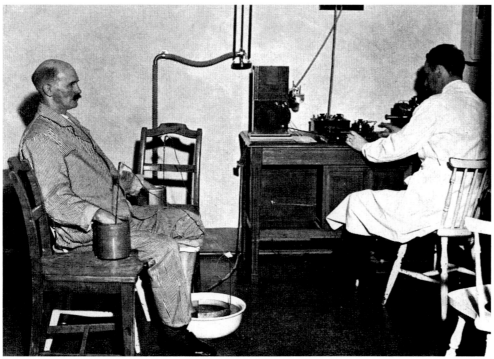

71:9

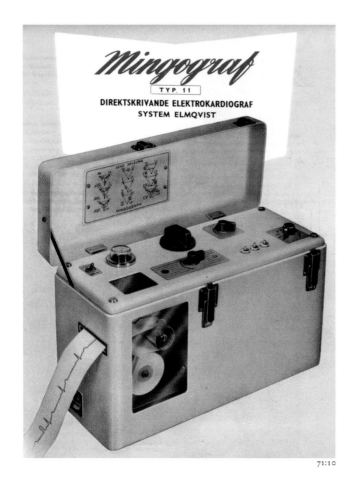

Due to our unique jet principle (frequency response up to 800—900 c/s!) our recorders are the only existing types giving accurate and true electrocardiograms, heart sounds, blood pressure recordings etc. in direct-writing.

MINGOGRAF TYPE 11

1-channel electrocardiograph for ECG-leads I, II, III, AVR, AVF, AVL, CR, CF and CV. Extremely easy to handle. Clear, eye-appealing, blue-black tracing on red-ruled-paper. 3 paper speeds: 25, 50 a. 100 mm/sec.

First scientifically true electrocardiogram in direct-writing! Weight 12 kg.

MINGOGRAF TYPE 21

2-channel apparatus: ECG simultaneously with Heart Sounds. One channel similar to Mingograf type 11 and the other specially designed for heart sound recording in 7 different frequency ranges up to 800 c/s. Built-in calibrating device.

The first heart sounds in direct-writing! Weight 16 kg.

Rune Elmquist's (1906–1996) direct-writing inkjet apparatus (the "Mingograf") is introduced in 1952 and represents a major advance in the technology for recording fast biomedical signals. With a glass capillary only 0.01 mm in diameter, the inkjet method produces a true representation of signals up to a frequency of about 900 c/s. The illustrations show the first model of the device and its principle of operation.

1 Galvanometer
2 Düse
3 Düsenstrahl
4 Verstärker
5 Schreibflüssigkeit
6 Pumpe

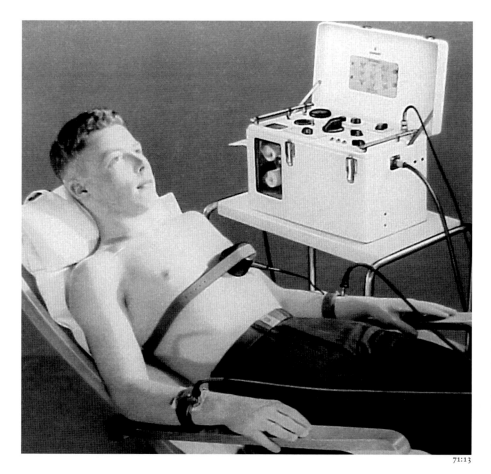

Heart sound registration using the first model of the Mingograf from 1952.

A four channel Mingograf introduced in 1955, in use during a cardiac catheterisation at the Karolinska Hospital in Stockholm in 1961.

71:13

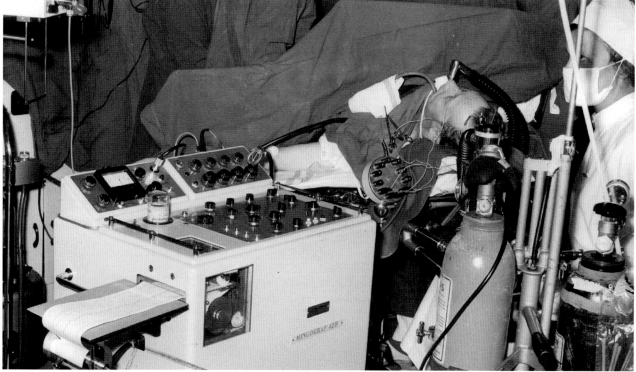

71:14

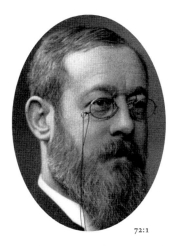

Josef von Mering (1849–1908) performs the laboratory work that proves the hypnotic action of diethylbarbituric acid. This compound had been synthesised a decade before, but it is the insightful reasoning of Emil Fischer (1852–1919), as presented in the beginning of their paper (reproduced here), that leads them to this seminal discovery.

72:1

Die Therapie der Gegenwart

1903   herausgegeben von Prof. Dr. G. Klemperer   März
in Berlin.

Ueber eine neue Klasse von Schlafmitteln.

Von Emil Fischer und J. v. Mering.

Fast ebenso dunkel wie das Wesen des natürlichen Schlafes ist trotz der nicht geringen Zahl von synthetischen Schlafmitteln der Zusammenhang zwischen chemischer Constitution und pharmakologischer Wirkung. Die seit der Einführung des Chloralhydrats in den Arzneischatz durch Liebreich im Jahre 1869 aufgefundenen Hypnotica ordnen sich chronologisch in folgende Reihe: Urethan, Paraldehyd, Amylenhydrat, Sulfonal, Trional und Chloralformamid; dazu sind in neuerer Zeit das Dormiol und endlich das Hedonal oder Methylpropylcarbinol-Urethan gekommen. Betrachtet man die Structurformeln der angeführten Stoffe, so ergiebt sich ein so grosser Unterschied, dass die schlafmachende Wirkung offenbar ganz verschiedenen Atomgruppen zukommt. Nach der chemischen Zusammensetzung lassen sich die genannten Mittel in 4 Klassen eintheilen. Zu dem Chloralhydrat gehören selbstverständlich sein directes Derivat, das Chloralformamid (Chloralamid) und aller Wahrscheinlichkeit nach auch der Paraldehyd, der ja nichts weiter ist als die polymere Form des Acetaldehyds, von dem das Chloralhydrat abgeleitet wird. Eine zweite Klasse repräsentirt das Amylenhydrat oder tertiärer Amylalkohol von folgender Structur

$$CH_3\!\!-\!\!C\!\!-\!\!OH$$
$$CH_3 \quad C_2H_5$$

in welchem ausser der Alkoholgruppe das mit drei Alkyl verbundene Kohlenstoffatom der Träger der schlafmachenden Wirkung zu sein scheint.

Ein Mittelding zwischen dieser ersten und zweiten Klasse bildet das Dormiol, welches die Combination von Chloralhydrat und Amylenhydrat ist. Die dritte Klasse repräsentirt das Urethan und sein Derivat, das Hedonal und die vierte Klasse endlich bilden die schwefelhaltigen Disulfone, von denen das Trional folgende Structur besitzt.

$$CH_3 \quad C_2H_5 \!\!-\!\! C \!\!-\!\! SO_2\!\cdot\!C_2H_5$$
$$SO_2\!\cdot\!C_2H_5$$

Sie haben mit dem Amylenhydrat eine gewisse Aehnlichkeit, denn das Centrum des Moleküls ist hier ein Kohlenstoffatom, das mit zwei Alkyl und zwei sehr fest haftenden Sulfonresten verknüpft ist. Weiterhin ist dem Amylenhydrat und den Disulfonen die Anwesenheit des Aethyls gemeinsam. Durch die Beobachtungen von Thierfelder und dem Einen von uns,[1] die später von Baumann und Kast,[2] sowie von Schneegans und dem Einen von uns[3] wesentlich vervollständigt wurden, wissen wir, dass von der Anzahl der Aethylgruppen die schlafmachende Wirkung der Alkohole und Disulfone stark beeinflusst wird.

Auf Grund dieser Betrachtungen schien es uns interessant, andere Stoffe, die ein mit mehreren Aethylgruppen beladenes und tertiär oder quaternär gebundenes Kohlenstoffatom enthalten, auf die schlafmachende Wirkung zu prüfen, und es ist uns in der That gelungen, eine neue grosse Klasse von Schlafmitteln dieser Art aufzufinden. Beide sind Harnstoffderivate. Die einen leiten sich ab von den Dialkylessigsäuren; als Repräsentant derselben führen wir die Diäthylverbindung an, welche folgende Structur hat:

$$C_2H_5 \quad H$$
$$C_2H_5 \!\!-\!\! C \!\!-\!\! CO\!-\!NH\!-\!CO\!-\!NH_2$$

und deshalb als Diaethylacetylharnstoff zu bezeichnen ist.

Die anderen sind Abkömmlinge der Diaethylmalonsäure mit cyklischer Structur des stickstoffhaltigen Theiles.

Als wichtigsten Körper dieser Gruppe nennen wir den Diaethylmalonylharnstoff mit der Structurformel

$$C_2H_5 \quad\quad CO\!-\!NH$$
$$C \quad\quad\quad\quad CO$$
$$C_2H_5 \quad\quad CO\!-\!NH$$

Durch Verbesserung der synthetischen Methoden ist es uns möglich gewesen, nicht allein zahlreiche Glieder der beiden erwähnten Klassen, sondern auch andere ähnliche Derivate der Dialkylmalonsäuren der pharmakologischen Untersuchung zugänglich zu machen und so einige überraschende Beziehungen zwischen chemischer Constitution und schlaferregender Wirkung festzustellen. Die folgende Zusammenstellung der Beobachtungen am Hunde ist nach chemischen Gesichtspunkten geordnet.

[1] Zeitschrift f. physiolog. Chemie 9, 511 (1885).
[2] Zeitschrift für physiol. Chem. 14, 52 (1889).
[3] Therapeutische Monatshefte 1892, 327.

13

72:2

F ISCHER was born in 1852 in Euskirchen, the son of a successful businessman. Instead of entering the family business as desired by his father, he started to study at the University of Bonn. After a year he moved to Strasbourg, where Baeyer (72.1) influenced him to take up chemistry. In 1874 he took his Ph.D. and subsequently during his distinguished career came to hold the chair of chemistry in Erlangen, Würzburg and from 1892 in Berlin. Fischer's work on purines and sugars started in the early 1880s and culminated with the Nobel Prize in Chemistry in 1902. However, by 1899 he had already started his important work on proteins and amino acids. The death of two of his three sons during the First World War left Fischer devastated. Together with a serious illness, this contributed to his death in 1919.

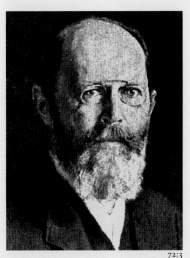

Emil Fischer

72:3

Ueber eine neue Klasse von Schlafmitteln.

DIE THERAPIE DER GEGENWART. BERLIN, WIEN: URBAN & SCHWARZENBERG; 1903; 44:97.

FISCHER AND von Mering investigate the hypnotic effect of various derivatives of barbituric acid and related substances. The reaction of dogs that have been given a few grams of the substance to be tested in the morning is followed through the day. The compound 5,5-diethylbarbituric acid ($(C_2H_5)_2—CH—CO—NH—CO—NH_2$) turns out to be a strong hypnotic. In man less than 1 g dissolved in a warm cup of tea is sufficient to produce adequate sleep within half an hour. With no known side effects seen, the authors report that the drug is already available as "Veronal" from the company E. Merck.

IN PERSPECTIVE:
Scheele and Bergman discovered uric acid in urine (72.2) and in 1834 Mitscherlich determined its correct formula (72.3). A few years later Liebig and Wöhler investigated its properties in some detail (72.4) and in 1882 Horbaczewski succeeded in synthesising the substance (72.5). The study of uric acid led Fischer to purine research. After two decades he had explored the subject thoroughly, having synthesised about 130 purine derivatives. He found that purine ($C_5N_4H_4$) was a heterocyclic compound and that uric acid was an oxide of purine. In 1864 Baeyer had prepared barbituric acid from hydrurilic acid and showed it on hydrolysis to form urea and malonic acid (72.6). Conrad and Guthzeit synthesised barbituric acid derivatives and also prepared "Veronal" (72.7), but they were unaware of the hypnotic effects of the substance. Fischer's work on purines had a lasting impact on basic and clinical biochemistry and on the pharmaceutical industry (72.8)(72.9) (72.10). His introduction of barbitone ("Veronal") as a hypnotic agent is a major contribution to clinical anaesthesiology (72.11).

72.1 Partington JR. *A History of Chemistry*. Vol. IV Mansfield Centre: Martino Fine Books; 1999. p775.
72.2 Scheele CW. Undersökning om Blåse-stenen. *Kungl Vet Handl* 1776; 37:327 and Bergman T. Tillägning Om Blåse-stenen. *Kungl Vet Handl* 1776; 37:333. See also ref 72.1 p333 and #21 Scheele page 120.
72.3 Mitscherlich E. Analyse kohlenstoffhaltige Verbindungen. *Ann Phys* 1834; 33:331.
72.4 von Liebig J, Wöhler F. Untersuchung über die Natur der Harnsäure. *Ann Pharm* 1838; 26:241.
72.5 Horbaczewski J. Synthese der Harnsäure. *Ber Deutsch Chem Gesell* 1882; 15(2):2678.
72.6 Baeyer A. *Gesammelte Werke*. Brunswick; 1905. See also ref. 72.1 p777.
72.7 Conrad M, Guthzeit M. Ueber Barbitursäurederivate. *Ber Deutsch Chem Gesell* 1882; 15(2):2845.
72.8 Lister JH. *The Purines*. John Wiley & Sons; 1996.
72.9 Simmons HA, Stone TW. *Purines: Basic and Clinical Aspects*. Kluwer Academic Publisher; 1991.
72.10 Daly JW, Manganiello V, Jacobson KA. *Purines in Cellular Signalling: Target for New Drugs*. Springer Verlag; 1990.
72.11 Stoelting RK. *Pharmacology and Physiology of Anesthetic Practice*. Chapter 4 Lippincott Williams & Wilkins Publ.; 1999.

Fischer and Mering conclude their investigation by stating that 1 gram of the hypnotic substance "diaethylacetylharnstoff" (which they named "Veronal") in a cup of tea produces sleep in man in about half an hour and that no side effects can be observed in short-term use (on the top of the next page).

18. Diaethylmalonylthioharnstoff

$$\begin{array}{c}C_2H_5\\ \\C_2H_5\end{array}\!\!>\!\!C\!<\!\!\begin{array}{c}CO-NH\\ \\CO-NH\end{array}\!\!>\!\!CS$$

Ein Hund von 7 kg erhält 1 g. Eine Stunde später schläft er tief, reagirt auf keine Reize und stirbt nach 8 Stunden.

Aus vorstehenden Beobachtungen ergeben sich folgende Beziehungen zwischen chemischer Structur und hypnotischer Wirkung in dieser Klasse. Säuren und Amide sind wirkungslos. Zur Erzeugung von Schlaf ist die Harnstoffgruppe erforderlich, aber sie genügt allein nicht. Es muss dazu kommen ihre Combination mit einem Reste, der mehrere kohlenstoffreiche Alkyle enthält. Der einfachste Fall dieser Art ist gegeben in den Harnstoffderivaten der Diäthyl- und Dipropylessigsäure (I. No. 1 und 2). Ungleich stärker wird aber die hypnotische Wirkung bei der cyklischen Anordnung der Harnstoffgruppe in den Derivaten der Dialkylmalonsäure. Hier ist dann weiter die Natur des Alkyls von wesentlicher Bedeutung. Die Wirkung, welche beim Dimethyl (III. No. 6) ganz fehlt, ist gering beim Methylaethyl (7), steigt beim Methylpropyl (8), wird recht stark beim Diaethyl (9) und erreicht ihren Höhepunkt beim Dipropyl (11). Beim Diisobutyl (12) steht sie ungefähr auf gleicher Stufe wie bei Diaethyl und beim Diisoamyl (13) ist sie wieder recht schwach. Das Dibenzylderivat (14) scheint ganz inactiv zu sein, was aber auch zum Theil durch die Schwerlöslichkeit bedingt sein kann.

Auffallend ist die Giftigkeit von CC-Diaethyl-N-Methylmalonylharnstoff (15), welcher sich von No. 9 nur dadurch unterscheidet, dass das eine Stickstoffatom noch ein Methyl bindet. Dies erinnert an den bekannten physiologischen Unterschied zwischen Acetanilid und seiner Methylverbindung (Exalgin) oder zwischen Phenacetin und Methylphenacetin.

Auffallend ist, dass die ringförmige Anordnung der Harnstoffgruppe in dem Diäthylhydantoin (C. I. 3) gegenüber dem Diäthylacetylharnstoff (C. I. 1) keine Verstärkung, sondern eine Abschwächung der Wirkung hervorruft.

Wie sehr selbst kleine Aenderungen an dem Molekül die pharmakologische Activität beeinflussen können, zeigen am deutlichsten die drei letzten Beispiele. Beim Diaethylmalonsäureureïd (C. III. 16) ist der stickstoffhaltige Ring des Diaethylmalonylharnstoffs (9) durch einfache Wasseranlagerung aufgespalten. Das genügt, um den Körper ganz wirkungslos zu machen. Das Gleiche

gilt für Dipropylmalonylguanidin (17), wo der Sauerstoff des Harnstoffrestes durch die NH-Gruppe ersetzt ist. Dem Diaethylmalonylthioharnstoff (18) endlich giebt die Anwesenheit des Schwefels einen ausgesprochen giftigen Charakter.

Aus der Reihe der zuvor besprochenen Präparate treten durch ihre hypnotische Wirkung Diaethylacetylharnstoff

$$\begin{array}{c}C_2H_5\\C_2H_5\end{array}\!\!>\!\!CH-CO-NH-CO-NH_2$$

Diaethylmalonylharnstoff

$$\begin{array}{c}C_2H_5\\ \\C_2H_5\end{array}\!\!>\!\!C\!<\!\!\begin{array}{c}CO-NH\\ \\CO-NH\end{array}\!\!>\!\!CO$$

Dipropylmalonylharnstoff

$$\begin{array}{c}C_3H_7\\ \\C_3H_7\end{array}\!\!>\!\!C\!<\!\!\begin{array}{c}CO-NH\\ \\CO-NH\end{array}\!\!>\!\!CO$$

so stark in den Vordergrund, dass ihre Prüfung am Menschen angezeigt erschien.

Dabei hat sich nun ergeben, dass der Diaethylacethylharnstoff an hypnotischer Kraft ungefähr dem Sulfonal gleich steht, dass ferner der Dipropylmalonylharnstoff etwa viermal so stark ist, aber nicht selten eine auffallend lange Nachwirkung hat.

In der Mitte zwischen Beiden steht der Diaethylmalonylharnstoff und übertrifft demnach an Intensität der Wirkung auch noch alle bisher gebräuchlichen Schlafmittel. Da die Substanz relativ leicht herzustellen ist und in Bezug auf Geschmack und Löslichkeit Vorzüge besitzt, so scheint sie von den Gliedern der neuen Klasse für den praktischen Gebrauch am meisten geeignet. Mit Rücksicht auf die allzu unbequeme chemische Bezeichnung schlagen wir dafür den Namen „Veronal" vor.

Das Veronal[1]) ist ein schön crystallisirender farbloser Stoff, der bei 191⁰ (Corr.) schmilzt, schwach bitter schmeckt, sich in ungefähr 12 Theilen kochendem Wasser und in 145 Theilen Wasser von 20⁰ löst.

Bei einfacher Schlaflosigkeit genügt in der Regel 0,5 g. Zur Bekämpfung von Agrypnie, die mit stärkeren Erregungszuständen einhergeht, kann man die Dosis bis 1 g steigern. Bei schwächlichen Personen, z. B. Frauen kommt man manchmal schon mit 0,3 g aus. Zur Erzielung von Schlaf sind demnach Dosen von 0,3—0,5—0,75—1 g erforderlich. Mehr als 1 g zu geben, dürfte selten indicirt sein.

Wird das Veronal in Lösung gegeben, so tritt der gewünschte Effect in etwa ½ Stunde ein. Am meisten empfiehlt sich, das gepulverte Mittel in einer Tasse warmen Thees durch

---

[1]) Das Präparat wird von der Firma E. Merck in Darmstadt in den Handel gebracht.

Umrühren zu lösen. Das Präparat wird übrigens auch im festen Zustand von den meisten Personen mit oder ohne Oblate gerne genommen.

Bei den bisherigen klinischen Beobachtungen haben sich unangenehme Nebenwirkungen nicht gezeigt; ob solche bei längerem und aus-

gedehntem Gebrauch auftreten können, muss die weitere therapeutische Untersuchung lehren.

Das Resultat unserer Versuche ist derart, dass wir kein Bedenken tragen, das Veronal den Klinikern und Aerzten zur Prüfung seines therapeutischen Werthes bei Schlaflosigkeit zu übergeben.

72:5

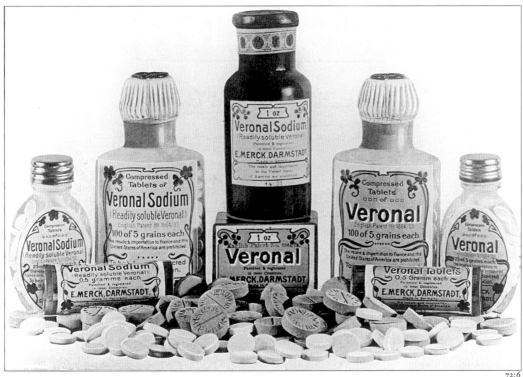

72:6

Advertisements for Veronal from the period 1908–1910.

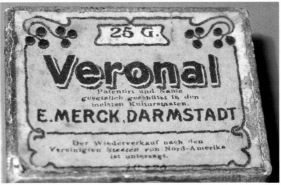

72:7

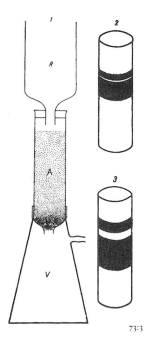

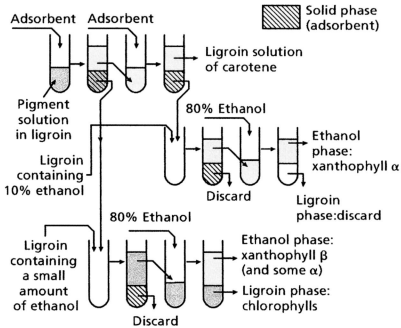

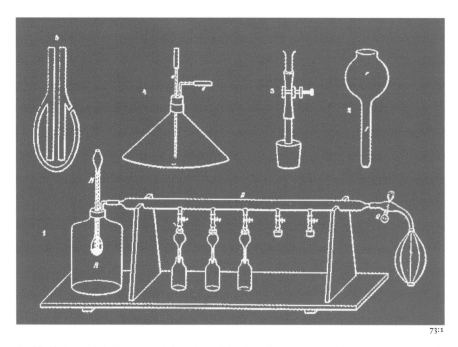

73:1

Mikhail Tswett's (1872–1919) drawing of the first chromatographic arrangement and the first chromatograms (right) and also his pioneering conception of a multicolumn device fitted with a pressure system (above).

73:3

Adsorbent   Adsorbent

Solid phase (adsorbent)

Ligroin solution of carotene

Pigment solution in ligroin

Ligroin containing 10% ethanol

80% Ethanol

Ethanol phase: xanthophyll α

Discard

Ligroin phase:discard

80% Ethanol

Ligroin containing a small amount of ethanol

Ethanol phase: xanthophyll β (and some α)

Discard

Ligroin phase: chlorophylls

73:2

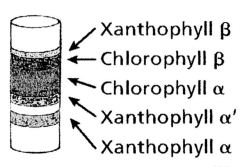

Xanthophyll β
Chlorophyll β
Chlorophyll α
Xanthophyll α'
Xanthophyll α

73:4

A separation scheme (left) reproducing the adsorptive precipitation and extraction method described by Tswett and the chromatographic separation of plant pigments obtained, as depicted by him.

TSWETT was born in 1872 in Asti, Italy, the only child of a previously high-ranking Russian official (73.1)(73.2). He spent his childhood in Lausanne and entered the University of Geneva in 1891 to study mathematics and physics. On completing his thesis on plant physiology in 1896 he went to St Petersburg, where he published the first observations on chlorophyll that later lead him to the invention of chromatography. Unable to find a position there, he moved in 1901 to Warsaw to work as a laboratory assistant at the Plant Anatomy and Physiology Department. In 1915, due to the chaotic conditions of the First World War, he had to leave Warsaw and after short periods in Moscow and Tartu (Estonia) he finally settled as professor at Voronezh University. Two years later in 1919, he died of a progressive heart disease. He was known as a man of principles, vivacious with a gentle humour.

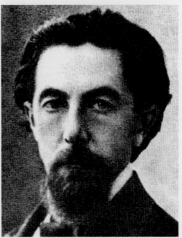

Mikhail Semenovich Tswett   73:5

On a New Category of Adsorption Phenomena and its Application to Biochemical Analysis.

TR VARSHAV OBSHCH ESTESTVOISPYT OTD BIOL 1903; 14:20.

THIS PAPER (73.3) is the first clear account of the ideas behind the chromatographic technique. Tswett uses powder of inulin (a polysaccharide) to filtrate a ligroin (a volatile hydrocarbon mixture) solution of chlorophyll to separate out carotene. He notes the rings of green and yellow appearing along the column and proposes "the possibility of developing a new method of physical separation of different substances dissolved in organic liquids" "based on the ability of the solutes to form physical adsorption compounds with different mineral and organic solids" (73.1)(73.3).

IN PERSPECTIVE:
Runge, who is also noteworthy for his discovery of phenol (73.4), studied synthetic dyestuffs around 1850 and in the process produced radial colour patterns, the forerunners of paper chromatograms (73.5). Goppelsroeder developed "capillary analysis" with paper strips (73.6) and applied the technique to clinical medicine (73.7). He took 507 urea samples from 178 patients with different diseases and carefully described the 1,874 bands appearing on the paper strips. Tswett introduced the term "chromatography" in 1906 (73.8) and summarised his findings on 126 different adsorbents in a major monograph in 1910 (73.9). He clearly envisioned the wide range of applicability of his technique and also made many observations and comments pointing to later developments (73.1). However, Tswett's work was all but forgotten till around 1930, when Kuhn's studies on carotene and vitamins (73.10) awoke interest in chromatography and led to its subsequent rapid development (73.11).

73.1 Sakodynskii KI. *Michael Tswett Life and work*. Carlo Erba Instrumentazione Milano; 1983. See also Sakodynskii KI. *J Chromatogr* 1981; 220:1.

73.2 Ettre LS. *M.S.Tswett and the Invention of Chromatography*. LC-GC Europe 1, September 2003.

73.3 Hesse G, Weil H. *Michael Tswett's first paper on chromatography*. M.Woelm Eschwege; 1954, a translation and reprint of the Russian publication.

73.4 Runge F. Ueber einige Produkte der Steinkohlendestillation. *Ann Phys* 1834; 31:65 and p513 and *Ann Phys* 1834; 32:308. See also #54 Lister page 282 for phenol in antiseptic surgery.

73.5 Runge F. *Zur Farbenchemie*. München; 1850.

73.6 Goppelsroeder F. *Über Capillar-Analyse und ihre verschiedenen Anwendung sowie über das Emporsteigen der Farbstoffe in den Pflanzen*. Wien: Selbstvlg; 1888.

73.7 Goppelsroeder F. *Studien über die anwendung der Capillaranalyse*. I. Bei Harnuntersuchungen. II. Bei vitalen Tinktionsversuchen. Basel: E.Birkhäuser; 1904.

73.8 Tswett MS. Physical chemical studies on chlorophyll adsorption. *Ber Dt Bot Ges*. 1906;24:316 and p384. Translated in Strain HH, Sherma J. *J Chem Ed* 1967; 44:235. See also ref. 73.1.

73.9 Tswett MS. *Chromofilli v Rastitelnom i Zhivotnom Mire* (Chromophylls in the Plant and Animal Kingdom) Warsaw: Karbasnikov Publishers; 1910.

73.10 Kuhn R, Lederer E. Zerlegung des Carotins in seine Komponente. *Dt Chem Ges* 1931; 64B:1349.

73.11 Gehrke CW, Wixom RL, Bayer E. Editors. *Chromatography—a Century of Discovery 1900–2000*. Amsterdam: Elsevier; 2001. See also #84 Martin page 434.

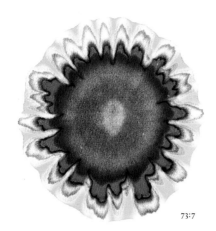

73:7

Friedlieb Runge's (1795–1867) interest in dye chemistry leads him to study reactions on the surface of paper and to prepare the first paper chromatograms. He publishes a book for artists (the title page is shown right) with original colour samples (some of which are shown on the opposite page). The beautiful patterns are obtained through, as he says, "chemical interaction". The ink chromatogram at the top of this page is produced in 1955, following Runge's instructions, as a centennial tribute to his achievements.

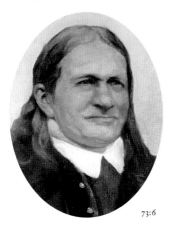

73:6

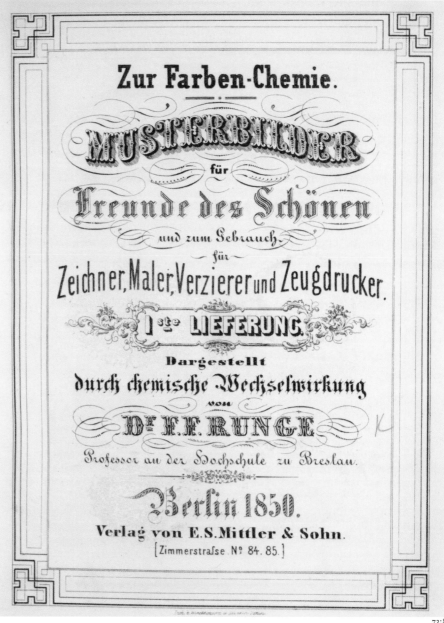

Zur Farben-Chemie.

MUSTERBILDER

für

Freunde des Schönen

und zum Gebrauch

für

Zeichner, Maler, Verzierer und Zeugdrucker.

I^{ste} LIEFERUNG

Dargestellt

durch chemische Wechselwirkung

von

Dr. F.F. RUNGE

Professor an der Hochschule zu Breslau.

Berlin 1850.

Verlag von E.S. Mittler & Sohn.

[Zimmerstraße No. 84. 85.]

73:8

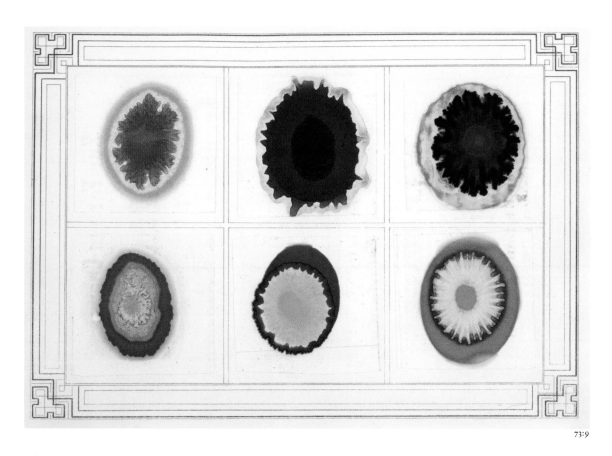

73:9

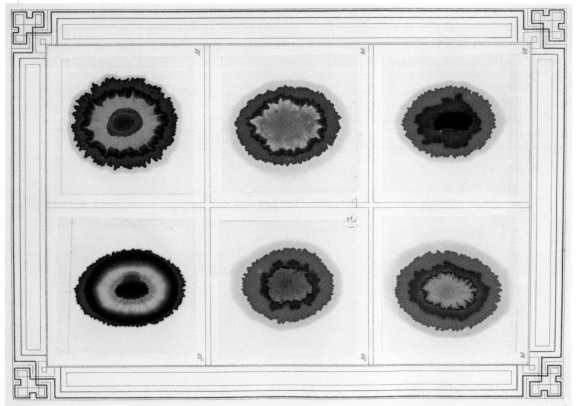

73:10

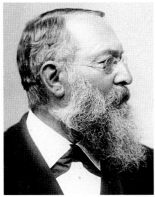
In 1861 Friedrich Goppelsroeder (1837–1919) and Christian Friedrich Schönbein (1799–1868) (see 77:4) discover the usefulness of the colour bands of different chemical reactions in porous media for separation purposes. Four decades later Goppelsroeder uses paper strips ("capillary analysis") to introduce the technique in clinical medicine. The table shows part of his observations of some 1,874 colour bands produced from 507 urea samples taken from 178 patients.

Anzahl der einzelnen mit den 507 Harnproben nebst ihrer auf die jeweilige

TAFEL 16.

Krankheiten.	Anzahl der Patienten	Anzahl der Harnproben	Gesammt-Zahl der beobachteten Zonen.	Farblose Zonen a. Anzahl.	b. In % der gesammtzahl =100%	gelblicher Hochschein bis sehr hell gelblich. a.	b.	gelblich bis lebhaft gelb. a.	b.	bräunliches Gelb bis bräunlich und lebhaft braun. a.	b.
I Kreislauforgane											
1. Aorteninsufficienz	1	3	8	—		2	25%	2	25%	2	25%
2. Degeneratio cordis	1	4	14	5,5	39,3%	6,5	46,4	2	14,3		—
3. Degeneratio cordis senilis	1	4	19	—		7	37	4	21	4	21
4. Vitium cordis	6	27	116	29,5	25,4	40,5	34,9	18	15,5	10	8,6
II Atmungsorgane											
5. Bronchiektasia	1	3	10	1	10	3	30	1,5	15	2	20
6. Bronchitis	7	18	67	22	32,8	28	41,8	13	19,4	3	4,4
7. Bronchitis acuta	5	6	23	8,5	37	4,5	19,6	8	34,8	1	4,3
8. Bronchitis apicis	1	4	11	5	45,4	3	27,3	1	9	1	9
9. Bronchitis chronica	2	6	24	5	20,9	12	50	7	29,1	—	—
10. Bronchitis chronica Emphysema pulmonum	5	11	38	7	18	16	42	7	18,4	4	10,5
11. Bronchitis foetida	1	2	6	2,5	41,7	1,5	25	2	33,3	—	—
12. Bronchitis Gastroptosis	1	3	19	—	—	5	26,3	4	21	3	15,8
13. Carcinoma mammae	1	5	25	9,5	38	3	12	6,5	26	4	16
14. Emphysema	1	1	4	3	75	—	—	1	25	—	—
15. Haemoptoë	1	3	12	4,5	37,5	6,5	54,1	1	8,3	—	—
16. Haemoptoë Phthisis pulmonum	1	1	2	1	50	1	50	—	—	—	—
17. Laryngitis acuta	1	1	4	2	50	2	50	—	—	—	—
18. Phthisis pulmonum	19	71	263	60,5	23	86,5	32,8	60	22,8	30,5	11,6
19. Phthisis pulmonum incipiens	1	1	2	1	50	1	50	—	—	—	—
20. Pleuritis. Bronchitis	2	7	24	2,5	10,4	11,5	48	3	12,5	3	12,5

73:12

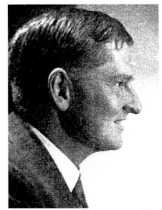

73:13

5. Rosaschein bis lebhaft Rosa.		6. Rötlicher Schein bis Ziegelrot.		7. Gefärbte Criställchen in der Eintauchs-Zone.		8. Farblose glänzende Criställchen in der Eintauchs-Zone.		9. Perlmutterglanz der Eintauchszone.		10. Fettiges Anfühlen der Eintauchszone.		11. Spiessige Gebilde in der obersten Zone.		12. Runde Gebilde in der obersten Zone.	
a.	b.	a.	b.	a.	b.	a.	b.	a.	b.	a.	b.	a.	b.	a.	b.
2	25%	—	—	—	—	—	—	—	—	—	—	—	—	—	—
—	—	—	—	—	—	—	—	—	—	—	—	(3)	(21,4%)	—	—
4	21	—	—	—	—	—	—	—	—	—	—	—	—	—	—
15	13	3	2,6%	(4)	(3,4%)	(1)	(0,8%)	—	—	—	—	(6)	(5,1)	(2)	(1,6%)
2,5	25	—	—	—	—	—	—	—	—	—	—	—	—	(1)	(10)
—	—	—	—	(1)	(1,5)	(1)	(1,5)	(1)	(1,5)	—	—	(2)	(3)	(1)	(1,5)
—	—	1	4,3	(1)	(4,3)	—	—	—	—	—	—	(1)	(4,3)	(1)	(4,3)
1	9	—	—	—	—	—	—	—	—	—	—	—	—	—	—
—	—	—	—	—	—	—	—	—	—	—	—	—	—	—	—
4	10,5	—	—	—	—	(1,5)	(4)	—	—	—	—	(1)	(2,6)	(1)	(2,6)
—	—	—	—	—	—	—	—	—	—	—	—	—	—	—	—
3	15,8	4	21	—	—	—	—	—	—	(1)	(5,2)	—	—	—	—
1	4	1	4	(1)	(4)	—	—	—	—	—	—	(1)	(4)	—	—

73:14

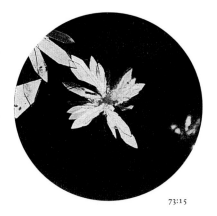

73:15

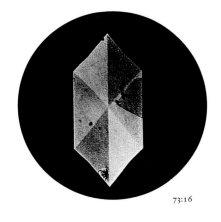

73:16

In 1931 Richard Kuhn (1900–1967) reintroduces chromatography and develops it into a powerful analytical technique. This allows him to isolate and to determine the properties of carotenoids and vitamins. The pictures show alfa-carotine and beta-carotine (right), as first described by Kuhn.

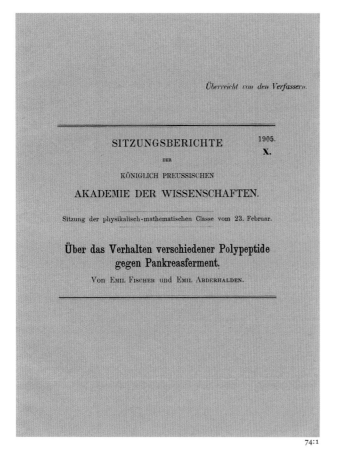

SITZUNGSBERICHTE 1905.
X.

DER

KÖNIGLICH PREUSSISCHEN

AKADEMIE DER WISSENSCHAFTEN.

Sitzung der physikalisch-mathematischen Classe vom 23. Februar.

Über das Verhalten verschiedener Polypeptide gegen Pankreasferment.

Von Emil Fischer und Emil Abderhalden.

74:1

Emil Fischer (1852–1919) and Emil Abderhalden (1877–1950) investigate the properties of polypeptides as compared to those of the pancreatic juice. They find that the substances can have many similar characteristics. The study is made possible by the success of Ivan Pavlov (1849–1936) in obtaining sufficiently pure pancreatic juice from dogs.

Über das Verhalten verschiedener Polypeptide gegen Pankreasferment.

Von Emil Fischer und Emil Abderhalden.

Nach Beobachtungen von E. Fischer und P. Bergell[1] zeigen die künstlichen Dipeptide den Fermenten des Pankreas gegenüber scharfe Unterschiede. Die einen, wie Glycylglycin, werden nicht in nachweisbarer Menge angegriffen, während andere, wie das Glycyl-l-Tyrosin, dadurch eine rasche Spaltung in die Componenten erfahren. Besonders interessant gestaltete sich der Versuch beim racemischen Leucylalanin; denn die Hydrolyse erfolgt hier asymmetrisch, d. h. sie beschränkt sich auf den einen optisch-activen Componenten des Racemkörpers. Die Ausdehnung dieser Untersuchungen auf die complicirteren Polypeptide wurde damals durch die schlechte Beschaffenheit des käuflichen Pankreasfermentes und die dadurch bedingte Schwierigkeit, die Producte der Hydrolyse zu isoliren, verhindert. Durch die Güte des Hrn. Prof. Pawlow in St. Petersburg sind wir inzwischen in den Besitz von reinem Pankreassaft, der von Hunden mittelst einer Pankreasfistel entnommen war, gelangt, und wir haben mit Hülfe dieses überaus wirksamen Fermentes eine ganze Reihe von Polypeptiden prüfen können. Wir fassen die Resultate in folgende kurze Übersicht zusammen:

Hydrolysirbar	Nicht hydrolysirbar
Glycyl-l-Tyrosin	Leucylprolin
Leucyl-l-Tyrosin	Glycylphenylalanin
Dialanylcystin	Glycylglycin
Dileucylcystin	Diglycylglycin
*Alanylleucylglycin	Triglycylglycin
Tetraglycylglycin	
Triglycylglycinester	
(Curtius' Biuretbase)	

[1] Ber. d. D. chem. Ges. 36, 2592 (1903) und 37, 3103 (1904).

74:2

FISCHER was born in 1852 in Euskirchen, the son of a successful businessman. Instead of entering the family business as desired by his father, he started to study at the University of Bonn. After a year he transferred to Strasbourg, where Baeyer (74.1) influenced him to take up chemistry. In 1874 he took his Ph.D. and subsequently during his distinguished career came to hold the chair of chemistry in Erlangen, Würzburg and from 1892 in Berlin. Fischer's work on purines and sugars started in the early 1880s and culminated with the Nobel Prize in Chemistry in 1902. However, by 1899 he had already started his important work on proteins and amino acids. The death of two of his three sons during the First World War left Fischer devastated. Together with a serious illness, this contributed to his death in 1919.

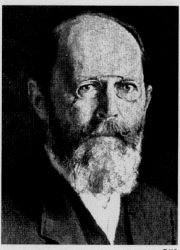

Emil Fischer   74:3

Untersuchungen über Aminosäuren, Polypeptide und Proteine (1899–1906).

BERLIN: SPRINGER; 1906.

IN THIS 770 page book, Fischer collects his results from seven years of research on the structure, synthesis and properties of amino acids, peptides and proteins. In 74 papers, some written in collaboration with Suzuki, Abderhalden and Warburg, he reports on new methods of separating and identifying amino acids and the discovery of new types, the cyclic proline and oxyproline. Fischer further identifies the peptide bond—CONH—and shows that it can link amino acids into longer chains of polypeptides. He studies the relationship between pancreatic juice just obtained by Pavlov (74.2) and the polypeptides (74.3) and finds that some polypeptides can have many characteristics similar to natural proteins.

IN PERSPECTIVE:
Fischer was just concluding his work on sugars and purines (74.4) when in 1899 he turned his attention to the structure of proteins. After publishing the book cited above, Fischer continued his work on proteins and polypeptides for another decade (74.5). In 1907 he obtained a polypeptide with a molecular weight of 1213 and in 1914 he succeeded in synthesising the first nucleic acid (74.6). A few years later he summarised his work on the synthesis of about 100 polypeptides (74.7). Fischer was well aware of the complexity of proteins and predicted that his substances represented only a tiny fraction of the number of possible structures to be found in natural proteins. In 1920, a year after Fischer's death, Staudinger introduced the concept of macromolecules (74.8) and started the research on polymers that would eventually transform the practice of medicine and most other walks of life.

74.1 See ref. 72.1.
74.2 Pavlov IP. *Physiology of Digestion*. Nobel Lecture Stockholm; 1904.
74.3 Fischer E, Abderhalden E. Über das Verhalten verschiedener Polypeptide gegen Pankreasferment. *Sitzb d K Pr Akad Wiss* 1905; I:290.
74.4 Fischer E. *Untersuchungen über Kohlenhydrate und Fermente (1884 –1908)* Berlin: Springer; 1909.
74.5 Hoesch K. Emil Fischer Sein Leben und sein Werk. *Ber Dtsch Chem Ges* 1921:54
74.6 Fischer E. Über phosphorsäureester des Methylglucosides und Theophyllinglucosids. *Sitz d k Pr Akad Wiss* 1914; II:905.
74.7 Fischer E. Isomerie der Polypeptide. *Sitz d k Pr Akad Wiss* 1916; II:990.
74.8 See #78 Staudinger page 400.

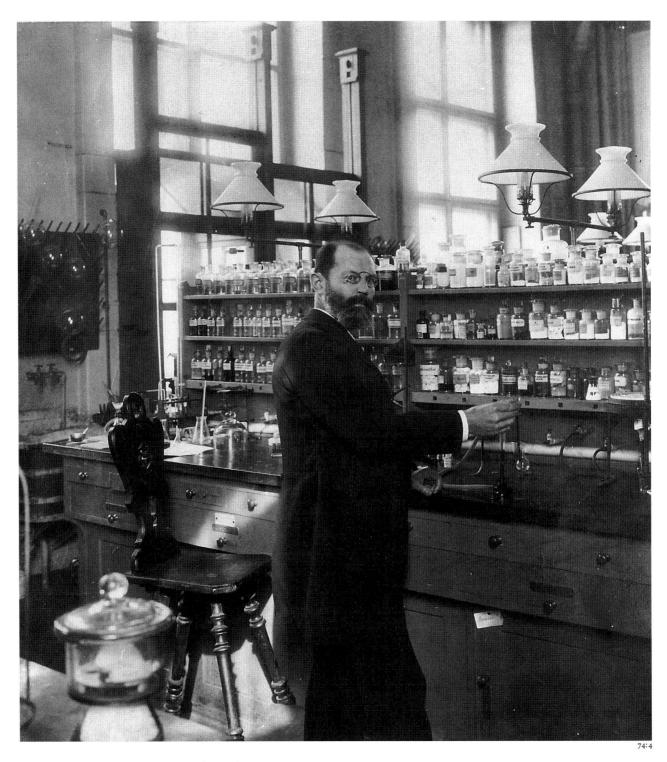

Emil Fischer in his laboratory in Berlin in about 1900.

74:4

BERICHTE
DER DEUTSCHEN
CHEMISCHEN GESELLSCHAFT

VIERUNDFÜNFZIGSTER JAHRGANG
(1921)
SONDERHEFT

EMIL FISCHER

Sein Leben und sein Werk

Im Auftrage
der Deutschen Chemischen Gesellschaft

dargestellt von

KURT HOESCH

BERLIN
EIGENTUM DER DEUTSCHEN CHEMISCHEN GESELLSCHAFT
„VERLAG CHEMIE" G. M. B. H., BERLIN UND LEIPZIG
1921

74:5

Inhaltsverzeichnis.

74:6

74:7

A presentation of Fischer's life and work, published by the German Chemical Society in 1921, shows the extraordinary extent and originality of his research. Many of his findings have been of fundamental importance for subsequent advances in biology and medicine. Under the heading "physiological and medical contributions" (page 240) one finds the landmark paper cited in #72 for its importance in the development of clinical anaesthesiology.

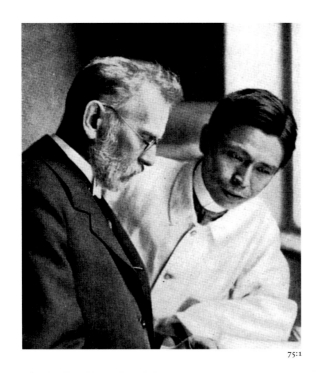

Paul Ehrlich (1854–1915) with his assistant Sachahiro Hata (1873–1938), who joins Ehrlich's research group in 1909 and almost immediately rediscovers a previously studied but rejected substance called "606". After extensive tests (a table summarising typical experimental results appears below) this substance is proven to be an efficient agent against syphilis and other spirochetal and trympanosomal infections. The announcement of the arsenic-based drug (see its formula) to the world under the name Salvarsan in 1910 marks the beginning of the modern era of chemotherapy. The news is first received with considerable scepticism, but soon the demand for the substance can only be met by large scale production at the Höchst Chemical Works.

$$As\!=\!\!=\!\!=\!\!As$$

NH$_2$ — OH   OH — NH$_2$

75:1   75:2

Tabelle XIII. Heilversuch mit Dioxydiamidarsenobenzol.

Maus	Nr. / Gewicht	Kontrolle: 1 / 14	2 / 21	3 / 14	4 / 14	5 / 14	6 / 14	7 / 15	8 / 16	9 / 16	10 / 19
	Infektion: je 0,2 ccm pro Maus von einer Blutverdünnung (Spirillenzahl ½), intraperitoneal.										
I. Anfall 1. Tag	Spirillenzahl. / Dose pro 20 g	$+(\frac{1}{10})$	$+(\frac{1}{10})$	$+(\frac{1}{10})$ 1:1000	+w. 1:1000	+w. 1:1500	+w. 1:1500	$+(\frac{1}{10})$ 1:2000	+w. 1:2000	$+(\frac{1}{5})$ 1:3000	+w. 1:3000
	2. Tag	+(2)	+(2—3)	—	—	—	—	—	—	$+(\frac{1}{2})$	$+(\frac{1}{10})$
	3. Tag (Dose)	+(10)	++	—	—1:1000	—	—1:1500	—	—1:2000	+w.	—1:3000
	4. Tag	—	—	—	—	—	—	—	—		
	5. Tag (Dose)	—	—	—	—	—	—	—1:2000	—1:2000	—1:3000	—1:3000
	6. Tag	—	—	—	—	—	—				
I. Rezidiv	Am Tage	7.	7.	20.	0	14.	0	16.	0	8.	0
	Dauer (Tage)	3	5	2		2		3		1	
	Höchste Spirillenzahl	+	+	+w.		+		+		+w.	
II. Rezidiv	Am Tage	13.	14.	23.		18.		22.		11.	
	Dauer (Tage)	3	5	3		3		2		1	
	Höchste Spirillenzahl	+	+	+		+		+		+s.w.	
III. Rezidiv	Am Tage	19.	21.	27.		24.		30.		15.	
	Dauer (Tage)	1	2	5		1		2		2	
	Höchste Spirillenzahl	+	+w.	+		+s.w.		+		+w.	
IV. Rezidiv	Am Tage	21.	26.	33.		26.		36.		21.	
	Dauer (Tage)	1	3	3		1		2		1	
	Höchste Spirillenzahl	+	+	+w.		+w.		+		+	
V. Rezidiv	Am Tage	27.	32.	64.		35.		47.		29.	
	Dauer (Tage)	1	4	2		1		1		2	
	Höchste Spirillenzahl	+w.	+	+		+w.		+w.		+	
VI. Rezidiv	Am Tage	kein Rezidiv mehr	kein Rezidiv mehr	kein Rezidiv mehr		43.		52.		41.	
	Dauer (Tage)					1		1		1	
	Höchste Spirillenzahl					+s.w.		+w.		+w.	
	Bemerkungen				dauernd frei		dauernd frei	kein Rezidiv mehr	dauernd frei	kein Rezidiv mehr	dauernd frei

75:3

EHRLICH was born in 1854 in Strehlen (now in Poland), the son of an innkeeper. He was educated in Breslau and later at the Universities of Strasbourg, Freiburg im Breisgau and Leipzig, where he received his doctorate in 1878. Ehrlich was appointed by Koch (75.1) as director of the new Institute of Infectious Diseases in Berlin in 1890. From 1899 he directed the Institute of Experimental Therapy in Frankfurt and also began his work on chemotherapy (75.2). Ehrlich became an honorary member of some 80 foreign academies and received the Nobel Prize in Medicine in 1908 for his work on immunity (75.3). He was a kind, modest and somewhat absent-minded person (75.4). An extremely heavy workload all his life, incessant cigar smoking and irregular eating habits all contributed to the stroke that ended his life in 1915.

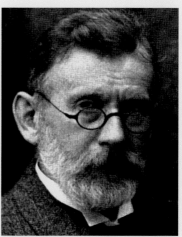

Paul Ehrlich   75:4

Die experimentelle Chemotherapie der Spirillosen (Syphilis, Rückfalls- fieber, Hühnerspirillose, Frambösie).

BERLIN: SPRINGER J; 1910.

EHRLICH AND his assistant Hata report the work leading them to the substance "606" (hydrochloride of dioxy-diamino-arseno-benzene) which, under the name "Salvarsan", was found to be highly effective against syphilis and other spirochetal and trympanosomal infections. Ehrich had found the correct formula of arsanilic acid and was then able to synthesise and test new compounds derived from it against these infections. Due to the oversight of an assistant, "Salvarsan" was set aside as being ineffective in 1907, but the careful work of Hata revealed the true potential of the substance.

IN PERSPECTIVE:
Although Paracelsus back in 1553 recommended mercury compounds for the treatment of syphilis (75.2), Ehrlich's work, using the novel concept of highly specific drug action (75.3), was accepted only after much opposition (75.4). Ehrlich collaborated with the chemical industry to produce the substances that he then tested in his exhaustive systematic trials. By contrast, Hoffmann at F Bayer & Co discovered "aspirin" (acetyl salicylic acid) by chance (75.5) and similarly Cade just happened to notice the therapeutic effect of lithium in manic patients (75.6). Believing that he could isolate a poison in the urine of psychiatrically ill patients he hit upon the remarkable effects of lithium urate. In another major drug discovery, Kuhn demonstrated in 1957 that a tricyclic compound (imipramine) could act as an antidepressant by blocking a neurotransmitter (serotonin) in the brain (75.7). Modern versions of neurotransmitter blockers such as fluoxetine (Prozac) (75.8) are widely used today. Early efforts to treat schizophrenia relied on barbiturates (75.9)(75.10) and it was experimentation with hypnotics in 1952 that led to the chance discovery of the first antipsychotic drug, chlorpromazine (75.10)(75.11).

75.1 See #61 Koch page 316.
75.2 Paracelsus: *Von der frantzösischen Kranckheit drey Bücher*. Frankfurt a.M.;1553. See also #3 Paracelsus page 32.
75.3 Himmelweit F. editor. *The Collected Papers of Paul Ehrlich* 3 vols. London: Pergamon Press; 1956–1960.
75.4 Marquardt M. *Paul Ehrlich*. London: William Heinemann Medical books Ltd; 1949.
75.5 Eichengrun A. 50 Jahre Aspirin. *Pharmazie* 1949; 4:582.
75.6 Cade J. Lithium salts in the treatment of psychotic excitement. *Med J Austral* 1949; 36:349.
75.7 Kuhn R. Über die behandlung depressiver zustande mit enine miminodiben zylderivat (G22355) *Schweiz Med Wochenschn* 1957; 87:1135.
75.8 Wong DT, Bymaster FP, Engleman EA. Prozac (Fluoxetine Lilly 110140) the first selective serotonine uptake inhibitor and an antidepressant drug: twenty years since its first publication. *Life Sciences* 1995; 57:411.
75.9 Kläsi J. Ueber die therapeutische anwendung der "dauernarkose" mittels somnifens bei schizophrenen *Zeitsch Gesamt. Neurol Psych* 1922; 74:557.
75.10 Lehmann HE, Ban TA. The History of Psychopharmacology of Schizophrenia. *Can J Psych* 1997; 42:152.
75.11 Delay J, Deniker P, Harl JM. Traitment des états d'excitation et d'agitation par une méthode médicamenteuse derivée de l'hibernothérapie (part 2) *Ann Med-psychol* 1952; 110:267.

Entwicklung von Schankern.

a

b

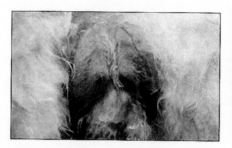

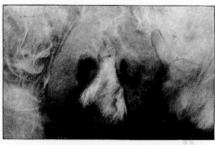

3 Wochen nach Infektion.
Kleine Knötchenbildung unter der Haut.

6 Wochen nach Infektion.
Deutliche Bildung von kleinen Schankern.

c

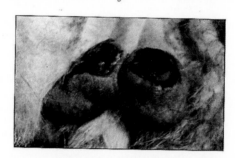

11 Wochen nach Infektion.
Vollständig ausgebildeter Schanker (Kontrolle Nr. IV).

Behandeltes Kaninchen Nr. VI.

d

e

Striking demonstrations of the result of Salvarsan treatment. Right, chancre due to a syphilitic infection in the rabbit and on the opposite page a spirill infection in the hen.

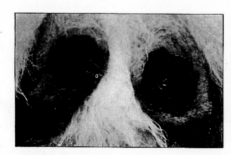

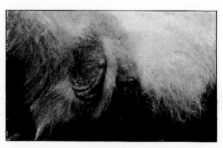

Behandlungstag.

18 Tage später.

75:5

388

a

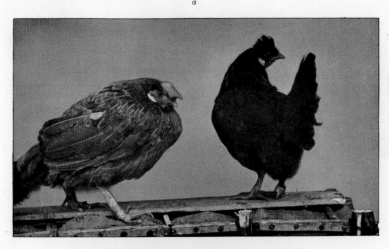

4 Tage nach Infektion.

Unbehandelt.   Behandelt 2 Tage nach Infektion.

b   *c*

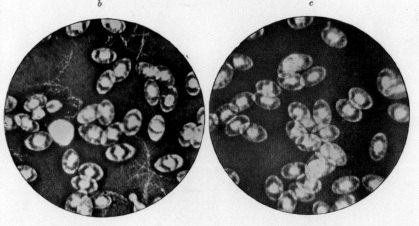

Kontrolle mit Spirillen.   Behandeltes Huhn.
                                      Spirillenfrei!

75:6

Below left, the combined fever graph of thirty cases of relapsing fever, to be compared with the combined fever graph of twenty cases of relapsing fever treated after day five with intravenous Salvarsan (right).

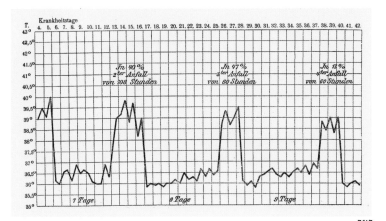

75:7

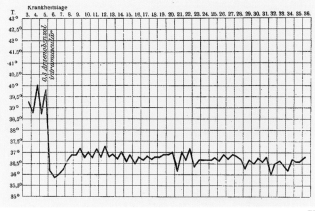

75:8

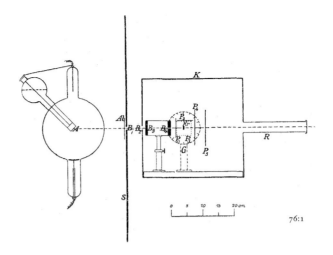

Max von Laue's (1879–1960) experimental setup when he observes the first X-ray diffraction pattern. Knowing the lattice constant of the copper sulphate crystal studied, Laue calculates the wavelength of the X-rays from the diffraction image (shown right) using a method well established in optical diffraction theory. The result agrees with other less precise earlier determinations of the wavelength of the X-rays.

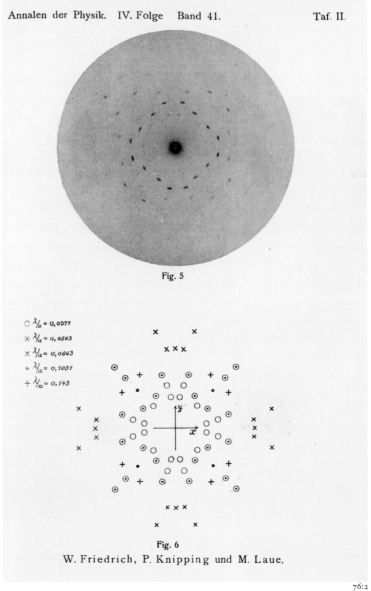

Annalen der Physik. IV. Folge Band 41. Taf. II.

Fig. 5

$\lambda/\alpha = 0,0377$
$\lambda/\alpha = 0,0563$
$\lambda/\alpha = 0,0663$
$\lambda/\alpha = 0,1051$
$\lambda/\alpha = 0,143$

Fig. 6

W. Friedrich, P. Knipping und M. Laue.

Laue was born in Pfaffendorf in 1879, the son of a military administrator. He began studying mathematics, physics and chemistry at the University of Strasbourg in 1898 and obtained his doctorate in 1903 in Berlin. In 1909 he moved to the theoretical physics department of Sommerfeld (76.1) in Munich where he made the discovery of X-ray diffraction, which was rewarded with the Nobel Prize in Physics in 1914. Laue showed great courage and kept his integrity during the Nazi years. After the Second World War he was director of the Fritz Haber Institute for Physical Chemistry and his impeccable character and sound judgement allowed him to exert great influence on the postwar rebuilding of German science. At heart a religious man, he loved outdoor activities and high speeds, but never had an accident until the fatal collision that took his life a few month after his retirement in 1959.

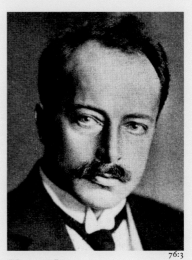

Max von Laue   76:3

Interferenzerscheinungen bei Röntgenstrahlen. Theoretischer Teil, Experimenteller Teil.

Ann d Phys Leipzig: J. A. Barth; 1913; 41:971.

Laue (writing the theoretical part) and his assistants Knipping and Friedrich (describing the experiments) report on the observation of diffraction patterns registered on photographic plates when copper sulphate crystals are exposed to X-rays. Laue notes the similarity between the patterns observed and those seen in optical diffraction according to Fraunhofer (76.2). Also he finds that the wavelength of the X-rays calculated from the lattice constant is in rough agreement with values expected from other work just reported (76.1).

IN PERSPECTIVE:
Laue's experiments were based on his insight, based on density considerations, that crystal lattices (76.3), had dimensions of the order 10^{-8} cm, while the wavelength of X-rays was around 10^{-8}–10^{-9} cm (76.1). He soon demonstrated that the diffraction pattern could be used to determine lattice dimensions of zinc sulphide accurately (76.4). Quantitative X-ray crystallography was immediately taken up by father and son W.H. Bragg and W.L. Bragg (76.5)(76.6). Starting with an NaCl crystal, the analysis was soon reduced to a standard procedure and later applied to a variety of complex substances (76.7). In combination with computerised Fourier analysis (76.8), the technique eventually led to the structural determination of many important biological molecules such as DNA (Watson, Crick, Wilkins 1953), vitamin B-12 (Hodgkin 1955), insulin (Sanger 1955), haemoglobin and myoglobin (Perutz, Kendrew 1960) (76.9). It also contributed greatly to advances in other fields of importance in medicine such as polymer science and microelectronics. Since 1971 synchrotron radiation, a powerful X-ray source first observed in 1947, has also been available for the studies of biological systems (76.10).

76.1 Sommerfeld A. Über der Beugung der Röntgenstrahlen. *Ann d Phys* 1912; 38:473.
76.2 Born M, Wolf E. *Principles of Optics.* Chapt. 8 and Chapt. 11. 7th ed. Cambridge: Cambridge University Press; 1999.
76.3 Bravais A. Mémoire sur les systèmes formés par des points distribué régulièrement sur un plan ou dans l'espace. *J École Pol* 1850; 19:1.
76.4 Laue M. Eine quantitative Prüfung der Theorie für die Interferenzerscheinungen bei Röntgenstrahlen. *Ann d Phys* 1913; 41:989.
76.5 Bragg WH. X-rays and Crystals. *Nature* 1913; 90:360 and p572.
76.6 Bragg WH, Bragg WL. *X rays and crystal structure.* G Bell and Sons; 1915.
76.7 Bragg WL. *X-ray Crystallograpy. Readings from Scientific American. Lasers and Light.* San Francisco: W. H. Freeman and Co; 1969. p161.
76.8 See # 32 Fourier page 176 and ref.32.8.
76.9 The birth of molecular biology. *New Scientist.* Special issue 1987;114(No 1561):38.
76.10 Rosenbaum G, Homles KC, Witz J. Synchroton radiation as a source for x-ray diffraction. *Nature* 1971; 230:434.

Father William Henry Bragg (1862–1942) and his son William Lawrence Bragg (1890–1971) are shown together in the photograph below. Soon after Laue's report on X-ray diffraction, they develop an X-ray spectrometer, shown on the right, and eventually turn the X-ray diffraction technique into a routine method for structural analysis of solids.

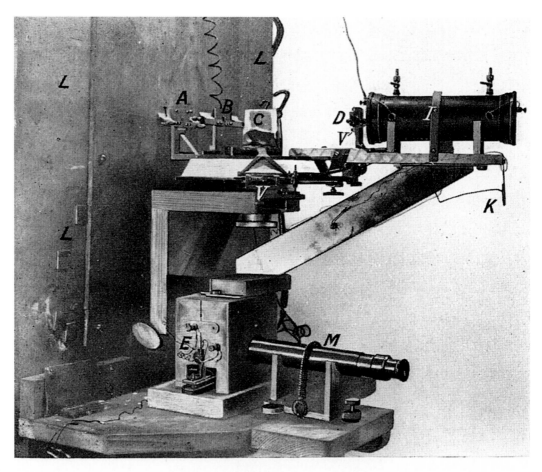

X-RAY SPECTROMETER.

LLL,	Lead box.	*V*,	Vernier of crystal table.
A, B, D,	Slits.	*V'*,	Vernier of ionisation chamber.
C,	Crystal.	*K*,	Earthing key.
I,	Ionisation chamber.	*E*,	Electroscope.
	M,	Microscope.	

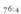

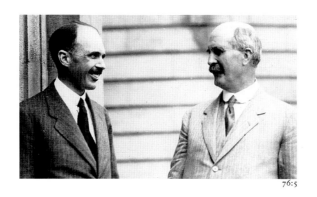

392

CHAPTER VII.

THE ANALYSIS OF CRYSTAL STRUCTURE. PT. I.

THERE are three types of faces which are more frequently developed on cubic crystals than any others. If a crystal grows regularly with faces of one of these types, it becomes a cube, a rhombic dodecahedron or an octahedron, according as to whether the faces have indices of the form {100} {110} or {111}. Faces with more complicated indices are comparatively uncommon on cubic crystals, and in making an examination of the crystal with the X-ray spectrometer, these simple faces are naturally the first to be investigated.

Fig. 26 shows the results of the examination of two cubic crystals. These are potassium and sodium chloride, whose very strong resemblance to each other suggests that the crystals are built up in the same way. They are two examples of a series of cubic crystals believed to be isomorphous, which have the composition RX, R being one of the alkaline metals lithium, sodium, potassium, rubidium, caesium, and X one of the haloids fluorine, chloride, bromine and iodine.

It is clear that the spectra given by corresponding

faces of the two crystals strongly resemble each other.

Moreover, we can in the following way institute a quantitative and a closer comparison, which brings out the identity of the structure.

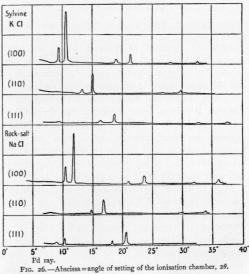

FIG. 26.—Abscissa=angle of setting of the ionisation chamber, 2θ.

For each face the wave length and the spacing of the crystal planes parallel to that face are connected by the equation

$$n\lambda = 2d \sin \theta.$$

76:6

Father and son Bragg first use the X-ray spectrometer to study the structure of two simple cubic crystals, sodium chloride and potassium chloride. They establish the relation between the distance of the lattice planes and the wavelength of the X-ray, known as the Bragg criterion (appearing at the bottom of the right-hand page reproduced above). The many lines in the powder X-ray patterns on the photographic strips correspond to the Bragg criteria for the different lattice planes of the two crystals.

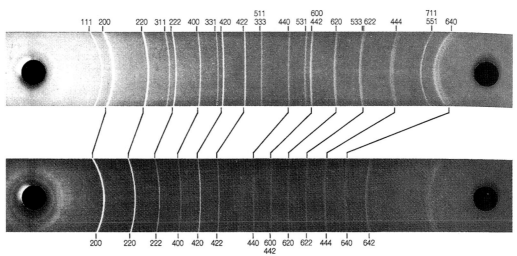

76:7

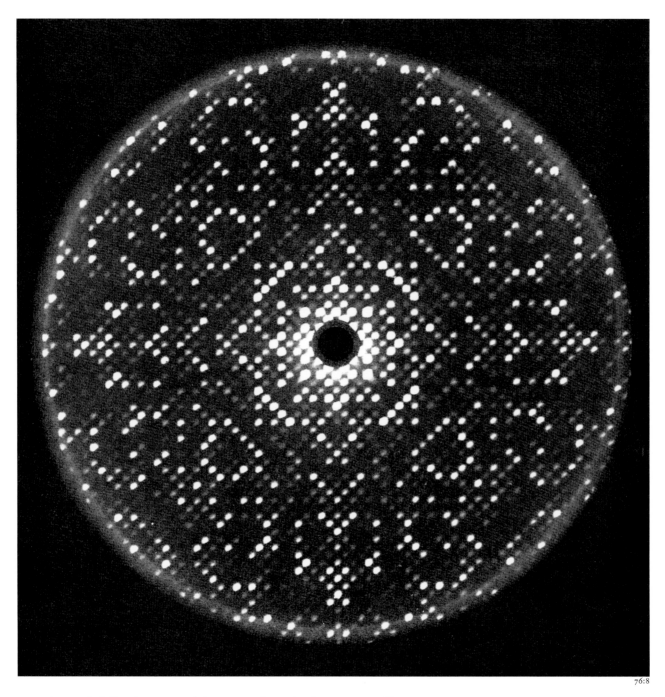

76:8

In 1965 David Phillips (1924–1999) determines the molecular structure of lysozym, the first enzyme to be analysed using X-ray diffraction. Patterns such as the one shown above reveal that the structure is made up of 1,950 atoms and has a size of about 40 Å.

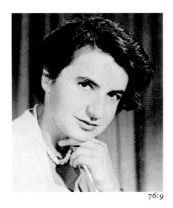

76:9

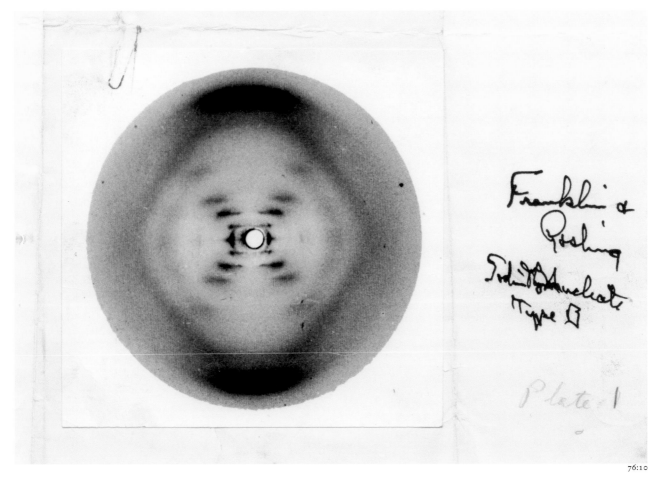

*Franklin &
Gosling
Sodium Thymonucleate
Type B*

Plate 1

76:10

1952 sees Rosalind Franklin (1920–1958),
working with Raymond Gosling, obtain the famous X-ray diffraction image of B-form DNA
which a year later plays a key role in the determination of the structure of the molecule. The
diffractogram shown here was sent to Linus
Pauling (1901–1994), at the time the leading
expert on complex molecular structures. Pauling, whose note appears on the right, was also
busy working on and close to solving the DNA
structure problem (see #88).

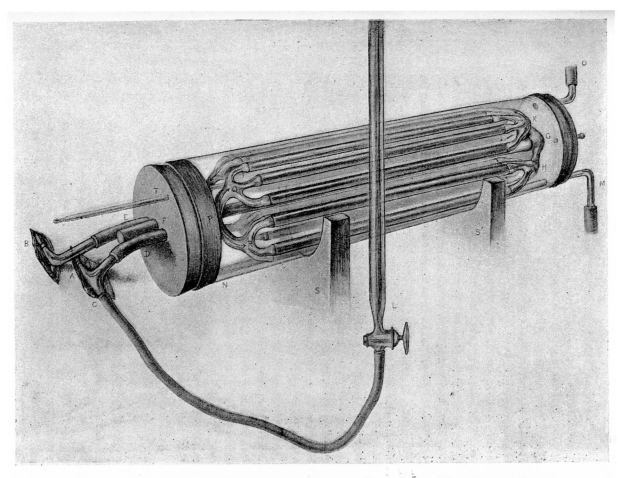

FIG. 1 PERSPECTIVE VIEW OF VIVIDIFFUSION APPARATUS; EARLIER FORM WITH SIXTEEN TUBES

A, arterial cannula; *B*, venous cannula; *C*, side tube for introduction of hirudin; *D*, inflow tube; *E*, outlet tube; *F, G*, supporting rod attached at *H* and *K* to branched U-tubes; *L*, burette for hirudin; *M, N*, tube for filling and emptying liquid in outer jacket; *O*, air outlet; *P*, dichotomous branching point of inflow tube; *Q* and *R*, quadruple branching points of same; *S, S′*, wooden supports; *T*, thermometer. At each of the points *H* and *K* the blood is collected from four tubes into one, bending around to the back, and there redividing into four return flow tubes. Arrows show the direction of flow.

77:1

The dialyser ("vividifusion") apparatus of John Abel (1857–1938). The walls of the sixteen parallel tubes are made of 0.05–0.1 mm thick collodion membranes and hirudin extracted from leaches is used as an anticoagulant. In animal experiments Abel finds that the clearance of salicylic acid following an intravenous injection of sodium salicylate is comparable to that of normal kidneys.

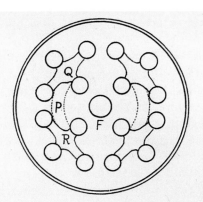

FIG. 2. CROSS SECTION OF APPARATUS SHOWN IN FIGURE 1

F, central supporting rod; *P*, point of dichotomous branching of system of blood tubes; *Q* and *R*, quadruple branch points. The sixteen small circles show the arrangement of the celloidin tubes; the blood flows up left-hand eight and down in the remainder.

77:2

ABEL was born on a farm near Cleveland Ohio in 1857. He graduated with a Ph.D. from the University of Michigan in 1883 before going to Germany for further education. After studies in Leipzig, Würzburg and Heidelberg, he received his M.D. from the University of Strasbourg in 1888. He returned to America and became a lecturer in materia medica and pharmacology at the University of Michigan. In 1893 he was appointed professor of pharmacology at the John Hopkins University, where he remained till his retirement in 1932. In his manners and ascetic habits of research, Abel emulated German professors. His emphasis on the importance of chemistry in medicine (77.1) significantly influenced the development of biochemistry and pharmacology in the United States.

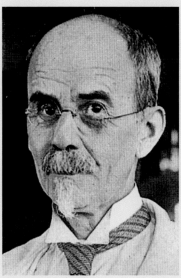

John Jacob Abel 77:3

On the Removal of diffusible Substances from the circulating Blood of living Animals by Dialysis.

J PHARM EXP THERAP 1914; 5(3): 275.

TOGETHER WITH collaborators Rowntree and Turner, Abel describes his "vividifusion" apparatus. This dialysis apparatus is made up of "celloidin" (or collodion (77.2)) tubes assembled in parallel. He explains how to prepare tubes that are about 40 cm long and 8 mm in diameter and present a 0.05-0.1 mm thick diffusion barrier. Abel uses hirudin (77.3) as an anticoagulant and when arterial blood is shunted through a device with 32 tubes, the removal of salicylic acid following an intravenous injection of sodium salicylate is reported to be comparable to the normal excretion of the kidneys. Using a saline solution of sufficiently low salt content, no detrimental effects of the treatment are observed even when dialysing for about ten hours.

IN PERSPECTIVE:
In 1846 Schönbein produced cellulose nitrate by treating paper with nitric and sulphuric acids (77.2). He called this substance guncotton (Schiesswolle), but it was also commonly called pyroxylin. Collodion (or celloidin) was a solution of pyroxylin in alcohol and ether. Archer introduced collodion in 1851 to improve on the first photographic process (77.4). It was used by Fick to produce a barrier for the diffusion process (77.5) and also became one of the first materials of the plastics industry (77.6). Abel prepared hirudin extract from leeches (hirudo medicinalis) that excrete the substance to prevent blood clotting. Although hirudin had been used in connection with blood-letting since antiquity, it was first characterised biochemically in 1955 (77.3). It is still an interesting anti-thrombotic substance of significant use and future potential (77.7). Based on Abel's work, Haas performed the first human haemodialysis in 1924 (77.8) and was also the first to introduce heparin into the procedure (77.9)(77.10). Two decades later Kolff built a large surface area device that quickly gained clinical acceptance (77.11).

77.1 Abel JJ. *Chemistry in relation to biology & medicine with especial reference to insulin & other hormones*. The Willard Gibbs Lecture 1927. Baltimore; 1939.

77.2 Partington JR. *A History of Chemistry* Vol. IV Mansfield Centre: Martino fine books; 1999. p195.

77.3 Markwart F. Untersuchungen über Hirudin. *Naturwissenschaften* 1955; 42:537.

77.4 See #38 Daguerre page 202 and ref 38.4 p 197.

77.5 See ref. 46.8 and #63 Van't Hoff page 324.

77.6 Hyatt JW, Hyatt IS. *Improvement in Treating and Moulding Pyroxyline*. US Patent 105,338 1870. See also #80 Carothers page 410.

77.7 Sohn JH, et al. Current status of the anticoagulant hirudin: its biotechnological production and clinical practice. *Appl. Microb. Biotech.* 2001; 57:606.

77.8 Haas G. Versuche der Blutauswaschung am Lebenden mit Hilfe der Dialyse. *Klin. Wochenschr.* 1925; 4(1): 13.

77.9 Haas G. Über Blutauswaschung. *Klin Wochenschr.* 1928; 7(29):1356.

77.10 Paskalev DN. Georg Haas (1886–1971) The forgotten hemodialysis pioneer. *Dialysis & Transplantation.* 2001; 30(12):828.

77.11 See #86 Kolff page 444.

IX. SUMMARY

1. A method has been devised by which diffusible constituents may be removed from the blood of a living animal, which does not involve any procedure prejudicial to life.

2. Two animals have made rapid and complete recovery after being subjected to the procedure for two and three hours respectively.

3. The method has been shown to be available for collecting from the blood, under the ordinary conditions of physiological experimentation, substances present only in small amount at one time.

4. Several types of apparatus have been constructed adapted to various purposes, and full details as to methods of construction are given.

5. Experience has been accumulated on the use of hirudin, and the procedure adopted for the economical preparation of solutions of this active principle from leech heads is given in detail.

6. As an organ of elimination of abnormal substances (e.g., poisons), quantitative results obtained with salicylic acid show that the apparatus in its present form compares not unfavorably with the kidney. The direction of improvement is indicated and experiments in this direction are in progress.

7. Data as to the effect of the procedure on blood pressure are given. It is shown that general oedema in striking degree may result from neglect of certain precautions.

8. Material has been collected in large quantity for the study of the non-proteid amino-bodies present in the blood. The chemical separation of these bodies is in progress and only preliminary results are here given.

9. Directions in which the method may be utilized, both for the study of problems in physiological chemistry, and as a promising therapeutic agent, have been indicated.

77:5

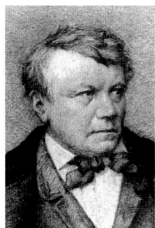

77:4

The conclusions of the dialyser experiments performed by Abel in 1913.

Christian Friedrich Schönbein (1799–1868) invents cellulose nitrate (also called guncotton or pyroxylin) and collodion in 1846. Collodion, or as Abel calls it celloidin, is a solution of pyroxylin in alcohol and ether. The usefulness of a thin film of this material as a diffusion barrier is first recognised by Adolf Fick (see #46).

Georg Haas (1886–1971) pioneers human haemodialysis in 1924 and also introduces heparin to the procedure in 1928. The drawing shows the principle of his "blood-wash" apparatus, where blood passes collodion tubes (in eight parallel cylinders) in contact with fluid from exchangeable glass vessels. The efficiency of the system is low and the procedure takes many hours. The picture below shows Haas sitting at the bedside of one of his four cases in 1926, while an assistant observes the blood flow through the system.

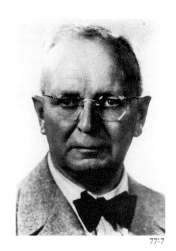

77:7

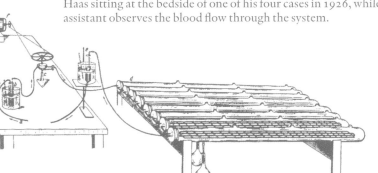

77:6

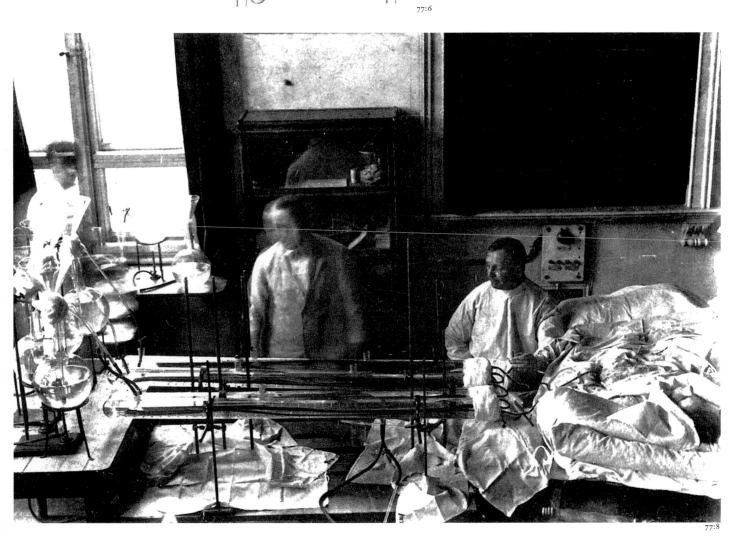

77:8

125. H. Staudinger: Über Polymerisation.

[Mitteilung aus dem Chem. Institut der Eidgen. Techn. Hochschule, Zürich.]

(Eingegangen am 13. März 1920.)

Vor einiger Zeit hat G. Schroeter[1]) interessante Ansichten über die Zusammensetzung von Polymerisationsprodukten, speziell über die Konstitution der polymeren Ketene veröffentlicht. Danach sollen diese Verbindungen Molekülverbindungen darstellen und sollen keine Cyclobutan-Derivate sein, wie früher angenommen wurde[2]); denn diese polymeren Ketene unterscheiden sich nach den Schroeterschen Untersuchungen in wesentlichen Punkten von Cyclobutan-Derivaten, die durch Synthese aus Aceton-dicarbonester-Derivaten zugänglich sind.

Die gleichen Ansichten über die Zusammensetzung von Polymerisationsprodukten hat schon im Jahre 1909 H. Hildebrand in einer im Thieleschen Laboratorium ausgeführten Dissertation ausgesprochen[3]), anschließend an eine Untersuchung über die Polymerisation des *asymm.* Diphenyl-äthylens. Das dimolekulare Polymerisationsprodukt soll nicht das Tetraphenyl-cyclobutan darstellen, sondern es soll eine Molekülverbindung sein, bei der Partialvalenzen den Zusammenhalt der ungesättigten Moleküle herbeiführen:

$$2\,(C_6H_5)_2\,C:CH_2$$

$$\rightarrow \quad \begin{array}{c} (C_6H_5)_2\,C\!-\!-\!CH_2 \\ \vdots \qquad \vdots \\ CH_2.\,C(C_6H_5)_2 \end{array} \quad \text{und nicht} \quad \begin{array}{c} (C_6H_5)_2\,C\!-\!-\!CH_2 \\ | \qquad | \\ CH_2.\,C(C_6H_5)_2 \end{array}$$

Solche Annahmen sind heute in der organischen Chemie sehr verlockend, nachdem eine große Anzahl gut charakterisierter Verbindungen, z. B. die Chinhydrone, nach den Untersuchungen von Pfeiffer[4]) als Molekülverbindungen, die durch Nebenvalenzen zusammengehalten werden, aufgefaßt werden. Und doch glaube ich, daß nach dem vorliegenden Beobachtungsmaterial solche Annahmen zur Erklärung des Entstehens der Polymerisationsprodukte nicht gemacht zu werden brauchen; vielmehr können die verschiedenartigsten Polymerisationsprodukte, wie ich im Folgenden zeigen möchte, durch normale Valenzformeln eine genügende Erklärung finden;

---

[1]) B. **49**, 2697 [1916].

[2]) Vergl. H. Staudinger, Die Ketene, Verlag F. Enke, Stuttgart 1912, 46.

[3]) H. Hildebrand, Über die Polymerisation des *asymm.* Diphenyläthylens, Dissert., Straßburg 1909.

[4]) A. **412**, 253 [1917]; **404**, 1 [1914].

78:1

The first page of Hermann Staudinger's (1881–1965) landmark paper on polymerisation, where he argues that molecules are bound together with covalent binding and do not merely, as previously assumed, form aggregates. He declares: "I do believe that the available observational material shows that such assumptions do not need to be made in order to explain the formation of polymerisation products; what is more, as I would like to show later, polymerisation products of the most varied types can be satisfactorily explained using normal valency formulae."

STAUDINGER was born in Worms in 1881. Working on his degree in chemistry in Strasbourg, he made his first major discovery (of ketenes) in 1907. This led to his appointment the same year as associate professor at the Technische Hochschule in Karlsruhe. In 1912 he became professor at the ETH in Zürich, where he did most of his pioneering work on macromolecular chemistry. From 1926 to his retirement in 1950 he was professor at the University of Freiburg in Breisgau. Staudinger clearly envisaged back in the 1930s the role of macromolecules in the function of life (78.1) It was therefore a fitting coincidence that the year 1953, when his work (with a bibliography of 644 entries) was recognised with the Nobel Prize in Chemistry, also marks the birth of molecular biology (78.2).

Über Polymerisation.

BERICHTE D DEUTSCH CHEM GESELLSCHAFT 1920; 53:1073.

STAUDINGER ARGUES that polymerisation of organic molecules results in long chains with the molecules bound together by a "primary", rather strong covalent binding. By considering various chain structures and their formation, he shows that there is no need to consider the alternative model proposed, that the molecules are bound only with "secondary" weak forces forming essentially only an aggregate.

IN PERSPECTIVE:
Staudinger's polymerisation theory and his notion of the macromolecule, which he introduced while working on synthetic rubbers (polyisoprene) (78.3), was confirmed when in 1926 the ultracentrifuge technique of Svedberg (78.4) demonstrated that many polymers and proteins (e.g. oxyhaemoglobin) had a much large molecular weight than expected (78.5). These findings and X-ray studies of the structure of natural materials (78.6) led to the acceptance of Staudinger's ideas and to many new plastics, all introduced during the 1930s (78.7). Also, although Goodyear had discovered the process of vulcanisation of rubber already in 1839, it now became possible to develop useful synthetic rubber materials such as the "Buna" types, which were produced on an industrial scale by copolymerisation of butadiene and styrene. Berzelius investigated silicon back in the 1820s and Ladenburg synthesised the first organic derivatives in the 1860s. From 1900 and for four decades Kipping made major contributions to silicon chemistry (78.8). Hyde's work on organosilicon polymers at Corning Glass Works (78.9) in the late 1930s initiated industrial research also at Dow Chemical and General Electric (GE) (78.10). By 1946 both GE and Dow Corning had facilities for the industrial production of silicones. Nowadays silicon rubber is an important component in many medical devices such as catheters, tubings, sealings and implants (78.11) (78.12).

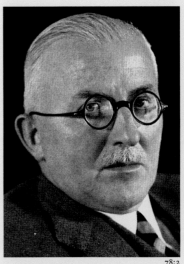

Hermann Staudinger
78:2

78.1 StaudingerH. Ueber die Makromolekulare Chemie. *Angew Chem.* 1936; 49:801.

78.2 See #88 Watson-Crick page 456.

78.3 Staudinger H, Fritschi J. Über Isopren und Kautschuks. 5.Mitt.: Über die Hydrierung des Kautschuks und über seine Konstitution. *Helv chim Acta* 1922; 5:285.

78.4 Svedberg T, Rinde H. The Ultra-Centrifuge, a new instrument for the determination of the size particle in amicroscopic colloids. *J Am Chem Soc* 1924; 46:2677.

78.5 Svedberg T, Fåhraeus R. A New Method for the Determination of the Molecular Weight of the Proteins. *J Am Chem Soc* 1926; 48:430.

78.6 Herzog RO, Jancke W, Polanyi M. Röntgen spectrographische Beobachtungen an Zellulose. *Z Phys* 1920; 3:343. and M. Polanyi: Das Röntgen-Faserdiagramm. *Z Phys* 1921; 7:149.

78.7 *Landmarks of the plastics industry 1862–1962* ICI Plastics Division 1962 and #80 Carothers page 410.

78.8 Kipping FS. Organic derivatives of silicon. *Proc Roy Soc A* 1937; 159:139 and ref. 78.10 chapt. 4.

78.9 Hyde JF, DeLong RC. Condensation Products of the Organo-silane Diols. *J Am Chem Soc* 1941; 63(5):1194.

78.10 Rochow EG. *An introduction to the chemistry of the silicones.* New York: J Wiley & Sons, Inc.; 1946.

78.11 Rochow EG. *Silicon and Silicones.* New York: Springer-Verlag; 1987.

78.12 Lane TH, Burns SA. Silica, silicon and silicones … unraveling the mystery, in: *Immunology of Silicones Current Topics in Microbiology and Immunology.* Potter M, Rose NR. editors. Berlin: Springer-Verlag; 1996. p210.

Staudinger applies his ideas about polymerisation to better understand the structure of cellulose. He investigates polyoxymethylene and finds it to be a simple model of cellulose. The photograph right illustrates the fibre-like appearance of the polymer. The X-ray diffraction pattern and the structure deduced from it are also shown.

The equipment and the reaction used by Staudinger to produce the synthetic rubber isoprene. His ideas about macromolecule chemistry grew out of his studies of natural and synthetic rubbers.

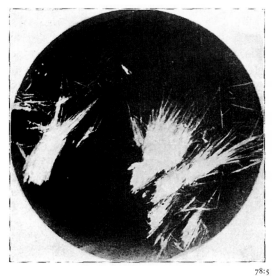

78:5

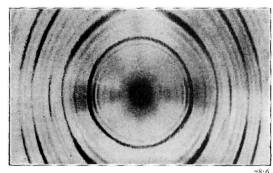

78:6

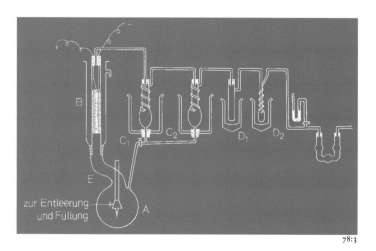

78:3

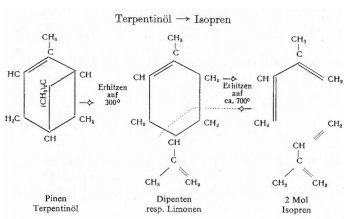

Terpentinöl → Isopren

Pinen
Terpentinöl

Dipenten
resp. Limonen

2 Mol
Isopren

78:4

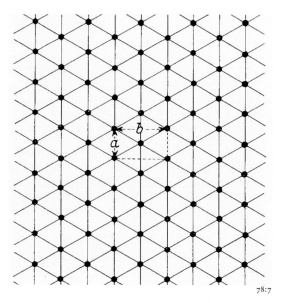

78:7

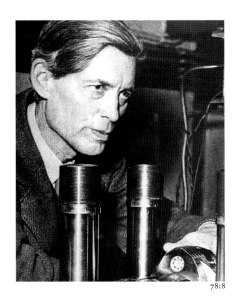

78:8

In 1926 Theodore Svedberg (1884–1971), using his newly invented ultra-centrifuge (the construction of the apparatus is shown in the drawing), determines the molecular weight of haemoglobin to be about 66,800, a value much larger than previously believed. This discovery lends important support to Staudinger's view on the mechanisms of polymerisation.

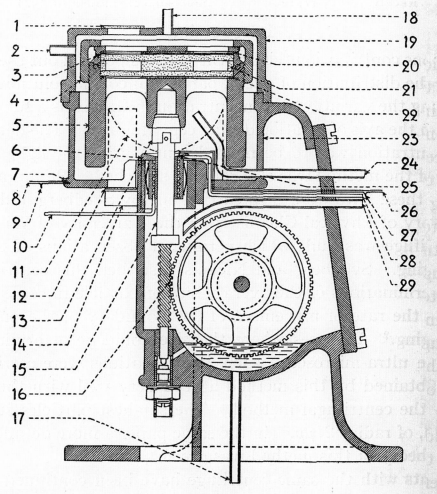

Fig. 1.

1, Upper window; 2, Hydrogen outlet; 3, Ebonite plate; 4, Lid of rotor; 5, Rotor; 6, Water-cooled spring bearing; 7–9, Thermocouple; 10, Water outlet; 11, Copper screen; 12, Lower window; 13, Carrying cone; 14, Reflecting prism; 15, Shaft of rotor; 16, Toothed wheel; 17, Oil outlet; 18, Hydrogen inlet; 19, Lid; 20, Rubber plate; 21, Cell; 22, Rubber plate; 23, Casing of centrifuge; 24, Hydrogen inlet; 25–27, Thermocouple; 28, Water inlet; 29, Oil inlet.

78:9

[CONTRIBUTION FROM THE RESEARCH LABORATORY, CORNING GLASS WORKS]

Condensation Products of the Organo-silane Diols

BY J. F. HYDE AND R. C. DeLONG

The hydrolysis of substituted organo-silicon halides is generally accompanied by dehydration to form complex condensation products containing siloxane linkages.[1,2,3,4] The extent and mode of the condensation is affected by the number of organic groups attached to the silicon. Thus, the mono-substituted compounds can form three-dimensional networks, with possible intermediate stages of dehydration in which thermo-setting properties are in evidence. The condensation of tri-substituted compounds is limited to the formation of dimers or ethers. The di-substituted compounds, on the other hand, should condense with the formation of chain molecules and should yield products having high molecular weights and possible thermoplastic characteristics. Although some polymers are described by Kipping and Murray[5] which seem to confirm this view, it appears that there is likewise a strong tendency toward the formation of cyclic structures.[4c] The lack of a clear understanding of the behavior of the substituted organo-silicon compounds and the possibility of producing useful resinous polymers from them led to an investigation of some of the disubstituted compounds, the results of which are described briefly in the present paper.

Discussion of Results

Liquid Hydrolysis Products.—The hydrolysis of the phenylethyl-, diethyl-, phenylmethyl-, dimethyl-, and diphenyl-dichlorosilanes, under mild conditions, results in the formation of relatively low molecular weight products. With one exception these products are liquids. The diphenyl compound forms a crystalline powder. A cyclic trimer appears definitely to be formed upon hydrolysis of the phenylethyldichlorosilane under the conditions described. Cyclic trimeric condensation products also appear to be present in the hydrolysis products of the diethyl and dimethyl compounds.

Resinous Polymers.—The removal of organic groups by hydrolysis or oxidation results in the

formation of additional siloxane linkages which contribute to the formation of higher polymers. When the hydrolysis products of the compounds containing phenyl groups are treated at elevated temperatures with aqueous hydrochloric acid, there is a gradual increase in the viscosity of the product which is accompanied by the evolution of benzene. If this treatment is continued sufficiently long the material reaches an extremely viscous tacky state but is fusible and readily soluble in toluene and other solvents. With still further treatment, gelation occurs and the product becomes infusible and insoluble but remains somewhat resilient. When air is passed through the hydrolysis products of the compounds containing alkyl groups at elevated temperatures, similar changes in viscosity occur and the resinification in this case is accompanied by the formation of aldehydes. Here also insoluble products result on longer treatment.

In the case of the phenylethyl compound, analysis and molecular weight of the polymer resulting from acid treatment just prior to gelation indicate that the cyclic trimeric rings have remained intact but have become joined together by the additional siloxane linkages formed by displacement of the phenyl groups.

The hydrolysis product of the phenylmethyl compound, when brought to a similar physical state by air treatment at elevated temperature, likewise appears to have approximately half of its di-substituted silicon atoms converted to mono-substituted silicon atoms by loss of methyl groups, a fact which is indicated by its increased silica residue. Upon acid treatment of the phenylmethyl hydrolysis product, however, gelation occurs with less loss of organic matter than would be expected from comparison with the behavior of the phenylethyl compound under similar conditions. The cyclic dimethyltrisiloxane, upon resinification, seems to gel when approximately one-fifth of the disubstituted silicon atoms are converted to mono-substituted atoms. In this case complications may be involved in the resinification. The point of gelation may be considerably affected by the compatibility of the polymers present. Opening of the ring may also be involved.

(1) Friedel, *Ann. chim. phys.*, [iv] 9, 5 (1866).
(2) Ladenburg, *Ann.*, 173, 143 (1874).
(3) Dilthey, *Ber.*, 38, 4132 (1905).
(4) Kipping and co-workers, (a) *J. Chem. Soc.*, 95, 302–314 (1909); (b) *ibid.*, 101, 2108–2166 (1912); (c) *ibid.*, 105, 484–500, 679–690 (1914); (d) *ibid.*, 107, 459–468 (1915).
(5) Kipping and Murray, *ibid.*, 1427–1431 (1928).

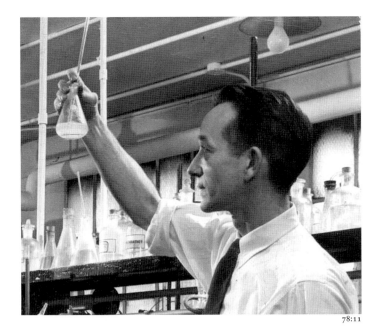

78:11

On the opposite page part of an important publication of James Franklin Hyde (1903–1999) from 1941 is reproduced. His work starts the industrial exploitation of organosilicon polymers, first at Corning Glass Works and from 1943 at the Dow Corning Corporation and at the General Electric Company. Hyde (shown in his laboratory) finds a way to convert silicon-containing compounds into silicones. Below, silicon rubber extrusion from the mid-1950s.

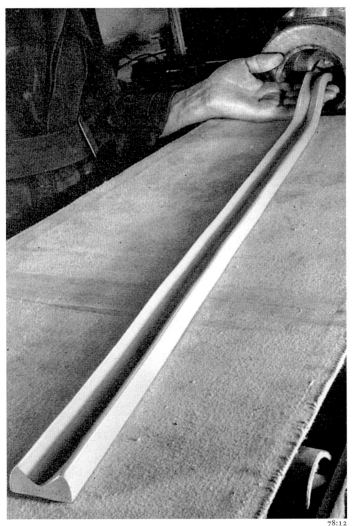

78:12

The mass spectrometer designed by
Francis Aston (1877–1945) with the discharge tube (B), the reservoir for the gas
to be analysed (C), the electromagnet
(M), the camera (W) and the pump (G).
The principle of the instrument is
shown in the drawing. The focusing at F
is achieved by selecting ions with the
slits S1, S2 and D and balancing the electrostatic deflection from plates P1 and
P2 against the magnetic deflection (O).

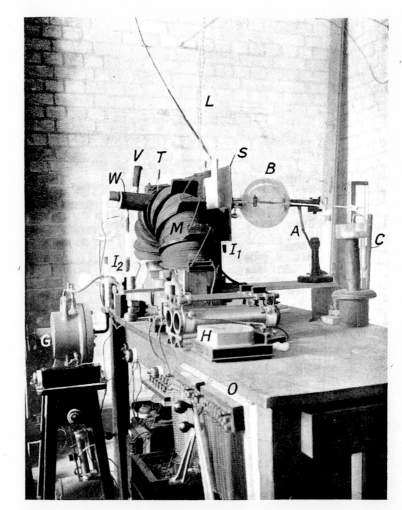

Photograph of the Original Mass-Spectrograph set up in the Cavendish
Laboratory in 1919.

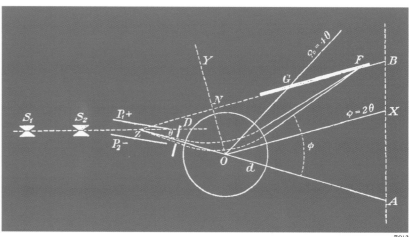

Francis William Aston

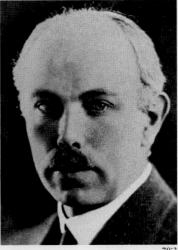

Francis William Aston

Aston was born in Harbonne in 1877. When he was fifteen he entered Mason's College in Birmingham to study chemistry. For a time he worked as a chemist in a brewery but in 1903 he returned to Birmingham to study physics. From 1910 to 1919, when Aston was elected to Trinity College in Cambridge, he was at the Cavendish Laboratory working for Thomson (79.1). Aston preferred to work alone and collaborated with others only when necessary to compensate for his fallibility as a theoretician. He received the Nobel Prize in Chemistry in 1922. Aston was a keen traveller, an avid sportsman, an accomplished amateur musician and a skilled photographer.

Isotopes.

London: E. Arnold & Co; 1922.

Aston describes his novel technique for obtaining a mass spectrograph. By balancing the magnetic deflection of the charged ions with an electrical field, he shows that focusing of the beam can be achieved at a certain spot. This improves the mass resolution of the instrument by an order of magnitude. He now explains the 20.2 average mass of neon as resulting from two isotopes (Greek: equal place) with masses 20 and 22, the first being ten times more abundant than the second. He reports on isotopes of many elements and introduces the concept that atomic masses are integral, with oxygen having the value of 16. Aston also presents the improved direct magnetic focusing technique invented by Dempster in 1918 (79.2).

IN PERSPECTIVE:
Double-focusing high resolution mass spectrometers (MS) were developed already in the 1930s using Dempster's invention. Mass separation using time of flight (TOF) discrimination, first proposed in 1946 (79.3), has been found to be well suited to biological research (79.4). Other techniques in MS instruments are a combination of a radio frequency electric field with a uniform magnetic field (ICR MS) or a static electric field (Quadrupole MS). ICR MS with Fourier analysis (79.5) provides the highest mass resolution and yields results for many ions simultaneously. New "soft" methods of ionisation have extended the use of MS to organic chemistry and molecular biology. Prominent among these soft methods are the matrix-assisted laser desorption and ionisation (MALDI MS) (79.6)(79.7) and the electrospray ionisation techniques (ESI MS) (79.7). Mass spectrometers were first combined in a practical way with a gas chromatograph (GC)(79.8) in the early 1960s (79.9), thereby making it possible to determine the structure of prostaglandines (79.10). Such combination instruments (GC-MS) as well as tandem mass spectrometers (MS-MS) are now common and powerful tools in many research applications.

79.1 See #69 Thomson page 356.
79.2 Dempster AJ. A new method of positive ray analysis. *Phys Rev* 1918; 11:316.
79.3 Stephens WE. A Pulsed Mass Spectrometer with Time dispersion. *Phys Rev* 1946; 69:691.
79.4 Cotter RJ. Time of Fligt Mass Spectrometry: Instrumentation and Applications in biological research. *Am Chem Soc* Washington DC 1997; p13.
79.5 See #32 Fourier page 176 and also compare with #96 Lauterbur page 498.
79.6 Tanaka K. *The origin of macromolecule ionization by laser irradiation.* Nobel Lecture Stockholm; 2002.
79.7 Fenn JB. *Electrospray for molecular elephants.* Nobel Lecture Stockholm; 2002.
79.8 See #84 Martin page 434 and also #73 Tswett page 376.
79.9 Ryhage R. Efficiency of molecule separators used in gas chromatograph-mass spectrometer applications. *Arkiv Kemi* 1967; 26:305.
79.10 Bergström S. *The prostaglandins: from the laboratory to the clinic.* Nobel Lecture Stockholm; 1982.

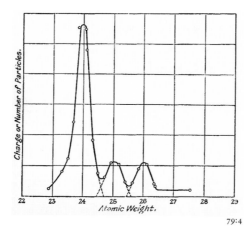

79:4

In 1918 Arthur Dempster (1886–1950) designs a mass spectrograph for ion beams of low and well-defined velocity. The apparatus (that he is seen adjusting in the photograph) is based solely on magnetic deflection (see the drawing of its principle of operation, right). With this instrument he is able to resolve the three isotopes of magnesium, as is demonstrated by the three peaks in the mass spectrograph (top diagram).

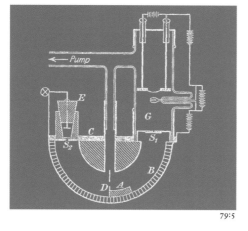

79:5

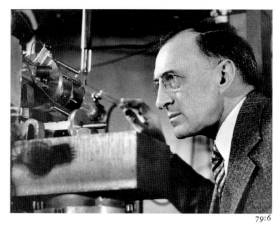

79:6

Mass spectra obtained by Aston showing (registration I) the separation of the two isotopes of neon, the abundant one with a mass of 20 (intense line) and the ten-times less abundant one with a mass of 22 (weak line).

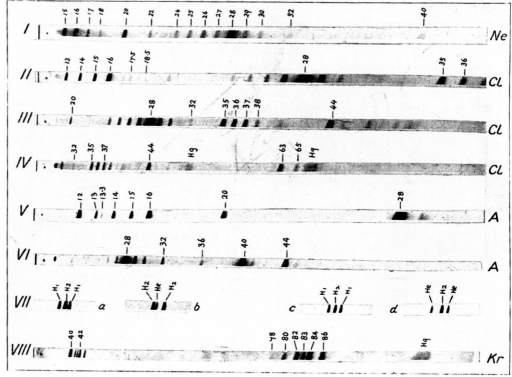

79:7

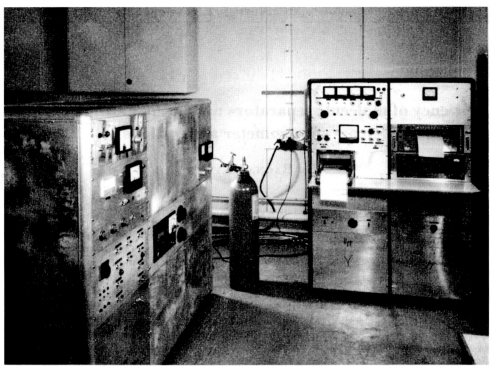

79:8

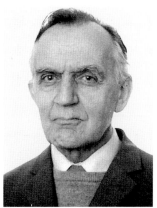

79:10

Ragnar Ryhage (1919–1994) develops a new instrument in 1967, a combined gas chromatograph and mass spectrometer (GC-MS). As a first application, the apparatus is used to determine the structure of prostaglandin, the hormone-like substances that participate in a wide range of body functions.

Left, Ryhage (on the right) sitting together with Sune Bergström (1916–2004), who is awarded the Nobel Prize in Medicine in 1982 for his work on prostaglandin.

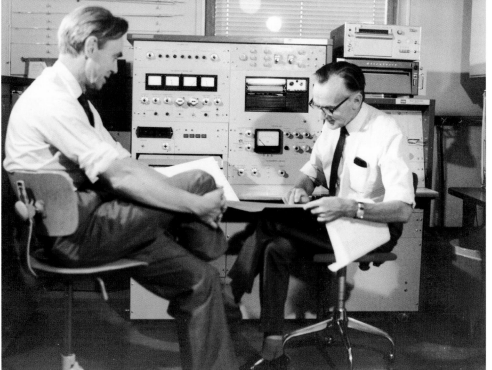

79:9

[CONTRIBUTION No. 11 FROM THE EXPERIMENTAL STATION OF E. I. DU PONT DE NEMOURS AND COMPANY]

STUDIES ON POLYMERIZATION AND RING FORMATION.
II. POLY-ESTERS

BY WALLACE H. CAROTHERS AND J. A. ARVIN

RECEIVED APRIL 13, 1929   PUBLISHED AUGUST 7, 1929

An example of a bi-bifunctional reaction is found in the reaction between a dibasic acid and a dihydric alcohol, $HOOC—R'—COOH + HO—R''—OH$, which, if it is conducted so as to involve both functional groups of each reactant, must lead to an ester having the structural unit, $—OC—R'—CO—O—R''—O— = —R—$.   In accordance with the thesis developed in the previous paper, esters formed in this way will be polymeric unless the number of atoms in the chain of the structural unit is less than seven. In this paper esters are described in which the number of atoms in the chain of the structural unit is 7, 8, 9, 10, 11, 12, 14, 15, 16, 18 and 22 atoms.   All these esters are highly polymeric, and, although some of them have been prepared by various methods, no monomeric form of any of them has as yet been isolated.

Preparation of the Esters

The following method was used for the preparation of the solid esters whose properties are listed in the table.   The acid together with a 5% excess of the glycol was placed in a Claisen flask provided with a receiver and condenser, and the flask was heated in a metal-bath.   At about 160° (bath temperature) reaction set in.   Water distilled off freely during the first hour (temp., 175–185°) and very slowly if at all during the succeeding two hours at the same temperature.   The receiver was now changed, the flask provided with a very fine capillary and heating continued under a good vacuum (usually less than 0.2 mm.) for about three hours, the temperature of the bath being raised to 200–250°.   During this period little or no distillate collected (provided only a 5% excess of glycol was used).   The residue, which was a slightly dark and, at 150°, more or less viscous liquid, was poured from the flask.   The amount of this residue corresponded with the theoretical (based on the acid used), and the amount of water actually collected approached the calculated more closely the larger the sample used (60–90%).   The esters were purified by crystallization.

Ethylene malonate was prepared by heating ethyl malonate and glycol in the same fashion.   There was some decomposition (evolution of gas) when the residue was heated to 240° *in vacuo*.   This residue was a thick sirup which could not be induced to crystallize.   It was dissolved in acetone, filtered and heated for several hours at 175–190° in high vacuum.   Nothing corresponding to a monomeric ethylene malonate was found on redistilling the distillates from this preparation.

The preparation and properties of some esters not included in the table are described in the Experimental Part of this paper.

Structure of the Esters

The conclusion that these compounds are esters and that they contain the structural unit —R— indicated above follows directly from the method of preparation and is supported by the analytical data and chemi-

CAROTHERS was born in 1896 in Burlington, Iowa. After studying chemistry he graduated from Tarkio College in 1920 and two years later he enrolled at the University of Illinois in Urbana. Carothers received his Ph.D. in 1924 and after a short stay as an assistant he accepted a teaching position offered to him at Harvard University. In 1928, keen on doing research, he gladly accepted the offer to head the newly established research centre at DuPont. Here Carothers soon achieved major success but his mental illness, aggravated by excessive drinking habits and the untimely death of his sister, all contributed to a deep depression that ended with his suicide at the age of only forty-one. At the time of his death his wife, whom Carothers had married the year before, was expecting their baby.

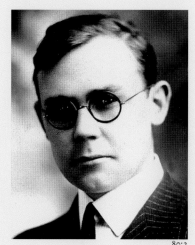

Wallace Hume Carothers

Studies on Polymerisation and Ring Formation. II Poly-Esters.

J Am Chem Soc 1929; 51(8):2560.

CAROTHERS AND Arvin report on the preparation and characterisation of a large number of esters. The experiments follow from theoretical considerations presented by Carothers in a preceding paper (80.1), which in turn is largely based on the results of Staudinger (80.2). Carothers discusses the properties and structures of the esters, determines their molecular weights and finds that all are highly polymeric.

IN PERSPECTIVE:

The first man-made plastic was invented in 1862 by Parkes using cellulose nitrate (pyroxine) with camphor as the plasticiser (80.3). Following Parkes, Hyatt replaced ether in collodion with camphor and produced the first commercial thermoplastic (celluloid) (80.4). Baekeland developed the first entirely synthetic mouldable plastic in 1909 (bakelite) (80.5). The cited work soon led to the discovery of how to obtain fibres of esters, but in 1935 it was found that polyamide (nylon) fibres had much better mechanical and chemical properties. DuPont launched nylon commercially in 1938. Other plastics from the 1930s include polystyrene, polymethyl methacrylate (plexiglas), mouldable polyvinylchloride (PVC), polyurethane and terafluorethylene polymers (PTFE, teflon). Also, in 1933 Gibson discovered that polyethylene could be formed at high pressures. Two decades later, Ziegler was able to produced high-density polyethylene at normal pressures by using special catalysts (80.6). Soon Natta employed a process similar to Ziegler's to make polypropylene for the first time (80.7). For four decades Flory investigated theoretically the spatial configuration of macromolecules (80.8) and also modelled the characteristics of a liquid crystal state (80.9) well before it was first produced synthetically in 1968 (80.10). Today, clinical medicine is inconceivable without many of the plastics mentioned above and liquid crystal technology is common in display applications.

80.1 Carothers WH. Studies on polymerization and ring formation. I An introduction to the general theory of condensation polymers. J Am Chem Soc 1929; 51(8):2548.

80.2 See #78 Staudinger page 400.

80.3 See ref. 78.7.

80.4 See #77 Abel page 396 and ref. 77.6.

80.5 Morris PJ. Polymer Pioneers. A popular history of the science and technology of large molecules. Philadelphia: Center for the History of Chemistry; 1986. p39. Also see ref. 78.7 p13.

80.6 Ziegler K. Consequences and Development of an Invention. Nobel Lecture Stockholm; 1963.

80.7 Natta G. From the Stereospecific Polymerisation to the Assymetric Autocatalytic Synthesis. Nobel Lecture Stockholm; 1963.

80.8 Flory PJ. Spatial Configuration of Macromolecular Chains. Nobel Lecture Stockholm; 1974.

80.9 Flory PJ. Phase Equilibria in Solutions of Rod-like Particles. Proc Roy Soc A 1956; 234: 60.

80.10 Kwolek SL. Wholly aromatic carbocyclic polycarbonate fiber having orientation angle of less than about 45 degrees. US Patent 3,819,587 1974.

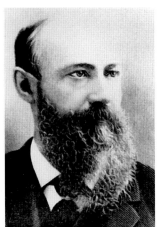

80:3

In 1861 Alexander Parkes (1813–1890) invents the first man-made plastic "Parkesine", which is made up of pyroxine (collodion) with camphor as a plasticiser. He unveils his invention at the Great International Exhibition in London in 1862 and is awarded a prize, as shown by the announcement reproduced here.

John Wesley Hyatt (1837–1920) develops the ideas of Parkes into a commercial enterprise. Together with his brother Isaiah, he founds the Celluloid Manufacturing Company in 1871. The picture shows their factory in Newark in 1875.

PRIZE MEDAL.

INTERNATIONAL EXHIBITION, 1862. CLASS IV.
OFFICIAL CATALOGUE, No. 1112.

PARKESINE.

A new material and manufacture now exhibited for the first time, has from its valuable properties induced the Inventor to Patent the discovery in England and France, and to devote his attention for the last ten years to the development of the capabilities and application of this beautiful substance to the Arts. In the Case are shown a few illustrations of the numerous purposes for which it may be applied, such as Medallions, Salvers, Hollow Ware, Tubes, Buttons, Combs, Knife Handles, Pierced and Fret Work, Inlaid Work, Bookbinding, Card Cases, Boxes, Pens, Penholders, &c.,—these have been produced solely by the exhibitor (as Samples), not having yet arranged a systematic manufacture for the material. It can be made Hard as Ivory, Transparent or Opaque, of any degree of Flexibility, and is also Waterproof; may be of the most Brilliant Colours, can be used in the Solid, Plastic or Fluid State, may be worked in Dies and Pressure, as Metals, may be Cast or used as a Coating to a great variety of substances; can be spread or worked in a similar manner to India Rubber, and has stood exposure to the atmosphere for years without change or decomposition. And by the system of ornamentation Patented by HENRY PARKES in 1861, the most perfect imitation of Tortoise-shell, Woods, and an endless variety of effects can be produced. Specimens of which may be seen in the Case.

Patentee and Exhibitor,
ALEX. PARKES,
BIRMINGHAM.

80:5

80:4

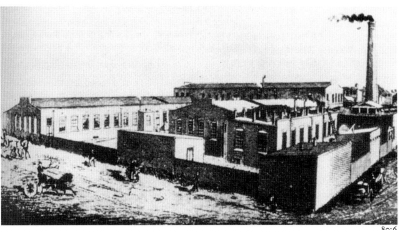

80:6

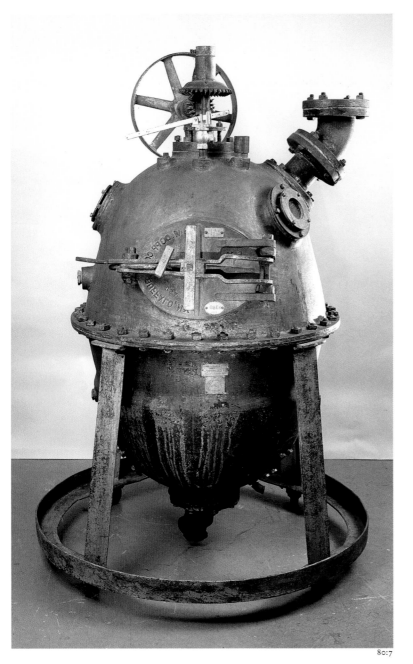

80:7

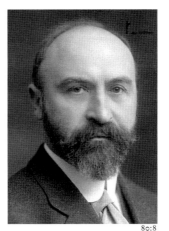

80:8

In 1907 Leo Bakeland (1863–1944) applies for a patent to protect his process for making phenol-formaldehyde resins using controlled pressure and heating. His original apparatus, the "Bakelizer", was called the "Old Faithful" and is shown in the photograph on the left.

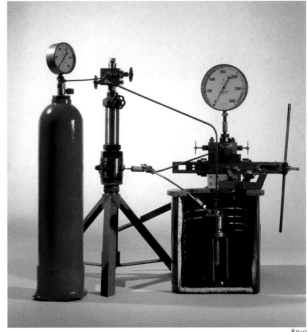

80:9

The apparatus used in 1933 by Reginald Oswald Gibson (1902–1983) when making the chance discovery of polyethylene. The compound was the unexpected find in an experiment where ethylene and benzaldehyde were combined at 170°C and at a pressure of 1,700 atm.

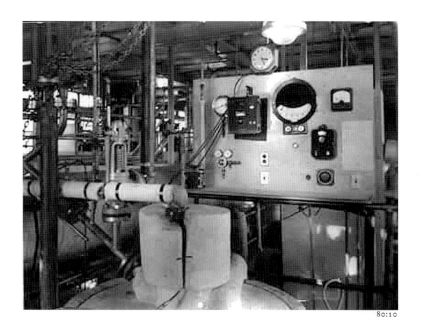

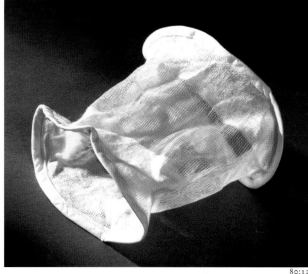

A sample made from the first experimental nylon (polyamide), from 1935.

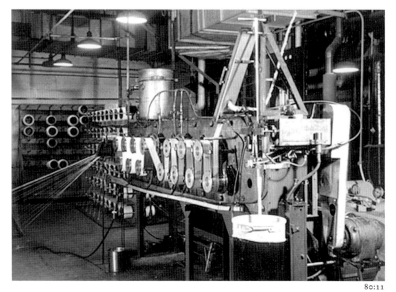

The equipment used at the factory of Du Pont in 1937 for producing nylon fibres. Pictures show the polymerisation apparatus (top) and the drawing machine and creel.

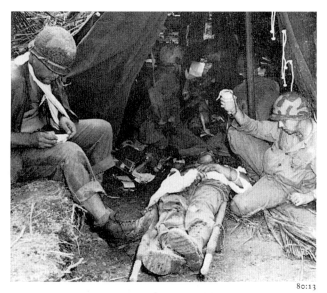

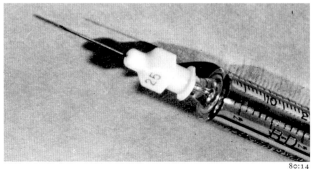

The first health care uses of nylon. Tents and litters of nylon prove superior in field use during the Second World War, particularly in hot and humid environments. A hypodermic needle moulded of Du Pont zytel nylon from 1952. On the opposite page, the introduction of nylon sutures in 1939. The sutures are sold in sealed glass tubes containing an antiseptic solution.

Du Pont Nylon Steps Into Surgery

The new sutures have some outstanding advantages

By P. F. Ziegler

Director of Research, Bauer & Black

THE surgical technique of closing wounds and ligating hemorrhages with threads of varying compositions had its crude beginning in dim, prehistoric times. In many of the very earliest writings allusions are made to this practice, but whether this drama of surgical progress began to unfold on some Arabian plain, in Egypt, or in densely populated India, available records leave us in some doubt.

Comprehensive writings on surgery make their appearance early in history, and one of the first is credited to the Indian surgeon Susruta, about 600 B. C. This writer recommends for suturing and ligating, materials such as cotton, strips of leather, fiber from the bark of trees, and animal sinews. Galen, in the first century, mentions the use of silk, and from this time on frequent references can be found to techniques and materials. The interesting fact to be observed, however, is that, while manufacture and processing have made giant strides, the base materials for present-day sutures have been essentially unchanged in two thousand years—that is, unchanged until the magic of modern chemistry produced a significantly different suture material, for nylon, recently produced by du Pont, has taken its place as a new tool with which the surgical profession can combat disease.

A study of the history of the suture reveals glimpses of the struggle of man to acquire a controlled technique of healing which cannot but heighten anyone's appreciation of the modern means now readily available for arresting hemorrhage and closing wounds safely. Today's ligature and suture materials, with the technique for their use, represent a heritage whose value to mankind cannot be overestimated. A sense of this value is enriched by glimpses of the long, long journey from darkness to light.

RELATED PROBLEMS

Before the age of asepsis, any means designed to stop hemorrhage and to close wounds was surrounded by numerous hazards. Bacteria native to or acquired by the ligature or suture material were buried with it in the patients' tissue; a terrifically high percentage of

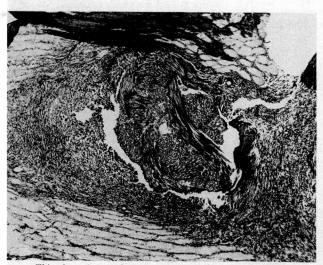

This photomicrograph—75 x magnification—shows a No. 1 serum-proof braided silk suture embedded eight days in the muscle of a dog. Note the relatively large area of inflamed tissue around this suture.

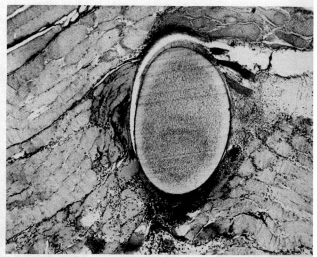

The same magnification of a No. 2 undyed nylon suture embedded two days in the muscle. You will note that the area of inflammation surrounding this suture is smaller, with less exudate showing.

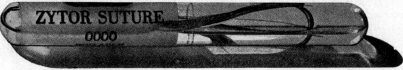

[14]

Sutures made of nylon are sold in sealed glass tubes containing an antiseptic solution to insure a sterile condition. The nylon is dyed a solid color; it helps in locating a suture in a wound.

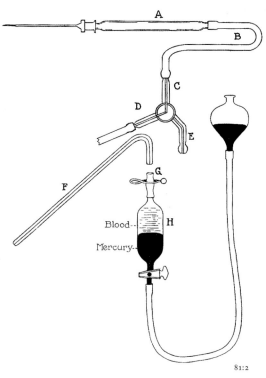

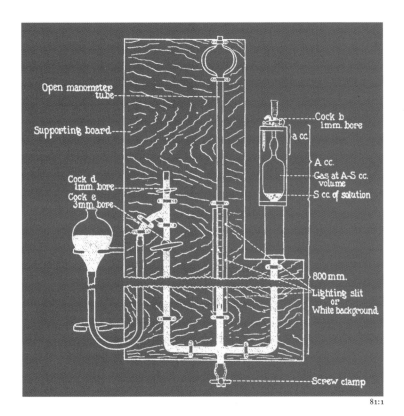

Illustrations of blood-handling techniques and the manometric method of blood gas analysis introduced by Donald van Slyke (1883–1971) in 1924. It soon replaced the volumetric methods that had been in use for more than half a century.

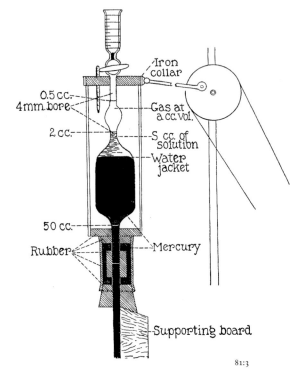

V AN SLYKE was born in 1883 in Pike (N.Y.). He received a B.Sc. in chemistry and in 1907 a Ph.D. in organic chemistry, both from the University of Michigan. He then worked as a research chemist at the Rockefeller Institute for Medical Research until he was appointed chief chemist at the Hospital of the Rockefeller Institute in 1914. He was elected to the National Academy of Sciences in 1921. Van Slyke moved to Brookhaven National Laboratory in 1949 where he remained active doing research almost until his death in 1971.

Quantitative Clinical Chemistry, Vol. I Interpretations, Vol. II Methods.

BALTIMORE: THE WILLIAMS AND WILKINS CO; 1931–1932.

IN THIS comprehensive work (a total of about 2,200 pages) written together with Peters, Van Slyke defines the state of the art in clinical chemistry. The first volume discusses the physiological role of substances of importance in clinical chemistry and its significance in diagnoses and therapy. The second volume presents the methodology and equipment needed to make the observations, the interpretation of which is dealt with in the first volume.

IN PERSPECTIVE:

The sciences of clinical chemistry can be traced back at least to Van Helmont and Boyle (81.1). Based on the work of Arrhenius and Oswald (81.2), Henderson and Hasselbach established the acid-base properties of the blood (81.3)(81.4). Blood gases were first measured with volumetric techniques (81.3) but from the 1930s the manometric technique of Van Slyke (81.5) was in general use, mostly to prevent metabolic acidosis in the newly introduced insulin treatment of diabetes. In the 1950s the observation of respiratory acidosis in polio patients led to the development of new sensor technology for pH (Astrup), oxygen (Clark) and carbon dioxide (Stow and Severinghaus) (81.3). Blood volumes needed for an analysis were reduced more than tenfold by the pioneering work of Bang (81.6) and by three further orders of magnitude by Scholander (81.7). Early titrimetric and gravimetric procedures were largely replaced during the 1920s by colorimetry and in the 1940s by photometry. Spectrophotometry, flame photometry and atomic absorption spectroscopy have since much improved the analysis of most elements. In the 1940s Natelson developed new highly sensitive analytical methods (81.8) and the radioimmunoassay technique of Berson and Yalow in 1959 made it possible to measure specific proteins and hormones at exceptionally low concentrations (81.9). The introduction of many new and useful tests led to a drastic need to speed up the processing of samples. The automation technology introduced by Skeggs (81.10) has become the indispensable backbone of modern clinical chemistry laboratories.

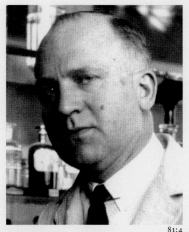

Donald Dexter Van Slyke

81:4

81.1 Rosenfeld L. *Four Centuries of Clinical Chemistry*. G & B Science Pub; 1999. See also #8. Van Helmont page 60, #14 Boyle page 88, #37 Magnus page 196, #39 Liebig page 208, #49 Kirchoff page 258, #51 Hoppe-Seyler page 268, #59 Bert page 304 and #62 Arrhenius page 320.
81.2 Ostwald WF. Die dissociation des Wassers. *Z phys Chem* 1893; 11:521.
81.3 Ref. 14.8.
81.4 Henderson LJ.: *Blood*. New Haven: Yale University Press; 1928 and ref. 62.9.
81.5 Van Slyke DD, Sendroy Jr J. Manometric analysis of gas mixtures. I The determination, by simple absorption, of carbon dioxide, oxygen and nitrogen in mixtures of these gases. *J Biol Chem*. 1932; 95:509. See also the cited work above.
81.6 Bang I. *Methoden zur mikrobestimmung einiger blutesandteile*. Wiesbaden: J.F.Bergman; 1916.
81.7 Scholander PF, Irving L. Micro blood gas analysis in fractions of a cubic millimeter of blood. *J Biol Chem* 1947; 169:561 and p551.
81.8 Natelson S, Lugovoy JK, Pincus JB. Determination of micro quatities of citric acid in biological fluids. *J Biol Chem* 1947; 170:597.
81.9 Yalow RS, Berson SA. Assay of Plasma Insulin in human subjects aby Immunological Methods. *Nature* 1959; 184:1648. See also ref. 70.8.
81.10 Skeggs LT. Principles of automatic chemical analysis. *Stand Methods Clin Chem* 1965; 5:31.

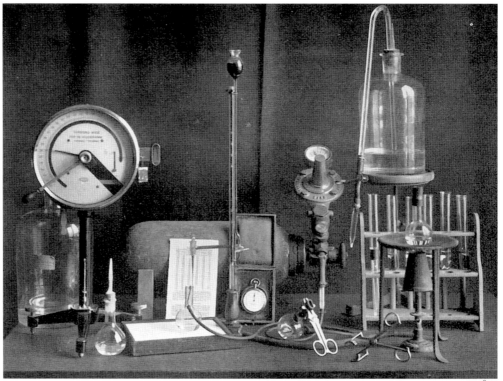

81:5

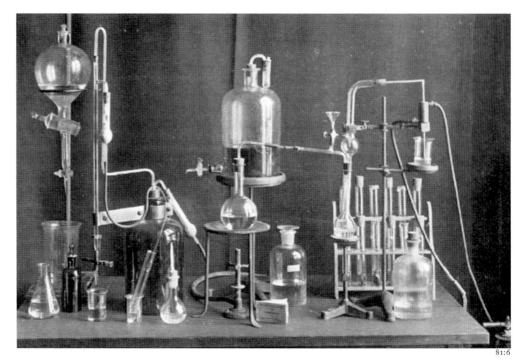

81:6

In 1916 Ivar Bang (1869–1918) introduces new analytic techniques that require only a tenth of the blood volume previously needed in clinical chemistry. The illustrations show Bang's apparatus for microdetermination of blood glucose and lipid levels (top) and for improved micro-Kjeldahl analysis of blood urea nitrogen (bottom).

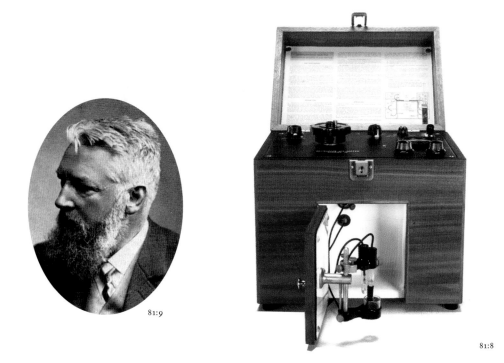

81:9

81:8

1893 sees Wilhelm Ostwald (1853–1932) publish the first investigation on the dissociation of water. His work lays the foundation of all future hydrogen ion (pH) measuring instruments, such as the one shown here from 1934.

The micro-Scholander technique of blood handling is introduced in 1947 and reduces a thousand fold the volume of blood previously needed for chemical analysis.

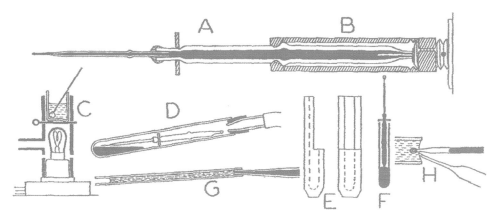

FIG. 1. *A*, extraction tube with sealed on burette needle. *B*, steel yoke holding extraction chamber tight against fiber bearing for micro plunger; *C*, lamp for keeping wax melted and for drying reagents in extraction tube; *D*, evacuation of extraction tube with attached needle; *E*, wooden holders for centrifuge; *F*, centrifuge tube with extraction chamber unit ready for centrifugation; *G*, transfer of blood sample by means of capillary hung on to the tip of the burette needle; *H*, cutting off wax cap in acid with drawn out, broken off glass rod.

81:7

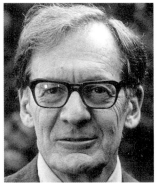

81:10

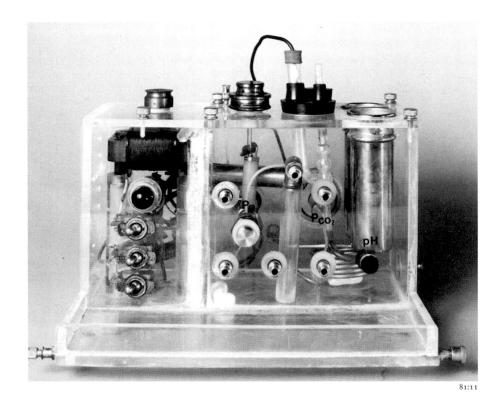

81:11

John Severinghaus and the first 3-electrode blood-gas apparatus with a Beckman/Clark oxygen electrode, a Stow/Severinghaus carbon dioxide electrode and a McInnes/Belcher pH electrode. It takes about a decade to develop a fully automated system. The first, built by Radiometer A/S in 1973, is shown below.

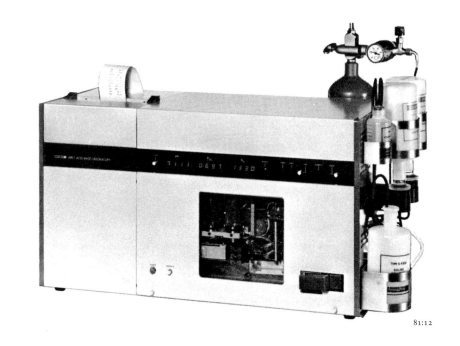

81:12

RADIOBIOLOGY

Assay of Plasma Insulin in Human Subjects by Immunological Methods

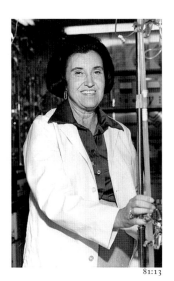

81:13

In 1959 Solomon Berson (1919–1972) and Rosalyn Yalow (shown here in her laboratory) conceive the radioimmunoassay technique, which makes it possible to measure specific proteins and hormones at exceptionally low concentrations. The text reports their results from the first study involving human insulin.

The introduction of many useful tests in clinical chemistry drastically increases the volume of analysis to be performed. In the mid-1950s Leonard Skeggs (1918–1997) starts work on the automation techniques that are now an indispensable part of all clinical chemistry laboratories. The diagram from an important paper of Skeggs in 1965 shows the principle proposed by him for a multiple analytic system that would eliminate what he called the "train of test tubes".

WE have previously reported on the immuno-assay of beef insulin and certain other animal insulins, employing antiserums from human subjects treated with commercial mixtures of beef and pork insulin[1]. The insulin-binding antibodies present in these antiserums do not form precipitable complexes with insulin, but with the use of insulin labelled with iodine-131 the complexes are readily demonstrable by paper chromatography and electrophoresis[2]. Beef, pork, sheep and horse insulins can be assayed quantitatively by measurement of the degree of competitive inhibition of binding of any insulin labelled with iodine-131[1-3]. As might have been anticipated, however, human insulin competes too weakly in systems employing human antiserum to be measurable at concentrations which obtain *in vivo*. Furthermore, the lack of availability of significant quantities of pure human insulin precludes its use as an antigen for animal immunization. However, in the present work, it has been found that human insulin cross-reacts strongly with insulin-binding antibodies in guinea pigs immunized with crystalline beef insulin, and that guinea pig anti-beef insulin serum has characteristics suitable for the detection and measurement of human insulin at concentrations which exist in the plasma of normal fasting subjects.

81:14

Multiple Analytical Systems

There is considerable advantage in combining two or more methods within a single flow circuit. For example, urea nitrogen and glucose

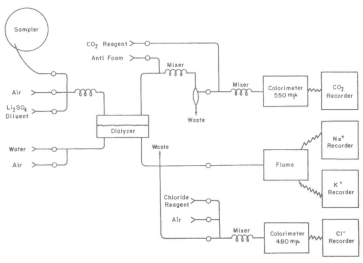

FIG. 3. Flow diagram of the method for the determination of sodium, potassium, chloride, and carbon dioxide.

are very often combined and run as one method yielding two results from a single sample. Creatinine and urea nitrogen have also been combined, as well as calcium and phosphorus.

81:15

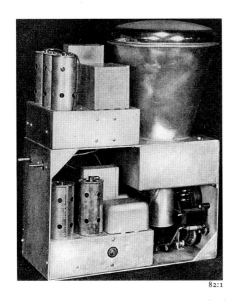

82:1

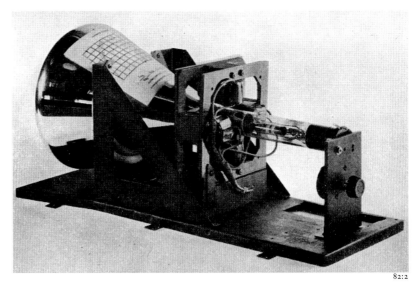

82:2

The block diagram of the experimental television system tested in New York in 1931. The camera ("iconoscope") and the receiver ("kinescope") are both based on cathode ray tube technology, as is apparent from the photographs.

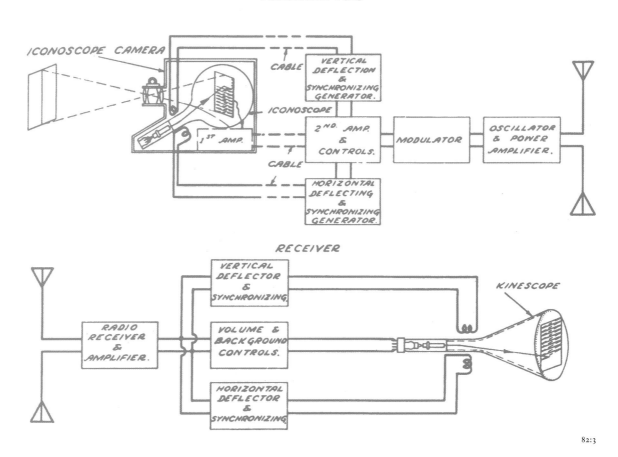

82:3

Vladimir Kozma Zworykin

ZWORYKIN was born in Mourom, Russia, in 1899, the son of an affluent family. He graduated in St. Petersburg and studied at the Collège de France in Paris before emigrating to the United States in 1919. While working for Westinghouse, he earned a Ph.D. in physics at the University of Pittsburgh and also invented electronic television components and systems. The Radio Corporation of America (RCA) was interested in exploiting these inventions and in 1929 Zworykin was named director of their electronics research laboratory. After retiring from RCA in 1954, he directed the Medical Electronics Center at the Rockefeller University. He died in 1982, having received numerous awards for his work on television systems.

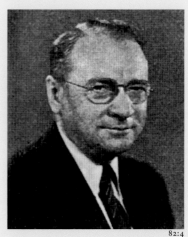

82:4

Vladimir Kozma Zworykin

Television.

J FRANKLIN INSTITUTE 1934; 217(1):1.

ZWORYKIN DESCRIBES a new, truly electrical television system where the visual image is translated into an electrical signal by a vacuum tube called an "iconoscope" (82.1). This device is "a virtual electric eye and consists of a photo-sensitive mosaic corresponding to the retina of the human eye, and a moving electron beam representing the nerve of the eye". Then the "kinescope" (cathode ray tube (82.2)) reproduces the image with an electron beam scanning over a fluorescent screen. The paper details the characteristics of the system and its components, shows pictures of the equipment and gives examples of transmitted images.

IN PERSPECTIVE:
Electro-mechanical systems for image transmission were proposed by LeBlanc, Lucas and Nipkow during the 1880s and built by Baird in 1925 (82.3). In 1908 Swinton suggested that an all-electronic television system could be built using scanned electron beams both in the camera and the display unit (82.4). Farnsworth (82.5) and Zworykin (82.6) invented the electronic television almost simultaneously. RCA first operated its system in 1932 (82.7). Based on experiences from the work on television, Zworykin designed the first scanning electron microscope (82.8) and reading aids for the blind (82.9). Also, by the early 1950s the image intensifiers could be used to greatly facilitate the visual evaluation of X-ray images (82.10). Closed-circuit television was introduced for the teaching of surgery in 1949 (82.10). Clinical monitoring of patients first became a reality when, in the 1960s, the widespread public use of television brought component costs down. Although liquid crystal displays (82.11) and plasma displays (82.12) are now preferred whenever compactness, very high resolution or low power consumption is required, television-based systems are still standard for clinical monitoring of the patient or when following medical procedures in real time.

82.1 Zworykin VK, Morton GA. *Television. The electronics of image transmission*. New York: J Wiley; 1940.
82.2 Braun F. Ueber ein Verfahren zur Demonstration und zum Studium des zeitlichen Verlaufes variabler Ströme. *Ann Phys Chem* 1897; 60:552.
82.3 Dinsdale A. *Television*. London: Sir I.Pitman & Sons; 1926.
82.4 Cambell-Swinton AA. Distant Electrical Vision. *Nature* 1908; 78:151. See also ref. 82.1 p225.
82.5 Farnsworth PT. *Television system*. US Patent 1,773,980 1930. (filed 1927) also ref. 82.1 p230.
82.6 Zworykin VK. *Television system*. US Patent 2,141,059 1938. (filed 1923)
82.7 Zworykin VK. Description of an experimental television system and the kinescope. *Proc IRE* 1933; 21(12): 1655.
82.8 See ref. 83.7.
82.9 Zworykin VK, Flory LE, Pike WS. *Research on reading aids for the blind*. J Frankl Inst May 1949. p483.
82.10 Zworykin VK. *Television techniques in biology and medicine*. In: Adv Biol Med Phys Vol.V Lawrence JH, Tobias CA. editors. New York: Academic Press; 1957.
82.11 See ref. 80.9 and ref. 80.10.
82.12 Bitzer DL, Slottow HG. *Principles and Applications of the Plasma Display Panel*. Proc.1968 Microelectr. Symp.IEEE. St Louis; 1968.

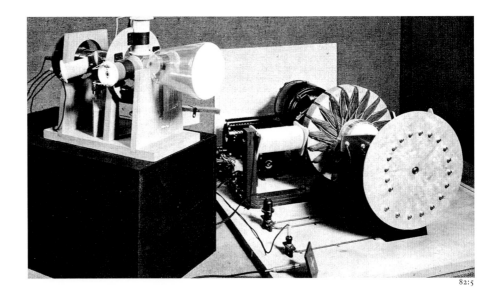

82:5

A model of an early television receiver built in Germany around 1906 using the cathode ray tube invented by Ferdinand Braun (1850–1918) in 1897.

A diagram of the principle of "distant electrical vision", the first entirely electrical television system proposed in 1908 by A Cambell-Swinton.

Philo Farnsworth (1906–1971) standing next to his television apparatus. In 1927 he applies for a patent for the invention of a dissector tube for electronic image generation and eight years later he is awarded the priority of invention for the electronic television.

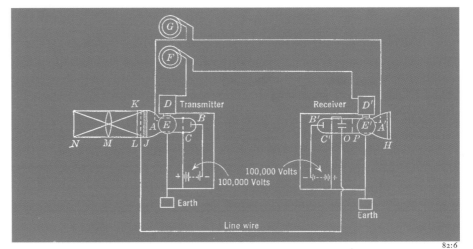

82:6

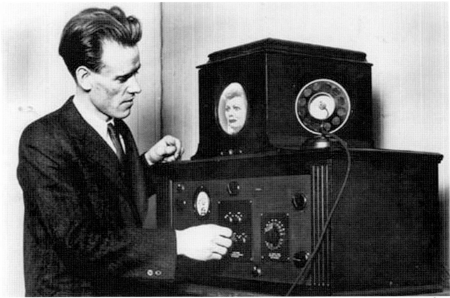

82:7

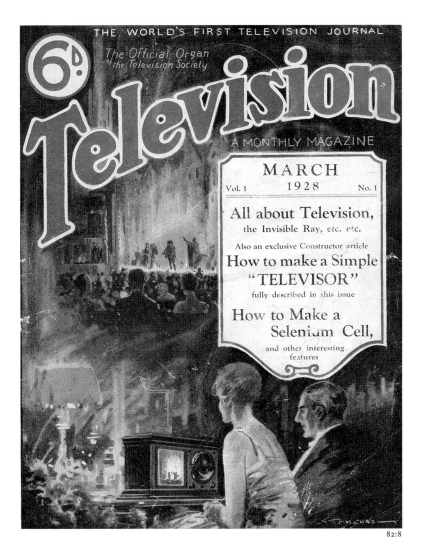

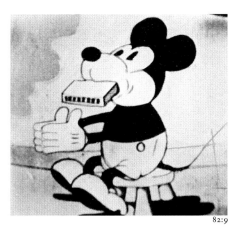

Cover of the first issue of the first television magazine that appeared in 1928.

A well-known Disney character shown by the experimental television system of 1931 and the chassis of the television receiver shown in picture 82:2. The mirror in the lid allows the viewer to see the television ("kinescope") screen.

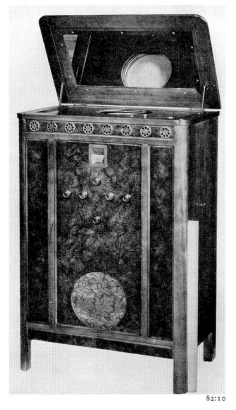

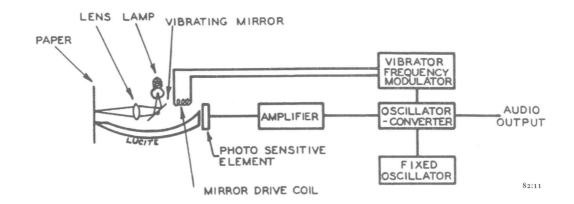

LENS LAMP VIBRATING MIRROR

PAPER

VIBRATOR
FREQUENCY
MODULATOR

AMPLIFIER

OSCILLATOR
-CONVERTER

AUDIO
OUTPUT

LUCITE

PHOTO SENSITIVE
ELEMENT

FIXED
OSCILLATOR

MIRROR DRIVE COIL

82:11

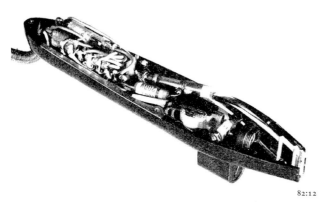

82:12

In 1949 Vladimir Zworykin (1889–1982) develops a reading device for the blind using a system employing optical scanning and electronic signal processing. The scanning head and its principle of operation are shown together with the considerable bulk of electronics needed for letter recognition. The system also includes a sound generating system that can articulate the letters.

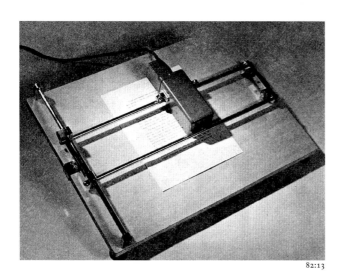

82:13

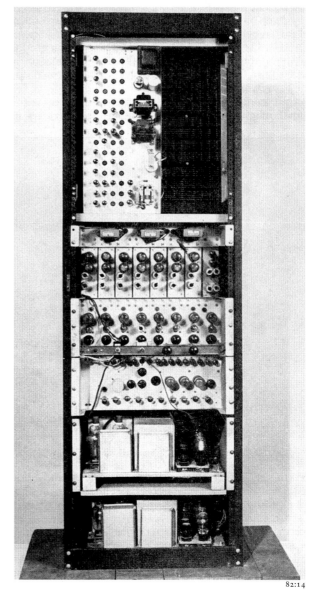

82:14

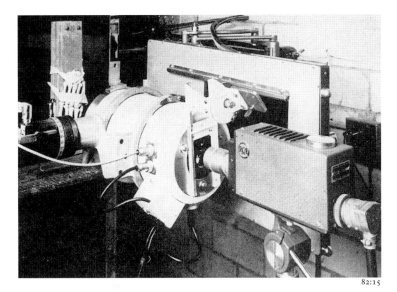

82:15

The building blocks and the implementation of a television system for fluoroscopy in the mid-1950s.

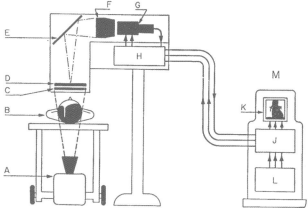

FIG. 33. Use of high-sensitivity television system for fluoroscopy (A, X-ray tube; B, patient; C, wafer grid; D, fluorescent screen; E, mirror; F, lens; G, image orthicon; H, preamplifier; K, viewing screen; J, amplifier; L, sweep generator)

82:16

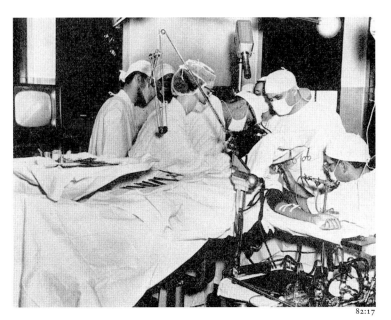

82:17

In 1949 television is used for the first time for teaching surgery. The picture shows a TV Eye camera transmitting an ear fenestration operation in Pittsburgh in the mid-1950s.

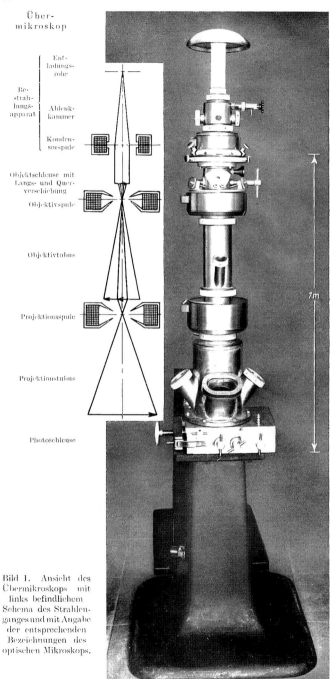

Ent-
ladungs-
rohr

Be-
strah-
lungs-
apparat

Ablenk-
kammer

Kondensor-
spule

Objektschleuse mit
Langs- und Quer-
verschiebung

Objektivspule

Objektivtubus

Projektionsspule

Projektionstubus

Photoschleuse

7 m

Bild 1. Ansicht des
Übermikroskops mit
links befindlichem
Schema des Strahlen-
ganges und mit Angabe
der entsprechenden
Bezeichnungen des
optischen Mikroskops.

Mikro-
skopier-
lampe

Zeit- und
Moment-
verschluß

Be-
leuch-
tungs-
apparat

Kon-
densor

Zentrierbarer
Objekttisch mit
Grobtrieb

Objektiv

Tubus

Photookular

Photoauszug

Aufnahmekassette

83:1

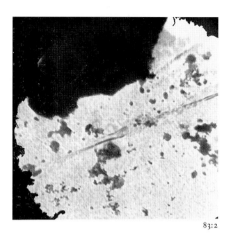

83:2

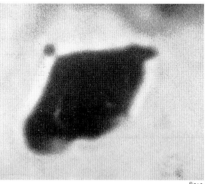

83:3

The first prototype electron microscope, having a magnification of about 30,000, is built in 1938. The functional parts are explained with the analogous optical microscope elements shown on the left. The photographs show a direct comparison between optical (bottom) and electron microscope images of a thin film of colloid silver particles.

RUSKA was born in Heidelberg in 1906. He completed his technical training at Brown-Boveri and Siemens & Halske and entered the Technical College of Berlin in 1927. As a student working on cathode ray oscilloscopes, he invented a superior magnetic lens for focusing electrons (83.1). After receiving his doctorate, Ruska worked at Fernseh Ltd on television receivers and photoelectric cells but returned to Siemens & Halske three years later to build the "supermicroscope" at the newly established laboratory for Electron Optics. From 1955 until his retirement in 1974, he headed the Institute for Electron Microscopy at the Fritz Haber Institute in Berlin. Two years before his death in 1988, he was awarded the Nobel Prize in Physics.

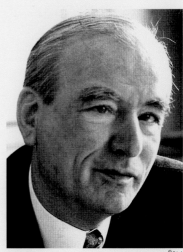

Ernst Ruska 83:4

Vorläufige Mitteilung über Fortschritte im Bau und in der Leistung des Übermikroskopes.

WISS VERÖFFENT A D SIEMENS-WERKEN
BERLIN: SPRINGER J; 1938; 17:99.

TOGETHER WITH von Borries, Ruska presents preliminary results obtained with a prototype electron microscope having a resolution of about 10^{-5} m at 80 kV. Images such as those of bacteria at 20,400 times magnification illustrate the performance of the instrument. The improved magnification of 30,000 is achieved with better design and the use of materials with more suitable magnetic properties than those previously employed in the laboratory models (83.2). The authors predict that, with advances in magnetic lens design and more stable electronics, further significant improvements could be achieved.

IN PERSPECTIVE:

De Broglie's concept that particles could be treated as waves (83.3) and the subsequent development of quantum physics laid the foundation for many of the technical advances of the 1930s, including the electron microscope. In 1934, Marton was the first to use electron microscopy to study biological samples (83.4) and, a decade later, improved sample preparation techniques allowed a more general application of the instrument to biomedical problems (83.5). In 1938 von Ardenne operated the first scanned Transmission Electron Microscope (83.6) and four years later Zworykin invented the Scanning Electron Microscope (SEM) (83.7). During the 1950s Oatley and his students gradually improved the SEM design (83.8) and, with advances in detector technology (83.9), the first commercial instruments were produced in 1965 (83.10). Today there are more than fifty thousand SEM units worldwide, revealing structure and topography down to dimensions of about 25×10^{-10} m. TEMs can have around ten times better resolution and give views on a truly atomic scale. Nowdays, the local composition of the sample can also be determined from connected instrumentation analysing the secondary events produced by the electron beam/target interaction. Both SEM and TEM techniques are fundamental tools of biomedical research (83.11).

83.1 Ruska E, Knoll M. Die Magnetische Sammelspule fuer schnellen Elektronenstrahlen. *Z techn Phys* 1931; 12:389 and p448. See also ref. 64.9.

83.2 Knoll M, Ruska E. Beitrag zur geometerischen Elektronenoptik I und II. *Ann Phys* 1932; 12:607 and p641.

83.3 De Broglie L. *Recherches sur la theorie des quanta.* These Paris: Masson & Cie; 1924.

83.4 Marton L. Electron microscopy of biological objects. *Phys Rev* 1934; 46(2):527. See also ref. 83.5 p501.

83.5 The Beginnings of Electron Microscopy. In: *Advances in Electronics and Electron Physics.* Hawkes PW. Editor. Academic Press; 1985. p167 and p43.

83.6 von Ardenne M. Das Elektronen-Rastermikroskop. *Z Phys* 1938; 109:553. See also ref. 83.5 p1.

83.7 Zworykin VK, Hillier J, Snyder RL. *A scanning electron microscope.* ASTM Bull 1942; 117:15.

83.8 Oatley CW.: *The Scanning Electron Microscope.* Cambridge: Cambridge University Press; 1972. also see ref. 83.5 p443.

83.9 Everhart TE, Thornley RF. Wide-band detector for micro-microampere low-energy electron currents. *J Sci Instrum* 1960; 3 7:246.

83.10 Stewart AD, Snelling MA. A new scanning electron microscope. *Proc 3rd Eur Conf Electron Microscopy Prague*; 1965. p55.

83.11 *Electron Microscopy in Medicine and Biology.* Gupta PD, Yamamoto H. editors. Science Publ. Inc; 2000.

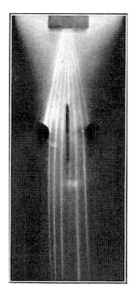
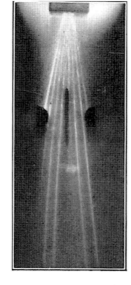
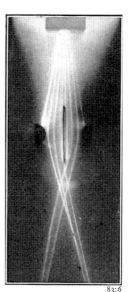

Visualisation of electron beams when manipulated in analogy to optical rays, from the very first report on electron microscopy in 1932.

83:6

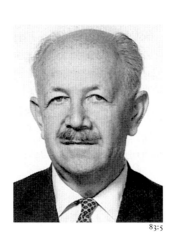

83:5

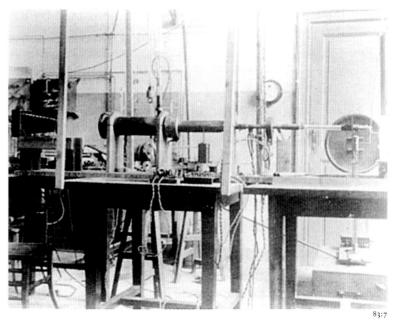

83:7

In 1934 Ladislaus Marton (1901–1979) is the first to use electron microscopy for studying a biological sample. His microscope is shown here, together with the first electron micrograph of a bacteriological specimen obtained by him in 1937.

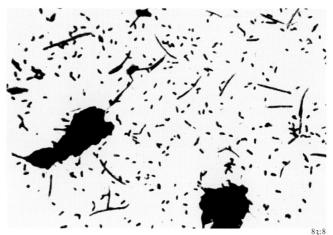

83:8

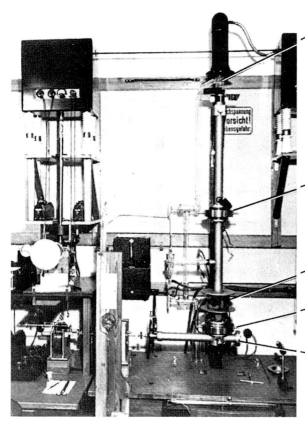

electron directional
radiator
(60 keV)

1. reduction lens

deflection system
(x-y direction)

2. reduction lens

exchangeable electron
collector unit
(e.g. photographic
recording of the image)

83:9

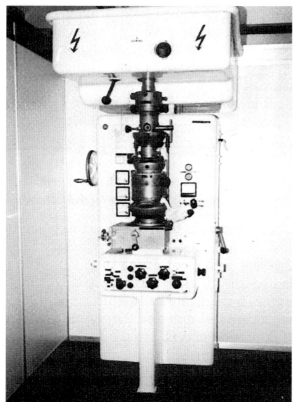

83:10

Manfred von Ardenne (1907–1997)
builds the first scanning transmission
microscope (see top picture) in 1938.
Two years later he takes the first stereo-
scopic images with this instrument.

The first commercial, series-produced
electron microscope is released by
Siemens AG in 1939.

Vladimir Zworykin (1889–1982) invents the scanning electron microscope in 1942. The block diagram and the instruments are shown together with an image obtained showing an etched nickel surface at about 500 Å resolution.

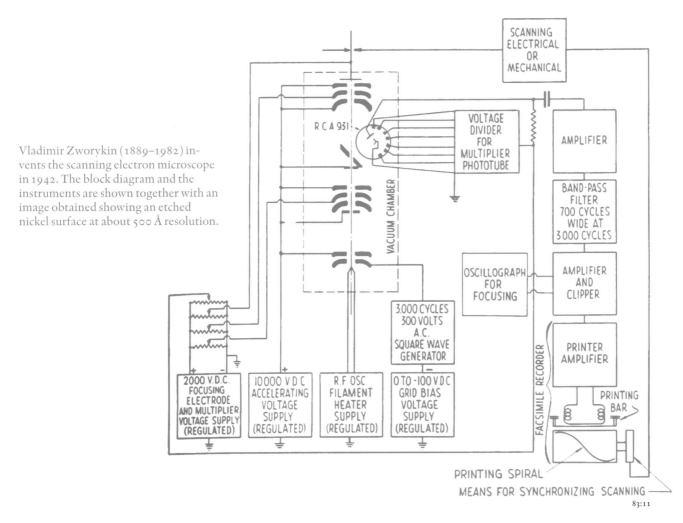

83:11

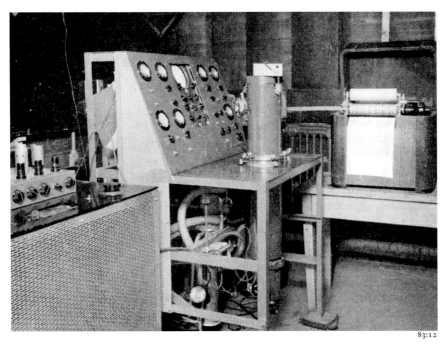

83:12

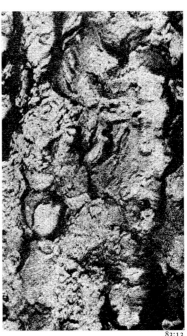

83:13

A major advance in the preparation of bio-medical samples for electron microscopy is the development in the early 1950s of the ultramicrotome technique, which could produce serial ultrathin (20–100 Å) sections of plastic-embedded or frozen samples. The pictures show the device and a cross section view of the photoreceptors from the compound eye of a moth, a difficult sample to prepare.

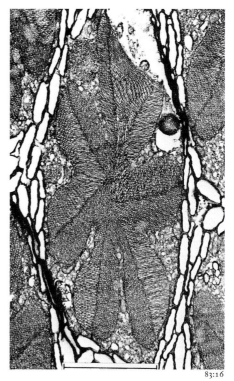

83:16

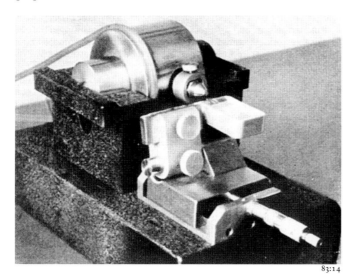

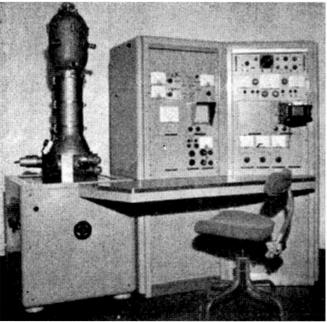

83:14

83:15

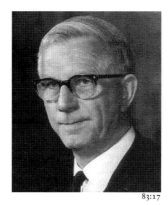

83:17

Charles Oatley (1904–1996) heads a research team in Cambridge that for almost two decades persistently advances the technology of scanning electron microscopy. Their work leads in 1965 to the introduction of the first commercially produced unit, the Stereoscan. The picture shows the prototype of this instrument from 1964.

151. A NEW FORM OF CHROMATOGRAM EMPLOYING TWO LIQUID PHASES

1. A THEORY OF CHROMATOGRAPHY

2. APPLICATION TO THE MICRO-DETERMINATION OF THE HIGHER MONOAMINO-ACIDS IN PROTEINS

By A. J. P. MARTIN AND R. L. M. SYNGE

From the Wool Industries Research Association, Torridon, Headingley, Leeds

(*Received 19 November 1941*)

INTRODUCTION

IN most forms of counter-current extraction column the very small drop required for the rapid attainment of equilibrium, and hence for high efficiencies, cannot be used owing to the difficulty of preventing it moving in the wrong direction. In the case of a solid, however, for any reasonable size of particle a filter will prevent movement in any undesired direction. Consideration of such facts led us to try absorbing water in silica gel etc., and then using the water-saturated solid as one phase of a chromatogram, the other being some fluid immiscible with water, the silica acting merely as mechanical support. Separations in a chromatogram of this type thus depend upon differences in the partition between two liquid phases of the substances to be separated, and not, as in all previously described chromatograms, on differences in adsorption between liquid and solid phases.

The difficulties of using chromatograms are very greatly lessened when the substances to be separated are coloured, or if colourless can be made visible. Various methods have been used for this [cf. Zechmeister & Cholnoky, 1936; Cook, 1941], though none of these was suitable for our problems. As the substances which we desired to separate were acids, and water was one of our phases, we were able to obtain visual evidence of the presence of any of these acids by adding a suitable indicator to the water with which the gel was saturated.

In the present paper we present an approximate theory of chromatographic separations, and describe an application of the new chromatogram to the micro-determination of the higher monoamino-acids in protein hydrolysates. This method is based on the partition of acetamino-acids between chloroform and water phases, and supersedes the macro-method described by us [Martin & Synge, 1941, 1], being rapid and economical both of materials and of apparatus.

Work is in progress, using ethyl acetate as the less polar phase in the chromatogram, on the separation of the acetyl derivatives of most of the other naturally occurring amino-acids, and the method promises also to be of use in analogous separations of simple peptides.

We wish to stress, however, that the possible field of usefulness of the new chromatogram is by no means confined to protein chemistry. By employing suitable phase pairs, many other substances should be separable. Where water is suitable as one of the phases, an indicator may be used to render visible the separation of organic acids or bases. Even where this is not possible, as with

(1358)

MARTIN was born in 1910 in London. He came to Cambridge University in 1929 with the intention of becoming a chemical engineer but eventually specialised in biochemistry. After graduating in 1932, he worked at the Dunn Nutritional Laboratory but left six years later to join Wool Industries Research Association at Leeds. Here, in collaboration with Synge, he developed the method of partition chromatography. Martin was appointed head of the Division of Physical Chemistry at the National Institute of Medical Research in 1952 and in the same year shared the Nobel Prize in Chemistry with Synge. Martin died in 2002.

A New Form of Chromatogram employing Two Liquid Phases.

1. A THEORY OF CHROMATOGRAPHY 2. APPLICATION TO THE MICRO-DETERMINATION OF THE HIGHER MONOAMINO-ACIDS IN PROTEINS. BIOCHEM J 1941; 35:1358.

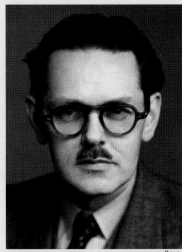

Archer J. P. Martin

84:2

MARTIN AND Synge present a theory of chromatographic separations using the "theoretical plate" concept and show that a chromatogram employing the partition of solutes between two liquid phases, one mobile (chloroform) and one stationary (water), exhibits about a 500 times higher separation efficiency than the best extraction and distillation columns. Silica prepared with methyl-orange in water as column packing is used as the stationary phase for separating monoamino-acids. It is noted that small particle diameter and high pressure over the column increase its efficiency. The general applicability of the method using suitable phase pairs and the fact that "the mobile phase need not be a liquid but may be a vapour" is pointed out.

IN PERSPECTIVE:

Partition chromatography quickly overtook the absorption methods introduced by Tswett (84.1). In paper chromatography, invented in 1944 (84.2), two solvents produce separation in a perpendicular direction on the sheet of a paper that acts as the stationary support. This technique was later replaced by thin-layer chromatography and various forms of electrophoresis (84.3). Size-exclusion chromatography (SEC), where separation is achieved based on molecular size, was introduced in 1959 (84.4) and is still an important technique. Specific interactions between biochemical compounds or between specific ions are the bases of affinity and ion exchange chromatography (IEC) (84.5). New packing materials and higher column pressures (a favourable design already suggested in the work cited above) led to high-performance liquid chromatography (HPLC) (84.6). Gas-liquid chromatography (GLC), also suggested in the original publication, was first announced by Martin in his Nobel Lecture (84.7). It is now among the most widely-used analytical techniques in the world. GLC with support coated open tubular (SCOT) capillary columns (84.8) provides very high separation efficiencies in small volumes. Gas chromatography and liquid chromatography, in combination with mass spectrometry or infrared spectroscopy, offer powerful techniques for the separation and identification of biomedical substances and molecules (84.9).

84.1 See #73 Tswett page 376.
84.2 Consden R, Gordon AH, Martin AJP. Quantitative Analysis of Proteins: A Partition Chromatographic Method Using Paper. *Biochem J* 1944; 38:224. See also ref. 73.5, ref. 73.6, and ref. 73.7.
84.3 Ettre LS, Kalász H. *The Story of Thin-layer Chromatography*. LC*GC North America 2001; 19:712.
84.4 Porath J, Flodin P. Gel filtration: A method for desalting and group separation. *Nature* 1959; 183:1657.
84.5 Sanger F. *The chemistry of insulin*. Nobel Lecture Stockholm; 1958. for the importance of IEC and paper chromatography in the determination of the amino acid sequence of insulin.
84.6 Ettre LS. Evolution of Liquid Chromatography: A Historical Overview. In: Horváth C. editor. *High-Performance Liquid Chromatography* Vol. I. New York: Academic Press; 1980.
84.7 Martin AJP. *The development of partition chromatography*. Nobel Lecture Stockholm; 1952.
84.8 Bente PF, Zenner EH, Dandeneau RD. *Silica chromatographic column*. US Patent 4,293,415 1981.
84.9 *A Century of Separation Science*. Issaq HJ. editor. New York: M.Dekker; 2002. See also #79 Aston page 406 and #97 Wagner-West page 504.

Qualitative Analysis of Proteins: a Partition Chromatographic Method Using Paper

By R. CONSDEN, A. H. GORDON AND A. J. P. MARTIN, *Wool Industries Research Association, Torridon, Headingley, Leeds*, 6

(*Received* 13 *May* 1944)

Gordon, Martin & Synge (1943*b*) attempted to separate amino-acids on a silica gel partition chromatogram, but found it impracticable owing to adsorption by the silica of various amino-acids.

They obtained, however, good separations by using cellulose in the form of strips of filter paper. Following further work along these lines, the present paper describes a qualitative micro-analytical technique for proteins. Using only 200 μg. of wool, it is possible by this method to demonstrate the presence of all the amino-acids which have been shown to be there by other methods.

The method is rather similar to the 'capillary analysis' method of Schönbein and Goppelsroeder (reviewed by Rheinboldt, 1925) except that the separation depends on the differences in partition coefficient between the mobile phase and water-saturated cellulose, instead of differences in adsorption by the cellulose. That adsorption of the amino-acids by the cellulose plays no significant part is seen from Table 1, where the partition coefficient calculated from the rates of movement of the bands are compared with those found directly by England & Cohn (1935). Too much stress should not be laid upon the agreement of these figures, which are based upon an assumed water content of the saturated cellulose and the assumption that the ratio of the weight of *n*-butanol to paper is constant in all parts of the strip. This assumption does not hold accurately. Nevertheless, the conclusion seems justified that the cellulose is playing the role of an inert support.

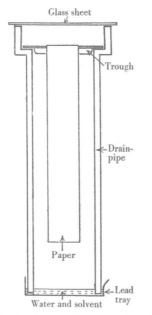

Fig. 3. Elevation of small trough in drain-pipe. 84:3

84:4

Two-dimensional chromatogram of a wool hydrolysate (180 μg.) on Whatman no. 1 sheet. Hydrolysate applied at circle. Run with collidine for 3 days in direction AB, then in direction AC with phenol for 27 hr. in an atmosphere of coal gas and NH_3 (produced from a 0·3 % NH_3 solution). The filter employed in photographing renders the yellow proline spot scarcely visible. (Photography by J. Manby, photographer to the University of Leeds.)

84:4

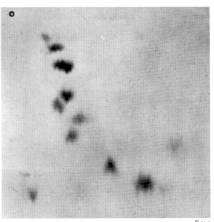

84:4

This paper from 1944 presents the modern technique of paper chromatography. The illustrations show an example of its use and a drawing of the simple apparatus employed. Paper chromatography has subsequently played a significant role in the progress of molecular biology, i.e. in the determination of the amino acid sequence of insulin. For more information on the work of Schönbein and Goppelsroeder mentioned in the introductory section of the paper, see #73 and #77.

436

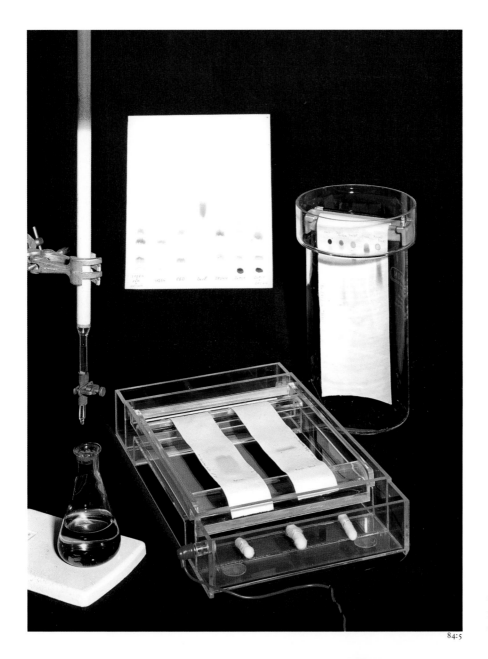

84:5

Chromatographic apparatus, including paper chromatographic equipment from the late 1940s.

Martin recognises, back in 1941, that gas can be used to great advantage as the mobile phase in chromatography. However, serious work is first described, quite casually, in his Nobel Lecture of 1952. The picture shows a gaschromatograph from the early 1960s.

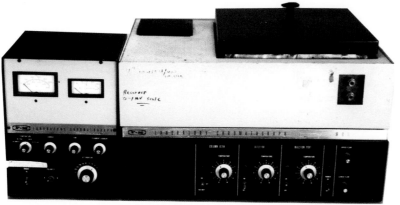

84:6

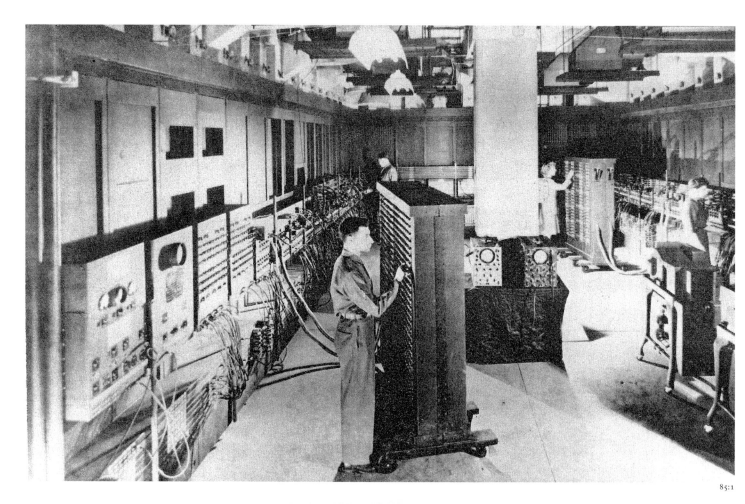

The ENIAC (electronic numerical integrator and computer) is built in 1945 by John Presper Eckert (1919–1995) and John William Mauchly (1907–1980). It is the first large-scale general-purpose electronic digital computer. Weighting 30 tons and consuming 170 kW energy, the machin makes 5,000 additions and 300 multiplications per second. As is shown by the two photographs, the program is set up using a table on wheels that is pushed around in the room.

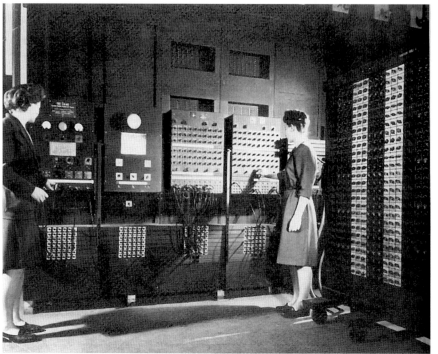

ECKERT was born in 1919 in Philadelphia. He graduated in 1941 from the Moore School of Electrical Engineering at the University of Pennsylvania. While teaching there he met and became friends with Mauchly. Mauchly, a physicist who was born in Cincinnati in 1907, had an interest in weather forecasting and was looking to improve the capacity of calculators. He wrote a proposal for a superior electronic computer (85.1) and, with the financial support of the US Army, he and Eckert were able to complete the ENIAC (Electronic Integrator and Computer) in 1946. In 1948 they started up the Eckert-Mauchly Computer Corporation, which produced the first UNIVAC (Universal Automatic Computer) machine in 1951. After selling the company, both men worked as directors in the computer industry they had founded. Mauchly died in 1980, with Eckert surviving him by fifteen years.

Description of the ENIAC and Comments on Electronic Digital Computing Machines.

NATIONAL DEFENSE RESEARCH COMMITTEE 1945.

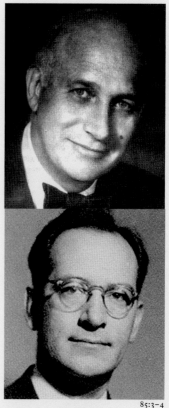

85:3–4

John Presper Eckert
John William Mauchly

THIS FIRST presentation of the ENIAC is co-authored by Brainerd, the project administrator, and Goldstein, the military mentor of the project. While Mauchly contributes the overall design philosophy, it is Eckert's engineering skills, along with his insistence on a wide margin of error for each component and on a modular design, which achieve sufficient reliability of function. Out of a total of almost 18,000 vacuum tubes, on average only 20 fail each day and these can be quickly found and replaced. The ENIAC weighs 30 tons and consumes 170 kW of energy. The program is set on switches and the machine carries out 5,000 additions and 300 multiplications per second.

IN PERSPECTIVE:
Schikard described a mechanical calculator in 1623, but Pascal built the first device, which is still extant (85.2). In 1703 Leibniz introduced binary arithmetics (85.3) and in 1854 Boole developed the two-valued algebra used today in all computer programming (85.4). At bout the same time Babbage conceived an "analytical engine" (85.5)(85.6) with many features of modern computers, but it took another century before Zuse, Stibitz and Aiken built the first programmable electromechanical computers (85.6)(85.7). Remarkably, the ENIAC remained in use for ten years, even though the UNIVAC was already about 20 times faster. In 1948 Bardeen and Brattain invented the transistor (85.8) and a decade later Kilby and Noyce designed the first integrated circuit (85.9). When Intel introduced the 4004 microprocessor chip in 1971, a computation power similar to the ENIAC was placed on a 5 mm² surface. Multi-channel cochlear implants (85.10) and artificial vision systems (85.11) are just two recent examples where advanced microelectronics and software provide help to the sensorily impaired patient.

85.1 Mauchly JW. The use of high speed vacuum tube devices for calculating. In: *The Origins of digital Computers: Selected Papers*. Randell B. editor. Berlin: Springer; 1973. p329.

85.2 Pascal B. *Oeuvres* 5 vols. 1779. Machine Arithmétique. Vol.4 1645. p7.

85.3 Leibniz GW. *Opera Omnia* 6 vols. 1768. Explication de l'arithmétique binaire. Vol. III 1703. p390.

85.4 Boole G. *An investigation of the laws of thought, on which are founded the mathematical theories of logic and probabilities.* London; 1854.

85.5 Menabrea LF. *Sketch of the Analytical Engine invented by Charles Babbage.* London; 1843.

85.6 Hooke DH, Norman JM. *Origins of Cyberspace. A Library on the History of Computing, Networking, and Telecommunications.* Novato: historyofscience.com; 2001.

85.7 Ref. 85.6 presents the genealogy of the first general-pupose programmable digital computers, as well as much other useful historic material up to 1990.

85.8 Bardeen J, Brattain WH. The Transistor, A Semi-Conductor Triode. *Phys Rev* 1948; 74 (2):230.

85.9 Kilby JS. Turning potential into realities: *The invention of the integrated circuit.* Nobel Lecture Stockholm; 2000.

85.10 Clark GM. Cochlear implants in the third millennium. *Am J Otol* 1999; 20:4.

85.11 Dobelle WmH. Artificial Vision for the Blind by Connecting a Television Camera to the Visual Cortex. *ASAIO J* 2000; 46:3.

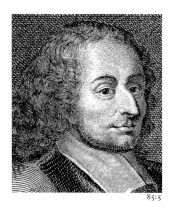

85:5

The first mechanical calculator was designed by Wilhelm Schickard (1592–1635) around 1623, but the first device still extant today was built by Blaise Pascal (1623–1662) in 1645. Pascal's portrait and his drawing of the calculator are shown.

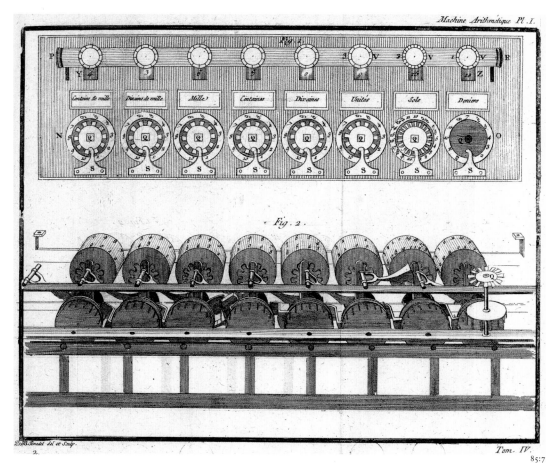

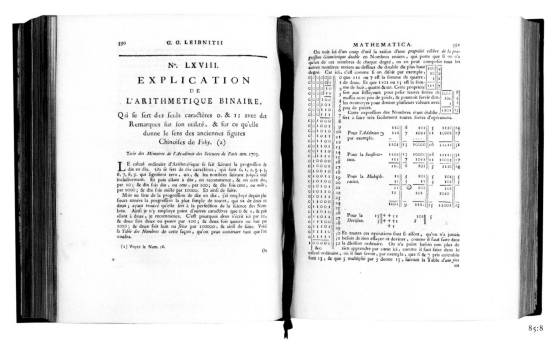

85:7

Wilhelm Leibniz (1646–1716) not only invents a mechanical calculator for multiplication, he also conceives differential calculus and in 1703 introduces binary arithmetic, the foundation of all calculations performed by modern computers. The first pages of this pioneering publication are reproduced here.

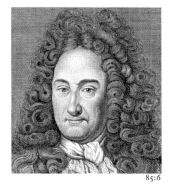

85:6

85:8

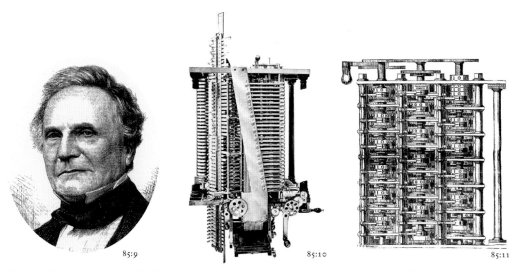

85:9   85:10   85:11

During the 1830s Charles Babbage (1791–1871) builds mechanical calculators with structure and concepts remarkably similar to modern computers. Only parts of his designs have survived for posterity. The picture on the right shows a portion of his Difference Engine I from 1832 and the picture in the middle depicts a model of the mill and the printing parts of his Analytical Engine from the late 1830s.

Helmut Schreyer (1912–1984) and Konrad Zuse (1910–1975) are shown in this picture while working on the Z1 computer in 1936. The Z1 is an electro-mechanical device and the world's first digital computer.

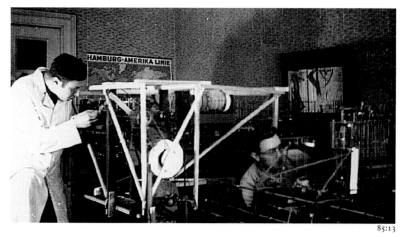

85:13

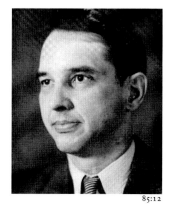

85:12

Around 1940 John Atanasoff (1903–1995) builds an electronic digital computer. The device is never fully operational but influences Mauchly when he designs the structure of the ENIAC.

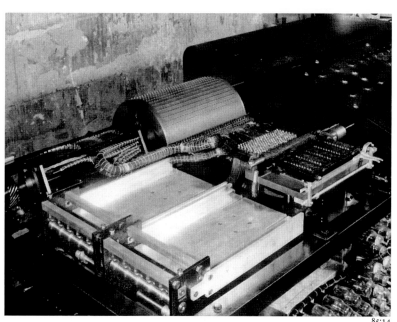

85:14

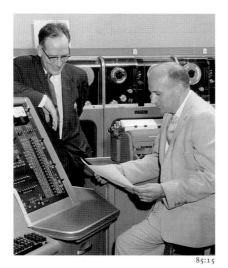

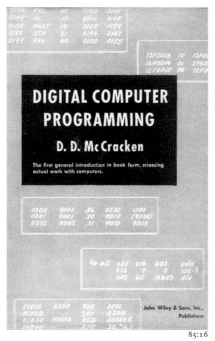

The Transistor,
A Semi-Conductor Triode

J. BARDEEN AND W. H. BRATTAIN

Bell Telephone Laboratories, Murray Hill, New Jersey
June 25, 1948

A THREE–ELEMENT electronic device which util-
izes a newly discovered principle involving a semi-
conductor as the basic element is described. It may be
employed as an amplifier, oscillator, and for other purposes for which vacuum tubes are ordinarily used. The
device consists of three electrodes placed on a block of
germanium[1] as shown schematically in Fig. 1. Two, called
the emitter and collector, are of the point-contact rectifier
type and are placed in close proximity (separation $\sim$.005
to .025 cm) on the upper surface. The third is a large area
low resistance contact on the base.

The germanium is prepared in the same way as that
used for high back-voltage rectifiers.[2] In this form it is an
N-type or excess semi-conductor with a resistivity of the
order of 10 ohm cm. In the original studies, the upper surface was subjected to an additional anodic oxidation in a
glycol borate solution[3] after it had been ground and etched
in the usual way. The oxide is washed off and plays no
direct role. It has since been found that other surface
treatments are equally effective. Both tungsten and phos-
phor bronze points have been used. The collector point
may be electrically formed by passing large currents in the
reverse direction.

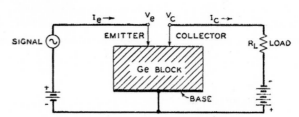

FIG. 1. Schematic of semi-conductor triode.

Mauchly (left) and Eckert at the console of a UNIVAC
I machine. The UNIVAC (universal automatic computer) is about twenty times faster than the ENIAC.
It is introduced in 1951 by Eckert and Mauchly's Electronic Control Company.

The first book from 1957, giving a general introduction to computer programming.

The beginning of the famous paper of John Bardeen
(1908–1991) and Walter Brattain (1902–1987)
reporting the invention of the transistor.

The first integrated circuit is built by Jack Kilby a
decade after the invention of the transistor. It is an
electronic oscillator system about 1.5×11 mm in size.

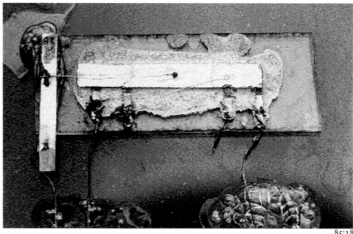

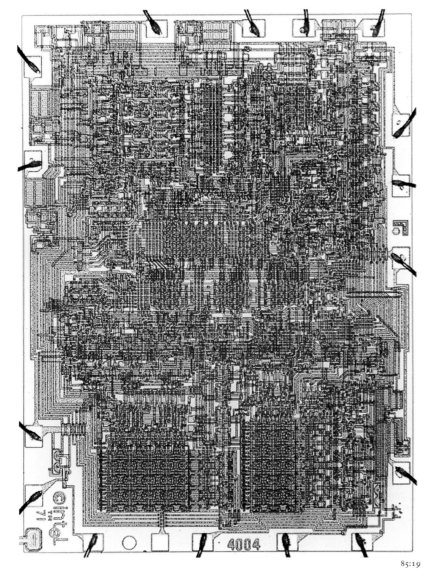

85:19

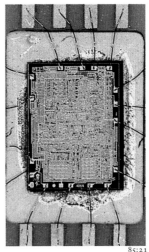

85:21

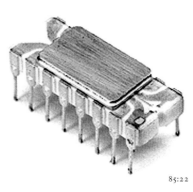

85:22

The circuitry (in two different magnifications) of the Intel 4004, the first microprocessor chip produced. When introduced in 1971 this central processing unit places a computation power similar to the ENIAC on a 5 mm² surface.

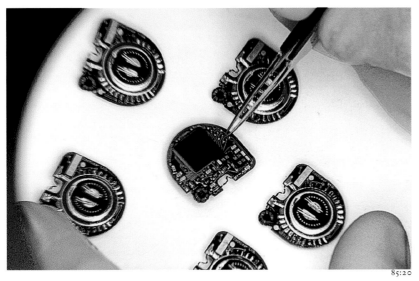

85:20

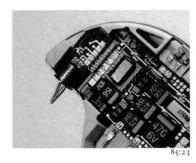

85:23

Two applications exemplifying the uses of microelectronics and microprocessors in modern medicine. Left, the microelectronic part of a sophisticated cochlear implant hearing aid and on the right, part of the electronics in an advanced pacemaker for cardiac support.

DE
KUNSTMATIGE
NIER

W. J. KOLFF

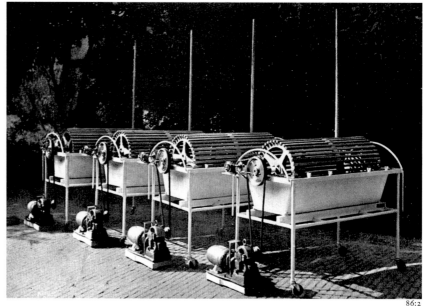

86:1

86:2

The title page of Willem Kolff's thesis, where he describes in detail the construction and use of a new large surface area artificial kidney. The illustrations show the principle of operation of the apparatus and a photograph of the first units built. Using cellophane tubing wound around a rotating drum that is partially immersed in dialysing fluid, Kolff treats fifteen patients. Although all of them die as a result of uraemia, the equipment and the procedure are soon acknowledged as a major advance.

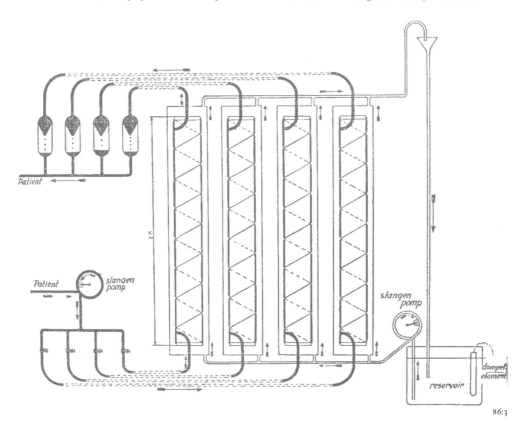

86:3

KOLFF was born in Leiden in 1911 and decided to follow in his father's footsteps and become a physician. After receiving his M.D. from the University of Leiden in 1938 he started postgraduate work at the University of Groningen but in 1940, when the Netherlands was occupied, he moved to the municipal hospital of Kampen, where he developed the first crude artificial kidney in 1943 (86.1). He received his Ph.D. in 1946 on the thesis cited below and joined the research staff of the Cleveland Clinic Foundation in 1950. Kolff moved to the University of Utah in 1967, where he was appointed professor of surgery and director of the Institute of Biomedical Engineering, a position he held until his retirement in 1986.

De Kunstmatige Nier.

KAMPEN: DRUKKERIJ KOK JH; 1946.

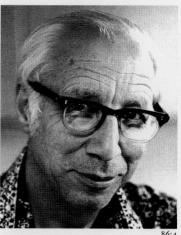

Willem Johan Kolff
86:4

KOLFF'S THESIS presents in some detail the design of the artificial kidney and gives case reports for the first fifteen patients treated between March 1943 and July 1944. The dialysis machine is made up of cellophane tubings wound around a rotating drum that is partially immersed in a dialysing fluid. Among the problems encountered are bleeding due to the administration of heparin, difficulties in cannulating the patients, maintaining undamaged vessels and restoring the proper electrolyte balance. The deaths (all patients died) are reported to be a consequence of uraemia and not due to the dialysis procedure.

IN PERSPECTIVE:

Kolff's work was based on Abel's "vividifusion" technique from 1913 (86.2), the discovery in 1908 and subsequent development of the cellophane membrane (86.3) and the new anticoagulant, heparin (86.4). Kolff's dialyser machine proved a success and led to renewed interest in peritoneal lavage (86.5), a technique for treating uraemia that first became viable in the 1980s, when newly designed peritoneal catheters could be left permanently in place. Today both synthetic and cellulose-based membranes are available for tailoring haemodialysis therapy (86.6) and heparin levels can be accurately controlled. Gibbon performed the first open heart surgery in 1953, but as early as 1938 he used membrane technology to oxygenate venous blood (86.7). More recently, extracorporeal membrane oxygenation (ECMO) has been introduced as a cardiopulmonary support, primarily in neonatal intensive care units (86.8). Kolff was instrumental in the development of heart-lung machines (86.9), circulation assist devices (86.10) and the Jarvik-7 artificial heart (86.11)(86.12), which was first implanted into a human in 1982. Today kidney and heart transplants are attractive alternatives to the use of artificial organs for treating severe renal or circulatory failure.

86.1 Kolff WJ, Berk HJ. The Artificial Kidney: A Dialyzer with a Great Area. *Acta med Scand* 1944; 117:121.

86.2 See #77 Abel page 396 particularly ref. 77.9. Also ref. 63.3, ref. 63.4 and ref. 46.8.

86.3 Charch DH. *Moistureproof Material*. US Patent 1,737,187 1929. (Filed 1927)

86.4 Murray DWG, et al. Heparin and the thrombosis of veins following injury. *Surgery* 1937; 2:163.

86.5 Kolff WJ. *New Ways of Treating Uraemia*. London: J & A Churchill Ltd; 1947.

86.6 Cheung AK, Leypoldt JK. The Hemodialysis Membranes: A Historical Perspective, Current State, and future Prospect. *Seminars in Nephrology*. 1997; 17(3):196.

86.7 Gibbon JH. An oxygenator with a large surface-volume ratio. *J Lab Clin Med* 1939; 24:1192.

86.8 Bartlett RH, et al. Exctracorporeal membrane oxygenation (ECMO) cardiopulmonary support in infancy. *Trans Am Soc Artif Intern Organs* 1976; 22:80.

86.9 Dubbleman CP. Attempts to Design an Artificial Heart-Lung Apparatus for the Human Adult (thesis). *Acta Physiol Parm Neerlandica* 1953; 2:1.

86.10 Kolff WJ. *Artificial Organs*. New York: John Wiley & Sons; 1976.

86.11 Jarvik RK. The Total Artificial Heart. *Scientific American* 1981; 244 (1):74.

86.12 Kolff WJ. The Artificial Heart. *Encyclopedia of Human Biology*. Vol.I Academic Press Inc; 1991. p386.

Nils Alwall (1904–1986) starts the first clinic specialised in dialysis in 1947. He pioneers the ultrafiltration technique and introduces the principle of hemofiltration. The picture on the right shows him at work in around 1960. Five years later he invents the plate dialyser, which in 1972 leads to the introduction of the first all-plastic disposable dialyser unit (shown below).

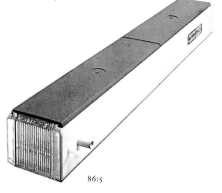

86:5

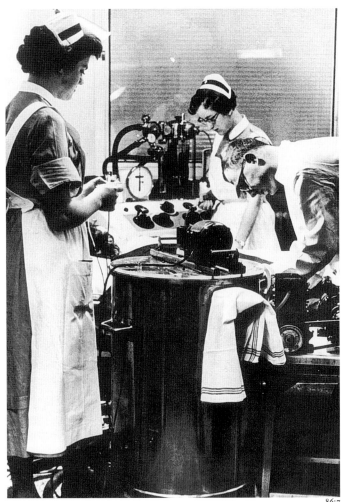

86:7

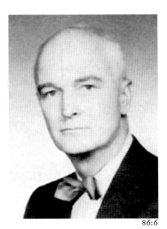

86:6

John Gibbon (1903–1973) develops the first efficient artificial oxygenator in 1938. The device shown here is his second design, which has a large surface-volume ratio.

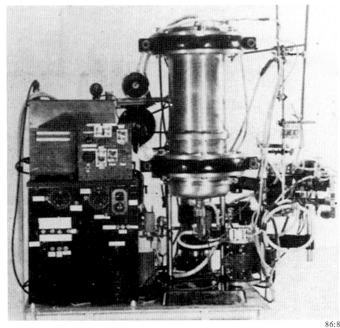

86:8

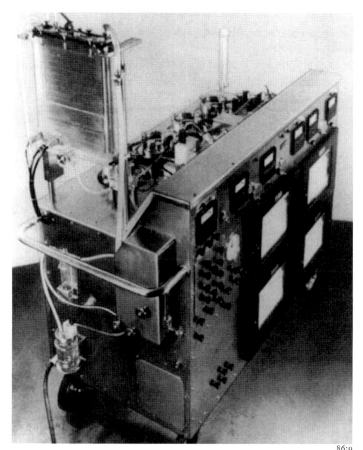

86:9

Gibbon also pioneers the development of heart-lung machines. In 1949 he designs the first prototype unit, which is then built by IBM Corp. His second apparatus, shown in the photographs, is successfully used at the first heart bypass surgery that takes place on 6 May 1953. The picture below left is taken on this occasion.

A heart-lung machine from the late 1950s constructed by Dennis Melrose, who in 1955 introduces a method of injecting potassium citrate and then potassium chloride to stop the beating of the heart, thereby greatly facilitating the work of the surgeon.

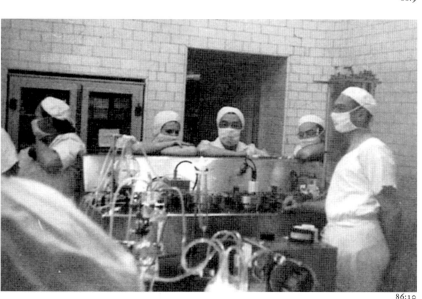

86:10

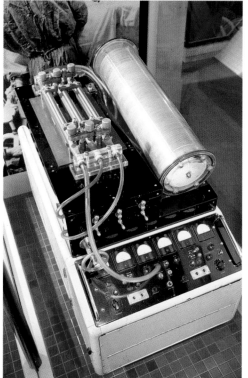

86:11

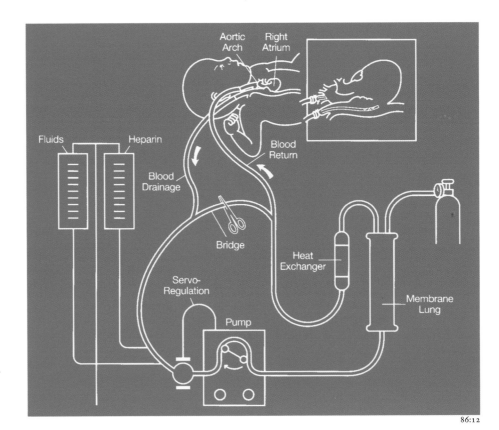

The principle of an ECMO (extra corporeal membrane oxygenation) procedure and a photograph (taken 1981) showing the original clinical implementation. The method is introduced in 1975 by Robert Bartlett for the temporary treatment of neonates with lungs unable to provide gas exchange adequately.

86:12

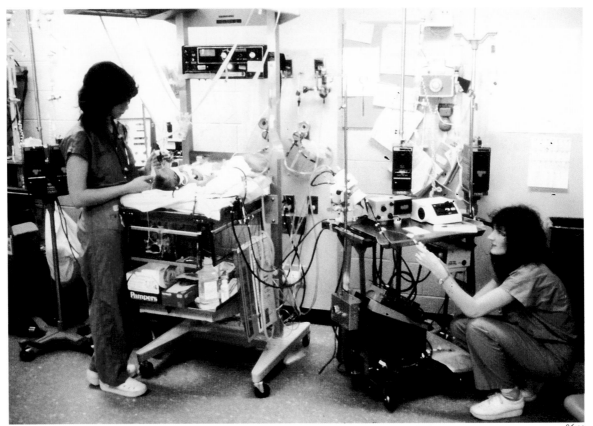

86:13

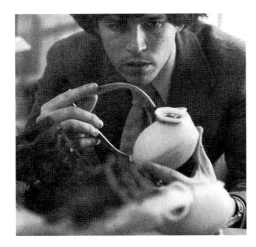

86:14

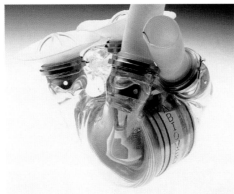

86:15

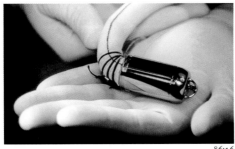

86:16

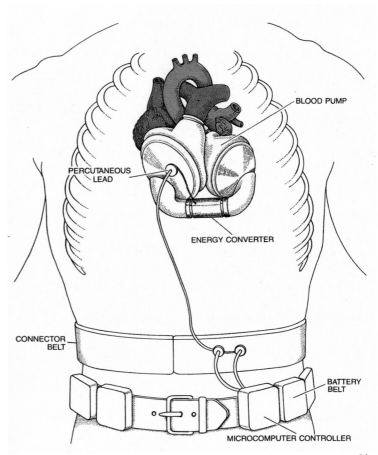

BLOOD PUMP

PERCUTANEOUS LEAD

ENERGY CONVERTER

CONNECTOR BELT

BATTERY BELT

MICROCOMPUTER CONTROLLER

86:17

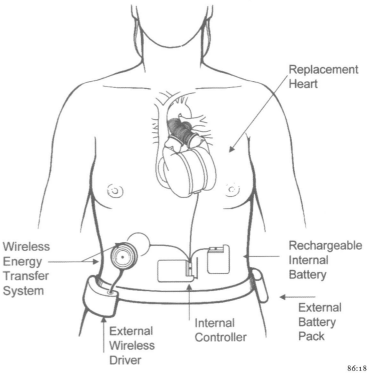

Replacement Heart

Wireless Energy Transfer System

Rechargeable Internal Battery

External Battery Pack

External Wireless Driver

Internal Controller

86:18

Robert Jarvik with his prototype artificial heart in 1973. In 1981, one year before his Jarvik-7 artificial heart was implanted into a human, Jarvik proposes a prospective artificial heart system shown by the drawing (upper right). His idea can be compared to a recent experimental device, the AbioCor artificial heart, shown in the middle picture and to the principle of its use explained by the diagram (right). The Jarvik 2000 device held in a hand is an experimental electrically powered axial flow pump, to be placed in the left ventricle as a bridge to subsequent transplant surgery.

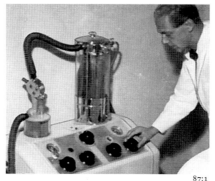

87:1

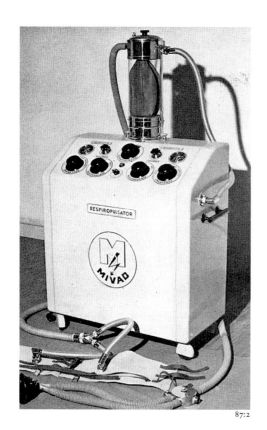

87:2

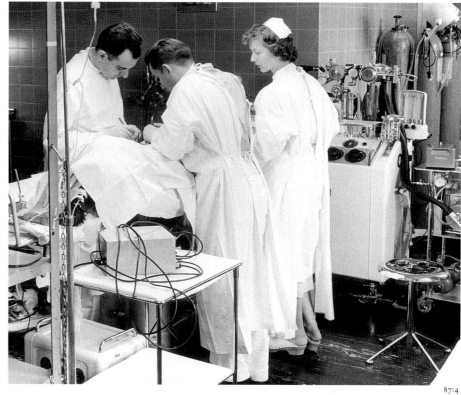

87:4

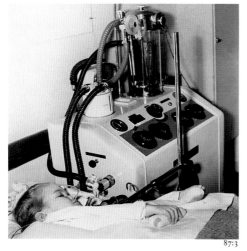

87:3

In 1950 Carl-Gunnar Engström (1912–1987) invents a respirator that allows efficient control of the gas volume delivered to the patient and also allows for active exhalation. It can be used both for adults and children and it is the first apparatus suitable for long-term ventilation as well as for use during anaesthesia. The device is introduced internationally in Copenhagen in 1951 and soon plays a major role when combating the severe polio epidemic that erupts in Denmark a year later. The photographs show Engström adjusting one of the first production units, the device in use on a child and in the operating room.

Carl-Gunnar Engström

ENGSTRÖM was born in Oskarshamn in 1912. After studying at Karolinska Institutet, he received his M.D. in 1941 and started to work at Epidemisjukhuset in Stockholm. While treating a patient suffering from poliomyelitis, he recognised the advantage of providing controlled insufflation volume and active expiration and designed a new respirator to achieve these objectives (87.1). Engström became convinced, through frequent blood gas analysis, that respiratory insufficiency was also a major problem (87.2) in diseases of other aetiology than poliomyelitis. His respirator came to good use in 1952, when a major polio epidemic erupted in Denmark (87.3). Engström's pioneering work on the use of ventilators in thoracic surgery and in intensive care is summed up in his thesis from 1963 (87.4).

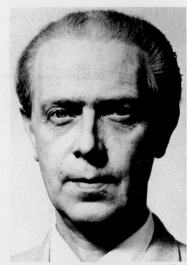

Carl-Gunnar Engström   87:5

Treatment of Bulbar Poliomyelitis by Special Postural Drainage.

THE SECOND INTERNATIONAL POLIOMYELITIS CONFERENCE COPENHAGEN 1951. PHILADELPHIA: J. B. LIPPINCOTT CO.; 1952. P429.

ENGSTRÖM INTRODUCES his new respirator by stating in the conclusion of this paper: "In order to make it possible to apply the suggested prone postural drainage in cases of bulbar poliomyelitis accompanied by respiratory paralysis, a new aggregate for artificial respiration also applicable to the prone position was constructed. This unit gives active exhalation but also can be synchronised to give active inhalation by the use of a face mask or a tracheal cannula."

IN PERSPECTIVE:
In 1543, Vesalius performed the first intubation, followed by artificial ventilation of a sow (87.5). Subsequently, respiration experiments were made primarily to clarify the physiology of breathing but later also to develop resuscitation techniques and to improve the delivery of inhalation anaesthetics (87.5). The risk of overdistending the lungs with excessive pressure was soon recognised (87.6) and devices were developed that instead produced a negative pressure around the whole body (iron lungs) (87.7)(87.8) or just around the thorax (cuirass ventilators) (87.9). In a paper following the one cited above, Engström and Svanborg report clinical cases showing how inadequate cuirass respirators could be for polio patients (87.2). Controlled volume positive pressure respirators also enabled the first prolonged treatment of patients with serious lung impairment (87.10). Mechanical respirators were able to provide some information on lung physiology (87.4)(87.10), but it was with the introduction in the 1970s of ventilators with electronic control (87.11) that these features could be clinically exploited. Today more than a hundred thousand ventilators are in use, many with advanced breathing modalities and some providing information on lung mechanics and, together with gas analysers, on the efficiency of the gas-exchange process.

87.1 Engström C-G. *Dubbelverkande respirator.* Svensk Patent 141554 1953. (Filed 1950).
87.2 Engström C-G, Svanborg NA. *The Importance of CO$_2$ Retension by Respiratory Insufficiency Caused by Poliomyelitis.* Same reference as the landmark paper cited p431.
87.3 Lassen HCA. *Management of Life-Threatening Poliomyelitis* Copenhagen 1952–1956. London: E & S Livinstone Ltd.; 1956. See also ref. 14.8 Chap. XVII.
87.4 Engström C-G. The clinical application of prolonged controlled ventilation: with special reference to a method developed by the author. *Acta Anaesth Scand* Suppl 13 1963.
87.5 See ref. 1.6 Liber VII (the last two pages) also #11 Hooke page 72, #23 Kite page 128, #47 Snow page 248 and #57 Trendelenburg page 294 and references 57.9–57.11.
87.6 Leroy D'Etoilles JJJ. Reserches sur l'asphyxie. *J Physiol* 1827; 7:45.
87.7 Woillez E. Sur le spirophore, appareil de sauvetage pour les asphyxiés principalement pour les noyés et les enfants nouveaunés. *C R Acad Sci* 1876; 82:1447. Also see *Scientific American* 1876; XXXV(25).
87.8 Drinker P, Shaw LA. An apparatus for prolonged administration of artificial respiration. I. A design for adults and children. *J Clin Invest* 1929; 7:229.
87.9 Eisenmenger R. Therapeutic application of supra-abdominal suction and compressed air in relation to respiration and circulation. *Wien med Wochenschr* 1939; 89:1032.
87.10 Norlander OP. The use of respirators in anaesthesia and surgery. *Acta Anaesth Scand* Suppl 30 1968.
87.11 Nordström L. On automatic ventilation. *Acta Anaesth Scand* Suppl 47 1972.

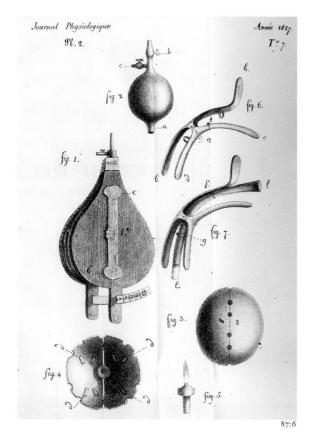

In 1827 Jean Leroy d'Etoilles (1798–1860), recognising the risks associated with high pressure in the lungs, constructs a bellows that can limit the pressure produced during artificial ventilation.

The "iron lung" concept of ventilation is introduced in 1876 by Eugéne Woillez (1811–1882). The device, the "Spirophore", creates a negative pressure (suction) around the body, reducing the risk of overdistending the lungs. An interesting feature of the device (see the announcement reproduced from the Scientific American magazine from the same year) is a rod that is resting on the chest of the patient to indicate its movements and thereby the efficiency of the ventilation provided.

Scientific American.

chest, the walls of which are seen to rise as in normal life. The ribs separate, the sternum is pushed up 0·393 inch at least (indicated by the movable rod which rests on it). Further, the epigastrum, and even the abdomen below, present an inspiratory projection, which shows that the enlargement of the chest is effected during this artificial inspiration not merely by the raising of the ribs and the sternum, but also

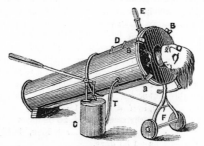

by the descent of the diaphragm. All returns to the former position when the lever is raised again. These complete respiratory movements may be repeated fifteen to eighteen times in a minute, as in a living man.

By means of a tube fixed into the windpipe of the body, and communicating with a graduated reservoir of air over a vessel of water, M. Woillez has measured the quantity of air which thus penetrates into the chest at each pressure of the lever. He finds that this is, on an average, 1¾ pints; whereas the physiological average is only $\frac{7}{10}$ pint. More than 22 gallons of air can be made to traverse the lungs of the asphyxiated person in ten minutes.

It is easy, then, to see the advantages presented by this apparatus for treatment of the asphyxiated, especially drowning persons and new born infants. In all cases of asphyxia by vitiated or insufficient air, or by certain poisonings, in paralysis of the respiratory muscles, in most dysphoric affections, in asphyxia by bronchial mucosities, and that due to inhalations of chloroform, and lastly, in determining some cases of apparent death, the spirophore may be used to produce an efficacious artificial respiration.

This respiration is without danger to the lungs, which are not liable to rupture, however strong the action of the lever. This innocuity is due to the fact that the force of penetration of the air into the lungs is never superior in this case (as also in the case of normal life) to the weight of the atmosphere.

THE SPIROPHORE.

This apparatus was recently described to the Paris Academy by M. Woillez. It is for restoring asphyxiated persons, especially such as have been in danger of drowning, and new born infants. We are indebted to the *Journal de Pharmacie et de Chimie* for the annexed engraving of the apparatus. It consists of a cylinder of sheet iron closed at one end and open at the other. The case is large enough to receive the body to be treated, which is let down into it as far as the head, which remains outside. A tightly fitting diaphragm closes the aperture about the neck. A strong air pump, C, containing more than four and a half gallons of air, is situated outside of the case, and communicates with it by a thick tube, T. It is worked by means of a lever, the descent of which produces aspiration of the air confined about the body. The raising of the lever again restores the abstracted air to the case. A transparent piece of glass, D, on the upper part of the cylinder enables one to see the chest and abdomen of the patient, and a movable rod, E, sliding in a vertical tube, is made to rest on the sternum.

M. Woillez states that he has made several experiments with the apparatus, the general results of which are as follows: When a human body is inclosed as described, and the lever quickly lowered, a vacuum is produced round the body, and immediately the external air penetrates into the

The Importance of CO_2 Retention by Respiratory Insufficiency Caused by Poliomyelitis

C.-G. ENGSTRÖM, M.D., and N. A. SVANBORG, M.D.

What ought to be stressed especially are those cases of respiratory paralysis where by the given methods we have stated hypoventilation and CO_2 retention with a successive deterioration of the general condition, which deterioration was neutralized by change of respirator. Theoretically it might be indicated to try an alkali therapy in order to bring these patients through a critical stage of the disease.

In these cases we first used a cuirass (Freiberger type) respirator, which was changed to a Sahlin type respirator if underventilation occurred. In some cases none of the respirators gave sufficient ventilation. The cuirass respirator, which in chronic cases usually gives sufficient ventilation often has been unsuitable for acute cases.

Interpretations of the signs in the charts:
General condition:
    uninfluenced: —
    slightly influenced: +
    moderately influenced: ++
    strongly influenced: +++
Patient moribund: m
Respirator I = type Freiberger (cuirass type)
Respirator II = type Sahlin

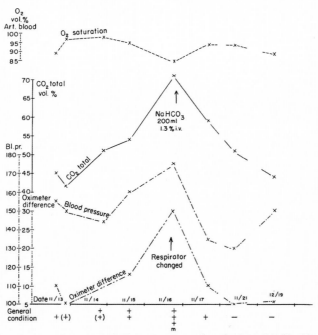

Chart 1. Girl, 17 years old, previously sound; 11/10/1950 fell ill with poliomyelitis with comparatively slow proceeding respiratory paralysis; 11/13 bad diaphragm and thorax breathing in afternoon. Rising blood pressure. She was given extra O_2 by Radnor catheter and was placed in a Freiberger respirator. General condition at first better, but then deterioration in the following days. On 11/16 the patient was in a coma and in the afternoon considered moribund. Patient was removed to another respirator (Sahlin type) and after a while was given NaHCO-200 ml. 1.3%-solution intravenous. Within a couple of hours the general condition was obviously better. Afterwards successively proceeding recovery; 11/18 uninfluenced, clear and lucid. Blood pressure satisfactory. Continuing good general condition. Pulmonary x-ray 11/16 satisfactory. Electrocardiogram 11/13 satisfactory.

Clinical cases of poliomyelitis, monitored with regular blood gas determinations, make Engström realise that carbon dioxide retention is also a major problem in diseases of other aetiology. He also finds (see part of his scientific exhibit from 1951 shown) that the cuirass type of ventilator (similar to iron lungs but only covering the thorax) often fails to provide adequate carbon dioxide elimination. These observations soon lead not only to his improved mechanical ventilator, but also to new technologies for blood gas determinations that can be used in routine clinical work (see #81).

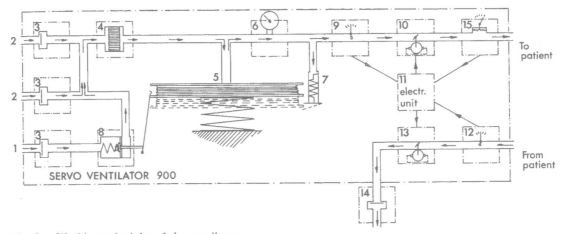

Fig. 2.—Working principles of the ventilator.

1. Air intake from a high pressure source
2. Gas intake from flow regulating devices
3. One way valve
4. Gas filter
5. Springloaded bellows
6. Manometer measuring pressure in the bellows
7. Excess and safety valve
8. "On demand" valve
9. Inspiratory flow-meter
10. Inspiratory choke valve
11. Electronic unit
12. Expiratory flow-meter
13. Expiratory choke valve
14. One way valve
15. Electronic pressure meter, measuring airway pressure

87:9

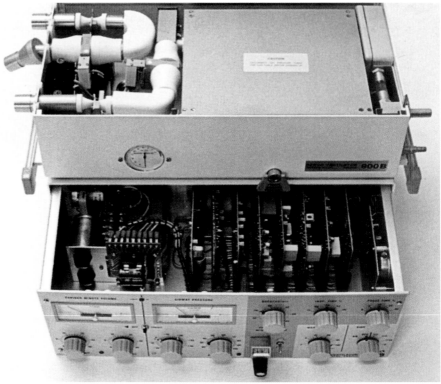

87:10

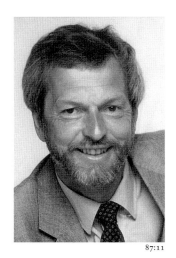

87:11

In 1971 Sven-Gunnar Olson introduces the first electrically controlled ventilator (the Servo Ventilator 900). The illustrations on the opposite page show the device and its principle of operation. The electrical system not only controls both the inspiratory and the expiratory phases of breathing, it also provides, as is shown by the tracings (top right), signals for airway pressure and flow during the entire breathing cycle. These features make it possible, for the first time, to monitor continuously the patient's lung mechanical parameters, information of significant diagnostic value.

A picture showing the Engström ventilator and carbon dioxide analyser (seen on top of the ventilator) built three decades after the introduction of the first original model. The device uses microprocessor technology to monitor physiological parameters of the ventilated patient such as lung mechanics, gas exchange and energy expenditure. It is also capable of adapting to the variable respiratory effort of the patient, always maintaining a pre-set ventilation level.

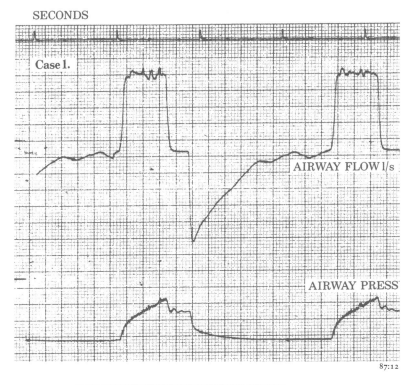

SECONDS

Case 1.

AIRWAY FLOW l/s

AIRWAY PRESS

87:12

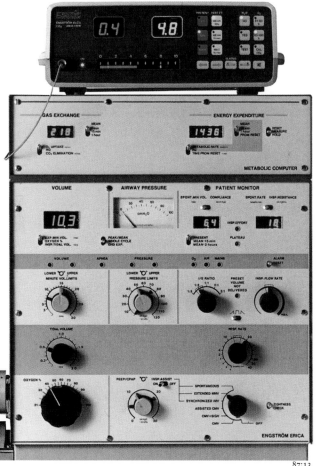

87:13

equipment, and to Dr. G. E. R. Deacon and the captain and officers of R.R.S. *Discovery II* for their part in making the observations.

[1] Young, F. B., Gerrard, H., and Jevons, W., *Phil. Mag.*, **40**, 149 (1920).

[2] Longuet-Higgins, M. S., *Mon. Not. Roy. Astro. Soc., Geophys. Supp.*, **5**, 285 (1949).

[3] Von Arx, W. S., Woods Hole Papers in Phys. Oceanog. Meteor., **11** (3) (1950).

[4] Ekman, V. W., *Arkiv. Mat. Astron. Fysik.* (Stockholm), **2** (11) (1905).

Franklin Crick   *J. D. Wats*

MOLECULAR STRUCTURE OF NUCLEIC ACIDS

A Structure for Deoxyribose Nucleic Acid

WE wish to suggest a structure for the salt of deoxyribose nucleic acid (D.N.A.). This structure has novel features which are of considerable biological interest.

A structure for nucleic acid has already been proposed by Pauling and Corey[1]. They kindly made their manuscript available to us in advance of publication. Their model consists of three intertwined chains, with the phosphates near the fibre axis, and the bases on the outside. In our opinion, this structure is unsatisfactory for two reasons : (1) We believe that the material which gives the X-ray diagrams is the salt, not the free acid. Without the acidic hydrogen atoms it is not clear what forces would hold the structure together, especially as the negatively charged phosphates near the axis will repel each other. (2) Some of the van der Waals distances appear to be too small.

Another three-chain structure has also been suggested by Fraser (in the press). In his model the phosphates are on the outside and the bases on the inside, linked together by hydrogen bonds. This structure as described is rather ill-defined, and for this reason we shall not comment on it.

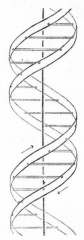

We wish to put forward a radically different structure for the salt of deoxyribose nucleic acid. This structure has two helical chains each coiled round the same axis (see diagram). We have made the usual chemical assumptions, namely, that each chain consists of phosphate diester groups joining β-D-deoxyribofuranose residues with 3′,5′ linkages. The two chains (but not their bases) are related by a dyad perpendicular to the fibre axis. Both chains follow right-handed helices, but owing to the dyad the sequences of the atoms in the two chains run in opposite directions. Each chain loosely resembles Furberg's[2] model No. 1; that is, the bases are on the inside of the helix and the phosphates on the outside. The configuration of the sugar and the atoms near it is close to Furberg's 'standard configuration', the sugar being roughly perpendicular to the attached base. There

This figure is purely diagrammatic. The two ribbons symbolize the two phosphate—sugar chains, and the horizontal rods the pairs of bases holding the chains together. The vertical line marks the fibre axis.

is a residue on each chain every 3·4 A. in the z-direction. We have assumed an angle of 36° between adjacent residues in the same chain, so that the structure repeats after 10 residues on each chain, that is, after 34 A. The distance of a phosphorus atom from the fibre axis is 10 A. As the phosphates are on the outside, cations have easy access to them.

The structure is an open one, and its water content is rather high. At lower water contents we would expect the bases to tilt so that the structure could become more compact.

The novel feature of the structure is the manner in which the two chains are held together by the purine and pyrimidine bases. The planes of the bases are perpendicular to the fibre axis. They are joined together in pairs, a single base from one chain being hydrogen-bonded to a single base from the other chain, so that the two lie side by side with identical z-co-ordinates. One of the pair must be a purine and the other a pyrimidine for bonding to occur. The hydrogen bonds are made as follows : purine position 1 to pyrimidine position 1 ; purine position 6 to pyrimidine position 6.

If it is assumed that the bases only occur in the structure in the most plausible tautomeric forms (that is, with the keto rather than the enol configurations) it is found that only specific pairs of bases can bond together. These pairs are : adenine (purine) with thymine (pyrimidine), and guanine (purine) with cytosine (pyrimidine).

In other words, if an adenine forms one member of a pair, on either chain, then on these assumptions the other member must be thymine ; similarly for guanine and cytosine. The sequence of bases on a single chain does not appear to be restricted in any way. However, if only specific pairs of bases can be formed, it follows that if the sequence of bases on one chain is given, then the sequence on the other chain is automatically determined.

It has been found experimentally[3,4] that the ratio of the amounts of adenine to thymine, and the ratio of guanine to cytosine, are always very close to unity for deoxyribose nucleic acid.

It is probably impossible to build this structure with a ribose sugar in place of the deoxyribose, as the extra oxygen atom would make too close a van der Waals contact.

The previously published X-ray data[5,6] on deoxyribose nucleic acid are insufficient for a rigorous test of our structure. So far as we can tell, it is roughly compatible with the experimental data, but it must be regarded as unproved until it has been checked against more exact results. Some of these are given in the following communications. We were not aware of the details of the results presented there when we devised our structure, which rests mainly though not entirely on published experimental data and stereochemical arguments.

It has not escaped our notice that the specific pairing we have postulated immediately suggests a possible copying mechanism for the genetic material.

Full details of the structure, including the conditions assumed in building it, together with a set of co-ordinates for the atoms, will be published elsewhere.

We are much indebted to Dr. Jerry Donohue for constant advice and criticism, especially on interatomic distances. We have also been stimulated by a knowledge of the general nature of the unpublished experimental results and ideas of Dr. M. H. F. Wilkins, Dr. R. E. Franklin and their co-workers at

The seminal paper on the structure of the DNA (deoxyribonucleic acid) molecule. The proposed configuration is made up of two helical ribbons of alternating sugar and phosphate. Purine-pyrimidine base pairs attached to the sugar bind the ribbons together by hydrogen bonding.

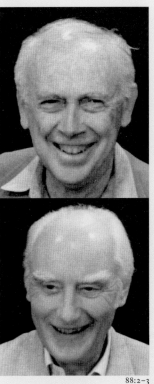

88:2–3

James D Watson
Francis H Crick

WATSON was born in Chicago in 1928 and obtained his Ph.D. in zoology from the University of Indiana. In 1951 he moved to the Cavendish Laboratory in Cambridge and, in collaboration with Crick, worked out the structure of DNA. He subsequently directed the Cold Spring Harbor Laboratory of Quantitative Biology and from 1988 to 1992 also headed the National Center for Human Genome Research at the NIH. Crick was born in 1916 near Northampton and held a B.Sc. in physics from University College London. After developing radar devices during World War II, he was working on his thesis when he became involved with the DNA structure problem. In 1976 he moved to the Salk Institute and turned his research interest to the functioning of the brain. In 1962 Watson and Crick shared the Nobel Prize in Medicine with Wilkins.

A Structure for Deoxyribose Nucleic Acid.

NATURE 1953; 171:737.

WATSON AND Crick present the correct structure of the DNA molecule. They describe the geometry of two helix chains of alternating sugar and phosphate. Along the chains two purine and two pyrimidine bases are bound to the sugar and the chains are held together by the hydrogen bonding between the purine-pyrimidine base pairs (adenin—thymine and guanine—cytosine). They also observe "that the specific paring we have postulated immediately suggests a possible copying mechanism for the genetic material". A month later they explained this mechanism in more detail (88.1).

IN PERSPECTIVE:
Avery had shown in 1944 that DNA was the carrier of genetic material (88.2). In a series of studies Chargaff, using the new technique of paper chromatography (88.3), found that purines and pyrimidines occurred in equal amounts in DNA (88.4). Proteins with helix structures had been described by Pauling in 1951 (88.5) and Furberg had already suggested a DNA configuration with a helix chain having bases bound to sugar inside and phosphates outside (88.6). Following pioneering work on the X-ray diffraction of DNA by Wilkins (88.7), the outstanding crystallographic techniques of Franklin (88.8) played a decisive and much discussed role in the events leading up to the discovery by Watson and Crick of the precise nature of the DNA structure (88.9). Since then the many landmarks of molecular biology have included understanding genetic coding, the production of recombinant DNA and monoclonal antibodies and the invention of the polymerase chain reaction (PCR) method of multiplying DNA. In 1990 the Human Genome Project was launched and the initial sequencing and analysis of the human genome were presented in 2001 (88.10).

88.1 Watson JD, Crick FH. Genetic implications of the structure of deoxyribonucleic acid. *Nature* 1953; 171:964.
88.2 Avery OT, MacLeod CM, McCarty M. Studies on the Chemical Nature of the Substance Inducing Transformation of Pneumococcal Types: Induction of Transformation by a Desoxyribonucleic Acid Fraction Isolated from Pneumococcus Type III. *J Exp Med* 1944; 79(1):137.
88.3 See #84 Martin page 434 and ref. 84.2.
88.4 Chagraff E, et al. The composition of the desoxyribonucleic acid of salmon sperm. *J Biol Chem* 1951; 192:223.
88.5 Pauling L, Corey RB. Atomic Coordinates and Structure Factors for Two Helical Configurations of Polypeptide Chains. *Proc Nat Acad Sci* 1951; 37(5):235 and also p251, p256, p272 and p282.
88.6 Furberg SV. On the Structure of Nucleic Acids. *Acta Chem Scand* 1952; 6:634.
88.7 Wilkins MHF, Stokes AR, Wilson HR. Molecular Structure of Deoxypentose Nucleic Acid. *Nature* 1953; 171:738.
88.8 Franklin RE, Gosling RG. Molecular Configuration in Sodium Thymonucleate. *Nature* 1953; 171:740.
88.9 Judson HF. *The Eigth Day of Creation*. New York: Simon & Schuster; 1979.
88.10 The International Human Genome Sequencing Consortium: Initial sequencing and analysis of the human genome. *Nature* 2001; 409:860. The Celera Genomics Sequencing Team: The sequence of the human genome. *Science* February 16 2001. p1304.

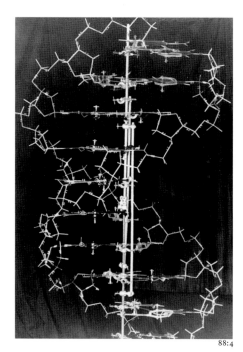

88:4

The original model of the DNA molecule and the explanation of the genetic implications of the specific pairing of the ribbons. In the landmark publication on the DNA structure, James Watson and Francis Crick (1916–2004) only hint at "a possible copying mechanism for the genetic material" (see illustration 88:1).

GENETICAL IMPLICATIONS OF THE STRUCTURE OF DEOXYRIBONUCLEIC ACID

By J. D. WATSON and F. H. C. CRICK

Medical Research Council Unit for the Study of the Molecular Structure of Biological Systems, Cavendish Laboratory, Cambridge

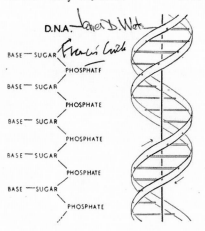

Fig. 1. Chemical formula of a single chain of deoxyribonucleic acid

Fig. 2. This figure is purely diagrammatic. The two ribbons symbolize the two phosphate-sugar chains, and the horizontal rods the pairs of bases holding the chains together. The vertical line marks the fibre axis

THE importance of deoxyribonucleic acid (DNA) within living cells is undisputed. It is found in all dividing cells, largely if not entirely in the nucleus, where it is an essential constituent of the chromosomes. Many lines of evidence indicate that it is the carrier of a part of (if not all) the genetic specificity of the chromosomes and thus of the gene itself.

Until now, however, no evidence has been presented to show how it might carry out the essential operation required of a genetic material, that of exact self-duplication.

We have recently proposed a structure[1] for the salt of deoxyribonucleic acid which, if correct, immediately suggests a mechanism for its self-duplication. X-ray evidence obtained by the workers at King's College, London[2], and presented at the same time, gives qualitative support to our structure and is incompatible with all previously proposed structures[3]. Though the structure will not be completely proved until a more extensive comparison has been made with the X-ray data, we now feel sufficient confidence in its general correctness to discuss its genetical implications. In doing so we are assuming that fibres of the salt of deoxyribonucleic acid are not artefacts arising in the method of preparation, since it has been shown by Wilkins and his co-workers that similar X-ray patterns are obtained from both the isolated fibres and certain intact biological materials such as sperm head and bacteriophage particles[2,4].

The chemical formula of deoxyribonucleic acid is now well established. The molecule is a very long chain, the backbone of which consists of a regular alternation of sugar and phosphate groups, as shown in Fig. 1. To each sugar is attached a nitrogenous base, which can be of four different types. (We have considered 5-methyl cytosine to be equivalent to cytosine, since either can fit equally well into our structure.) Two of the possible bases—adenine and guanine—are purines, and the other two—thymine and cytosine—are pyrimidines. So far as is known, the sequence of bases along the chain is irregular. The monomer unit, consisting of phosphate, sugar and base, is known as a nucleotide.

The first feature of our structure which is of biological interest is that it consists not of one chain, but of two. These two chains are both coiled around a common fibre axis, as is shown diagrammatically in Fig. 2. It has often been assumed that since there was only one chain in the chemical formula there would only be one in the structural unit. However, the density, taken with the X-ray evidence[2], suggests very strongly that there are two.

The other biologically important feature is the manner in which the two chains are held together. This is done by hydrogen bonds between the bases, as shown schematically in Fig. 3. The bases are joined together in pairs, a single base from one chain being hydrogen-bonded to a single base from the other. The important point is that only certain pairs of bases will fit into the structure. One member of a pair must be a purine and the other a pyrimidine in order to bridge between the two chains. If a pair consisted of two purines, for example, there would not be room for it.

We believe that the bases will be present almost entirely in their most probable tautomeric forms. If this is true, the conditions for forming hydrogen bonds are more restrictive, and the only pairs of bases possible are :

adenine with thymine ;
guanine with cytosine.

The way in which these are joined together is shown in Figs. 4 and 5. A given pair can be either way round. Adenine, for example, can occur on either chain ; but when it does, its partner on the other chain must always be thymine.

This pairing is strongly supported by the recent analytical results[5], which show that for all sources of deoxyribonucleic acid examined the amount of adenine is close to the amount of thymine, and the amount of guanine close to the amount of cytosine, although the cross-ratio (the ratio of adenine to guanine) can vary from one source to another. Indeed, if the sequence of bases on one chain is irregular, it is difficult to explain these analytical results except by the sort of pairing we have suggested.

The phosphate-sugar backbone of our model is completely regular, but any sequence of the pairs of bases can fit into the structure. It follows that in a long molecule many different permutations are possible, and it therefore seems likely that the precise sequence of the bases is the code which carries the genetical information. If the actual order of the

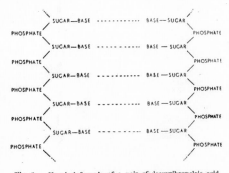

Fig. 3. Chemical formula of a pair of deoxyribonucleic acid chains. The hydrogen bonding is symbolized by dotted lines

88:5

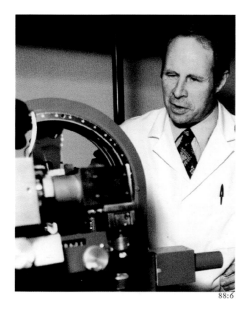

88:6

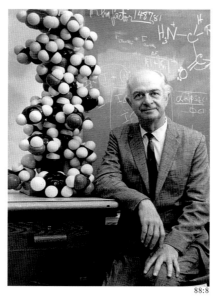

88:8

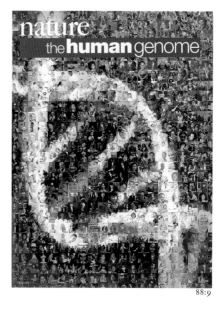

88:9

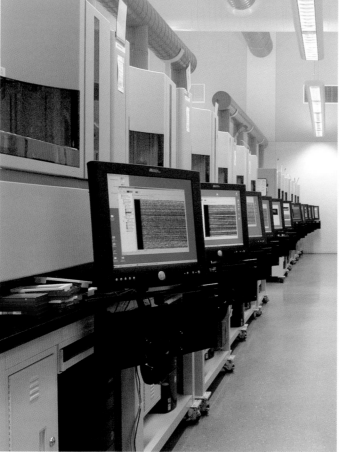

88:7

In 1951 Linus Pauling (1901–1994) (middle photograph) develops a helix model for polypeptides that match the known diffraction data for the alpha-keratin fibre. His work, and that of Sven Furberg (1920–1983) (left) the following year, set the conceptual stage for the subsequent discovery of the structure and function of DNA.

The February 2001 cover of the magazine Nature announcing the results of the International Human Genome Mapping Consortium.

A line of fully automated DNA analysers at the Broad Institute, one of the major facilities engaged in genome sequencing (including the work on the human genome). The instruments are loaded with prepared sequencing products for capillary electrophoresis and analysis. They run round the clock, every day of the year, for maximal throughput.

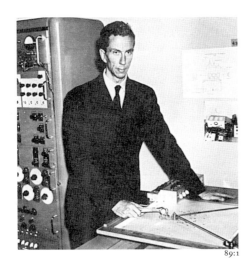

89:1

In 1953 Gunnar Fant introduces a much improved speech synthesiser named OVE I. The device reproduces speech by generating vowels (sounds from an open vocal tract), where two of the most prominent resonance frequencies of the vocal tract can be manually adjusted. Right, a comparison between a spoken sentence "I love you" (top) and the synthesised version produced by OVE I. In both cases the diagrams show frequency content and intensity of the sounds as a function of time.

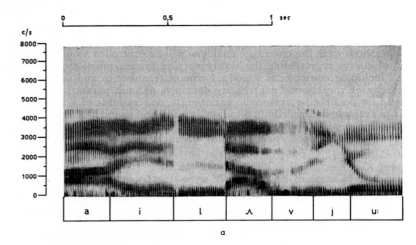

a

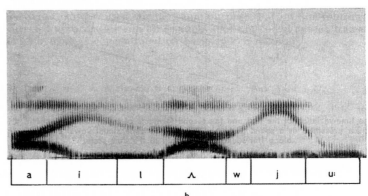

b

Fig. 3. Time-frequency-intensity spectrograms of the sentence "I love you". Sonagraph analyzer.

a) Spoken by Swedish male subject.

b) Manual reproduction of the same sentence with the resonance analogue, Ove, and the spoken sentence as an audible reference. The following variables were utilized: on-off of primary voice source, the voice fundamental, the first formant and the second formant. The third formant was kept constant.

The synthesized sentence was of a good intelligibility. Observe the general differences between spectrograms a) and b). The 4th and the 5th formants of the spoken sentence do not contribute anything to the intelligibility. The abrupt change of the spectral pattern in some of the boundaries between adjacent sounds of speech a) is not essential for the intelligibility of the synthetically reproduced sentence, which shows smoother transitions. Observe also the correct reproduction of sound intensity variations within the syllables of the synthesized sentence, i. e. the reduced intensity of the consonantal sound patches. This is obtained with no other intensity control than that which follows from the combined filter action of the synthesizer in analogy to the actual vocal tract transmission process. The overall changes in sound intensity is largely a function of formant frequencies and the voice fundamental. The complete preservation of these natural relationships in Ove represents an advantage compared to other synthesizers, e. g. those of references[12], [15].

IVA 24 (1953): 8

89:2

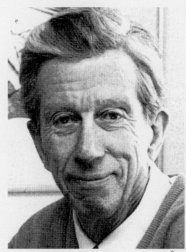

Gunnar Fant

89:3

FANT was born in 1919 in Nyköping Sweden and started his studies in Electrical Engineering at the Royal Institute of Technology (KTH) in Stockholm in 1938. After graduating in 1945, he worked at the acoustic laboratory of the Ericsson Telephone Company for four years. Having spent the following two years at the acoustic laboratory of the Massachusetts Institute of Technology, he returned to KTH to head the newly established Speech Transmission Laboratory (STL). In 1966 a personal chair was created for him there as professor at the Department of Speech Communication and Music Acoustics. Fant, who retired in 1987, is a member of several Swedish and foreign scientific academies and has been honoured with more than a dozen awards for his pioneering work in speech communication and related areas.

Speech Communication Research.

IVA (THE ROYAL SWEDISH ACADEMY OF ENGINEERING SCIENCES) 1953; 24(8):331. STOCKHOLM: ESSELTE; 1954.

FANT REPORTS first on recent advances made in analysing and synthesising speech. He then presents the research directed by him at the STL, with an emphasis on the newly developed "OVE I" speech synthesiser. This electronic device is a "formant" (a resonance characteristic of the vocal tract) synthesiser for vowels, where the frequency position of the two most prominent formants could be manually adjusted. Vowels, some voiced consonants and simple sentences composed of voiced sounds are reported to have been reproduced with reasonably good quality. The device is considered an advance compared to previous synthesisers (89.1) (89.2).

IN PERSPECTIVE:
Until the mid 1930s only mechanical devices had been built for speech generation (89.3). At that time Dudley started work at the Bell Laboratories on the Voice Coder (Vocoder), which by 1939 had evolved into the Voice Operation Demonstrator (Voder) (89.2). The Voder was an electronic speech frequency analyser connected to a speech synthesiser with some manual keyboard control of the intensity and tone quality. Speech characterisation through frequency mapping (sonography) was developed during the 1940s into a powerful tool (89.4). By manipulating these sonographs and using a Pattern Play Back unit that could generate sounds from the sonograph, perception and information content of speech could be studied in some detail (89.5)(89.6)(89.7). During the 1970s advances in computer technology allowed several text-to-speech systems to be developed (89.8)(89.9). Subsequently, these systems were made into commercial products that could be used as aids for the blind and those with speech impairments. Combining text-to-speech technology with optical scanners and pattern recognition software, Kurzweil introduced the first reading machine for the blind in 1976 (89.10).

89.1 Fant G. *Acoustic Analysis and Synthesis of Speech with Applications to Swedish*. Ericsson Technics 1959; 1:3.

89.2 Dudley H, Reiss RR, Watkins SSA. A Synthetic Speaker. *J Franklin Inst* 1939; 227:739 and ref. 25.9.

89.3 See #25 Kempelen page 138 and on sound and hearing see #13 Kircher page 82 and #26 Volta page 144.

89.4 Potter RK, Kopp GA, Green HC. *Visible Speech*. New York: D.Van Nostrand Co.; 1947.

89.5 Cooper FS, et al. Some Experiments on the Perception of Synthetic Speech Sounds. *J Acoust Soc Am* 1952; 24:597.

89.6 Lawrence W. The synthesis of speech from signals which have a low information rate. In: *Communication Theory*. Jackson W. editor. Symposium on "Applications of Communication Theory" London September 1952. London: Butterworth Scientific Publications; 1953. p460.

89.7 Peterson GE. *The information-bearing elements of speech*. p402 in main publication ref. 89.6.

89.8 Carlson R, Granström B. A text-to-speech system based on a phonetically oriented programming language — *Speech Transmission Laboratory report* QPSR1, 1975;1.

89.9 See ref 25.10.

89.10 Kurzweil R. The Kurzweil Reading Machine: a technical overview. In: *Science, Technology and the Handicapped*. Redden MR, Schwandt W. editors. AAAS Report 76-R-11 1976;3.

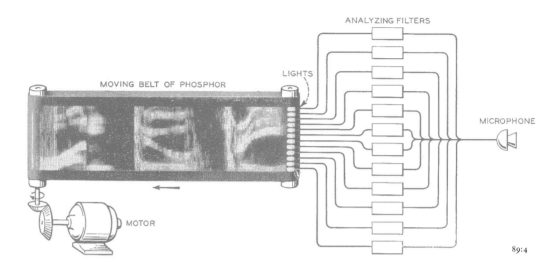

89:4

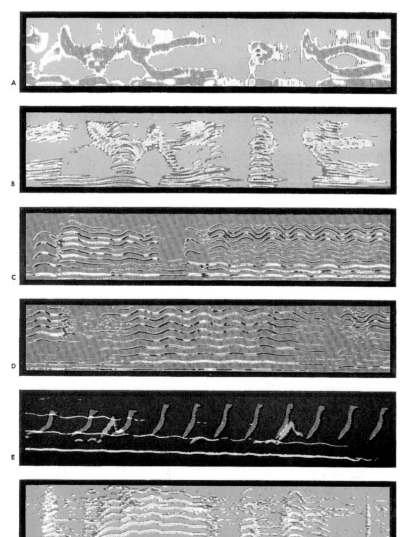

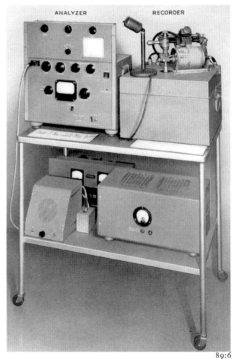

89:6

In the mid-1940s the invention of the sound spectrograph greatly advances the science of speech analysis and synthesis. The method of recording these spectrographs and the equipment employed are shown here, together with a number of examples ranging from simple words (A, B, F, D) to bird songs (E) and the sobs of Caruso (C).

89:5

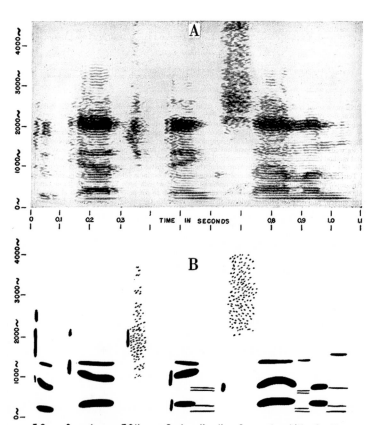

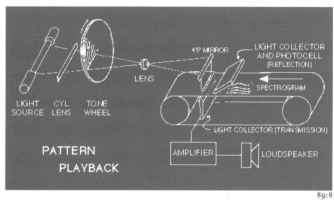

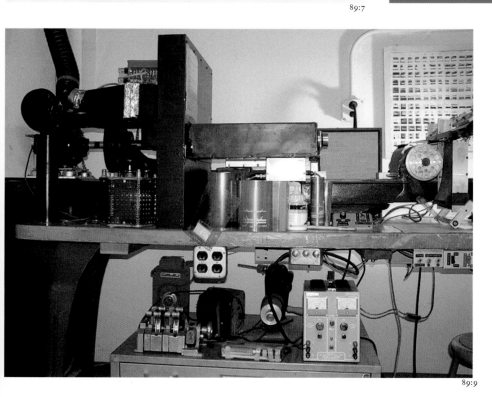

By manual manipulation of a sound spectrograph, an original recording (marked A) can be changed as regards the frequency/intensity content (marked B). The result can then be evaluated using the Pattern Playback unit (shown in the photograph), which produces sounds from a spectrograph by a method shown in the diagram. These techniques turn out to be most helpful in developing new methods of speech analysis and synthesis.

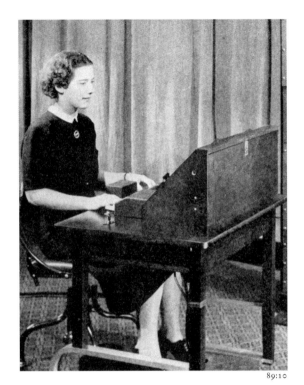

89:10

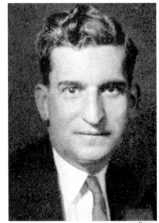

89:11

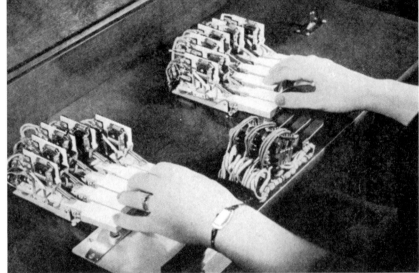

89:12

Homer Dudley (1896–1980)
pioneers electronic speech synthesis by introducing the VODER
(voice operation demonstrator)
at the World's Fair in New York in
1939. The device processes speech
using bandpass filter banks under
manual control, as shown in the
picture.

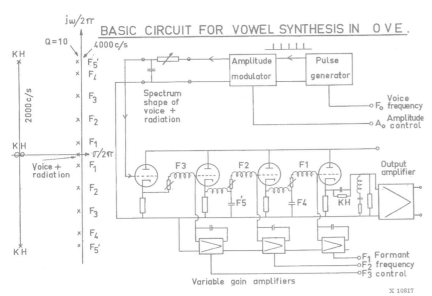

Fig. 47. Block diagram with circuit details of the vocal tract resonance analog incorporated in the Swedish speaking machines OVE I and II.

89:13

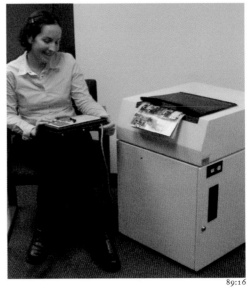

89:16

Ray Kuzweil's reading machine for the blind from 1976. This is the first device combining optical scanners, text-to-speech technology and pattern recognition software.

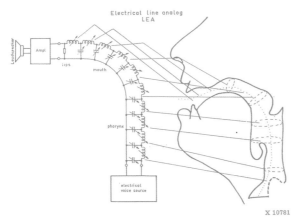

X 10781

Fig. 15. The electrical line analog LEA comprises 45 cascaded LC low-pass filters simulating the vocal cavities. LEA is a research tool for interrelating physiological and acoustic data on speech production.

89:14

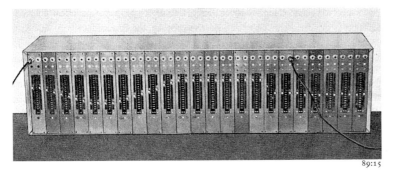

89:15

Key elements of the speech synthesiser OVE I and II built in the 1950s by Fant. The basic circuit diagram is shown here, together with the electric line analogue for modelling the characteristics of the human vocal tract.

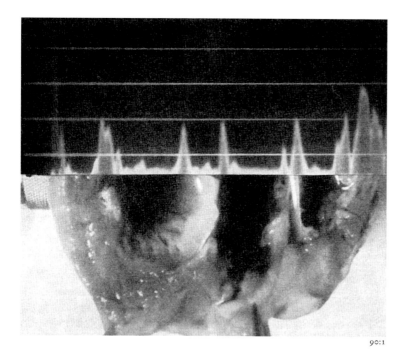

90:1

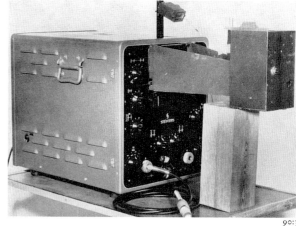

90:3

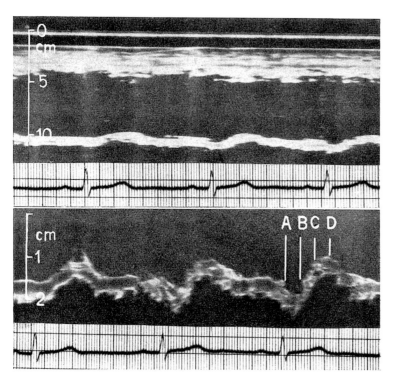

In 1954 Inge Edler (1911–2001) and Helmuth Hertz (1920–1980) introduce the technique of ultrasound echo cardiography. The equipment shown above, a "reflectoscope", is originally developed for industrial material testing applications (see #66). Top left, a display of the ultrasound echoes observed as the sound pulses bounce from the various internal structures of the heart. For comparison a crossectional view of the heart is shown just underneath and adjacent to the train of echoes. The image below shows ultrasound tracings in time (together with the ECG) and also gives their physiological interpretation.

Fig. 7. Top: General view. Bottom: Enlargement of the movements of the posterior wall of the heart. A–B indicates the isometric contraction when the wall moves 2–3 mm. in dorsal direction. B–C denotes the first part of the emptying phase, maximum ejection, when the wall rapidly moves in ventral direction. C–D denotes the final phase of emptying, reduced ejection, when the wall moves slowly in ventral direction.

90:2

Inge Edler, Carl Helmuth Hertz

E DLER was born in 1911 in Burlöv, Sweden. He started his medical studies at the University of Lund in 1930 and remained here until his retirement in 1977. From 1944 he carried out clinical work at the Department of Medicine at Malmö Allmänna Sjukhus and was later responsible for the cardiology laboratory there. From 1950 to 1960 Edler directed the cardiovascular laboratory of Lunds Lasarett. He was appointed head of the Department of Cardiology there in 1963. Hertz was born in 1920 in Berlin, and was related to the famous physicist Heinrich Hertz. He received his Ph.D. in physics from the University of Lund in 1956 and held the chair at the Department of Electrical Measurements from 1963 until his death in 1980. Edler and Hertz received many honours for their pioneering work in cardiological ultrasound diagnostics, including the 1977 Albert Lasker Clinical Medical Research Award.

The Use of Ultrasonic Reflectoscope for the Continuous Recording of the Movements of Heart Walls.

KUNGL FYSIOGRAFISKA SÄLLSKAPETS I LUND FÖRH 1954; 24(5):40.

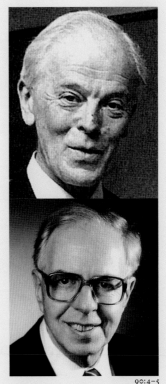

Inge Edler
Carl Helmuth Hertz

EDLER AND Hertz describe their equipment and how it can be used to produce ultrasonic pulse echoes from isolated hearts and from the hearts of human beings. A specially designed film camera attached to a reflectoscope operated at 2.5 MHz and designed for use in industrial material testing (90.1) is shown to be useful in detecting the blood-heart wall boundaries. Continuous recordings of the movements of the left ventricle wall in health and in disease and the left atrial wall in mitral stenosis are obtained.

IN PERSPECTIVE:
Although Langvin produced ultrasound waves for underwater exploration as early as 1916 (90.2) and both continuous and pulsed waves were used in material testing during the 1930s and 1940s (90.1), it was Wild who introduced echo-ranging in medical applications in 1950, first for tissue characterisation (90.3) and two years later for tumour detection (90.4). By the early 1960s ultrasound diagnostics had been successfully introduced not only in cardiology (90.5) but also in ophthalmology (90.6), brain diagnostics (90.7) and in obstetrics and gynaecology (90.8). The pulse echo technique was extended to two-dimensional registrations in 1967 (90.9) and during the following decade transesophageal echocardiography was developed (90.10). Imaging with Doppler techniques was invented in the mid 1950s by Satamura and was able not only to show the motion of structures but also the flow of blood (90.11). Over the years ultrasound diagnostics has undergone many technical refinements, improving methods and increasing the number of applications in clinical medicine. Today it rivals X-ray techniques as the most important of diagnostic modalities.

90.1 Sokolov SY. Ultrasonic oscillations and their applications. *Tech Phys* 1935; 2:1. See also ref. 66.6.

90.2 See #66 Curie page 338 and ref. 66.2 and also #40 Doppler page 212.

90.3 Wild JJ. The Use of Ultrasonic Pulses for the Measurement of Biological Tissue and the Detection of Tissue Density Changes. *Surgery* 1950; 27:183.

90.4 Wild JJ, Reid JM. The Effects of Biological Tissues on 15-mc Pulsed Ultrasound. *J Acoust Soc Am* 1953; 25(2): 270.

90.5 Edler I. Ultrasoundcardiography. *Acta Med Scand* Suppl. 1961; 170.

90.6 Oksala A, Lehtinen A. Diagnosis of Detachment of the Retina by Means of Ultrasound. *Acta Ophth* 1957; 35:461.

90.7 Leksell L. Echoencephalography. I Detection of Intracranial Complications following Head Injury. *Acta Chir Scand* 1956; 110:301.

90.8 Donald I, Brown TG. Demonstration of tissue interfaces within the body by ultrasonic echo sounding. *British J Radiol* 1961; 34:539.

90.9 Åsberg AG. Ultrasonic cinematography of the living heart. *Ultrasonics* 1967; 5:113.

90.10 Daniel WG, Mugge A. Transesophageal Echocardiography. *The New England J Med* May 1995. p1268.

90.11 Edler I, Lindström K. Ultrasonic doppler techniques in heart disease: II Clinical applications. In: *Proc first World Congress on Ultrasonic Diagnostics in Medicine*. Vienna 1969. Bock J, Ossonig K. editors. 1971. p455. See also #40 Doppler page 212.

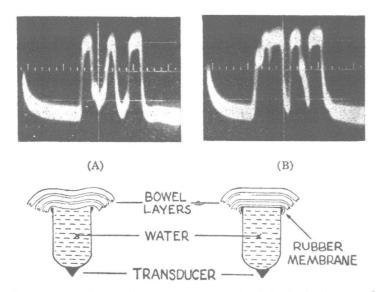

(A) (B)

In the first years of the 1950s John Wild pioneers the use of pulsed ultrasound beams for tissue characterisation. In 1952, together with John Reid, he measures the thickness of the bowel wall and also explores the potential of the method for diagnosing cancer of the brain. The illustrations show transducer designs and experimental results from these two early investigations.

FIG. 1. Method of measurement of biological tissues. (A) Echogram of three layers of dog's bowel placed over mouth of echoscope; (B) Rubber membrane interposed between water in chamber and the tissues. The effect of the rubber membrane on the echogram can be seen. The sound beam penetrated the rubber membrane (condom).

90:6

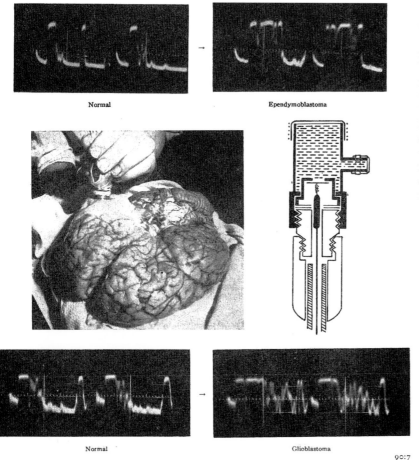

Normal

Ependymoblastoma

Cancer of the brain. Far left, two echograms of normal brain tissue approximately 1.4 cm thick. Right, two echograms of a piece of malignant tumor arising from the same brain. The tumor was reduced to half-thickness. Two pairs of echograms recorded with the echoscope (mid-right) on the whole brain (mid-left) are shown at the bottom. Normal echograms (bottom left) were taken from the opposite lobe of the brain from that occupied by the tumor. The greater number of echoes coming from the tumor can be seen in the echograms (bottom right).

Normal

Glioblastoma

90:7

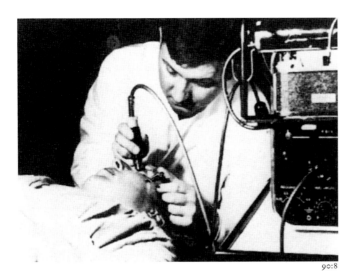
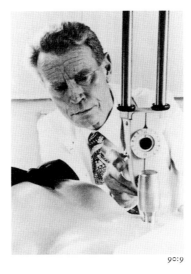

90:8 90:9

Early medical applications of ultrasound include intraocular foreign body detection and diagnoses of detachment of the retina, as demonstrated by Arvo Oksala in the mid-1950s (left), and obstetrical and gynaecological examinations introduced by Ian Donald in the mid-1960s (right).

Ultrasound Doppler techniques are introduced for medical diagnostics in the mid-1950s (see #40) and in 1969 Inge Edler and Kjell Lindström also show that the method is useful not only to observe moving structures but also blood flow, as is demonstrated by the chart shown here, taken from their paper.

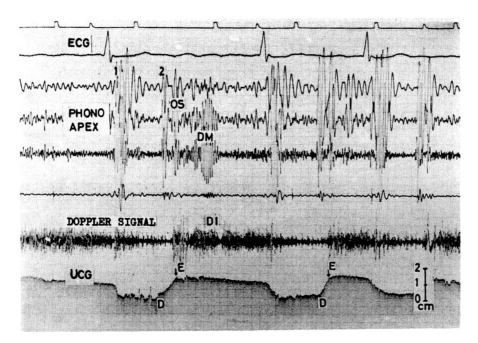

Figure 2: Tight mitral stenosis with atrial fibrillation. Simultaneous recording of ECG, Phonocardiogram taken from the apex, Doppler tracing and pulsed ultrasoundcardio-gram (UCG) of the movement of the anterior mitral leaflet. The transducer of the "Doppler detector" was applied in the third left interspace and the beam directed toward the mitral valve. The transducer of the pulsed ultrasound was applied in the fourth left interspace and the movement of the anterior mitral leaflet was recorded.

90:10

An Implantable Pacemaker for the Heart

SOMMAIRE: Description d'un régulateur compact, destiné à être implanté sous la peau au niveau de l'épigastre. Le générateur d'impulsion est composé d'un multivibrateur avec un transistor au silicium. L'amplitude des impulsions est d'environ 2 volts, leur durée est d'environ 1,5 milliseconde. Leur fréquence est constante et d'environ 80 pulsations par seconde. La source d'énergie est un petit accumulateur au cadmium-nickel, composé de deux séries interconnectées de cellules, de 60 mAh chacune.

ONE of the major problems in connection with the permanent use of pacemakers for the heart is the prevention of infection through the channel where the cable is brought out through the skin.

A compact pacemaker is described which is intended to be implanted subcutaneously in the epigastrium. The pulse generator consists of a repetitive blocking oscillator with a silicon transistor. The pulses are fed to the base-circuit of a second silicon transistor. The collector circuit of the second transistor is connected to the electrode over an RC network. The pulse height is about 2 V, and the pulse duration is about 1·5 msec. The pulse frequency is constant and about 80 pulse/sec.

The source of energy is a small nickel-cadmium accumulator consisting of two series-connected cells of 60 mAh each. The apparatus also contains a coil and a silicon diode, which form the secondary circuit of an inductive charging device. The primary circuit of this device consists of a 150 kc/s generator feeding a large diameter coil. This coil is placed over the pacemaker outside the skin, when the accumulator is charged.

The electrode cable had to be specially developed in order to withstand the movements in the body (about 10^5 bends every day).

Experience from animal experiments and one human case are reported.

R. Elmqvist and A. Senning,
Stockholm

91:1

Reproduction of the short announcement made in 1959 by Rune Elmqvist (1906–1996) and Åke Senning (1915–2000) of the first fully implanted pacemaker. The human case mentioned on the last line refers to the patient Arne Larsson, shown below at a later time holding his pacemaker. Larsson was an engineer and participated actively in the testing of the pacemaker design that was implanted. Larsson lived for another forty-two years and had five lead systems and twenty-two pulse generators (eleven different pacemaker models) during this time. His death was unrelated to his conduction system disease.

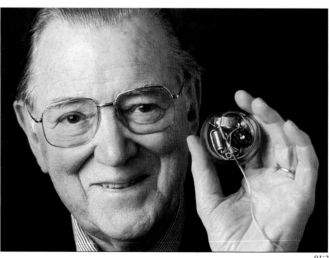

91:2

ELMQUIST was born in Lund, Sweden, in 1911. He studied but never practised medicine. A self-taught engineer who in 1948 had invented the direct writing ink jet ECG recorder (91.1), Elmqvist was appointed head of the laboratory of Järnhs Elektriska AB (later Elema-Schönander AB and Siemens-Elema AB) in Solna. From 1952 Elmqvist was director of the Electromedical Division and later also served as a board member. Senning was born in 1915 in Rättvik, Sweden. He studied medicine in Uppsala and in 1948 moved to Sabbatsbergs Hospital in Stockholm, where he helped develop the heart-lung machine (91.2). From 1956 he carried out pioneering cardiac surgery at Karolinska Sjukhuset. He moved in 1961 to head the Surgical Clinic of the University Hospital in Zürich.

An Implantable Pacemaker for the Heart.

PROCEEDINGS OF THE SECOND INTERNATIONAL CONFERENCE ON
MEDICAL ELECTRONICS PARIS 24–27 JUNE 1959. LONDON; 1960. P253.

IN THIS short communication Elmqvist and Senning describe a fully implantable pacemaker, designed according to their experiences from animal studies and from one human case (91.3). The device, which is shaped like a shoe polish tin, has a diameter of 55 mm and a thickness of 16 mm and is powered by a nickel-cadmium accumulator. With two silicon transistors that had recently became available, it generates 2 V pulses of 1.5 ms duration at a rate of about 80 per minute. It is implanted subcutaneously and has to be recharged by an induction coil placed over the pacemaker outside the skin.

IN PERSPECTIVE:
When McWilliam performed the first animal studies of cardiac pacing in 1889 (91.4), the electrophysiology of the heart had been under investigation for almost half a century (91.5). Hyman was the first to attempt therapy when in 1930 he developed "an artificial pacemaker" that delivered impulses to the right atrium through a needle across the chest wall (91.6). From experiences of open-heart surgery, endovenous stimulation of the sinoatrial node was introduced by Bigelow in 1950 (91.7). This work greatly influenced not only Senning but also Zoll, who demonstrated how to manage Stokes-Adams attacks using plate electrodes on the chest (91.8). In 1959 Greatbatch and Chardack implanted the first battery-operated pacemaker with a usability period of about five years (91.9) and subsequently new methods eliminated the absolute need for thoracotomy (91.10). The patient in the landmark paper cited survived more than twenty pacemakers over forty-two years and died of a malignancy in 2000 (91.3). Pacemakers today have sophisticated software, can adapt to the patient and may have a million times more transistor functions than the device implanted by Senning in 1958.

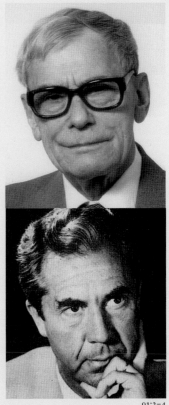

91:3–4

Rune Elmqvist
Åke Senning

91.1 See #71 Einthoven page 366 ref. 71.9.
91.2 Crafoord C, Norberg B, Senning Å. Clinical studies in extracorporeal circulation with a heart-lung machine *Acta Chir Scand* 1957; 112:220. See also #86 Kolff page 444 ref. 86.7 and ref. 86.9.
91.3 Larsson B, et al. Lessons From the First Patient with an Implanted Pacemaker: 1958–2001. *PACE* 2003; 26(1):114.
91.4 McWilliam JA. Electrical stimulation of the heart in man. *Brit Med J* 1889; 1:348 and ref. 23.10, 23.11.
91.5 Schechter DC. *Exploring the origins of electrical cardiac stimulation*. Minneapolis: Medtronic Inc.; 1983 and ref. 65.2, 65.3, 65.7. See also #23 Kite page 128.
91.6 Hyman AS. Resuscitation of the stopped heart by intracardial therapy. *Arch Int Med* 1930; 46:553.
91.7 Callaghan JC, Bigelow WG. An electrical artificial pacemaker for standstill of the heart. *Ann Surg* 1951; 134:8.
91.8 Zoll PM. Resuscitation of the heart in ventricular standstill by external electric stimulation. *New Engl J Med* 1952; 247:768.
91.9 Greatbatch W, Chardack WM. A transistorized implantable pacemaker for the long-term correction of complete atrioventricular block. *M Electron NEREM* 1959; 48:643.
91.10 Carlens E, et al. New method for atrial-triggered pacemaker treatment without thoracotomy. *J Thorac Cardiov Surg* 1965; 50:229.

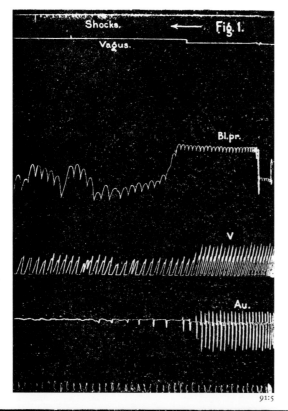

Fig. 1.

91:5

In 1889 John McWilliam (1857–1937), having just observed a case of cardiac failure and sudden death from ventricular fibrillation, decides to investigate the role of the autonomic nervous system in the genesis of sudden death. He studies whether electric shocks can reactivate the heart of a cat when depressed by vagal stimulation. The positive results obtained (shown here by two of his graphs) open up the field of cardiac resuscitation and pacing.

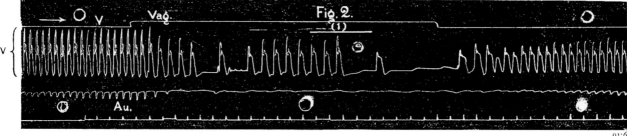

Fig. 2.

91:6

Albert Hyman (1893–1972) and his "artificial pacemaker", which delivers repetitive electric stimulation to the right atrium through a needle across the chest wall. He introduces this first attempt at therapy in 1930.

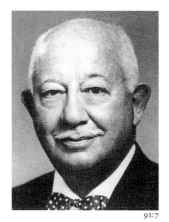

91:7

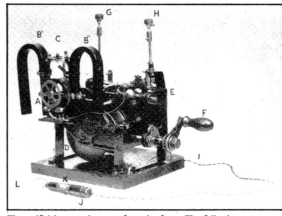

The artificial pacemaker seen from the front. The following important features are to be noted: A, magnetogenerator; B' and B'',companion magnet pieces; C, neon lamps; D, spring motor; E, ballistic governor; F, handle; G, impulse control; H, speed control; I, flexible electric cord; J, insulated handle; K, handle switch, and L, electrode needle.

91:8

Paul Zoll (1912–1999) makes a major advance in the first years of the 1950s by demonstrating that plate electrodes (see the picture of his equipment) on the chest can be used to manage the so called Stokes-Adams disease, which is characterised by sudden collapses into unconsciousness due to a disorder of heart rhythm.

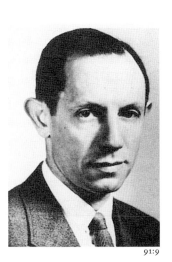

91:9

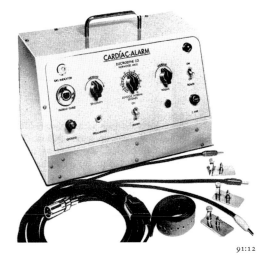

91:12

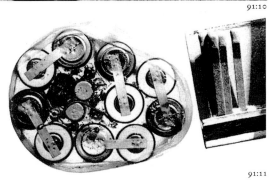

91:10

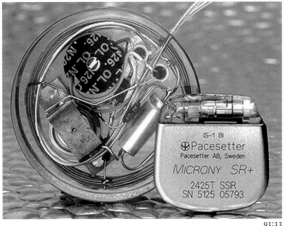

91:11

The original Greatbatch-Chardac pacemaker from 1959, shown separately bottom left and when insulated in a silicon rubber capsule, with the electrodes attached left. This, the first battery operated pacemaker, has a usability period of about five years.

The first pacemaker designed and implanted in 1958 by Elmqvist and Senning, as compared to a modern device that may have more than a million times more transistor functions and can operate adaptively with sophisticated sensors and software.

91:13

Stimulated Optical Radiation in Ruby

Schawlow and Townes[1] have proposed a technique for the generation of very monochromatic radiation in the infra-red optical region of the spectrum using an alkali vapour as the active medium. Javan[2] and Sanders[3] have discussed proposals involving electron-excited gaseous systems. In this laboratory an optical pumping technique has been successfully applied to a fluorescent solid resulting in the attainment of negative temperatures and stimulated optical emission at a wave-length of 6943 Å.; the active material used was ruby (chromium in corundum).

92:1

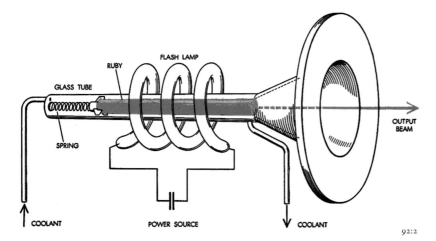

GLASS TUBE

RUBY

FLASH LAMP

SPRING

COOLANT

POWER SOURCE

OUTPUT BEAM

COOLANT

92:2

The concise introduction of Theodore Maiman's paper reporting the first observation of *LASER* (light amplification by stimulated emission of radiation) action.

A drawing explaining Maiman's ruby laser arrangement and a picture of the actual device. When the intensity of the pulses of the flash light (coiled around the ruby rod) exceeds a certain level, intense red light pulses, about 0.5 ms long, are observed leaving the ruby rod in the axial direction.

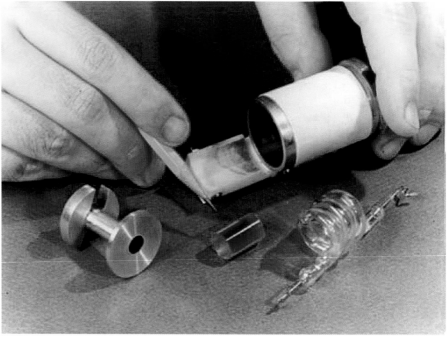

92:3

M AIMAN was born in 1927 in Los Angeles. He received a B.Sc. in engineering physics in 1949 from the University of Colorado and, after studying electrical engineering and physics, he obtained his Ph.D. from Stanford University in 1955. Maiman was employed as section head at Hughes Research Laboratories when he built the first LASER (Light Amplification by Stimulated Emission of Radiation) device in 1960. Two years later he founded his own company for developing and manufacturing lasers. He joined TRW Inc. in 1976 as director for new high-technology ventures and has subsequently also served as director of other companies and organisations engaged in promoting laser technology.

Stimulated Optical Radiation in Ruby.

NATURE 1960; 187:493.

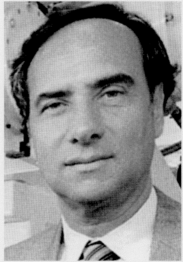

Theodore Maiman   92:4

MAIMAN DESCRIBES in this concise report the energy levels of pink ruby (aluminium oxide with 0.05% chromium), with particular emphasis on the three excited levels of the chromium atom. A ruby rod with polished and silvered ends is illuminated using a flash lamp to raise the atom to the excited states. When the flash pumping exceeds a certain level, Maiman observes laser action corresponding to the transition from the metastable excited state to the ground state. Pulses of an intense red beam of light are generated with a duration of about 0.5 ms.

IN PERSPECTIVE:

Einstein showed in 1917 that absorption and spontaneous emission of radiation must be accompanied by the phenomenon of stimulated emission (92.1). In 1954 Townes, Basov and Prokhorov reported observing this at microwave frequencies (92.2). Four years later Schawlow, Townes and Gould conceived systems operating at optical frequencies (92.3)(92.4). Soon after Maiman's report Javan, Bennett Jr and Herriott were able to demonstrate in a He-Ne gas discharge the first continuously operating laser (92.5)(92.6). Within a few years lasers were developed in many other media, notably in semiconductors (92.7). The argon ion laser (92.8) and the Nd-YAG laser (92.9) are used today for retinal surgery. Excimer (excited diatomic molecule) lasers evolved during the 1970s and produce high power, pulsed ultraviolet radiation that is suitable for the "cold", evaporative, removal of biological tissue. They are now the precise tool of refractive surgery (92.10). Photodynamic therapy, which uses laser light interaction with specific photosensitising drugs, has been found useful in certain cancer types of the lung, the skin and the aerodigestive tract (92.11). Laser-based systems are widely used in microscopic imaging and spectroscopy of biological materials down to the subcellular level, and laser Doppler methods play an important role in cardio-vascular diagnostics (92.12).

92.1   Einstein A. Zur Quantentheorie der Strahlung. *Physik Zeitschr* 1917; 18:121.

92.2   Townes CH. *Production of coherent radiation by atoms and molecules.* Nobel Lecture Stockholm; 1964.

92.3   Schawlow AI, Townes CH. Infrared and optical masers. *Phys Rev* 1958; 112:1940.

92.4   Gould G. *Light amplifying apparatus.* US Patent Application 804504 1959 approved as US Patent 4,053,845 Optically pumped laser amplifiers 1977.

92.5   Javan A, Bennett Jr WR, Herriott DR. Population inversion and continuous optical maser oscillation in a gas discharge containing a He-Ne mixture. *Phys Rev Lett* 1961; 6:106.

92.6   Bennett Jr WR. Background of an Inversion: The first gas laser. *IEEE J.Selected Topics in Quant.Electr.* 2000; 6(6):869.

92.7   Hall RN, et al. Coherent light emission from GaAs junctions. *Phys Rev Lett* 1962; 9:366.

92.8   Bennett Jr WR, et al. Superradiance, Excitation Mechanism, and Quasi-CW oscillations in the Visible Ar+laser. *Appl Phys Lett* 1964; 4(10):180.

92.9   Geusic JE, Marcos HM, Van Uitern LG. Laser Oscillation in Nd:doped yttrium aluminium, yttrium gallium and gadolinium garnets. *Appl Phys Lett* 1964; 4:182.

92.10   McGhee NJ, et al. editors. *Excimer Lasers in Ophthalmology, Principles and Practice.* Butterworth-Heinemann Medical; 1997.

92.11   Schuitmaker JJ, et al. Photodynamic therapy: a promising new modality for the treatment of cancer. *J Photochem Photobiol B Biology* 1996; 34(1):3.

92.12   See ref. 9.11, ref 49.9, ref. 40.7.

PHYSICAL REVIEW   VOLUME 112, NUMBER 6   DECEMBER 15, 1958

Infrared and Optical Masers

A. L. SCHAWLOW AND C. H. TOWNES*
Bell Telephone Laboratories, Murray Hill, New Jersey
(Received August 26, 1958)

The extension of maser techniques to the infrared and optical region is considered. It is shown that by using a resonant cavity of centimeter dimensions, having many resonant modes, maser oscillation at these wavelengths can be achieved by pumping with reasonable amounts of incoherent light. For wavelengths much shorter than those of the ultraviolet region, maser-type amplification appears to be quite impractical. Although use of a multimode cavity is suggested, a single mode may be selected by making only the end walls highly reflecting, and defining a suitably small angular aperture. Then extremely monochromatic and coherent light is produced. The design principles are illustrated by reference to a system using potassium vapor.

92:5

The abstract of the famous paper from 1958 by Arthur Swawlow (1921–1999) and Charles Townes predicting the theoretical possibility of producing optical MASER (or LASER replacing Microwave with Light in the acronym) action, for instance in a potassium vapour system.

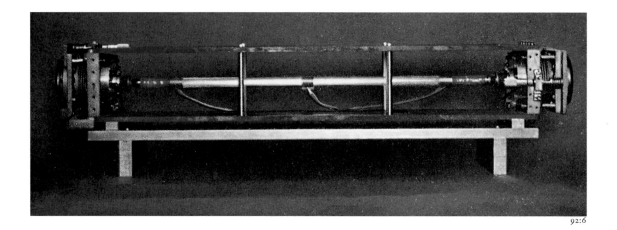

92:6

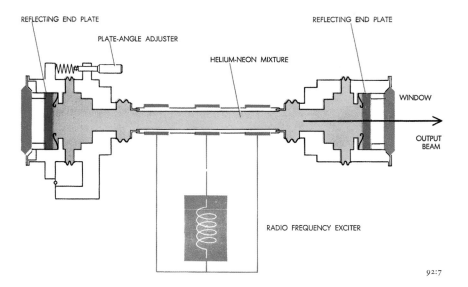

92:7

The first gas laser producing a continuous
beam of light is invented by William Bennett
Jr and Ali Javan in 1960. As is shown on the
opposite page in the diagram of their apparatus and in the picture of the actual device, they
excite a He-Ne gas mixture with a discharge
from a radio frequency source.

Below the inventors stand next to the laser.
From right to left, Bennett Jr and Javan, together with D R Herriott, who is in the process
of adjusting a mirror of the device.

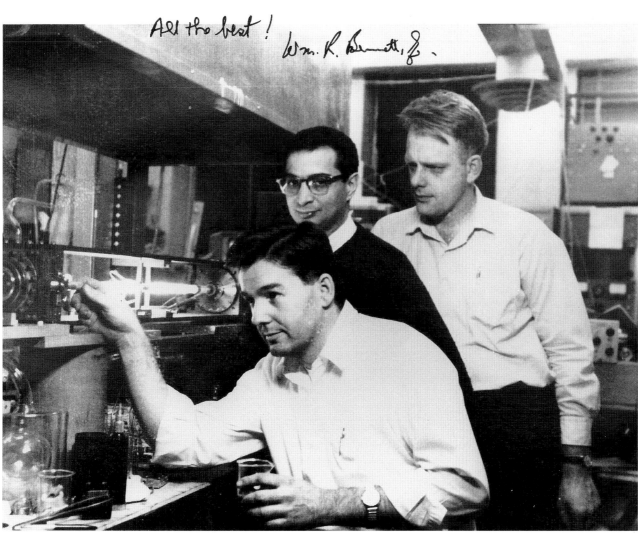

92:8

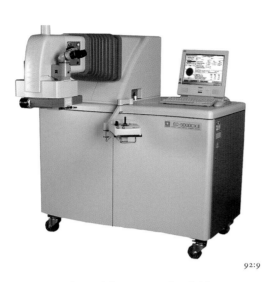

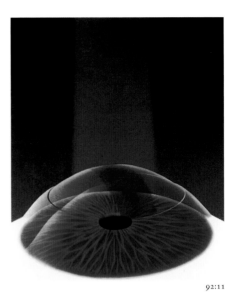

Excimer (exited diatomic molecule) lasers are invented during the 1970s and deliver high power pulsed ultra violet light that lends itself to "cold" evaporative removal of biological tissue. Modern units such as the one shown in the picture can be controlled with high precision and are the effective tools of refractive surgery, as illustrated by the ablated cornea in the photograph.

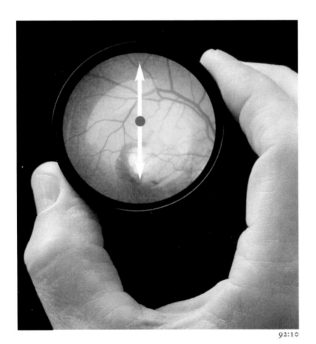

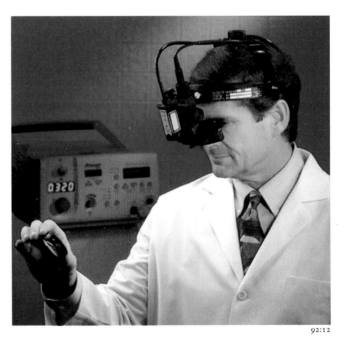

Laser Indirect Ophthalmoscopy with a frequency-doubled YAG laser allows the examination of the entire retina even in the presence of cataracts (for direct ophthalmoscopy that reveals only the more central portions of the retina, see #45). The equipment is frequently used in retinal detachment surgery and in photocoagulation procedures.

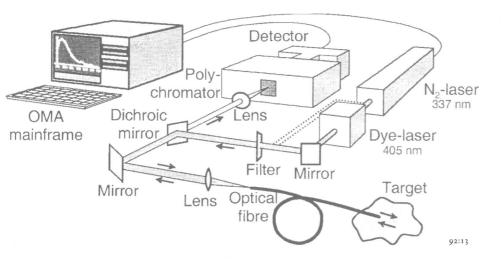

The schematic representation of a laser-based optical multichannel analyser (OMA) for in vivo fluorescence investigations of the skin. A nitrogen laser is pumping a dye laser that emits radiation at 405 nm, close to the wavelength of the peak fluorescence of skin. With suitable photosensitising agents (i.e. a substance called ALA) and laser irradiation at carefully selected wavelength(s), skin areas with basal cell carcinoma can be selectively targeted. The good results obtained with such a photodynamic therapy (PDT) are shown by the upper row of images in the illustration below. The corresponding skin perfusion images beneath are generated with laser Doppler techniques (LDPI) (see #40) and verify the success of the treatment.

92:13

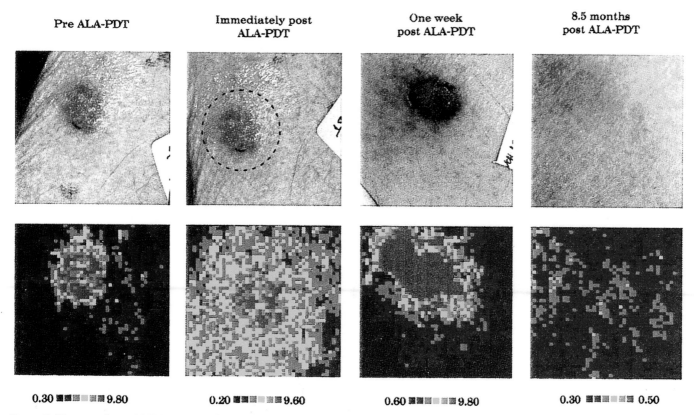

Figure 2. Photographs and LDPI pictures of a mixed superficial/nodular basal cell carcinoma on the arm of a 78-year-old male. The images were taken before treatment, immediately following treatment by laser light irradiation, 1 week and 8·5 months after the PDT procedure. The increased blood flow immediately after the treatment procedure has extended beyond the treatment area into the surrounding non-illuminated normal skin, indicating a recreation of vessels to supply the treated area with blood, as in an immediate inflammatory response. A week following the treatment, an inflammatory reaction is seen, with an extended blood perfusion limited to this area. Eight and a half months after the treatment the lesion is hardly visible and the blood perfusion was as high as in the normal surrounding skin. Note the different colour scales in the blood flow images.

92:14

Scand J Plast Reconstr Surg 3: 81–100, 1969

INTRA-OSSEOUS ANCHORAGE OF DENTAL PROSTHESES

I. *Experimental Studies*

P.-I. Brånemark, U. Breine, R. Adell, B. O. Hansson, J. Lindström and Å. Ohlsson

*From the Laboratory of Experimental Biology, Department of Anatomy, University of Gothenburg
and the Department of Plastic Surgery, Sahlgrenska Sjukhuset, Gothenburg, Sweden*

Abstract. An investigation of factors controlling healing and long term stability of intra-osseous titanium implants to restore masticatory function in dogs revealed that an integrity of the good anchorage of the implant requires: (1) Non-traumatic surgical preparation of soft and hard tissues and a mechanically and chemically clean implant. (2) Primary closure of the mucoperiosteal flap, to isolate the implant site from the oral cavity until a biological barrier has been reestablished. (3) Oral hygiene to prevent gingival inflammation. Provided these precautions are taken, it is possible to subject dental prostheses, connected to the implants, to unlimited masticatory load. With these precautions such implants were found to tolerate ordinary use in dogs for periods of more than 5 years without signs of tissue injury or other indications of rejection phenomena.

Macroscopic clinical investigation, stereomicroscopy, roentgenography and light microscopy of the implant site *in situ* and after removal from the body showed that the soft and hard tissues had accepted the implant and incorporated it without producing signs of tissue injury. In fact the bone appeared to grow into all the minute pits and impressions in the surface of the titanium implant, without any shielding layer of buffer tissue at all.

These findings indicate that dental prostheses can be successfully anchored intra-osseously in the dog suggesting that its possible clinical use in oral rehabilitation should be given unprejudiced consideration.

93:1

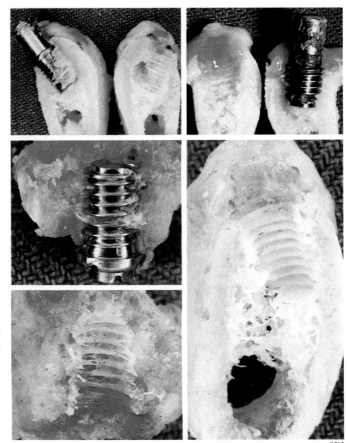

93:2

The abstract and illustration from the report of Per-Ingvar Brånemark and his colleagues on the first successful long term experiment with titanium implants for restoring masticatory function in dogs. After a five year period no tissue injury or rejection phenomena is observed.

B RÅNEMARK was born in Karlshamn, Sweden, in 1929. He studied medicine in Lund and received his M.D. there in 1956. Three years later he presented his thesis on vital microscopy of bone marrow (93.1). In 1960 he moved to the University of Gothenburg, where he became professor of anatomy in 1969. Brånemark holds more than thirty honorary positions throughout the world and his concept of osseointegration (structural and functional connection between living bone and an implant) has also lead to successful commercial enterprises.

Intra-osseous Anchorage of Dental Prostheses. I Experimental Studies.

SCAND J PLAST RECONSTR SURG 1969; 3:81.

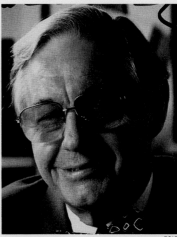

Per-Ingvar Brånemark

93:3

BRÅNEMARK AND his collaborators (Breine, Adell, Hansson, Lindström and Ohlsson) present five years' experience of intra-osseous titanium implants in twelve dogs. Firstly reviewing the literature, they find that not enough is known about the biological prerequisites for permanent anchorage of a prosthesis to bone tissue (93.2). Using X-ray investigations, stereo-microscopy and histological analysis, they find that titanium screws totally imbedded in the bone are mechanically very stable for several years, provided that the implant bed is prepared with a minimum of bone tissue damage and is sealed off from the oral cavity while the barrier function between implant and tissue is re-established. The authors declare their intention to explore the use of this technique in human prosthodontics.

IN PERSPECTIVE:
Titanium was discovered in 1791 by Gregor (93.3), but was only prepared in pure form by Hunter in 1901, because the metal's reactivity easily produced oxide layers on the surface. This property, however, partly explains why titanium and its alloys (TiAlV) are superior as regards corrosion resistance and biocompatibility, compared to other metal alloys used as implant materials such as stainless steel and the cobalt alloys (CoCrMo or CoNiCrMo) (93.4). Brånemark's studies of bone marrow (93.1)(93.5) led to the chance discovery of the favourable properties of titanium implants when embedded with proper techniques into bone tissue (93.6). From an early start in the mid 1970s, the method gained acceptance during the following decade and today more than a million people worldwide have received osseo-integrated titanium-anchored dental prostheses (93.7). The concept has also proved useful outside dentistry, particularly in reconstructive surgery and in the attachment of hearing aids and prostheses (93.8). Many key applications of implants rely on polymeric biomaterials (93.9), some with sophisticated properties such as bio-degradability and the ability to promote wound healing or bone formation (93.10). Major uses include components of the cardiovascular system (vessels and valves), substitutes for different type of tissues, ligaments and skin, and suture material.

93.1 Brånemark P-I. Vital microscopy of bone marrow in rabbit. *Scand J Lab Invest* 1959; 11 (Suppl. 38):1.

93.2 Adell R, et al. Intra-osseous anchorage of the dental prostheses. II Review of Clinical Approaches. *Scand J Plast Reconstr Surg* 1970; 4:19.

93.3 Gregor W. Beobachtungen und Versuche über den Menakanite, einen in Corwall (Kierchspiel Menaccan bei Falmouth) gefundenen magnetischen Sand. *Chem Ann.* (L von Crell) 1791; Bd.1.

93.4 Brunette DM, et al. editors. *Titanium in Medicine*. Springer Verlag; 2001.

93.5 Brånemark P-I, et al. Regeneration of bone marrow. A clinical and experimental study following removal of bone marrow by curettage. *Acta Anat* (Basel) 1964; 59:1.

93.6 Williams E. *A Matter of Balance*. Akademiförlaget; 1992.

93.7 Brånemark P-I, Zarb GA, Albrektsson T. editors. *Tissue-Integrated Prosthesis: Osseointegration in clinical Dentistry*. Chicago: Quintessence Publ. Inc.; 1985.

93.8 Williams E, Rydevik B, Brånemark P-I. editors. *From Molecule to Man; Facts and Hypotheses—Options and Opportunities*. Göteborg: The Institute of Applied Biology; 2000.

93.9 Shtilman MI. *Polymeric Biomaterials* Part I Polymer Implants. Brill Academic Publishers; 2003.

93.10 Hubbell J. Biomaterials in tissue engineering. *Biotechnology*. 1995; 13:565.

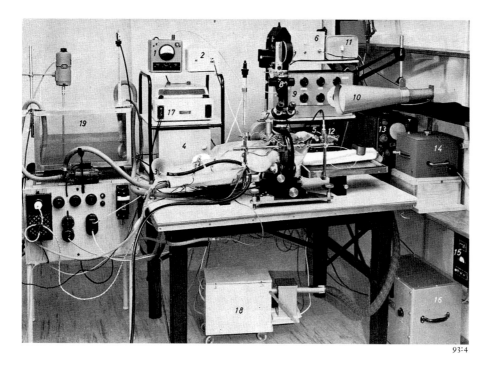

The chance discovery of the remarkable biocompatibility exhibited by titanium goes back to 1959 and early studies of the capillary blood flow in the bone marrow of rabbits. An overview of the experimental setup used by Brånemark in these investigations is shown together with the microscopic arrangement and a picture of the capillary bed in the bone marrow. Titanium was inadvertly used in some of the preparations to create a permanent microscopic field of view.

93:4

Fig. 29. General view of experimental set-up. 1 Exposure meter. 2 Respiration recorder. 3 Microphone of respiration recorder. 4 Blood pressure recorder. 5 Pressure chamber for blood pressure recorder. 6 Photometer with photocells 7 and 8. 9 Corpuscular flow velocity recorder. 10 Cathode ray tube for corpuscular flow velocity recorder. 11 Time marker. 12 Electronic switch. 13 Oscilloscope. 14 Oscilloscope camera. 15 Power unit for mercury lamp. 16 Main voltage stabiliser. 17 Temperature recorder. 18 Apparatus for supply of thermostatically controlled, moistened air. 19 Tyrode's solution.

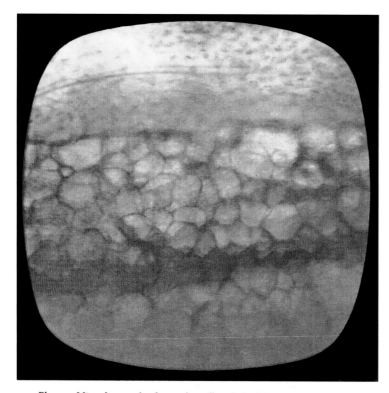

Plate 2. Microphotograph of typical capillary bed of bone marrow (×300).

93:5

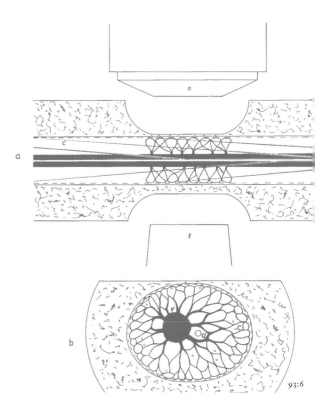

93:6

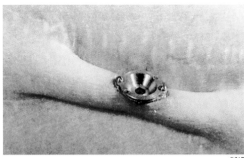

93:7

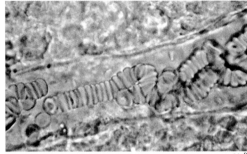

93:8

A titanium inspection chamber inserted in the upper arm for blood cell studies and a view of the cells in vivo, as obtained using the more recent microscopic and imaging equipment shown.

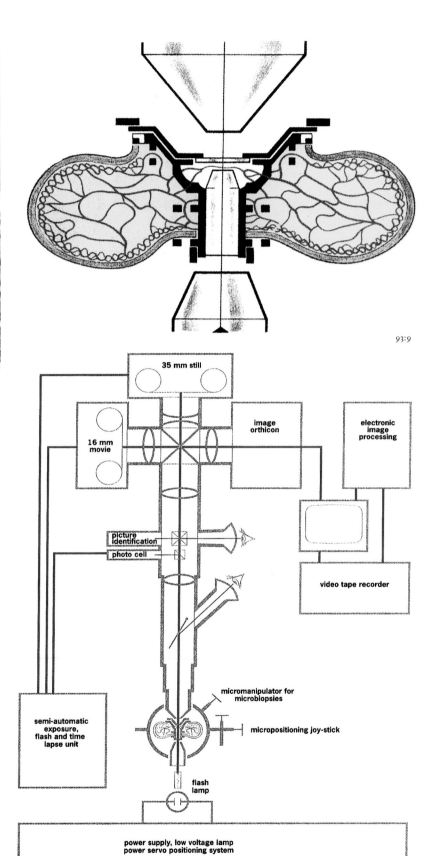

93:9

35 mm still

image orthicon

electronic image processing

16 mm movie

picture identification

photo cell

video tape recorder

micromanipulator for microbiopsies

micropositioning joy-stick

semi-automatic exposure, flash and time lapse unit

flash lamp

power supply, low voltage lamp power servo positioning system

93:10

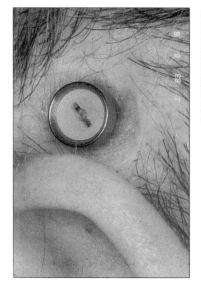

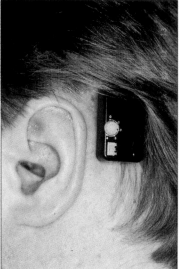

93:11

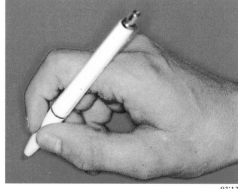

93:13

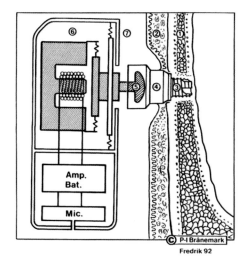

Fredrik 92

93:12

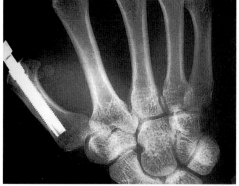

93:14

Fig. 19. Bone conduction hearing aids can be anchored with a fixture in the skull bone. The surgical procedure demands suitable bone preparation and careful trimming of the penetrated skin according to the method proposed by Hallén to avoid relative movement in the region of skin penetration.

A titanium fixture for anchoring bone conduction hearing aids.

An example of a titanium tissue anchored limb prosthesis. X-ray image showing the thumb prosthesis anchored to the skeleton and a picture of the prosthesis in use.

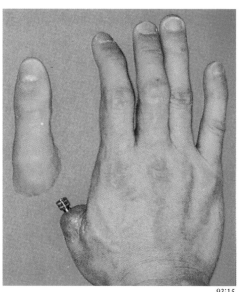

93:15

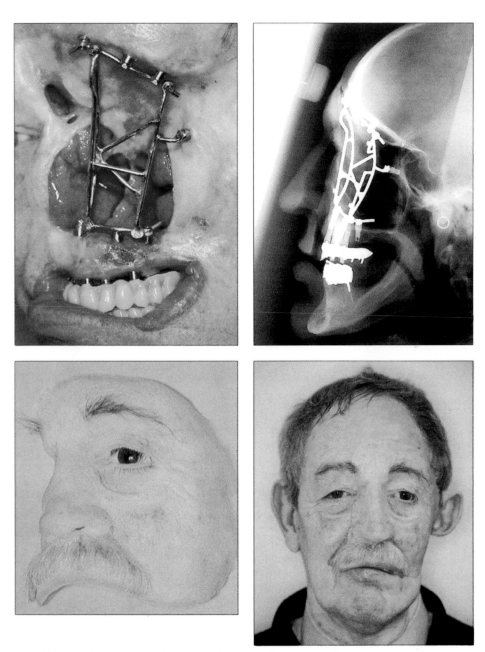

Fig. 20. Typical example of a large maxillofacial defect as a result of tumour resection, where the tissue has been irradiated. Following pre-operative hyperbaric oxygen treatment, the patient was reconstructed with an autologous bone transplant and titanium fixtures, which both anchor a facial prosthesis and provide permanent stability for an upper jaw bridge.

93:16

A large maxillofacial defect as a result of tumour resection, reconstructed with an autologous bone transplant and titanium fixtures that provide adequate stability for an upper jaw bridge.

Tumor Detection by Nuclear Magnetic Resonance

Raymond Damadian

Abstract. *Spin echo nuclear magnetic resonance measurements may be used as a method for discriminating between malignant tumors and normal tissue. Measurements of spin-lattice (T_1) and spin-spin (T_2) magnetic relaxation times were made in six normal tissues in the rat (muscle, kidney, stomach, intestine, brain, and liver) and in two malignant solid tumors, Walker sarcoma and Novikoff hepatoma. Relaxation times for the two malignant tumors were distinctly outside the range of values for the normal tissues studied, an indication that the malignant tissues were characterized by an increase in the motional freedom of tissue water molecules. The possibility of using magnetic relaxation methods for rapid discrimination between benign and malignant surgical specimens has also been considered. Spin-lattice relaxation times for two benign fibroadenomas were distinct from those for both malignant tissues and were the same as those of muscle.*

94:1

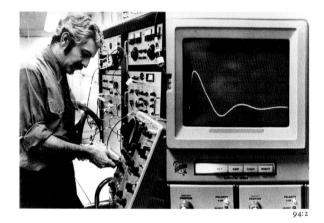

94:2

Raymond Damadian in his laboratory and the abstract of the paper, where he reports his discovery that NMR (nuclear magnetic resonance) techniques can differentiate between tumour and healthy tissue. In the NMR method a sample in a magnetic field is exposed to pulsed RF (radio frequency) radiation and the decaying signal emitted by the protons of the cellular water in response to the RF excitation is detected. According to the theory of this process developed by Felix Bloch (1905–1983) in 1946, the decay can be characterised by two time constants T1 and T2. The picture shows Damadian at his equipment. The part of his paper reporting the values of T1 and T2 for different types of tissue sample is also reproduced.

Table 2. Spin-lattice (T_1) and spin-spin (T_2) relaxation times (in seconds) in tumors.

Rat No.	Weight (g)	T_1	T_2
Walker sarcoma			
6	156	0.700	0.100
7	150	.750	.100
8	495	.794 (0.794)*	.100
9	233	.688	
10	255	.750	
Mean and S.E.		0.736 ± 0.022	.100
P		< .01†	
Novikoff hepatoma			
11	155	0.798	0.120
12	160	.852	.120
13	231	.827	.115
Mean and S.E.		0.826 ± 0.013	0.118 ±
P		< .01†	0.002
Fibroadenoma (benign)			
14		0.448	
15		.537	
Mean		.492	
Distilled water			
		2.691	
		2.690	
		2.640	
Mean and S.E.		2.677 ± 0.021	

* Spin-lattice relaxation time after the specimen stood overnight at room temperature.   † The *P* values are the probability estimates of the significance of the difference in the means of T_1 for the malignant tumor and for brain.

94:3

DAMADIAN was born in 1936 in Forest Hills, New York. He studied the violin at the Julliard School of Music, mathematics at the University of Wisconsin and in 1960 earned an M.D. from the Albert Einstein College of Medicine. After post-doctoral studies in biophysics at Harvard University, he joined the faculty at the State University of New York Downstate Medical Center in 1969. The nuclear magnetic resonance (NMR) studies cited below were carried out at the NMR Specialties Company in New Kensington. Damadian founded the FONAR company in 1978 for the manufacture of magnetic resonance imaging (MRI) scanners and he is still the president and chairman of this company.

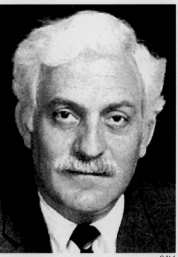

94:4

Raymond Damadian

Tumor Detection by Nuclear Magnetic Resonance.

SCIENCE 1971; 171:1151.

DAMADIAN REPORTS some characteristics of biological tissue studied by a pulsed NMR spectrometer. Tissue properties are determined, according to a technique introduced by Hahn in 1950 (94.1)(94.2), from the decay times of the radio frequency (RF) radiation that is emitted by the protons of the cellular water subsequent to a specific set of RF pulse excitations. It is shown that healthy tissue taken from the rectus muscle, liver, stomach, small intestine, kidney and brain of rats may exhibit significantly differing decay times, but also that malignant liver tissue (Novikoff hepatoma) is characterised by almost three times longer decay times than healthy liver tissue. A benign tumour (fibroadenomas) is found to have properties similar to that of the kidney.

IN PERSPECTIVE:

In 1938 Rabi conducted the first nuclear magnetic resonance experiment, demonstrating its use for determining nuclear magnetic moments in a lithium chloride molecular beam (94.3). In 1946 the phenomenon was observed in the solid state by Bloch (in water) and by Purcell (in paraffin) (94.4). Bloch's theory of NMR (94.5) explained the decay times as used by Damadian in the paper cited above. Since the magnetic field affecting the nucleus depends on the electron clouds around it, a "chemical shift" of the NMR resonance frequency can be used to examine molecular structure. For three decades, this was the foremost application of NMR. Many molecules and compounds were analysed in this way, some also of direct biological and medical interest (94.6). By the late 1960s attention turned specifically to the water-protein interaction within cells (94.7). Damadian's discovery paved the way for progress towards medical applications. Early methods and equipment for magnetic resonance imaging (MRI) (94.8)(94.9)(94.10) were soon replaced by new techniques capable of creating images rapidly and of good enough quality for clinical use (94.11).

94.1 Mattson J, Simon M. *The pioneers of NMR and magnetic resonance in medicine. The Story of MRI.* New York: Dean Books Co.; 1966. Chapt. 6 and Chapt. 3.

94.2 Hahn EL. Spin echoes. *Phys Rev* 1950; 80:580.

94.3 Rabi II, et al. A new method of measuring nuclear magnetic moment. *Phys Rev* 1938; 53:318. See also ref. 94.1 Chapt. 1.

94.4 Purcell EM, Torrey HC, Pound RV. Resonance absorption by nuclear magnetic moments in a solid. *Phys Rev* 1946; 69:37. See also ref. 94.1 Chapt. 3.

94.5 Bloch F. Nuclear induction. *Phys Rev* 1946; 70:478. See also ref. 94.1 Chapt.4.

94.6 Odeblad E. Nuclear magnetic resonance in biology and medicine. *Ztschr f med Isotopenforsch* 1956; 1:25.

94.7 Hazlewood CF, Nichols BL, Chamberlain NF. Evidence for existence of a minimum of two phases of ordered water in skeletal muscle. *Nature* 1969; 222:747.

94.8 Damadian RV. *Apparatus and method for detecting cancer in tissue.* US Patent 3,789,832 1974.

94.9 Damadian RV. Field Focusing Nuclear Magnetic Resonance (FONAR): Visualization of a Tumor in a Live Animal. *Science* 1976; 194:1430.

94.10 Damadian RV, Goldsmith M, Minkoff L. NMR in cancer: XVI Fonar image of the live human body. *Physiol Chem Phys* 1977; 194:1430.

94.11 See #96 Lauterbur page 498.

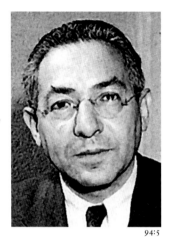
A New Method of Measuring Nuclear Magnetic Moment*

It is the purpose of this note to describe an experiment in which nuclear magnetic moment is measured very directly. The method is capable of very high precision and extension to a large number and variety of nuclei.

Consider a beam of molecules, such as LiCl, traversing a magnetic field which is sufficiently strong to decouple completely the nuclear spins from one another and from the molecular rotation. If a small oscillating magnetic field is applied at right angles to a much larger constant field, a re-orientation of the nuclear spin and magnetic moment with respect to the constant field will occur when the frequency of the oscillating field is close to the Larmor frequency of precession of the particular angular momentum vector in question. This precession frequency is given by

$$v = \mu H/hi = g(i)\mu_0 H/h. \quad (1)$$

To apply these ideas a beam of molecules in a $^1\Sigma$ state (no electronic moment) is spread by an inhomogeneous magnetic field and refocused onto a detector by a subsequent field, somewhat as in the experiment of Kellogg, Rabi and Zacharias.[1] As in that experiment the re-orienting field is placed in the region between the two magnets. The homogeneous field is produced by an electromagnet capable of supplying uniform fields up to 6000 gauss in a gap 6 mm wide and 5 cm long. In the gap is placed a loop of wire in the form of a hairpin (with its axis parallel to the direction of the beam) which is connected to a source of current at radiofrequency to produce the oscillating field at right angles to the steady field. If a re-orientation of a spin occurs in this field, the subsequent conditions in the second deflecting field are no longer correct for refocusing, and the intensity at the detector goes down. The experimental procedure is to vary the homogeneous field for some given value of the frequency of the oscillating field until the resonance is observed by a drop in intensity at the detector and a subsequent recovery when the resonance value is passed.

The re-orientation process is more accurately described as one in which transitions occur between the various magnetic levels given by the quantum number m_i of the particular angular momentum vector in question. An exact solution for the transition probability was given by Rabi[2, 3] for the case where the variable field rotates rather than oscillates. However, it is more convenient experimentally to use an oscillating field, in which case the transition probability is approximately the same for *weak* oscillating fields *near* the resonance frequency, except that ϑ is replaced by $\vartheta/2$ in Eq. (13). With this replacement and with passage to the limit of weak oscillating fields, the formula becomes for the case of $i = \frac{1}{2}$

$$P(\tfrac{1}{2}, -\tfrac{1}{2}) = \frac{\vartheta^2}{(1-q)^2 + q\vartheta^2} \sin^2 \{\pi tr[(1-q)^2 + q\vartheta^2]^{\frac{1}{2}}\}, \quad (2)$$

where ϑ is $\frac{1}{2}$ the ratio of the oscillating field to the steady field, q is the ratio of the Larmor frequency of Eq. (1) to the frequency r of the oscillating field. The denominator of the expression is the familiar resonance denominator. The formula is generalized to any spin i by formula (17).[2]

In the theory of this experiment, t, in Eq. (2), is replaced by L/v, where L is the length of the oscillating region of the field, and v is the molecular velocity. $P(\frac{1}{2}, -\frac{1}{2})$ must then be averaged over the Maxwellian distribution of velocities. However, the first term is not affected by the velocity distribution if t is long enough for many oscillations to take place. The average value of the $\sin^2$ term over the velocity distribution is approximately $\frac{1}{2}$.

To produce deflections of the weakly magnetic molecules sufficient to make the apparatus sensitive to this effect, the beam is made 245 cm long; the first deflecting field is 52 cm in length and the second 100 cm.

We have tried this experiment with LiCl and observed the resonance peaks of Li and Cl. The effects are very striking and the resonances sharp (Fig. 1). A full account of this experiment, together with the values of the nuclear moments, will be published when the homogeneous field is recalibrated.

I. I. RABI
J. R. ZACHARIAS
S. MILLMAN
P. KUSCH

Hunter College (J. R. Z.),
Columbia University,
New York, N. Y.
January 31, 1938.

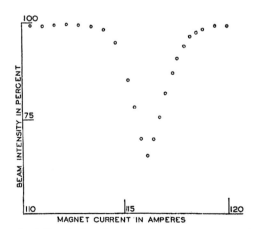

FIG. 1. Curve showing refocused beam intensity at various values of the homogeneous field. One ampere corresponds to about 18.4 gauss. The frequency of the oscillating field was held constant at 3.518×10^5 cycles per second.

* Publication assisted by the Ernest Kempton Adams Fund for Physical Research of Columbia University.
[1] Kellogg, Rabi and Zacharias, Phys. Rev. 50, 472 (1936).
[2] Rabi, Phys. Rev. 51, 652 (1937).
[3] C. J. Gorter, Physica 9, 995 (1936). We are very much indebted to Dr. Gorter who, when visiting our laboratory in September 1937, drew our attention to his stimulating experiments in which he attempted to measure nuclear moments by observing the rise in temperature of solids placed in a constant magnetic field on which an oscillating field was superimposed. Dr. F. Bloch has independently worked out similar ideas but for another purpose (unpublished).

94:6

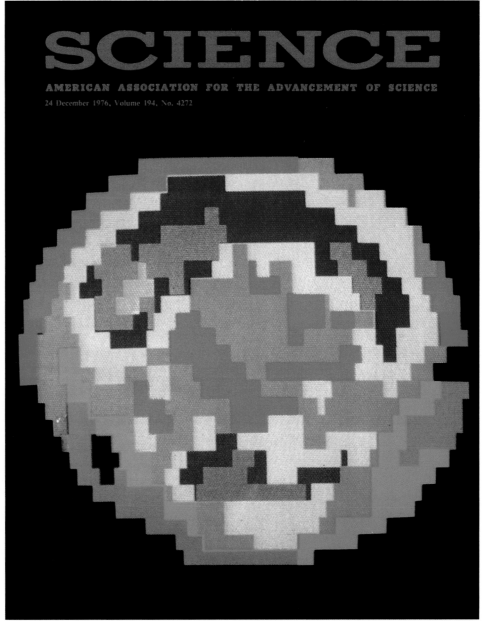

The cover of the magazine Science showing the first image of a tumour in a live animal obtained by Damadian in 1976 using the NMR technique developed by him. With a scanning aperture of 1 mm and the thorax diameter of the mouse being 13 mm, the image has poor resolution and overestimates the tumour size.

SCIENCE

AMERICAN ASSOCIATION FOR THE ADVANCEMENT OF SCIENCE

24 December 1976, Volume 194, No. 4272

94:7

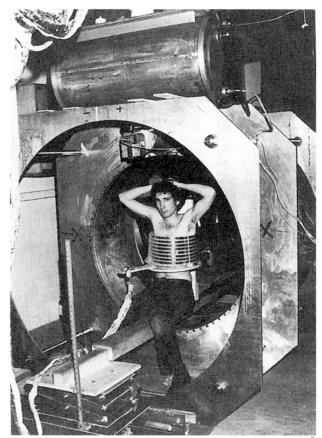

Lawrence Minkoff sitting in Damadian's whole body scanner, called "Indomitable", taking the first human NMR scan on 3 July 1977. It takes fourteen hours to prepare for the experiment and more than four hours to collect the 106 picture elements for the image shown below.

94:8

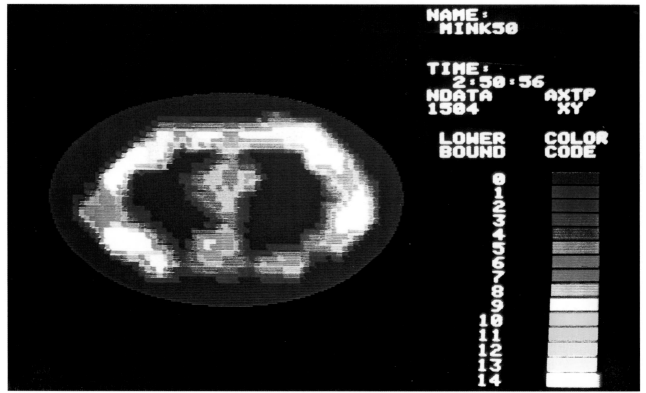

94:9

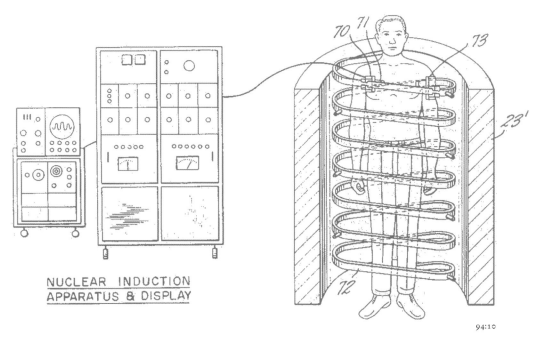

3,789,832

NUCLEAR INDUCTION
APPARATUS & DISPLAY

94:10

Drawing from Damadian's patent from 1974 showing a schematic representation of his FONAR (field focused nuclear magnetic resonance) whole body apparatus.

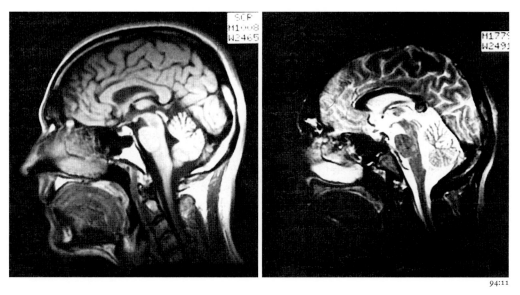

94:11

Modern MRI (magnetic resonance imaging) pictures of the same subject, illustrating the implications of using the two different decay time constants T1 (left) and T2 (right) for image formation. The mechanism behind T1 is the relaxation of the RF excited protons, while that of T2 is the relaxation due to exchange of excitation between protons. The markedly different images can be used in concert for diagnostic purposes.

1973, *British Journal of Radiology*, 46, 1016–1022

Computerized transverse axial scanning (tomography): Part I. Description of system

G. N. Hounsfield

Central Research Laboratories of EMI Limited, Hayes, Middlesex

(Received February, 1973 and in revised form July, 1973)

ABSTRACT

This article describes a technique in which X-ray transmission readings are taken through the head at a multitude of angles: from these data, absorption values of the material contained within the head are calculated on a computer and presented as a series of pictures of slices of the cranium. The system is approximately 100 times more sensitive than conventional X-ray systems to such an extent that variations in soft tissues of nearly similar density can be displayed.

For many years past, X-ray techniques have been developed along the same lines, namely the recording on photographic film of the shadow of the object to be viewed. Recently, it has been realized that this is not the most efficient method of utilizing all the information that can be obtained from the X-ray beam. Oldendorf (1961) carried out experiments based on principles similar to those described here, but it was not then fully realized that very high efficiencies could be achieved and so, picture reconstruction techniques were not fully developed.

As the exposure of the patient to X rays must be restricted, there is an upper limit to the number of photons that may be passed through the body during the examination, and so to the amount of information that can be obtained. It is, therefore, of great importance that the method of examination ensures that all the information obtained is fully utilized and interpreted with maximum efficiency.

In the conventional film technique a large proportion of the available information is lost in attempting to portray all the information from a three-dimensional body on a two-dimensional photographic plate, the image superimposing all objects from front to rear. In order that any one internal structure may be seen, it must clearly stand out against the variations of the materials in front and behind it.

The technique to be described divides the head into a series of slices, each being irradiated via its edges; the radiation is confined to the slice and for this reason, unlike conventional X-ray techniques, the information derived from any object within the slice is unaffected by variations in the material on either side of the slice. Data are processed and displayed by digital computer methods.

A report on this work was presented at the April 1972 Annual Congress of the British Institute of Radiology (Ambrose and Hounsfield, 1973). A short account has also appeared in the *New Scientist* (*Technology Review*), 1972.

PRINCIPLES OF THE METHOD

The aim of the system is to produce a series of images by a tomographic method as illustrated in Fig. 1. Each image shown at the bottom of the figure is derived from a particular slice.

In the actual equipment, the patient is scanned by a narrow beam of X rays. The X-ray tube, detectors, and collimators are fixed to a common frame, as shown in Fig. 2, those rays which pass through the head being detected by two collimated sensing devices (scintillation detectors) which always point towards the X-ray source. Both X-ray source and detectors scan across the patient's head linearly taking 160 readings of transmissions through the head as shown in scan 1 on the scanning sequence diagram (Fig. 3). At the end of the scan the scanning system is rotated 1 deg. and the process is repeated, as shown in scans 2 and 3. This continues for 180 deg. when 28,800 (180×160) readings of transmission will have been taken by each detector. These are stored in a disc file for processing by a mini computer. A picture is reconstructed from the data by the following method:

A separate detector measures the intensity of the X-ray source and the readings taken from this can be used to calculate absorption by the material along the X-ray beam path, where

$$\text{Absorption} = \log \frac{\text{Intensity of X rays at source}}{\text{Intensity of X rays at detector}}$$

If the body is divided into a series of small cubes each having a calculable value of absorption, then the sum of the absorption values of the cubes which are contained within the X-ray beam will equal the total absorption of the beam path. Each beam path, therefore, forms one of a series of 28,800 simultaneous equations, in which there are 6,400 variables and, providing that there are more equations than variables, then the values of each cube in the slice can be solved. In short there must be more X-ray readings than picture points.

95:1

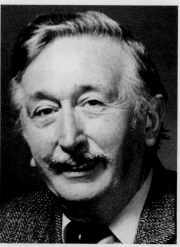

Godfrey Hounsfield   95:2

Hounsfield was born in a village in Nottinghamshire in 1919. During World War II, he joined the Royal Air Force, working as a radar mechanic and learning radio communication. After the war he received a diploma in electrical engineering from the Faraday House Electrical Engineering College in London. In 1951 he joined the staff of EMI where, among other assignments, he led the design of Britain's first all-transistor computer. While working on pattern recognition problems, he invented the computed axial tomography (CAT or just CT) technique. Hounsfield shared the 1979 Nobel Prize in Medicine with Cormack (95.1) for their development of computer-assisted tomography.

Computerized transverse axial scanning (tomography): Part I. Description of system.

Br J Radiol 1973; 46:1016.

Hounsfield describes a technique where a narrow collimated beam of X-rays scans through an object at a multitude of angles and the absorption of the material within the object is calculated. Each linear scan illuminates a slice of the object about 1 cm thick and creates 160 transmission values. With 180 rotations, each one degree, a total of 180×160=28,800 readings need to be processed. The absorption coefficient is determined with an accuracy of about 0.5%, making the device about 100 times more sensitive than conventional X-ray systems. This allows the display of variations in soft tissues of similar density. In clinical tests a picture of a slice made of 80×80 points takes about five minutes to generate.

IN PERSPECTIVE:

In 1933 Bartelink was the first to describe medical tomography (tomos = slice) (95.2). With an X-ray tube rigidly connected to the detector, he scanned a focused beam across the object, producing images of planes by discriminating out-of-focus areas. Oldendorf conducted tomographic experiments on a simple mechanical model using collimated gamma radiation and also showed how to reconstruct the interior of a slice of a very simple object (95.3). In the early 1960s Cormack carried out similar experiments, but in addition developed general mathematical tools for image reconstruction (95.4)(95.5). The first clinical study using X-ray CT was reported by Ambrose, who made brain scans in healthy and diseased states with the equipment described by Hounsfield (95.6). Today two- and three-dimensional images with up to fifty times the resolution described above can be created in around a second. More than 30,000 locations around the world use X-ray CT equipment and, together with MRI (95.7) and PET (95.8), it is one of the most powerful tools in medical diagnostics.

95.1 Cormack AM. *Early two-dimensional reconstruction and recent topics stemming from it.* Nobel Lecture Stockholm; 1979.

95.2 Bartelink DL. Röntgenschnitte. *Forschr Röntgenstr* 1933; 47:399.

95.3 Oldendorf WH. Isolated flying spot detection of radiodensity discontinuities-displaying the internal structural pattern of a complex object. *IRE Trans Bio-medical Electr* 1961; 8:68.

95.4 Cormack AM. Representation of a function by its line integrals, with some radiological applications. *J Appl Phys* 1963; 34:2722.

95.5 Cormack AM. Reconstruction of densities from their projections, with applications in radiological physics. *Physics in Medicine and Biology* 1973; 18:195. See also #96 Lauterbur page 498 and ref. 99.6.

95.6 Ambrose J. Computerized transverse axial scanning (tomography): Part 2. Clinical application. *Br J Radiol* 1973; 46:1023.

95.7 See #94 Damadian page 486, #96 Lauterbur page 498.

95.8 See #99 Phelps page 514.

Aus dem St. Canisius Ziekenhuis Nymwegen (Holland)

Röntgenschnitte

Von **D. L. Bartelink**

Mit 13 Abbildungen

Unsere normalen Röntgenbilder enthalten die Schatten aller zwischen Röhre und Platte gelegenen Gegenstände, wie man sagt: ,,übereinander projiziert". Dies hat wichtige praktische Folgen. In manchen Projektionen, z. B. des Felsenbeines, wird dessen Bild von Schatten aus anderen Tiefen des Kopfes störend überlagert. Dies gilt besonders in dem Falle, wo die schattengebenden Gebildeplatten näher liegen. Oft kann man dann nur noch die gröberen Umrisse erkennen, von der feineren Zeichnung aber nicht mehr entscheiden, ob sie von dem Felsenbeine herrührt und zu welchem Teile sie gehört.

Wenn es sich um die Fragestellung nach feineren Einzelheiten handelt, empfindet der Röntgenologe das Bedürfnis, ein Felsenbein isoliert darstellen zu können. Er nimmt dann die besonderen Projektionsrichtungen oder die Stereoskopie zu Hilfe. Der Meinung vieler Beobachter nach bleibt dabei aber meistens vieles zu wünschen übrig. Also ist es interessant, daß es möglich ist, zwar nicht absolut aber doch auf einem Umwege, Körperteile mittels Röntgenstrahlen m. w. isoliert abzubilden. Mit Hilfe eines besonderen Apparates ist man imstande, scharfe Bilder von flachen

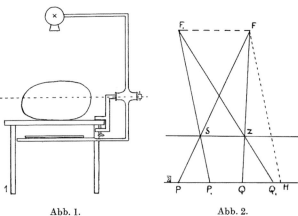

Abb. 1.   Abb. 2.

Schnitten (von beliebig großer Flächenausbreitung) des zu untersuchenden Körperteiles herzustellen, wobei alles außerhalb des Schnittes gelegene verwaschen erscheint. Den Namen Röntgenschnitte, wobei man vergleichsweise an Mikrotomschnitte denke, tragen solche Bilder insoweit zu recht, als sie eine ebene Schicht gleichmäßig scharf zeigen, insoweit zu unrecht, als an den Grenzen dieser Schicht auch noch gewisse Teile halbscharf mit abgebildet erscheinen. Im folgenden soll theoretisch gezeigt werden, daß es mechanisch tatsächlich gelingen kann, dieses Ziel zu erreichen.

Wenn man eine Röhre und eine Platte mittels eines Rahmens starr verbindet und dann während der Aufnahme den Rahmen um eine Achse senkrecht zum Zentralstrahl dreht (Abb. 1), so werden nur diejenigen Punkte eines Körpers (welchen man innerhalb des Rahmens aufgestellt hat und welcher die Drehung nicht mitmacht) auf der Platte scharf abgebildet, welche in der Verlängerung der obengenannten Achse liegen. Alle anderen Punkte des Körpers werden infolge der Projektionsverschiebung unscharf. Eine derartige, scharf abgebildete Linie hat nur einen beschränkten praktischen Wert.

Man kann aber auch eine Ebene scharf abbilden. In Abb. 2 sind dargestellt: F ein Röhrenfokus, P ein Punkt einer Platte und S ein Punkt in einem zu untersuchenden Körper, an welcher Stelle

95:3

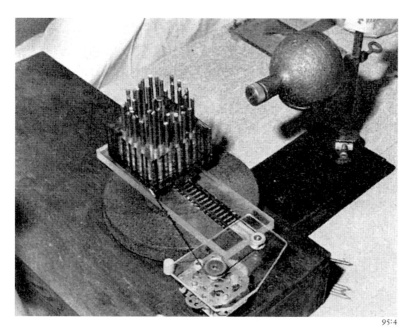

95:4

In 1961 W H Oldendorf demonstrates a tomographic recording and reconstruction technique using the simple mechanical model shown in the picture. The diagram of the experiment displays the model as rings of iron nails surrounding an iron and an aluminium nail. The system is rotated in a collimated beam of gamma radiation and the absorption is recorded. From these measurements the internal structure of the model and the position the aluminium nail are determined.

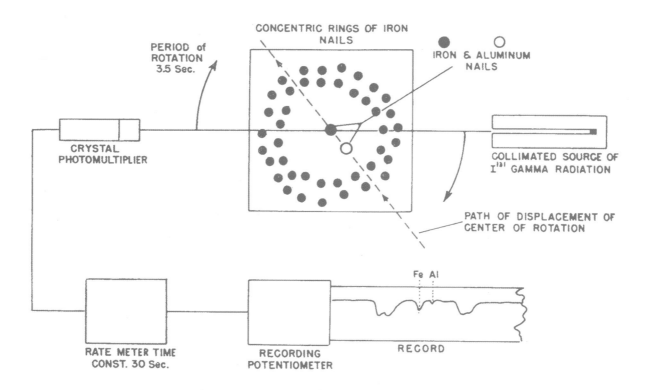

DIAGRAM OF A SIMPLE DEMONSTRATION MODEL OF A RADIODENSITY
DISCONTINUITY DETECTION SYSTEM

95:5

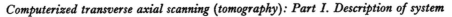

Computerized transverse axial scanning (tomography): Part I. Description of system

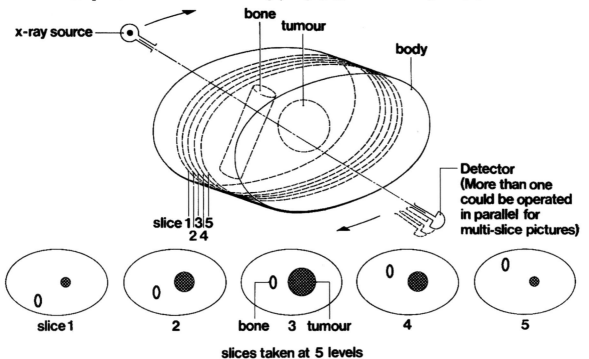

slices taken at 5 levels

FIG. 1.

Computerized transverse axial techniques on a body containing bone and tumour.

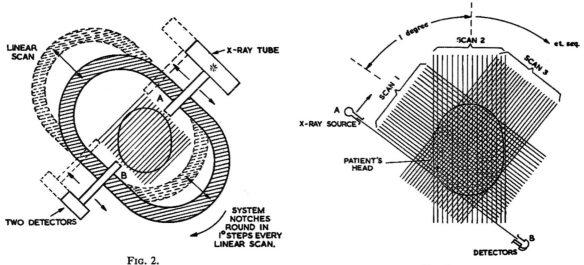

FIG. 2.

Motion of scanning frame and detectors for producing two continuous slices.

FIG. 3.

Simplified illustration of the scanning sequence.

1017

95:6

Illustrations from Hounsfield's paper in 1973 showing the method employed by the CT system to create an image. A collimated X-ray beam scans out a 1 cm thick slice by generating 160 transmission values. Then 180 rotations, each 1 degree, build up the total of 160 times 180 or 28,800 readings to be processed. The system is about 100 times more sensitive than conventional X-ray apparatus.

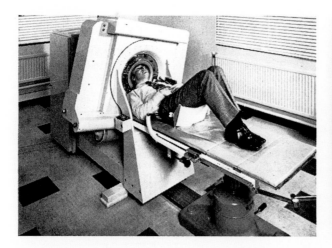

FIG. 5.
Illustration of the patient in position.

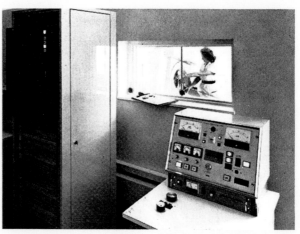

FIG. 6.
X-ray control console.

95:7

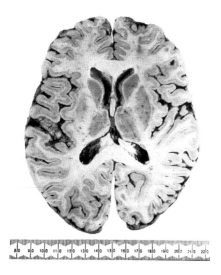

95:8

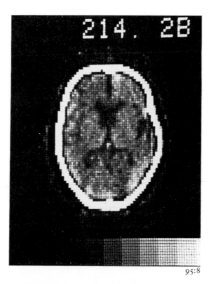

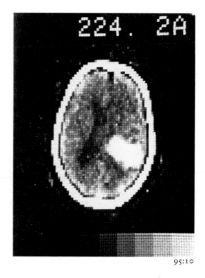

95:10

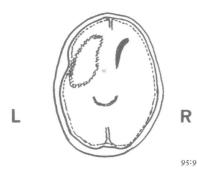

L   R

95:9

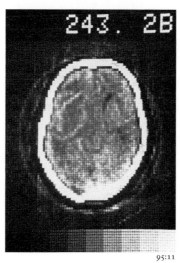

95:11

The pictures show the apparatus and some of the clinical results obtained. A section through a normal brain is shown with a scale for comparison and just to the right the corresponding CT image. The image 224 2A shows a haematoma, while the drawing clarifying the image 243 2B reveals a left inferior frontal tumour.

For Dr. Andras Gedeon with best regards Paul C. Lauterbur

Image Formation by Induced Local Interactions: Examples Employing Nuclear Magnetic Resonance

AN image of an object may be defined as a graphical representation of the spatial distribution of one or more of its properties. Image formation usually requires that the object interact with a matter or radiation field characterized by a wavelength comparable to or smaller than the smallest features to be distinguished, so that the region of interaction may be restricted and a resolved image generated.

This limitation on the wavelength of the field may be removed, and a new class of image generated, by taking advantage of induced local interactions. In the presence of a second field that restricts the interaction of the object with the first field to a limited region, the resolution becomes independent of wavelength, and is instead a function of the ratio of the normal width of the interaction to the shift produced by a gradient in the second field. Because the interaction may be regarded as a coupling of the two fields by the object, I propose that image formation by this technique be known as zeugmatography, from the Greek ζευγμα, "that which is used for joining".

The nature of the technique may be clarified by describing two simple examples. Nuclear magnetic resonance (NMR) zeugmatography was performed with 60 MHz (5 m) radiation and a static magnetic field gradient corresponding, for proton resonance, to about 700 Hz cm^{-1}. The test object consisted of two 1 mm inside diameter thin-walled glass capillaries of H_2O attached to the inside wall of a 4.2 mm inside diameter glass tube of D_2O. In the first experiment, both capillaries contained pure water. The proton resonance line width, in the absence of the transverse field gradient, was about 5 Hz. Assuming uniform signal strength across the region within the transmitter–receiver coil, the signal in the presence of a field gradient represents a one-dimensional projection of the H_2O content of the object, integrated over planes perpendicular to the gradient direction, as a function of the gradient coordinate (Fig. 1). One method of constructing a two-dimensional projected image of the object, as represented by its H_2O content, is to combine several projections, obtained by rotating the object about an axis perpendicular to the gradient direction (or, as in Fig. 1, rotating the gradient about the object), using one of the available methods for reconstruction of objects from their projections[1–5]. Fig. 2 was generated by an algorithm, similar to that of Gordon and Herman[4], applied to four projections, spaced as in Fig. 1, so as to construct a 20×20 image matrix. The representation shown was produced by shading within contours interpolated between the matrix points, and clearly reveals the locations and dimensions of the two columns of H_2O. In the second experiment, one capillary contained pure H_2O, and the other contained a 0.19 mM solution of $MnSO_4$ in H_2O. At low radio-frequency power (about 0.2 mgauss) the two capillaries gave nearly identical images in the

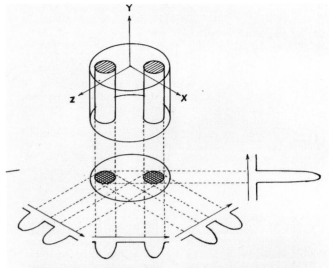

Fig. 1 Relationship between a three-dimensional object, its two-dimensional projection along the Y-axis, and four one-dimensional projections at 45° intervals in the XZ-plane. The arrows indicate the gradient directions.

Fig. 2 Proton nuclear magnetic resonance zeugmatogram of the object described in the text, using four relative orientations of object and gradients as diagrammed in Fig. 1.

96:2

Paul Lauterbur presents a novel and general approach to image formation (that he calls "zeugmatography"), where a point in an object is characterised through its joint interaction with two external fields. The method is demonstrated using NMR (nuclear magnetic resonance) techniques. A linear magnetic field gradient is imposed on two water-filled glass capillaries, and the protons of the water are also exposed to a radio frequency (RF) field. If the direction of the gradient is rotated relative to the object, a magnetic resonance image (MRI) can be built up. The continuation of the paper follows on page 500.

96:1

Lauterbur was born in 1929 in Sidney, Ohio. After obtaining a B.Sc. in chemistry from Case Institute of Technology, he worked at the Mellon Institute and at the Chemical Center Laboratories of the Army. In 1962 he received a Ph.D. in chemistry from the University of Pittsburgh and joined the faculty of the State University of New York at Stony Brook. Here Lauterbur worked on nuclear magnetic resonance (NMR) applications and developed magnetic resonance imaging (MRI). Since 1985 he has been Professor of Chemistry, Biophysics and Computational Biology at the University of Illinois in Chicago. Lauterbur shared the 2003 Nobel Prize in Medicine with Mansfield for discoveries concerning MRI.

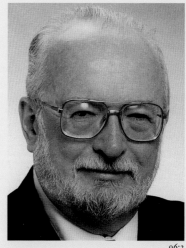

Paul Lauterbur 96:3

Image Formation by Induced Local Interactions: Examples Employing Nuclear Magnetic Resonance.

Nature 1973; 242:190.

Lauterbur presents a novel approach to image formation ("zeugmatography"), where a point in an object is characterised through its joint interaction with two external fields. The method is demonstrated by producing images of two water-filled glass capillaries using NMR techniques. First a linear magnetic field gradient is imposed on the object, and then the protons of the water are also exposed to a radio frequency (RF) field. Since the expected resonance frequency and relaxation times of the proton depend on the local magnetic field, the gradient creates a spatial "scan" of the NMR properties of the object. If the direction of the gradient is rotated relative to the object, a magnetic resonance image (MRI) can be built up. Lauterbur shows that adding a paramagnetic ion to the water changes the image. The appearance of the image depends also on which relaxation time is chosen to represent the NMR properties.

IN PERSPECTIVE:

From Rabi first observing NMR in 1938, the technique and the theory developed into a common tool for chemical studies (96.1)(96.2). The ability of NMR to differentiate between different biological tissues and make MRI possible was discovered by Damadian (96.3). Lauterbur's invention soon gave rise to work to improve image quality and to speed up image generation (96.4)(96.5). In 1976 Mansfield suggested the echo-planar imaging (EPI) technique (96.6)(96.7), where RF pulses with tailored frequency content allowed fast read-out from an entire object plane. This made real-time imaging possible at rates of more than 10 images per second. During the 1990s functional MRI (fMRI, visualises blood flow through the dependence of NMR on the oxygen content of blood) was developed for brain function studies (96.8)(96.9) and magnetised He-3 and Xenon-129 gases have also been used to produce images of the airways (96.10).

96.1 See #94 Damadian page 486 and especially ref. 94.1, ref. 94.2 and ref. 94.5.
96.2 Ramsey NF, Purcell EM. Interactions between nuclear spins in molecules. *Phys Rev* 1952; 85:143.
96.3 See #94 Damadian page 486.
96.4 Lauterbur PC, et al. Zeumatographic high-resolution nuclear magnetic resonance spectroscopy of chemical inhomogeneity within macroscopic objects. *J Am Chem Soc* 1975; 97:6866.
96.5 Kumar A, Welti D, Ernst RR. NMR Fourier Zeugmatography. *J Magn Res* 1975; 18:69.
96.6 Mansfield P, Maudsley AA. Planar spin imaging by NMR. *J Phys C: Solid State Phys* 1976; 9:L409.
96.7 Mansfield P, Maudsley AA, Bains T. Fast scan proton density imaging by NMR. *J Phys E: Sci Instr* 1976; 9:271.
96.8 Buxton RB. *An Introduction to Functional Magnetic Resonance Imaging.* Cambridge University Press; 2002.
96.9 McRobbie DW, et al. *MRI From Picture to Proton.* Cambridge University Press; 2003.
96.10 Albert MS, et al.: Biological magnetic resonance imaging using laser-polarized 129Xe. *Nature* 1994; 370:199. See also Klarreich E. Take a deep breath. *Nature* 2003; 424:873.

zeugmatogram (Fig. 3a). At a higher power level (about 1.6 mgauss), the pure water sample gave much more saturated signals than the sample whose spin-lattice relaxation time T_1 had been shortened by the addition of the paramagnetic Mn^{2+} ions, and its zeugmatographic image vanished at the contour level used in Fig. 3b. The sample region with long T_1 may be selectively emphasized (Fig. 3c) by constructing a difference zeugmatogram from those taken at different radio-frequency powers.

Applications of this technique to the study of various inhomogeneous objects, not necessarily restricted in size to those commonly studied by magnetic resonance spectroscopy, may be anticipated. The experiments outlined above demonstrate the ability of the technique to generate pictures of the distributions of stable isotopes, such as H and D, within an object. In the second experiment, relative intensities in an image were made to depend upon relative nuclear relaxation times. The variations in water contents and proton relaxation times among biological tissues should permit the generation, with field gradients large compared to internal magnetic inhomogeneities, of useful zeugmatographic images from the rather sharp water resonances of organisms, selectively picturing the various soft structures and tissues. A possible application of considerable interest at this time would be to the *in vivo* study of malignant tumours, which have been shown to give proton nuclear magnetic resonance signals with much longer water spin-lattice relaxation times than those in the corresponding normal tissues[6].

The basic zeugmatographic principle may be employed in many different ways, using a scanning technique, as described above, or transient methods. Variations on the experiment, to be described later, permit the generation of two- or three-dimensional images displaying chemical compositions, diffusion coefficients and other properties of objects measurable by spectroscopic techniques. Although applications employing nuclear magnetic resonance in liquid or liquid-like systems are simple and attractive because of the ease with which field gradients large enough to shift the narrow resonances by many line widths may be generated, NMR zeugmatography of solids, electron spin resonance zeugmatography, and analogous experiments in other regions of the spectrum should also be possible. Zeugmatographic techniques should find many useful applications in studies of the internal structures, states, and compositions of microscopic objects.

P. C. LAUTERBUR

Department of Chemistry,
State University of New York at Stony Brook,
Stony Brook, New York 11790

Received October 30, 1972; revised January 8, 1973.

[1] Bracewell, R. N., and Riddle, A. C., *Astrophys. J.*, **150**, 427 (1967).
[2] Vainshtein, B. K., *Soviet Physics–Crystallography*, **15**, 781 (1971).
[3] Ramachandran, G. N., and Lakshminarayan, A. V., *Proc. US Nat. Acad. Sci.*, **68**, 2236 (1971).
[4] Gordon, R., and Herman, G. T., *Comm. Assoc. Comput. Mach.*, **14**, 759 (1971).
[5] Klug, A., and Crowther, R. A., *Nature*, **238**, 435 (1972).
[6] Weisman, I. D., Bennett, L. H., Maxwell, Sr., L. R., Woods, M. W., and Burk, D., *Science*, **178**, 1288 (1972).

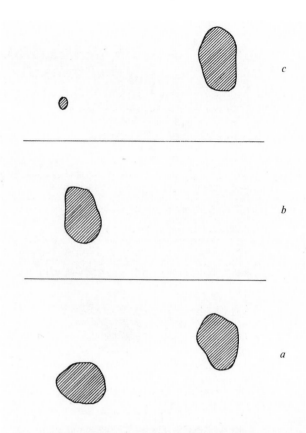

Fig. 3 Proton nuclear magnetic resonance zeugmatograms of an object containing regions with different relaxation times. a, Low power; b, high power; c, difference between a and b.

96:5

Continuation of Lauterbur's paper, where he further elucidates the properties of the new imaging method. By adding a paramagnetic ion to the water in one of the capillaries thereby changing its magnetic properties, the image of it changes dramatically. The appearance also depends on which relaxation time (see more on this #94) is chosen to represent the NMR characteristics of the object.

96:4

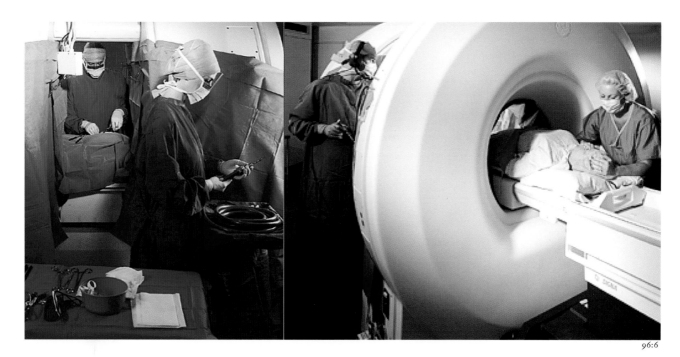

96:6

Open configuration MRI equipment introduced in the mid 1990s for image-guided therapy.

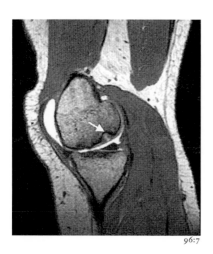

96:7

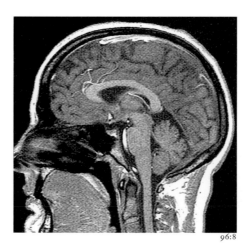

96:8

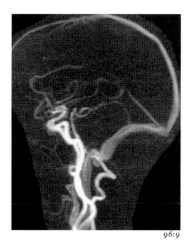

96:9

Examples of images obtained by sophisticated MRI techniques. Far left,
cartilage defect and bone erosion, in
the middle, thin slice near the mid of
the brain and right, a phase contrast
magnetic resonance angiography
(MRA) of the brain showing the arterial (intense) and venous (weak) circulation.

Functional NMR (fNMR) visualises blood flow rather than structure. Visualisation of cardiac flow velocity fields using 3D (three dimensional) phase contrast MRI and 3D visualisation software (top). From the flow velocity field the pressure fields can also be calculated and displayed, as is done below for the left ventricle.

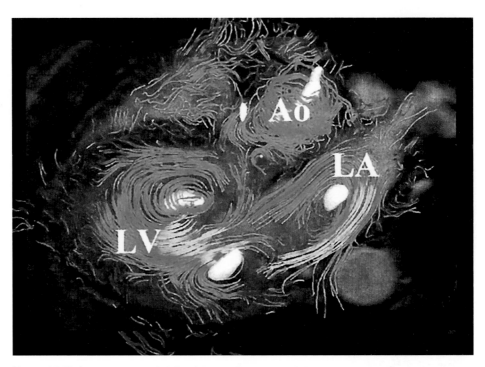

Figure 4.9 High vortex core probability (white surfaces) in the left atrium (LA), left ventricle (LV) and aorta (Ao) of a patient with dilated cardiomyopathy without valvular regurgitation at late-diastole. The velocity field is visualized using streamlines generated from a 2D plane

96:10

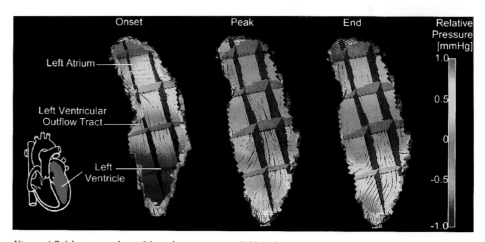

Figure 4.7 A long axis slice of the relative pressure field (color) and the velocity field (black streamlines) in the left side of the normal human heart at the onset, peak, and end of the early phase of diastolic inflow. A schematic drawing shows the orientation of the complete 3D volume

96:11

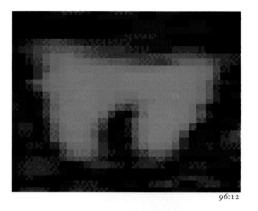

96:12

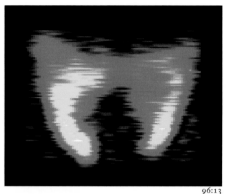

96:13

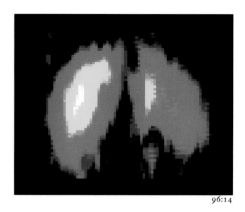

96:14

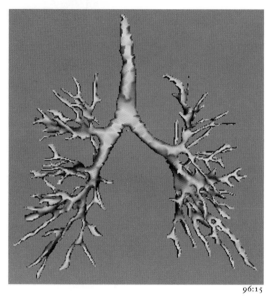

96:15

The first NMR picture (top left), taken in 1994 by Mitchell Albert of the air filling the rat lung, using specially prepared hyperpolarised (HP) gas with the ^{129}Xe isotope. The image top middle is taken of the same rat lung now with hyperpolarised ^{3}He isotope gas. The first NMR image of the air filling a healthy human lung as obtained using the hyperpolarised ^{3}He gas (top right).

Left, a three dimensional rendering of the airway tree created by stacking images of coronary slices of the lung obtained with the ^{3}He MRI technique. The in plane resolution is 1.8 mm and the slice thickness is 13 mm.

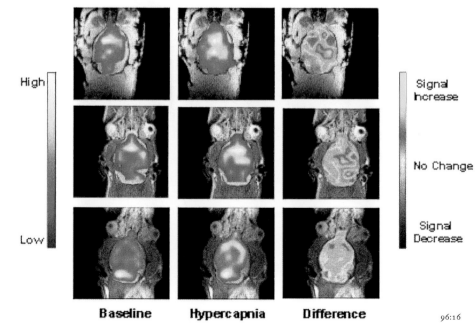

High

Low

Signal Increase

No Change

Signal Decrease

Baseline   **Hypercapnia**   **Difference**

96:16

A study demonstrating the effect of hypercapnia (excess carbon dioxide in blood) on the distribution of inhaled hyperpolarised (HP) ^{129}Xe in the rat brain. Left column, animals are ventilated with alternate breaths of HP ^{129}Xe gas and oxygen. Middle column, images acquired during the induction of hypercapnia, in which animals are ventilated with alternate breaths of HP ^{129}Xe gas and 5% carbon dioxide. Right column, difference images obtained by subtracting the baseline image from the image taken during hypercapnia.

Measurement of continuous distributions of ventilation-perfusion ratios: theory

PETER D. WAGNER, HERBERT A. SALTZMAN, AND JOHN B. WEST

Department of Medicine, University of California, San Diego, La Jolla, California 92037

WAGNER, PETER D., HERBERT A. SALTZMAN, AND JOHN B. WEST. *Measurement of continuous distributions of ventilation-perfusion ratios: theory.* J. Appl. Physiol. 36(5): 588–599. 1974.—Most previous descriptions of the distribution of ventilation-perfusion ratios ($\dot{V}_A/\dot{Q}$) divide the lungs into only two or three uniform compartments. However, an analysis which would result in definition of the position, shape, and dispersion of the distribution would be more realistic. We describe here such a technique, applicable both in health and disease, in which the characteristics of distributions containing up to three modes can be determined. In particular, areas with low but finite $\dot{V}_A/\dot{Q}$ ratios are separated from areas whose $\dot{V}_A/\dot{Q}$ ratio is zero (shunt), and regions with high $\dot{V}_A/\dot{Q}$ ratios are differentiated from regions that are unperfused (dead space). To perform the measurement, dextrose solution or saline is equilibrated with a mixture of several gases of different solubilities and then infused into a vein. After a steady state has been established, the concentrations of each gas are measured in the mixed arterial blood and mixed expired gas. The curve relating arterial concentration and solubility is transformed into a virtually continuous distribution of blood flow against $\dot{V}_A/\dot{Q}$, using techniques of numerical analysis. The relation between expired concentration and solubility is similarly converted into the distribution of ventilation. The numerical analysis technique has been tested against many artificial distributions of $\dot{V}_A/\dot{Q}$ ratios and these have all been accurately recovered.

The abstract of the paper presenting the multiple inert gas elimination technique (MIGET). A schematic illustration of the method is given in the drawing. Six to eight gases with different solubilities are dissolved in saline and infused in a vein. Arterial and mixed venous blood samples are drawn, together with a sample from the mixed expired gas. For each of the gases a retention and excretion ratio is calculated, as given by the formulae.

97:1

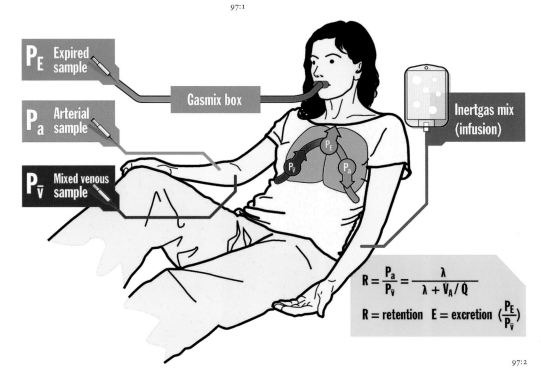

$$R = \frac{P_a}{P_{\bar{v}}} = \frac{\lambda}{\lambda + \dot{V}_A/\dot{Q}}$$

$$R = \text{retention} \quad E = \text{excretion} \left(\frac{P_E}{P_{\bar{v}}}\right)$$

97:2

WAGNER was born in Karachi in 1944, and obtained his M.D. from the University of Sydney in 1969. The following year he went to the University of California in San Diego, where he became a member of the faculty in 1973 and professor of medicine in 1984. Since 1999 he has also been the head of the Division of Physiology. West was born in 1928 in Adelaide and received his M.D. there in 1959. He obtained a Ph.D. from the University of London in 1960. From 1962 onwards West directed the Respiratory Research Group at the Postgraduate Medical School. He has been professor of medicine and physiology at the University of California in San Diego since 1969.

Measurement of continuous distributions of ventilation-perfusion ratios: theory

J APPL PHYSIOL 1974; 36(5):588.

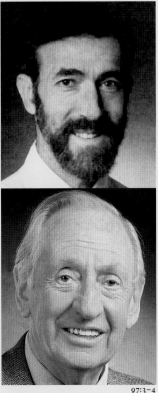

97:3-4

Peter Wagner
John West

WAGNER, WEST and Saltzman describe a method to determine the distribution functions for ventilation (V_A) and perfusion (Q) in the lungs. Six inert gases with different blood solubilities (ranging from sulphur hexafluoride to acetone) are dissolved in saline and infused into a peripheral vein. For a given lung compartment in steady state, the amount of gas eliminated (exhaled) and the amount retained (in the arterial blood) depends only on the ratio V_A/Q and the solubility of the gas. An iterative technique is used to find the V_A/Q ratios distributed over fifty compartments, which agree with the total measured elimination and retention for all the gases.

IN PERSPECTIVE:

In the late 1940s interest in positive pressure ventilation (97.1) led to studies of its effects on the circulatory system (97.2). The ventilation/perfusion (V_A/Q) conditions in the lungs were initially assessed with simple three compartment lung models (97.3). In the 1960s Lenfant developed the continuous V_A/Q distribution concept (97.4) and Farhi analysed inert gas exchange over the lungs (97.5). The method of Wagner and West relied on the development of a technique for simultaneous measurement of the blood concentrations of up to eight inert gases, some in very low concentrations (97.6). Other methods, using transient non-steady state conditions, have also been developed to study the gas exchange process. Thus, from the concentration variations of nitrogen and the respiratory gases during a single expiration, the inhomogeneity of the lung could be assessed (97.7)(97.8). Furthermore, topographic information on the distribution of ventilation and perfusion has also been obtainable since the early 1960s using radionuclides (97.9). More recently, using tomographic techniques (97.10), sophisticated images have been generated (97.11) showing both the ventilation (with inhaled Xe-133) and the perfusion distribution (with infused I-131 labelled macroaggregated albumin).

97.1 See #87 Engström page 450 and ref. 87.10.

97.2 Werkö L. The influence of positive pressure breathing on the circulation in man. *Acta med Scand.* 1947; 193:1.

97.3 Riley RL, Cournand A. Analysis of factors affecting partial pressures of oxygen and carbon dioxide in gas and blood of lungs: theory (methods). *J Appl Physiol* 1951; 4:77 and p102. See also ref. 6.6 and ref. 37.6.

97.4 Lenfant C, Okubo T. Distribution function of pulmonary blood flow and ventilation-perfusion ratio in man. *J Appl Physiol* 1968; 24:668.

97.5 Farhi LE. Elimination of inert gas by the lung. *Resp Phys* 1967; 3:1.

97.6 Wagner PD, Naumann PF, Laravuso RB. Simultaneous measurement of eight foreign gases in blood by gas chromatography. *J Appl Physiol* 1974; 36(5):600.

97.7 West JB, et al. Measurement of the ventilation perfusion ratio inequality in the lung by the analysis of a single expirate. *Clin Sci Lond* 1957; 16:529.

97.8 Okubo T, Lenfant C. Distribution function of lung volume and ventilation determined by lung N_2 washout. *J Appl Physiol* 1968; 24:658.

97.9 West JB, Dollery CT. Distribution of blood flow and ventilation-perfusion ratio in the lung, measured with radioactive CO_2. *J Appl Physiol* 1960; 15:405.

97.10 See #95 Hounsfield page 492.

97.11 Jaszczak RJ. Tomographic radiopharmaceutical imaging. *Proc IEEE* 1988; 76(9):1079.

FIG. 1. Examples of chromatograms of mixtures of eight (*A*) and six (*B*) gases. In each case, one gas (SF₆), is not detected by flame ionization detector, so only 7 and 5 peaks are seen, respectively. Elution time for halothane, the slowest gas, is 8 min (*A*, column temperature 160°C and carrier flow 30 ml/min) and 4 min (*B*, column temperature 170°C and carrier flow 50 ml/min). Note adequate separation of all gases in both cases.

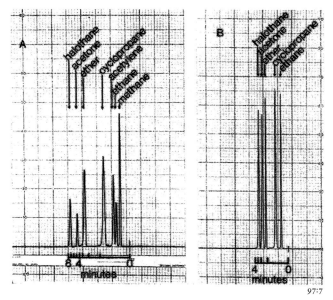

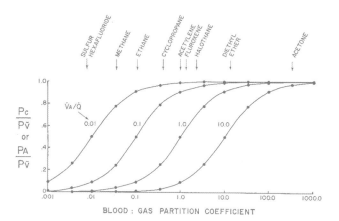

FIG. 1. Relationship between inert gas retention $Pc/P\bar{v}$ (or excretion $PA/P\bar{v}$) and blood-gas partition coefficient, using a logarithmic scale for the abscissa. Four curves are drawn, each for homogeneous lung units with different $\dot{V}A/\dot{Q}$ ratios. Note that the curves are all smooth and monotonic. Blood-gas partition coefficients for human blood at 37°C are also shown.

97:5

The samples taken according to the MIGET method shown in illustration 97:2 are equilibrated with helium and then analysed by gas chromatography. The result, obtained in about 8 minutes, is shown in the figure above. High sensitivity and good separation are seen for all gases.

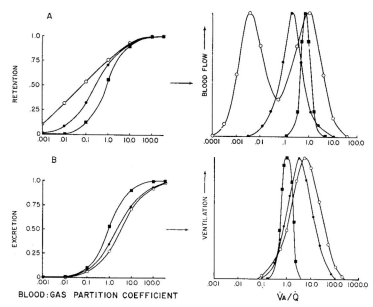

FIG. 2. *A:* relationships between inert gas retention and blood-gas partition coefficient in three examples of lungs with ventilation-perfusion inequality. Note the preservation of smoothness and monotonicity in each case. Corresponding distributions of blood flow are shown with the same symbols. *B:* relationships between inert gas excretion and blood-gas partition coefficient in the corresponding distributions of ventilation.

97:6

The excretion or retention ratios of entirely homogeneous lungs with their ventilation to perfusion ratio (VA/Q) as a parameter, starting with 0.01 far left and ending with 10.0 far right. Each trace is made up of the values of nine different gases (listed at the top of the graph) covering a very wide range of solubility (shown along the horizontal axis).

Left, three cases where the lungs are no longer homogenous, meaning that different compartments of a lung have different VA/Q ratios. The left column shows the three retention and excretion curves and the right column shows the resulting calculated distribution of perfusion (top right graph) and ventilation (bottom right graph) as a function of the VA/Q ratio of the lung compartments.

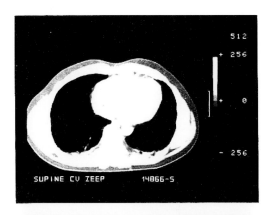

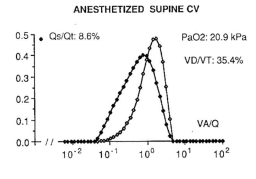

ANESTHETIZED SUPINE CV

Qs/Qt: 8.6%   PaO2: 20.9 kPa

VD/VT: 35.4%

VA/Q

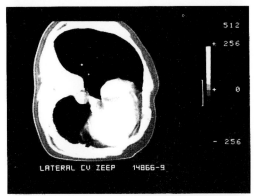

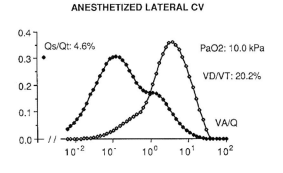

ANESTHETIZED LATERAL CV

Qs/Qt: 4.6%   PaO2: 10.0 kPa

VD/VT: 20.2%

VA/Q

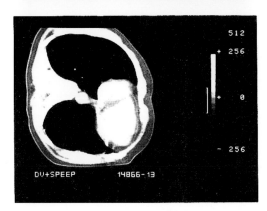

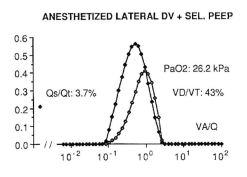

ANESTHETIZED LATERAL DV + SEL. PEEP

PaO2: 26.2 kPa

Qs/Qt: 3.7%   VD/VT: 43%

VA/Q

Figure 1:
Transverse CT scans of the chest and V_A/Q distributions (○ :ventilation, ● :blood flow, l/min) in a male patient (age 38, smoker) during anaesthesia and CV with ZEEP in the supine position (*upper panel*); lateral position (*middle panel*); and in the lateral position with DV+SPEEP (*lower panel*). Note the large amount of perfusion of regions with low V_A/Q ratios and the low PaO_2 during conventional ventilation in the lateral position. There is only a small shunt and the corresponding CT scan shows only a small amount of atelectasis in de-

pendent lung regions. During DV+SPEEP, the atelectatic regions have disappeared and there is a good match between the ventilation and perfusion distributions.

97:8

A comparison between CT imaging of the chest and the quantitative assessment of the ventilation/perfusion conditions using MIGET. A case of controlled ventilation (denoted in the figure by CV) during anaesthesia, with the patient in supine (top) and lateral (middle and lower) positions. The middle pair of images show that in the lateral position a significant portion of the lung is not properly ventilated (the blood flow curve is shifted to the left of the ventilation curve), resulting in decreased oxygenation. The bottom pair of images demonstrate that applying a positive pressure (SEL.PEEP) selectively to the dependent (lower lying) lung restores the overlap between the ventilation and the perfusion curves and re-establishes adequate oxygenation.

IEEE TRANSACTIONS ON COMMUNICATIONS, VOL. COM-22, NO. 5, MAY 1974

A Protocol for Packet Network Intercommunication

VINTON G. CERF AND ROBERT E. KAHN, MEMBER, IEEE

98:1

Abstract—A protocol that supports the sharing of resources that exist in different packet switching networks is presented. The protocol provides for variation in individual network packet sizes, transmission failures, sequencing, flow control, end-to-end error checking, and the creation and destruction of logical process-to-process connections. Some implementation issues are considered, and problems such as internetwork routing, accounting, and timeouts are exposed.

CONCLUSIONS

We have discussed some fundamental issues related to the interconnection of packet switching networks. In particular, we have described a simple but very powerful and flexible protocol which provides for variation in individual network packet sizes, transmission failures, sequencing, flow control, and the creation and destruction of process-to-process associations. We have considered some of the implementation issues that arise and found that the proposed protocol is implementable by HOST's of widely varying capacity.

The next important step is to produce a detailed specification of the protocol so that some initial experiments with it can be performed. These experiments are needed to determine some of the operational parameters (e.g., how often and how far out of order do packets actually

98:2

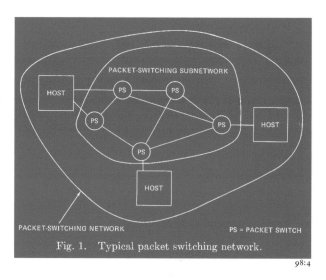

Fig. 1.   Typical packet switching network.

98:4

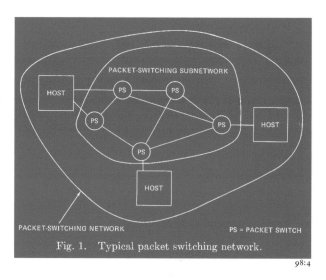

Fig. 2.   Three networks interconnected by two GATEWAYS.

In 1974 Vinton Cerf and Robert Kahn lay out the structure and protocol for intercommunication between different packet switching computer networks. This is the introduction of the internetwork protocol (IP).

(may be null)		Internetwork Header					
LOCAL HEADER	SOURCE	DESTINATION	SEQUENCE NO.	BYTE COUNT	FLAG FIELD	TEXT	CHECKSUM

Fig. 3.   Internetwork packet format (fields not shown to scale).

98:3

CERF was born in New Haven in 1943. After studying mathematics at Stanford University, he obtained his Ph.D. in computer science from the University of California in Los Angeles in 1972. He was with the Advanced Research Project Agency (ARPA) from 1976 to 1982, when he joined MCI, serving there since 2003 as senior vice president of Technology and Strategy. Kahn was born in Brooklyn in 1938. He received a B.E.E. from City College and his Ph.D. from Princeton University in 1964. He has worked at the Bell Telephone Laboratories and with Bolt Beranek and Newman Inc. After thirteen years at ARPA, in 1986 he founded the Corporation for National Research Initiatives, where he is now chairman and president.

A Protocol for Packet Network Intercommunication.

IEEE TRANS COMMUNICATIONS 1974; COM-22(5):637.

CERF AND Kahn lay out the structure and protocol necessary for intercommunication between different packet-switching computer networks. Each network with its transmission control programs (TCP) is interfaced by gateways to other networks. The format necessary for internet communication as permitted by the gateways is established from fundamental considerations and explained with great clarity. The resulting internetwork protocol (IP) is flexible and can support messaging between computer networks of widely varying character.

IN PERSPECTIVE:

Since the Peloponnesian war (431 BC), when optical signalling with torches first came into widespread use (98.1), military concerns have been an important driving force behind the development of communication technology. Hooke, when reading about the plight of the citizens of Vienna during the Turkish siege, proposed in 1684 a "way how to communicate one's mind at great distances" using signs and telescopes (98.2). Chappe put Hooke's idea into practice in 1794, when the desperate military situation after the French Revolution demanded rapid communication between Paris and Lille (98.3). More recently military concern for computer network vulnerability gave the impetus to the work cited above (98.4)(98.5). Health-related information exchange, from patients to professionals or among professionals, traditionally takes place through meetings or through point-to-point contacts and has been used to demonstrate the potential of advanced telemedicine (98.6)(98.7). However, many applications rely increasingly on the Internet (98.8). At the end of the 20th century an estimated 60 million adults used the internet to find health-related information (98.9). Confidentiality, security and data integrity remain major concerns (98.10)(98.11), but better informed patients are likely to take more responsibility for their health care decisions in the future, thereby fundamentally changing the role of the professionals and the way health care is delivered.

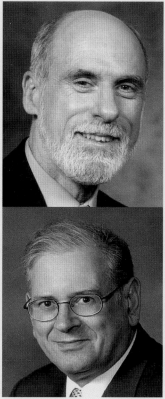

98:5-6

Vinton Cerf
Robert Kahn

98.1 Karass Th. *Geschichte der Telegraphie*. Teil 1. Braunschweig: F. Vieweg & Sohn; 1909. p27.

98.2 See ref. 38.3 p142.

98.3 Chappe I. *Histoire de la télégraphie*. Paris: chez l'auteur; 1824. See also ref. 85.6 p178–181.

98.4 Holzmann GJ, Pehrson B. *The Early History of Data Networks*. IEEE Computer Society Press; 1995. See also #85 Eckert-Mauchly page 438.

98.5 Lynch DC. Historical Evolution. In Lynch DC, Rose MT. editors. *Internet System Handbook*. Reading: Addison-Wesley Comp.; 1993.

98.6 Norris AC. *Essentials of Telemedicine and Telecare*. John Wiley & Sons; 2002.

98.7 Marescaux J, et al.: Transatlantic robot-assisted telesurgery. *Nature* 2001; 413:379.

98.8 Rusovick RM, Warner DJ. The globalization of interventional informatics through Internet mediated distributed medical intelligence. *New Medicine* 1998; 2:155.

98.9 Kaufmann M. The Internet: A reliable source? *Washington Post* February 16 1999. pZ17.

98.10 Silberg WM, Lundberg GD, Musacchio RA. Assessing, controlling and assuring the quality of medical information on the Internet. *JAMA* 1997; 277:1244.

98.11 Spielberg AR. On call and online: Socio-historical, legal and ethical implications of email for the patient-physician relationship. *JAMA* 1998; 280. See also ref. 4.11.

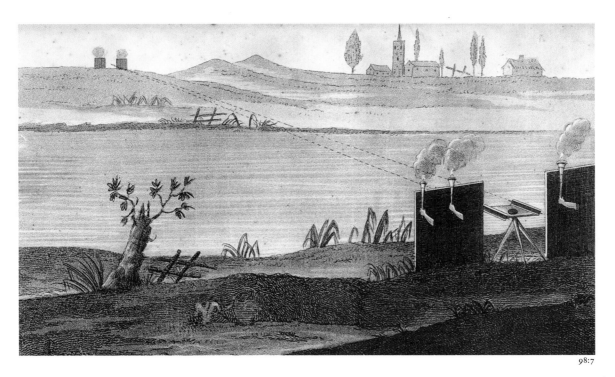

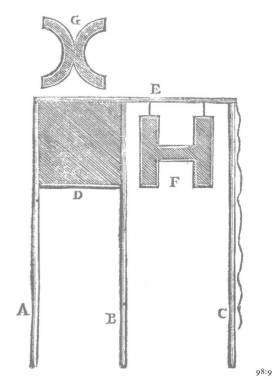

98:7

The torch system was used by the Greeks for communication during the Peloponnesian war of 430 BC. Two groups of torches, each having one to five units, could designate positions in a 5×5 matrix covering the entire Greek alphabet.

Dr. Hook's *Difcourfe to the* Royal Society, *May* 21. 1684. *fhewing a Way how to communicate one's Mind at great Diftances.*

THAT which I now propound, is what I have fome Years fince difcourfed of; but being then laid by, the great Siege of *Vienna*, the laft Year, by the *Turks*, did again revive in my Memory; and that was a Method of difcourfing at a Diftance, not by Sound, but by Sight. I fay therefore 'tis poffible to convey Intelligence from any one high and eminent Place, to any other that lies in Sight of it, tho' 30 or 40 Miles diftant, in as fhort a Time almoft, as a Man can write what he would have fent, and as fuddenly to receive an Anfwer, as he that receives it hath a
Mind

98:8

98:9

The plight of the citizens of Vienna during the Turkish siege of 1683 prompts Robert Hooke to propose a new method of communication using mechanical signs and telescopes to read them at a distance.

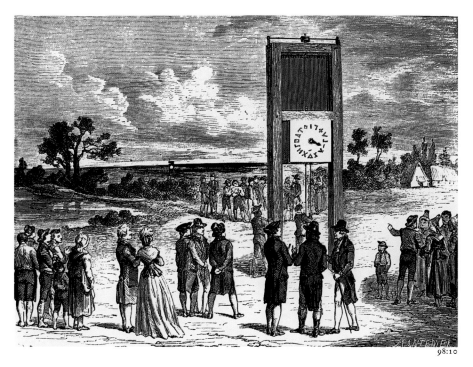

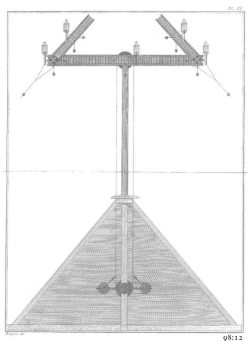

98:10

98:12

In 1791 Claude Chappe (1763-1805) constructs a telegraph based on two synchronised pendulum clocks, with numbers one to ten on the face of the clocks. When the pointer passes the number to be communicated, a sound signal alerts the receiving party. Each letter is given a certain number and can be transmitted in this way. A more practical device, the semaphore telegraph, was demonstrated by Chappe in 1793. It is rapidly taken into service between Paris and Lille to speed up communications, something badly needed in the desperate military situation of France after the French Revolution.

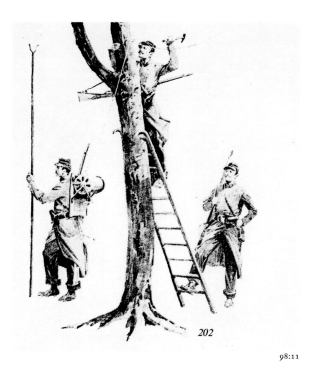

202

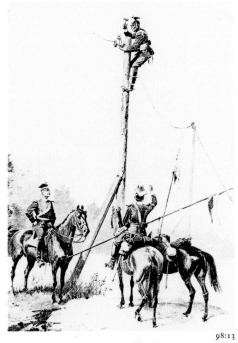

98:11

98:13

Another illustration of the importance of communications in wartime. The French telegraph corps setting up telegraph lines (left) that are cut down by Prussian troops (right) during the Franco-Prussian war of 1870-71.

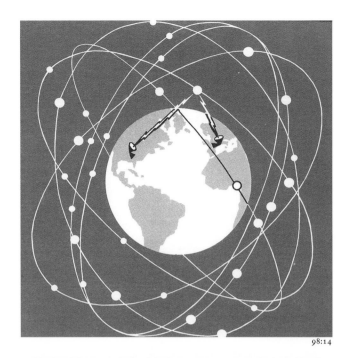

A large number of passive and active satellites are envisaged in the mid-1960s to provide complete telecommunication coverage for the whole earth.

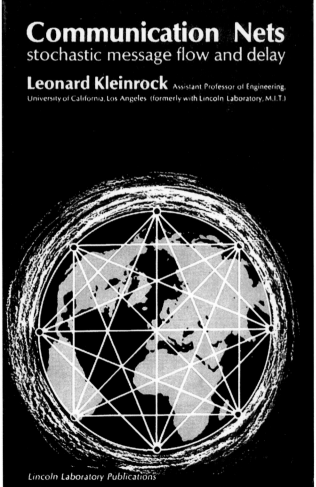

Communication Nets
stochastic message flow and delay

Leonard Kleinrock Assistant Professor of Engineering, University of California, Los Angeles (formerly with Lincoln Laboratory, M.I.T.)

Lincoln Laboratory Publications

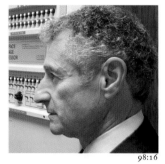

In 1964 Leonard Kleinrock provides the theoretical basis of computer networking and five years later his computer becomes the first node of the ARPANET, the precursor to the Internet of today.

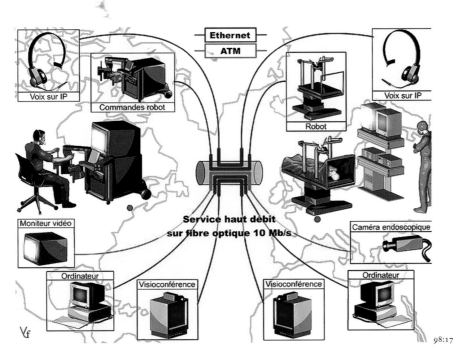

98:17

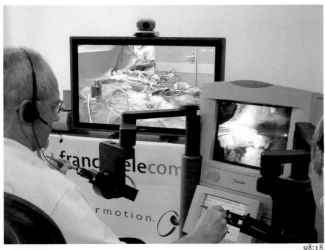

98:18

Images from the first transatlantic robot-assisted telesurgery in September 2001, initiated by Jacques Marescaux. The "Operation Lindbergh", as the project is called, lasts about an hour and is successfully performed by doctors in New York on a patient in Strasbourg, France. The building blocks of the technical systems are shown together with images from the operation in progress.

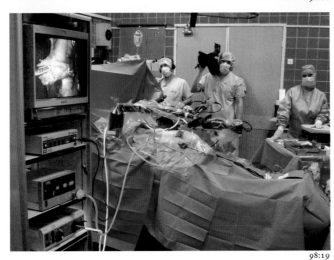

98:19

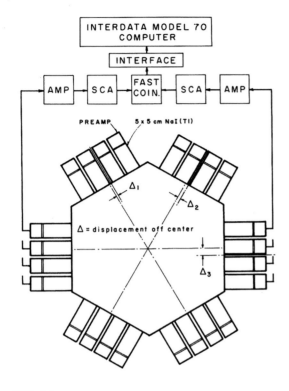

FIG. 11. Schematic illustration of prototype PETT.

99:1

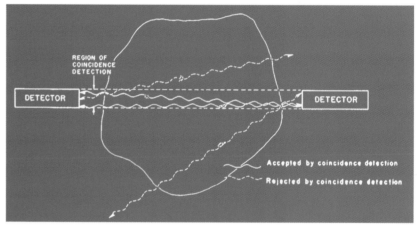

99:3

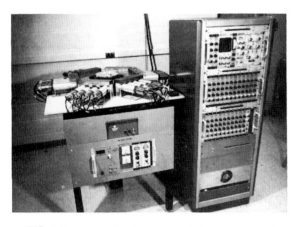

99:2

FIG. 12. Photograph of prototype PETT. Object examined (phantom or animal) is placed on computer-controlled turntable at center of hexagon. Axis of rotation is perpendicular to plane of hexagon. Phantom is shown on turntable.

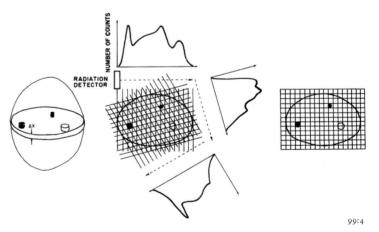

99:4

The schematics and a photograph of the prototype positron emission tomography (PET) device designed by Michael Phelps and co-workers in 1974. Objects marked with radionucleids emit a pair of high energy photons each time an electron positron pair is annihilated (see #69). Only photons that arrive at the detectors on each side of the object at the same time are accepted. This criterion corresponds to the collimation of the X-ray beam used in the CT method and greatly improves resolution in an image plane.

The scanning and image reconstruction systems illustrated above are similar to those employed by the CT and MRI techniques (see #95 and #96).

P HELPS was born in Cleveland in 1939. He received a Ph.D. in chemistry from Washington University, St. Louis in 1970. He stayed until 1975 as a member of the faculty of the School of Medicine, beginning his work on positron emission tomography (PET). After a short period at the University of Pennsylvania, Phelps moved to the University of California School of Medicine in 1976. Previously professor of biomathematics and of radiological sciences, since 1992 he has been head of the division of nuclear medicine and the department of molecular and medical pharmacology.

Application of Annihilation Coincidence Detection to Transaxial Reconstruction Tomography.

J NUCL MED 1975; 16(3):210.

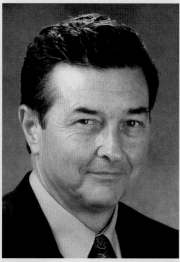

Michael Phelps 99:5

TOGETHER WITH Hoffman, Mullani and Ter-Pogossian, Phelps presents a prototype system of a positron emission transaxial tomograph. The device creates images of the distribution of positron-emitting radionucleids. When the positron (99.1) is annihilated, a pair of high energy photons is created. The new concept is to allow detection only of those photons that arrive at the detectors on each side of the object at the same time. This coincidence technique corresponds to the collimation of X-rays employed in computed tomography (CT) (99.2) and results in much-improved resolution within well-defined image planes. The imaging capability of the device is demonstrated in model and animal studies and is found to compare favourably with conventional scintillation cameras.

IN PERSPECTIVE:

Positron annihilation radiation was first used in medicine in the early 1950s for the localisation of brain tumours (99.3)(99.4). In the early 1970s tomographic (single plane) techniques were developed (99.5) and, with the invention of X-ray CT in 1973 (99.2), similar methods were also applied in PET devices (99.6). Over the years better detector configurations, increased numbers of detectors and new detector materials have steadily improved image quality and image access time (99.7). The development of new radiopharmaceuticals has been, and still is, of key importance in finding new applications of PET in medicine (99.8). Initially only ^{15}O labelled oxygen and carbon dioxide were available but nowadays specially designed mini-cyclotrons are used to produce many other radio-pharmaceuticals, including the important ^{14}C labelled deoxyglucose and ^{18}F labelled 2-fluorode-oxy-D-glucose (99.9). Major clinical uses of PET are tumour detection (also with whole body scans) and cardiac viability diagnosis. Another important area is the study of brain function in general, and the evaluation of Alzheimer's and Parkinson's diseases in particular (99.8). A combination instrument PET/CT that is able to produce both anatomical and biological (functional) images simultaneously has also been described (99.10).

99.1 See # 69 Thomson page 356 and ref. 69.7.

99.2 See # 95 Hounsfield page 492.

99.3 Wrenn Jr FR, Good ML, Handler P. The use of positron emitting radioisotopes for localization of brain tumors. *Science* 1951; 113:525.

99.4 Brownell GL, Sweet WH. Localisation of brain tumors with positron emitters. *Nucleonics* 1953; 11:40.

99.5 Burnham CA, Brownell GL. A multi-crystal positron camera. *IEEE Trans Nucl Sci* 1972; NS-19(3):201.

99.6 Chesler DA. Positron tomography and three dimensional reconstruction techniques. In Freedman GS. Editor. *Tomographic Imaging in Nuclear Medicine.* New York: Society of Nuclear Medicine; 1973. p176.

99.7 Nutt R. The History of Positron Emission Tomography. *Molecular Imaging and Biology* 2002; 4(1):11.

99.8 Phelps ME. Positron emission tomography provides molecular imaging of biological processes. *PNAS* 2000; 97(16):9226.

99.9 Reivich M, et al. The (^{18}F) fluorodeoxyglucose method for the measurement of local cerebral glucose utilization in man. *Circulation Research* 1979; 44:127.

99.10 Beyer T, et al. A combined PET/CT scanner for clinical oncology. *J Nucl Med* 2000; 41:1369.

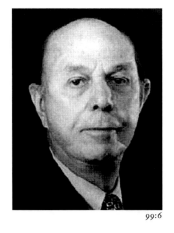

Positron annihilation methods are first applied in medicine in 1953 when Gordon Brownell designs an apparatus for localising brain tumours (see image 69:8). Following the introduction of tomographic techniques in the mid-1960s, Brownell builds the first tomographic PET imaging device (shown in the photograph) in 1969.

99:6

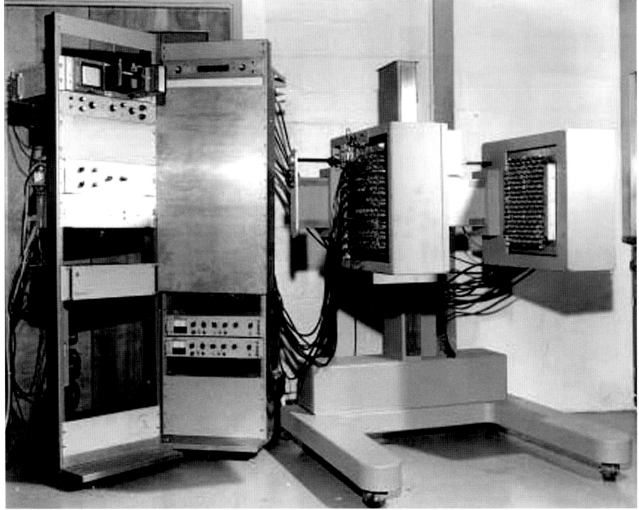

99:7

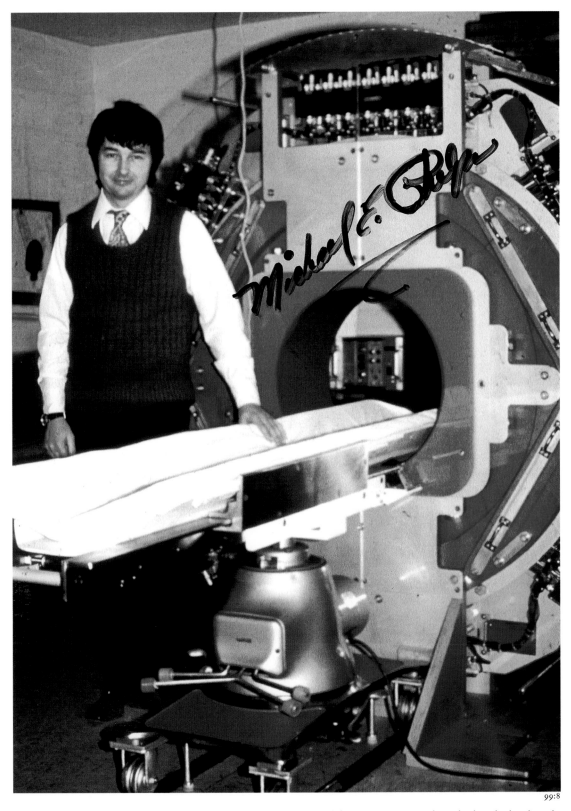

Michael Phelps with the PETT III apparatus, a development of the prototype unit described in the landmark paper from 1975. This device takes the first PET images of blood flow, glucose metabolism and bone scans using Fluorine 18 (^{18}F) as the radionucleid.

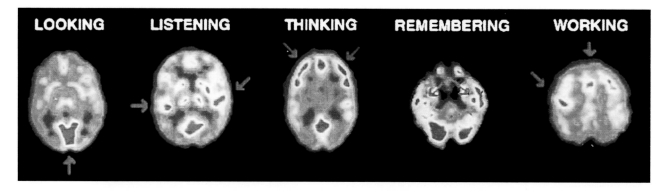

Fig. 3. PET studies of glucose metabolism to map human brain's response in performing different tasks. Subjects looking at a visual scene activated visual cortex (arrow), listening to a mystery story with language and music activated left and right auditory cortices (arrows), counting backwards from 100 by sevens activated frontal cortex (arrows), recalling previously learned objects activated hippocampus bilaterally (arrows), and touching thumb to fingers of

Illustration of the power of the PET technique for molecular imaging of biomedical processes. Top, glucose metabolism of the brain when performing different tasks and bottom the progression of Alzheimer's disease, with a comparison to the normal brain of a new-born baby.

On the opposing page (top) the PET images reveal the characteristics of early Parkinson's disease, while the conventional MRI image only shows the structure of the brain.

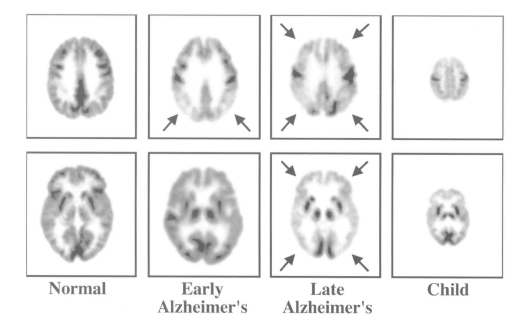

| Normal | Early Alzheimer's | Late Alzheimer's | Child |

Fig. 4. PET study of glucose metabolism in Alzheimer's disease. The "early Alzheimer's" is at stage of "questionable Alzheimer's disease" and illustrates characteristic metabolic deficits in parietal cortex (arrows) of the brain. In "late Alzheimer's," metabolic deficit has spread throughout areas of cortex (arrows), sparing subcortical (e.g., internal) structures (bottom image), and primary motor and sensory areas, such as visual (bottom image) and motor cortices (top image). At late stage disease, metabolic function in Alzheimer's is similar to that of newborn, shown to the far right, which underlies their similar behavior and functional capacity. MRI studies were normal.

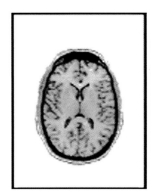
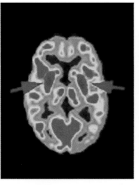
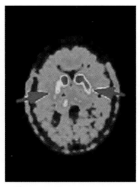
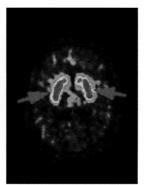

MRI
Human

**Glucose
Metabolism**

Pre-Synaptic

Post-Synaptic

99:11

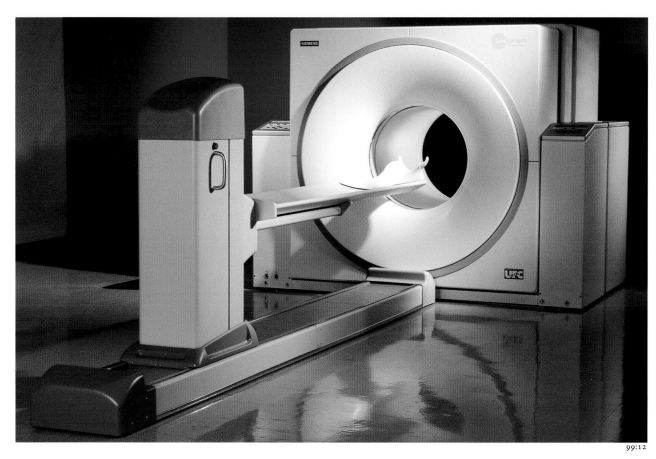

99:12

In 2000 the first combination instrument PET/CT (such as the one shown in the photograph) is introduced. The equipment simultaneously generates anatomical and biological (functional) images and is able to scan the whole body in about four minutes.

Timeline and topics at a glance

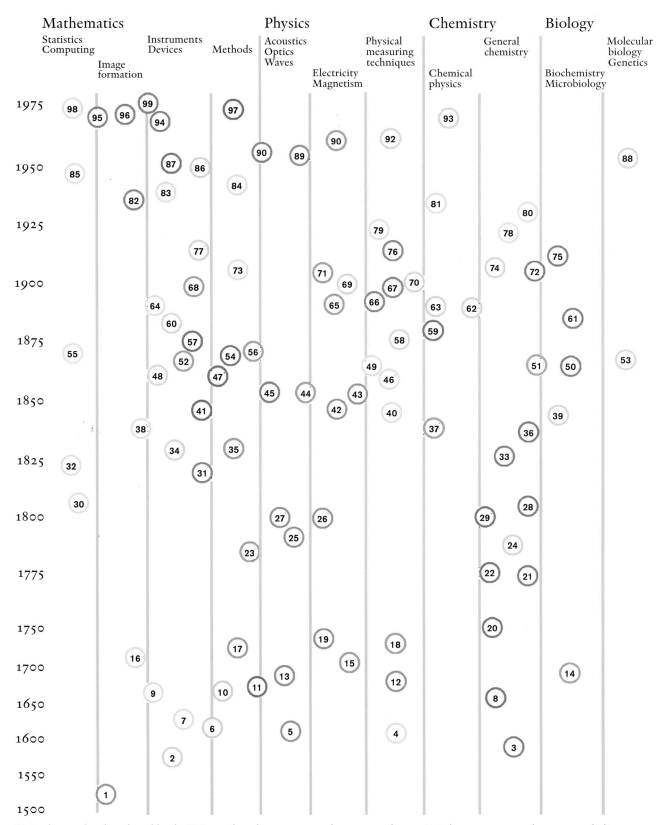

Mathematics

Statistics
Computing

Image
formation

Instruments
Devices

Methods

Physics

Acoustics
Optics
Waves

Electricity
Magnetism

Physical
measuring
techniques

Chemistry

Chemical
physics

General
chemistry

Biology

Biochemistry
Microbiology

Molecular
biology
Genetics

1975
1950
1925
1900
1875
1850
1825
1800
1775
1750
1700
1650
1600
1550
1500

■ Cardiovascular physiology, blood   ■ Lung physiology, gases, ventilation, anaesthesia   ■ Life processes, reproduction, metabolism, gas exchange   ■ Germs, theory of diseases, drugs   ■ Diagnostic methods and equipment   ■ Materials, equipment and methods for treating disease   ■ Basic materials and methods in clinical medicine and medical research   ■ Anatomy, muscle movement and electrophysiology, sensory physiology.

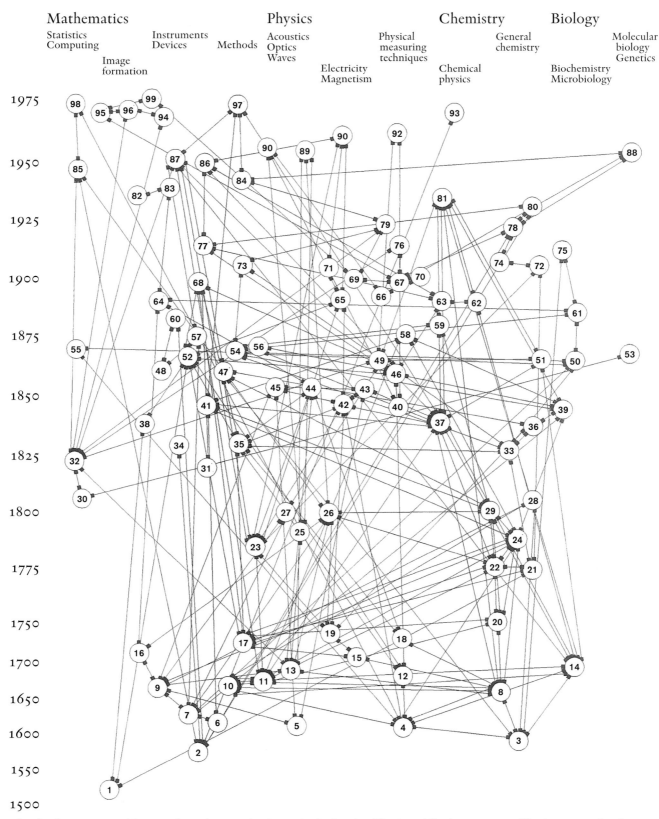

Graphical presentation of the interrelation between the ninety-nine landmark publications. A line between two publications means that they reference each other or that they are described with common references and involve closely associated topics or personalities.

1. **Dürer**, Albrecht

Hierinn sind begriffen vier Bücher von menschlicher Proportion.
[edited by Willibald Pirckheimer].
[Nuremberg, Hieronymus Andrea Formschneyder for Dürer's widow, 1528].
Folio—128 leaves and 4 double-page folding leaves. Illustrated throughout with 136 wood-cuts of full-length human figures and numerous smaller woodcut figures and diagrams in the text and on the folding leaves.

2. **Paré**, Ambroise

Les Oeuvres. Avec les figures, & portraicts, tant de l'Anatomie que des instruments de Chirurgie, & de plusieurs Monstres.
Paris, chez Gabriel Buon, 1575.
Folio—pp (20), 945, (46). Portrait of Paré and 295 woodcuts in the text.

3. **Paracelsus**, Theophrastus Philippus Aureolis Bombastus von Hohenheim

Der Buecher und Schrifften … Jetzt auffs new auss den Originalien, und Theophrasti eigner Handschrifft, soviel derselben zubekommen gewesen, auffs trewlichts und fleissigst an tag geben: Durch Ioannem Huserum.
In Ten Volumes and Two Appendices.
Basel, Conrad Waldkirch, 1589–1590.
4to—10 volumes comprising together 5372 pages. The authors' portrait is repeated in all volumes. For full collation see: Sudhoff 216–225a.

4. **Santorio**, Santorio

Methodi vitandorum errorum omnium, qui in arte medica contingunt libri quidecim, quorum principia sunt av auctoritate medicorum, & philosophorum principium desumpta, eaque omnia experimentis, & rationibus analyticis comprobata …
Venetiis, apud Fransicus Barilettus, 1603.
Folio—ff (6), 230, (16).

5. **Kepler**, Johannes

Ad Vitellionem Paralipomena, quibus Astronomiae Pars Optica traditur; potissimum de Artificiosa Observatione et Aestimatione Diametrorum deliquiorumque Solis et Lunae … De Modo Visionis et Humorum Oculi Usu.
Francofurti, apud Claudium Marnium & haeredes Joannis Aubrii, 1604.
4to—pp (16), 449, (18). One engraved plate with explanatory text, 2 folding tables; numerous diagrams in the text.

6. **Santorio**, Santorio

Ars de statica medica aphorismorum sectionibus septem comprehensa.
Venetiis, apud Nicolaum Polum, 1614.
12mo—ff (11), 1–84.

7. **Santorio**, Santorio

Commentaria in primam Fen primi libri Canonis Avicennae.
Venetiis, Jacobus Sarcina, 1625.
Folio—pp (8), columns 1–802, pp (10). Woodcuts in the text.

8. **Helmont**, Jean Baptiste van

Ortus Medicinae. Id est, initia physicae inaudita. Progressus medicinae novus, in morborum ultionum, ad vitam Longam … Editio nova, … multam partem adacutior reddiuta & exornation.
Amsterodami, apud Ludovicum Elzevirium, 1652.
4to—pp (34), 636, (2), [637]–652, 663–884 [mispaginated 894], (48) index. Frontispiece portrait of van Helmont and his son.

9. **Borel**, Pierre

De vero telescopii inventore, cum brevi omnium conspiciliorum historia … accessit etiam centuria Observationum microcospicarum [sic].
Hagae-Comitum, Ex typographia Adriani Vlacq, 1655.
4to—pp (12), 67, (1); pp 63, (1), 45, (5). One engraved folding plate, 2 engraved full-page portraits, numerous woodcuts in the text.

10. **Wren**, Christopher

'An Account of the Rise and Attempts, of a Way to conveigh Liquors immediately into the Mass of Blood.'
In: Philosophical Transactions, Num. 7, Monday, Decemb. 4. 1665, pp 128–130.
Oxford, A. & L. Lichfield for Ric. Davis, 1665.

11. **Hooke**, Robert

'An Account of an Experiment made by M. Hook, of Preserving Animals alive by Blowing through their Lungs with Bellows.'
In: Philosophical Transactions. Numb. 28. Monday, October 21, 1667. Pp 539–540.
London, printed by T.N. for John Martyn and Nathaniel Brooks, 1667.

12. **Borelli**, Giovanni Alfonso

De motu animalium. Pars prima [-altera].
Rome, Angeli Bernabo, 1680–81.
4to—pp (12), 376, (12); pp (4), 520. With 18 folding engraved plates.

13. **Kircher**, Athanasius

Neue Hall- und Thon-Kunst, oder Mechanische Gehaim-Verbindung der Kunst und Natur, durch Stimme und Hall-Wissenschafft gestifftet, worinn ingemein der Stimm, Thons, Hall- ind Schalles Natur, Eigenschafft, Krafft und Wunder-Würckung, auch deren geheime Ursachen, mit vielen neu- und ungemeinen Kunst-Wercken und Proben vorgestellt werden. In gleichem wie die Sprach- und Gehör-Instrumenta, Machinen und Kunst-Wercke, vorbildender Natur, zur Nachahmung, so wohl die Stimm, Hall- und Schall an weitentlegene Ort zu führen, als auch in abgesonderten Gehaim-Zimmern, auf kunstverborgenen Weise, vertreulich und ungefahr sich mit einander zu unterreden sollen verfertigt werden. Endlich wie solche schöne Erfindung zu Kriegs-Zeiten nutzlichen könneangebracht und gebrauchet werden. In unsere Teutsche Mutter-Sprach übersetzet von Agatho-Carione [pseudonym for Tobias Nisslen].
Nördlingen, gedruckt bey Friderich Schultes, in Verlegung Arnold Heylen, 1684.
Folio—pp (16), 162, (16). Engraved frontispiece, one engraved plate, 19 engravings and over 50 woodcut figures, diagrams and music in the text.

14. **Boyle**, Robert

Memoirs for the Natural History of the Human Blood, especially the Spirit of that Liquor.
London, Samuel Smith, 1683–84.
8vo—pp (16), 289, (7).

15. **Hauksbee**, Francis

Physico-Mechanical Experiments on Various Subjects. Containing an Account of several Surprizing Phenomena touching Light and Electricity, producible on the Attrition of Bodies. With many other Remarkable Appearances, not before observ'd. Together with the Explanations of all the Machines (the Figures of which are Curiously Engrav'd on Copper) and other Apparatus us'd in making the Experiments.
London, printed for the Author by R. Brugis, 1709.
4to—pp (14), 194. With 7 folding engraved plates numbered I–VII and one smaller plate facing page 160.

16. **Leeuwenhoek**, Antoni van

Opera Omnia, seu Arcana Naturae, ope exacitissimorum microscopiorum detecta, experimentis variis comprobata, Epistolis, ad varios illustres Viros … comprehensa & Quatuor Tomis distincta.
Lugduni Batavorum [Leiden], J. A. Langerak, 1722.
4to—in four volumes. The first Latin edition containing all of Leeuwenhoek's 165 letters numbered from 28 to 146 and I–XLVI. With 110 engraved plates and 117 engravings in the text.

17. **Hales**, Stephen

Statical Essays [vol. I.] Vegetable Staticks; or, An Account of Some Statical Experiments on the Sap of Vegetables … [vol. II.] Statical Essays: containing Haemastaticks; or, An Account of some Hydraulick and Hydrostatical Experiments made on the Blood and Blood-Vessels of Animals.
London, W. & J. Innys, and T. Woodward [vol. I], 1727; W. Innys and R. Manby, and T. Woodward [vol. II], 1733.
8vo—pp (7), vii, (2), 376, with 19 engraved plates; vol. II: pp xxii, (26), 361, (23).

18. **Bernoulli**, Daniel

Hydrodynamica, sive de viribus et motibus fluidorum commentarii.
Strassburg, Joh. Henr. Decker for Johann Reinhold Dulsecker, 1738.
4to—pp (8), 304. With 12 folding engraved plates.

19. **Jallabert**, Jean

Experiences sur l'electricité, avec quelques conjectures sur la cause de ses effets.
Geneve, Barrillot & Fils, 1748.
8vo—pp xii, (2) errata, 1–144, *129–*144, 145–304. With 3 folding engraved plates and one folding letterpress table.

20. **Black**, Joseph

'Experiments upon Magnesia alba, Quicklime, and some other Alcaline Substances.'
In: Essays and Observations, Physical and Literary, read before a Society in Edinburgh. Volume II, pp 157–225.
Edinburgh, G. Hamilton and J. Balfour, 1756.

21. **Scheele**, Carl Wilhelm

Chemische Abhandlung von der Luft und dem Feuer.

Nebst einem Vorbericht von Torbern Bergman.

Uppsala, printed by Johan Edman for Magnus Swederus, and Siegfried Lebrecht Crusius in Leipzig, 1777.

8vo—pp (2), iv (Vorrede), (16) Vorbericht, 155, (1). One folding engraved plate. A few copies has an inserted half-title leaf giving the name of the printer, Johan Edman, who is otherwise not mentioned in the book.

22. **Priestley**, Joseph

Experiments and Observations on Different Kinds of Air. Volumes I–III.

London, J. Johnson, 1774–1777.

8vo—Vol. I: pp (2), xxiii, (5), 324, (4). Double-page engraved frontispiece and one double-page plate; Vol. II: pp xliv, 399, (17), (4) adverts. Engraved frontispiece and 3 plates; Vol. III: pp xxxiv, (6), 411, (9), (4) adverts. Folding engraved frontispiece.

23. **Kite**, Charles

An Essay on the Recovery of the Apparently Dead.

London, C. Dilly, 1788.

8vo—pp xxvii, (1), 274, (2). With 3 engraved plates and 4 folding tables.

24. **Lavoisier**, Antoine-Laurent

'Premier Mémoire sur la Respiration des Animaux, par MM: Seguin et Lavoisier.'

In: Mémoires de l'Academie Royale des Sciences, 1789, pp 566–584.

Paris, (1793)

25. **Kempelen**, Wolfgang von

Mechanismus der menschlichen Sprache nebst der Beschreibung seiner sprechenden Maschine.

Wien, J.B. Degen, 1791.

8vo—pp (20), 456. Engraved frontispiece portrait, 26 engraved plates. and one folding table.

26. **Volta**, Alessandro

'On the Electricity excited by the mere Contact of Conducting Substances of Different Kinds.'

In: Philosophical Transactions 90 (1800), Part 2, pp 403–431, with one folding engraved plate, numbered XVII.

London, W. Bulmer for Peter Elmsley, 1800.

27. **Herschel**, Wilhelm

'XIII. Investigation of the Powers of the prismatic Colours to heat and illuminate Objects; with Remarks, that prove the different Refrangibility of radiant Heat. To which is added, an Inquiry into the Method of viewing the Sun advantageously, with Telescopes of large Apertures and high magnifying Powers; XIV. Experiments on the Refrangibility of the invisible Rays of the Sun; XV. Experiments on the solar, and on the terrestial Rays that occasion Heat; with a comparative View of the Laws into which Light and Heat, or rather the Rays which occasion them, are subject, in order to determine whether they are the same, or different.

In: Philisophical Transactions, of the Royal Society of London. For the Year MDCCC.

Part I. Pp 255–283, one engraved plate numbered X; pp 284–294, one plate numbered XI; pp 293–326, with 5 engraved plates numbered XII–XVI.

London, W. Bulmer and Co. and sold by Peter Elmsly, 1800.

28. **Davy**, Humphry

Researches, Chemical and Philosophical; chiefly concerning Nitrious Oxide, or Dephlogisticated Nitrious Air, and its Respiration.

London, printed for J. Johnson, by Biggs and Cottle, Bristol, 1800.

8vo—pp xvi, (2), 580, (2) errata. One engraved plate.

29. **Sertürner**, Friedrich

'Darstellung der reinen Mohnsäure (Opiumsäure) nebst einer chemischen Untersuchung des Opiums mit vorzüglicher Hinsicht auf einen darin neu entdeckten Stoff und die dahin gehörigen Bemerkungen.'

In: Journal der Pharmacie für Aerzte, Apotheker und Chemisten von D. Johann Bartholomäus Trommsdorff. 14. Band. Pp 47–93.

Leipzig, Siegfried Lebrecht Crusius, 1806.

30. **Legendre**, Adrien-Marie

Nouvelles Méthodes pour la Détermination des Orbites des Comètes; avec un Supplément contenant divers perfectionnemens de ces Méthodes et leur application aux deux Comètes de 1805.

Paris, Courcier, 1806.

4to—pp viii, 80. One engraved plate; Supplément aux Nouvelles Méthodes pour la détermination des Orbites des Comètes: pp 55, (1) blank.

31. **Laennec**, René Théophile Hyacinthe

De l'auscultation médiate, ou traité du diagnostic des maladies des poumons et du coeur,… Tome Premier [-Second].

Paris, J.-A. Brosson & J.S. Chaudé, 1819.

Volume I: pp (5), viii–xlviii, 456, (8), with 4 folding engraved plates numbered I–IV.

Volume II: pp xvi, 472.

32. **Fourier**, Jean Baptiste

Théorie Analytique de la Chaleur.

Paris, Firmin Didot, Père et Fils, 1822.

8vo—pp (4), xxii, 639, (1). With 2 engraved plates.

33. **Labarraque**, Antoine-Germain

De l'emploi des chlorures d'oxide de sodium et de chaux.

Paris, l'Auteur & Madame Huzard, 1825.

8vo—pp 48.

34. **Civiale**, Jean

De la Lithotritie, ou broiement de la pierre dans la vessie.

Paris, chez Béchet jeune, et Aillaud, 1827.

8vo—pp lx, 254; Rapport par Chaussier & Percy: pp 38; (12), (2) errata. With 5 very large folding plates and one folding letterpress table.

35. **Poiseuille**, Jean Léonard Marie

Recherches sur la force du coeur aortique.

Paris, de l'imprimerie de Didot le jeune, 1828.

4to—pp iv, [7]–44. One engraved plate.

36. **Dumas**, Jean Baptiste

'Recherches de chimie organique relatives à l'action du chlore sur l'alcool. Loi des substitutions ou métalepsie.' Lu à l'Académie des Sciences, le 13 janvier 1835.

In: Mémoires de l'Académie des Sciences. Pp (2) half-title, 7–44.

Paris, Firmin Didot frères et Cie, (1835).

37. **Magnus**, Heinrich Gustav

'Ueber die im Blute enthaltenen Gase, Sauerstoff, Stickstoff und Kohlensäure.'

In: Annalen der Physik und Chemie. Herausgegeben von J.C. Poggendorff. Band 40. Pp 583–606. One woodcut in the text.

Leipzig, Johann Ambrosius Barth, 1837.

38. **Daguerre**, Louis Jacques Mandé

Historique et description des procédés du Daguerréotype et du Diorama.

Paris, Lerebours – Susse Frères, 1839.

8vo—pp (4), 79, (1), (4) adverts. With 6 lithographed plates. There were several issues with different imprints, the first appeared in mid-August 1839 with the imprint of Alphonse Giroux et Cie.

39. **Liebig**, Justus von

Die organische Chemie in ihrer Anwendung auf Physiologie und Pathologie.

Braunschweig, Verlag von Friedrich Vieweg und Sohn, 1842.

8vo—pp xvi, (2), 342, (2) errata.

40. **Doppler**, Johann Christian

'Ueber das farbige Licht der Doppelsterne und einiger anderer Gestirne des Himmels.'

Abgedruckt K. Böhmischen Gesellschaft der Wissenschaften. Abhandlungen. V. Folge. Band 2, pp 465–482, with one plate.

Prag, Borrosch & André, 1842.

41. **Hutchinson**, John

'On the Capacity of the Lungs, and on the Respiratory Functions, with a View of establishing a Precise and Easy Method of detecting Disease by the Spirometer.'

In: Medico-Chirurgical Transactions, published by the Royal Medical and Chirurgical Society of London. Volume 29. Pp 137–252, with 28 diagrams (with figures) in the text.

London, Longman, Brown, Green, and Longmans, 1846.

42. **Du Bois-Reymond**, Emil

Untersuchungen über thierische Elektricität. Volume I--II:1-2.

Berlin, G. Reimer, 1848–1860, (1884).

8vo—Volume I. (1848): pp lvi, 743, (1) errata. With 6 folding engraved plates. Volume II:1. (1849): pp (6), 608. With 4 folding engraved plates numbered I–IV; Volume II:2. (1860, 1884): pp 579, with two engraved plates numbered V–VI (pp 385–579 with plate VI not published until 1884).

43. **Helmholtz**, Hermann von

'Messungen über den zeitlichen Verlauf der Zuckung animalischer Muskeln und die Fortpflanzungsgeschwindigkeit der Reizung in den Nerven.'

In: Archiv für Anatomie, Physiologie und

wissenschaftliche Medicin. Herausgegeben von Dr. Johannes Müller. Jahrgang 1850. Pp 276–364. With one folding lithographed plate (numbered Taf. VIII) with 7 figures.
Berlin, Veit et Comp., (1850).

44. Weber, Ernst Heinrich

'Ueber die Anwendung der Wellenlehre auf die Lehre vom Kreislaufe des Blutes und insbesondere auf die Pulslehre.'
In: Archiv für Anatomie, Physiologie und wissenschaftliche Medicin. Herausgegeben von Johannes Müller. Jahrgang 1851. Pp 497–546. One folding engraved plate numbered Taf. XX.
Berlin, Veit et Comp., (1851).

45. Helmholtz, Hermann von

Beschreibung eines Augen-Spiegels zur Untersuchung der Netzhaut im lebenden Auge.
Berlin, A. Förstner'sche Verlagsbuchhandlung, 1851.
8vo—pp 43, (5) incl. final blank leaf. One engraved plate.

46. Fick, Adolf

Die medicinische Physik. [Supplementband zu Müller-Pouillet's Lehrbuch der Physik — Für Mediziner].
Braunschweig, Friedrich Vieweg und Sohn, 1856.
8vo—Lieferung 1–6 issued in three parts as follows: pp xii, (2), 192, (2) adverts; pp (2), 193–384; pp 385–537, (1) errata, xiii–xiv.

47. Snow, John

On Choloroform and Other Anaesthetics: Their Action and Administration.
London, John Churchill, 1858.
8vo—pp viii, xliv, 443, (1). Wood-engraved figures in the text.

48. Czermak, Johann

'Physiologische Untersuchungen mit Garcia's Kehlkopfspiegel.'
In: Sitzungsberichte d. k. Akademie der Wissenschaften, mathematisch-naturwissenschaftliche Klasse, Wien, 29 (1858), pp 557–584.
Wien, 1858.

49. Kirchoff, Gustav Robert

'Untersuchungen über das Sonnenspectrum und die Spectren der chemischen Elemente.'
In: Abhandlungen der königl. Akademie der Wissenschaften zu Berlin. Physikalische Klasse. Part I, 1861: pp 63–95 with 3 plates (two folded lithographed plates (I–II) and one engraved plate (III); Part II, 1863: pp 4–16 with 2 folded lithographed plates numbered Ia and III.
Berlin, Königl. Akademie der Wissenschaften, in Commission bei F. Dümmler's Buchhandlung, 1861, 1863.

50. Pasteur, Louis

'Mémoire sur les corpuscules organisés qui existent dans l'atmosphère, examen de la doctrine des générations spontanées.'
In: Annales de Chimie et de Physique. Troisième Série 4. Tome LXIV. Pp 5–110. With 2 folding plates numbered Pl. I–II.
Paris, Victor Masson et fils, 1862.

51. Hoppe-Seyler, Felix

'Ueber das Verhalten des Blutfarbstoffe im Spectrum des Sonnenlichtes.'
In: Archiv für pathologische Anatomie und Physiologie und für klinische Medicin. Herausgegeben von Rudolf Virchow. Band 23. Zweite Folge: Dritter Band. Pp 446–449.
Berlin, Georg Reimer, 1862.

52. Marey, Etienne-Jules

Physiologie médicale de la circulation du sang basée sur l'étude graphique des mouvements du coeur et du pouls artériel avec application aux maladies de l'appareil circulatoire.
Paris, Adrien Delahaye, 1863.
8vo—pp viii, 569. With 235 figures in the text.

53. Mendel, Gregor

'Versuche über Pflanzen-Hybriden.'
In: Verhandlungen des naturforschenden Vereines in Brünn. IV. Band (1865), Abhandlungen: pp 3–47.
Brünn, Verlage des Vereines, Georg Gastl's Buchdruckerei, 1866.

54. Lister, Joseph

'On a New Method of Treating Compound Fracture, Abscess, etc, with Observations on the Conditions of Suppuration.'
In: The Lancet, 1867, volume I: March 16, pp 326–29; March 23, pp 357–59; March 30, pp 387–89; April 27, pp 507–09; Volume II; July 27, pp 95–6.
London, The Lancet, 1867.

55. Maxwell, James Clerk

'On Governors.'
In: Proceedings of the Royal Society of London, 16 (1868), p 270–283.
London, Taylor and Francis, 1868.

56. Fick, Adolf

'Ueber die Messung des Blutquantums in den Herzventrikeln.'
In: Verhandlungen der Physikal.-Medicin. Gesellschaft in Würzburg. Neue Folge. II. Band. [issued with]: Sitzungsberichte der physikalisch-medicinischen Gesellschaft zu Würzburg für das Gesellschaftsjahr 1870. Page xvi in XIV. Sitzung am 9. Juli 1870.
Würzburg, Stahel'schen Buch- und Kunsthandlung, 1872.

57. Trendelenburg, Friedrich

'Beiträge zu den Operationen an den Luftwegen.' [dated 6. December 1869].
In: Archiv für Klinische Chirurgie. Herausgegeben von B. von Langenbeck. Band 12. Pp 112–133. One lithographed plate numbered Taf. III.
Berlin, August Hirschwald, 1871.

58. Voit, Carl von

'Beschreibung eines Apparates zur Untersuchung der gasförmigen Ausscheidungen des Thierkörpers.'
In: Abhandlungen der Bayerischen Akademie der Wissenschaften zu München. Band XII, 1. Abth. pp (2) title, 219–271, (1) blank. With 3 folding lithographed plates: Taf. I–III.
München, 1876.

59. Bert, Paul

La pression barométrique. Recherches de physiologie expérimentale.
Paris, G. Masson, 1878.
8vo—pp (2) blank, (6), viii, 1168. With 89 figures in the text.

60. Nitze, Max

'Eine neue Beobachtungs- und Untersuchungsmethode für Harnröhre, Harnblase und Rectum.'
In: Wiener Medicinische Wochenschrift, Jahrgang 1879, columns 649–652, 688–691, 713–716, 776–782 and 806–810.
Wien, L.W. Seidel & Sohn, 1879.

61. Koch, Robert

'Zur Untersuchung von pathogenen Organismen.'
In: Mittheilungen aus dem kaiserlichen Gesundheitsamte. Erster Band.
Berlin, Verlag der Norddeutschen Buchdruckerei, 1881.
4to—pp 1–48, with 14 plates numbered I–XIV, with six photographic figures on each plate.

62. Arrhenius, Svante

Recherches sur la conductibilité galvanique des électrolytes. Premier – Second Partie.
Mémoire présenté a l'Academie Royale des Sciences de Suède le 6 Juin 1883. Bihang till Kongl. Svenska Vetenskaps-Akademiens Handlingar, Volume 8, No. 13, pp 1–63; No 14: pp 1–89.
Stockholm, P.A. Norstedt & Söner, 1884.

63. Van't hoff, Jacobus Henricus

Lois de l'équilibre chimique dans l'état dilué, gazeux ou dissous.
Mémoire présente a l'Academie Royale des Sciences de Suède le 14 Octobre 1885. Kongl. Svenska Vetenskaps-Akademiens Handlingar, Volume 21, No. 17: pp 1–58.
Stockholm, P. A. Norstedt & Söner, 1886.

64. Abbe, Ernst

Ueber Verbesserungen des Mikroskops mit Hilfe neuer Arten optischen Glases.
(Sonder-Abdruck aus den Sitzungsberichten der medicin.-naturw. Gesellschaft zu Jena. Sitzung vom 9. Juli 1886.)
Jena, Frommansche Buchdruckerei, (1886)
8vo—pp (1–24 facsimile in Moritz von Rohr, Ernst Abbes Apochromate. Jena, Carl Zeiss, 1936).

65. Waller, Augustus Désiré

'A Demonstration on Man of Electromotive Changes accompanying the Heart's Beat.'
In: The Journal of Physiology [London].

Edited by Michael Foster, Vol. VIII. 1887. Pp 229–234.

Cambridge, published by the proprietors, (1887).

66. **Curie**, Pierre [written with Jacques Curie]

'Dilatation électrique du Quartz.'

In: Journal de Physique, 2e Série, Tome VIII, 1889. Pp 149–168

Paris, Bureau de Journal de Physique, 1889.

67. **Röntgen**, Wilhelm Conrad

'Ueber eine neue Art von Strahlen (Vorläufige Mittheilung)' + 'Ueber eine neue Art von Strahlen. II. Mittheilung.'

In: Sitzungsberichte der physik.-med. Gesellschaft zu Würzburg. Jahrgang 1895, No 9: pp 132–141; Jahrgang 1896, No 1: pp 11–16 with one full-page halftone illustration of "Hand des Anatomen Geheimrath von Kölliker"; 1896, No 2: pp [17]–19.

Würzburg, Verlag der Stahel'schen Buchhandlung, 1896–97.

68. **Riva-Rocci**, Scipione

'Un Sfigmomanometro nuovo.'

In: Gazetta medica di Torino, 47 (1896), pp 981–996, 1001–1017.

Turin, 1896.

69. **Thomson**, Joseph John

'Cathode Rays.'

In: The London, Edinburgh, and Dublin Philosophical Magazine and Journal of Science. Vol XLIV. [Fifth Series.] October 1897. Pp 293–316, with 6 figures in the text.

London, Taylor and Francis, (1897).

70. **Curie**, Marie Sklodowska

'Rayon émis par les composés de l'uranium et du thorium.'

In: Comptes rendus hebdomadaires des Séances de l'Academie des Sciences, volume 126. Séance 12 April, 1898, pp 1101–1103.

Paris, Gauthier-Villars, 1898.

71. **Einthoven**, Willem

'Galvanometrische registratie van het menschelijk electrocardiogram.'

In: Herinnerungsbundel Professor S.S. Rosenstein, pp 101–106, with one plate (Pl. V.)

Leiden, Edouard Ijdo, 1902.

72. **Fischer**, Emil Hermann & J. von **Mering**

'Ueber eine neue Klasse von Schlafmitteln.'

In: Die Therapie der Gegenwart. Medicinisch-Chirurgische Rundschau für praktische Ärzte (44. Jahrgang.) Neueste Folge. V. Jahrgang. März, 1903. pp 97–101.

Berlin & Wien, Urban & Schwarzenberg, 1903.

73. **Tswett**, Mikhail Semenovich

'O novoy kategorii adsorptsionnykh yavleny i o primenenii ikh k biokhimicheskomu anal-izu' ["On a New Category of Adsorption Phenomena and on its Application to Biochemical Analysis."]

In: Trudy Varshavskago obshchestva estestvoispytatelei, Otd. Biol., Volume 14, (1903), pp 20–39.

Warshaw, 1905.

74. **Fischer**, Emil Hermann

Untersuchungen über Aminosäuren, Polypeptide und Proteine (1899–1906).

Berlin, Julius Springer, 1906.

8vo–pp x, (2), 770.

75. **Ehrlich**, Paul & Sahachiro **Hata**,

Die experimentelle Chemotherapie der Spirillosen (Syphilis, Rückfallfieber, Hühnerspirillose, Frambösie).

Berlin, Julius Springer, 1910.

8vo–pp viii, 164, (4) adverts. With 3 folding letterpress tables and 5 plates.

76. **Laue**, Max von, with W. Friedrich and P. Knipping

'Interferenzerscheinungen bei Röntgenstrahlen.'

In: Annalen der Physik. Vierte Folge. Band 41. No. 10 (1913), pp 971–988, with 4 plates with 10 figures and 2 figures in the text.

Leipzig, Johann Ambrosius Barth, 1913.

77. **Abel**, John Jacob (with Leonard G. Rowntree and B.B. Turner)

'On the Removal of diffusible Substances from the circulating Blood of living Animals by Dialysis.'

In: The Journal of Pharmacology and Experimental Therapeutics. Volume V, No. 3, January, 1914, pp 275–316, with 11 figures in the text.

Baltimore, Pharmacological Laboratory of the Johns Hopkins University, the Waverly Press, 1914.

78. **Staudinger**, Hermann

'Über polymerisation.' [signed Zürich, Juli 1919]

In: Berichte der Deutsche Chemische Gesellschaft, Jahrgang 53 (1920), pp 1073–1085.

Weinheim, Deutsche Chemische Gesellschaft, 1920.

79. **Aston**, Francis William

Isotopes.

London, Edward Arnold, 1922.

8vo–pp viii, 152. With 4 full-page plates and 21 figures in the text.

80. **Carothers**, Wallace H.

'Studies on Polymerization and Ring Formation. I. An Introduction to the General Theory of Condensation Polymers.' & [with J.A. Arwin] II. Poly-Esters.

In: The Journal of the American Chemical Society, vol. 51, August, 1929, No. 8. Pp 2548–2570.

Washington D.C., American Chemical Society, 1929.

81. **Van Slyke**, Donald Dexter & John P. **Peters**

Quantitative Clinical Chemistry. Volume I. Interpretations. —Volume II. Methods.

Baltimore, The Williams & Wilkins Company, 1931-1932.

Two volumes, pp xvi, 1264, (4) with 124 figures; volume II: pp xx, 957, (5), with 95 figures.

82. **Zworykin**, Vladimir Kozma

'Television' [presented, October 18, 1933].

In: Journal of The Franklin Institute devoted to Science and the Mechanic Arts, Vol. 217, January, 1834, No. 1. Pp 1–37, with 31 figures in the text.

Philadelphia, The Franklin Institute, 1934.

83. **Ruska**, Ernst & Bodo von **Borries**

'Vorläufige Mitteilung über Fortschritte im Bau und in der Leistung des Übermikroskopes.'

In: Wissenschaftliche Veröffentlichungen des Wernerwerkes der Siemens & Halske AG zu Siemensstadt, XVII. Band, 1. Heft, pp 99–196, with 7 illustrations in the text.

Berlin, Julius Springer, 1938.

84. **Martin**, Archer J.P. and R.L.M. **Synge**

'A New Form of Chromatogram employing Two Liquid Phases. 1. A Theory of Chromatography. 2. Application to the Micro-Determination of the Higher Monoamino-Acids in Proteins.'

In: Biochemical Journal, 35 (1941), 151, pp 1358–1368, with 3 figures in the text.

London, Biochemical Society, 1941.

85. **Eckert**, John Presper & John William **Mauchly**

Description of the ENIAC and Comments on Electronic Digital Computing Machines. – AMP Report 171:2R Moore School of Electrical Engineering, University of Pennsylvania. Restricted.

No place, distributed by the Applied Mathematical Panel, National Defense Reseach Committee, November 30, 1945.

4to–pp (82), with 3 folding plates, and diagrams in the text.

86. **Kolff**, Willem J.

De Kunstmatige Nier. Proefschrift ter Verkrijging van de Graad van Doctor … 16 Januari 1946, …

Kampen, J.H. Kok, (1946).

8vo–pp (4), 200. With more than 54 figures including 7 photo plates and frontispiece, and 4 folding tables and diagrams.

87. **Engström**, Carl-Gunnar

'Treatment of Bulbar Poliomyelitis by Special Postural Drainage.'

In: Poliomyelitis. Papers and Discussions Presented at the Second International Poliomyelitis Conference. Compiled and Edited for the International Poliomyelitis Congress. Pp 429–430 with 5 photo figures in the text.

Philadelphia, J. B. Lippincott Company, 1952.

88. **Watson**, James Dewey & Francis Harry Compton **Crick**,

'A Structure for Deoxyribose Nucleic Acid.'
In: Nature 171, No. 4356, April 25, 1953, pp 737–38.
London, The Nature, 1953.

89. **Fant**, Gunnar

'Speech Communication Research'.
In: IVA [The Royal Swedish Academy of Engineering Sciences] Tidskrift för Teknisk Vetenskaplig Forskning, 24, 8, pp 331–337, with 4 figures in the text.
Stockholm, Esselte, 1954.

90. **Edler**, Inge and Carl Helmuth **Hertz**

'The Use of Ultrasonic Reflectoscope for the Continuous Recording of the Movements of Heart Walls.'
In: Kungl. Fysiografiska Sällskapets i Lund Förhandlingar, Band 24, Nr 5, 1954, pp 40–58, with 11 figures in the text.
Lund, Gleerupska Universitetsbokhandeln, 1954

91. **Elmqvist**, Rune and Åke **Senning**

'An Implantable Pacemaker for the Heart.'
In: Medical Electronics. Proceedings of the Second International Conference on Medical Electronics Paris 24–27 June 1959. Edited by C.N. Smyth. Pp 253–254.
London, Iliffe & Sons Ltd., 1960.

92. **Maiman**, Theodore Harold

'Stimulated Optical Radiation in Ruby'.
In: Nature, Vol. 187, No. 4736, August 6, 1969, pp 493–494, with 2 figures in the text.
London, Macmillan & Co., 1960.

93. **Brånemark**, Per-Ingvar, with U. Breine, A. Adell, N.O. Hansson, J. Lindström and A. Ohlsson.

'Intra-Osseous Anchorage of Dental Prostheses. I. Experimental Studies.'
In: Scandinavian Journal of Plastic Reconstructive Surgery, 3 (1969), pp 81–100, with 19 figures in the text and one colour plate.
Stockholm, Almqvist & Wiksell Periodical Co., 1969.

94. **Damadian**, Raymond V.

'Tumor Detection by Nuclear Magnetic Resonance.'
In: Science, Volume 171, Number 3976, 19 March, 1971, pp 1151–1153.
Washington D.C., American Association for the Advancement of Science, 1971.

95. **Hounsfield**, Godfrey N.

'Computerized transverse axial scanning (tomography): Part I: Description of system.'
In: The British Journal of Radiology, Vol. 46, No. 552, December 1973, pp 1016–1022, with 10 figures in the text.
London, The British Institute of Radiology, 1973.

96. **Lauterbur**, Paul C.

'Image Formation by Induced Local Interactions: Examples Employing Nuclear Magnetic Resonance.'
In: Nature, Volume 242, No. 5394, March, 16, 1973, pp 190–191, with 2 figures.
London, Macmillan Journals Ltd., 1973.

97. **Wagner**, Peter D., Herbert A. **Saltzman**, and John B. **West**

'Measurement of continuous distributions of ventilation-perfusion ratios: theory.'
In: Journal of Applied Physiology, volume 36, No. 5, May 1974, pp 588–599, with 10 figures in the text.
Washington, D.C. American Physiological Society, 1974.

98. **Cerf**, Vinton G. and Robert E. **Kahn**

'A Protocol for Packet Network Intercommunication.'
In: IEEE Transactions on Communications, Volume Com-22, Number 5, May 1974, pp 637–648, with 11 figures and portraits of the authors.
New York, The Institute of Electrical and Electronics Engineers, Inc., 1974.

99. **Phelps**, Michael E. with Edward J. Hoffman, Noizar A. Mullani, and Michael M. Ter-Pogossian.

'Application on Annihilation Coincidence Detection to Transaxial Reconstruction Tomography'
In: Journal of Nuclear Medicine, March, 1975, Volume 16, Number 3, pp 210–224, with 19 figures in the text.
St. Louis, Missouri, Washington University School of Medicine, 1975.

1. *1:1* the landmark publication #1. *1:2* Painting in El Prado, Madrid Iván F. Durer. Képmuvészeti Alap Kiadóvállalata Budapest 1955. *1:3* Detail a painting by Jacopo de Barbari in Museo e Gallerie di Canpodimonte. Naples. *1:5* the second edition of reference 1.4 from 1538. *1:6* the landmark publication #1. *1:7* and *1:8* reference 1.4. *1:9–1:11* the landmark publication #1.

2. *2:1* the landmark publication #2. *2:2* Engraving by Horbeck. *2:3* reference 2.3. *2:4* reference 2.2. *2:5–2:7* reference 2.4. *2:8* reference 2.6.

3. *3:1* reference 3.2. *3:2* Hagelin O. Rare and important medical books in the library of the Swedish Society of Medicine. Stockholm 1989. *3:3* Portrait by A. Hirschvogel 1538. *3:4* Gesner C. The practise of the new and old phisicke ... Newly corrected and published in English by G Baker London 1599. *3:5* Ioannes Sambucus. Veterum aliquot ac recentium Medicorum Philosophorumque Icones C.Plantin Antwerp 1574. *3:6* reference 3.6. *3:7* reference 3.9. *3:8* reference 3.8. *3:9* and *3:10* reference 57.11.

4. *4:1–4:3* the landmark publication #4. *4.4* Engraving by Giacomo Piccini 1660. Castiglioni A. La vita e l'opera di Santorio Santorio Capodistriano. Bologna/Trieste 1920. *4:5* woodcut from Galen Works in Latin, Prefaces and edited by Joannes Rivirius Lyon 1528. Courtesy of Stephen Greenberg National Library of Medicine. Bethesda, MD *4:7* Aristotle collected scientific writings, Augsburg 1518–1520. *4:8* and *4:10* reference 4.3. *4:9* reference 4.6 and The Sjögren Library of the Royal Swedish Academy of Engineering Sciences. Stockholm. *4:11* reference 4.7. *4:12* and *4:13* Galerie hervorragender Ärzte und Naturforscher. Beilage zur Münchener medizinischen Wochenschrift. *4:14–4:17* reference 4.10.

5. *5:1* Repro- och fotoenheten /Kungliga biblioteket Stockholm from the landmark publication #5 *5:2* reference 5.2. *5:3* Opera Omnia Ed. Ch Frisch Frankfurt 1858–1871. *5:4* reference 5.6. *5:5* and *5:6* from reference 5:3. *5:7–5:10* reference 5.8. *5:11–5:13* details images in references 5.5 and 5.9. *5:14* and *5:15* reference 5.9. *5:16* and *5:17* reference 5.12.

6. *6:1–6:3* the landmark publication #7. *6:4* medal engraving by C.Rizzi 1765. The Wellcome Trust Medical Photographic Library. London. *6:5* and *6:6* the landmark publication #7. *6:7* reference 6.6. *6:8* and *6:10* from reference 7.10. *6:9* the Bibliothèque de l'Académie national de Médecine Paris. Courtesy of Marie Davaine. *6:12* and *6:13* reference 6.9. *6:11* reference 6.7. *6:14* and *6:15* from reference 6:11. *6:16* reference 6.10. Courtesy of Engström Medical AB Bromma Sweden (now GE Healthcare).

7. *7:1* the landmark publication #7. *7:2* and *7:3* reference 7.3. *7:4–7:6* the Museo Di Storia Della Scienza. Florence. *7:7* Engraving by Giacomo Piccini 1660, Castiglioni A. La vita e l'opera di Santorio Santorio Capodistriano Bologna/Trieste 1920. *7:8* and *7:10* Museum Gustavianum, Uppsala University Museum Uppsala. *7:9* Celsius A. Observationer om twänne beständiga grader på en Thermometer. Kungl.Sv.Vet.Handl. Jul–Sept. 1742. *7:11* reference 7.4. *7:12* reference 7.6. *7:13* Hirschfeld J. Galerie berühmter Kliniker und hervorragender Aerzte unserer Zeit ... Wien 1877. *7:14* and *7:15* reference 7.8. *7:16* and *7:17* reference 9.2. *7:18* reference 7.8. *7:19* and *7:20* reference 6.8. *7:21* courtesy of José Pessoa—Divisao de Documentacao Fotográfica do Instituto Portugues de Museus. Museum of Physics of the University of Coimbra. Portugal. *7:22* reference 7.10.

8. *8:1* and *8:3* reference 8.6. *8:2* and *8:4* reference 8.4. *8:5* detail from a portrait in the landmark publication #8. *8:6* and *8:7* reference 8.5. *8:8* the landmark publication #18. *8:10* reference 8.8. *8:9* the Medical Photographic Library of the Wellcome Trust. London. *8:11* taken from Silby E. A key to physic and the occult sciences. London 1810.

9. *9:1–9:3* the landmark publication #9. *9:4* Museé Goya. Castres and from Chabbert P. Pierre Borel (1620?–1671) Revue d'Histoire des Sciences. 1968; XXI(4): 303. *9:5* the Museo Di Storia Della Scienza. Florence. *9:6* and *9:7* reference 9.2. *9:8* the Museo Di Storia Della Scienza. Florence. *9:9* reference 9.6.

10. *10:1–10:4* reference 10.2. *10:5* detail from a portrait by Sir Godfrey Kneller. National Maritime Museum London. *10:6* and *10:7* Anel D. L'art de succer les playes sans servir de la bouche d'un homme. Trevoux 1720–1721. *10:8–10:9* the Medical Photographic Library of the Wellcome Trust. London. *10:10* the Science & Society Picture Library of the Science Museum London. *10:11* and *10:12* reference 10.10.

11. *11:1* the landmark publication #11. *11.2* No portrait exists of Robert Hooke. *11:3* Translation by Benjamin Farrington. Trans.Roy.Soc.S.Africa 1933;20(I). reference 1.6. *11:4* the landmark publication #11. *11:5* and *11:6* reference 11.5 and the English translation, Alembic Club Reprints No 17 1907.

12. *12:1* the landmark publication #12. *12:2* Lithograph by Pierre Vignéron, Vignéron et Doin. Gallerie Médicale 1825–1829 Paris. *12:3* and *12:4* the landmark publication #12. *12:5* Wilhelm Weber's Werke Band 6 Berlin 1894. Courtesy of Dr Roland Rappmann Bibliothek der RWTH Aachen. (Also in reference 12.8). *12:6* reference 12.11 and Musée de Beaune. Beaune (Cote-d'Or). Courtesy of Dominique Debrot.

13. *13:1* and *13:2* the landmark publication #13. *13:3* Detail from Giorgio de Sepius. Romani Collegii Musaeum Celeberrimum. Amsterdam 1678. *13:4–13:9* the landmark publication #13. *13:10* and *13:11* reference 13.1.

14. *14:1* and *14:2* the landmark publication #14. *14:3* Masson F. Robert Boyle. A biography. London 1914. *14:4* and *14:5* the landmark publication #14. *14:6* Hewson W. The Works. Ed.G.Gulliver London 1846. *14:7* Hewson W. Phil.Trans. Roy.Soc. 1770;60;368. *14:8* detail from a painting by J.G.Sandberg from Söderbaum H. Jac.Berzelius Band 2. Uppsala 1929. *14:9* reference 36.5 volume 6 page 67.

15. *15:1* and *15:2* the landmark publication #15. *15:4* reference 15.7. *15:5* reference 15.6. Kungl.Tekniska Högskolans Bibliotek Stockholm. *15:6* reference 15.9 memoire I. p 576. *15:7* reference 15.9 memoire II p610. *15:8* courtesy of Capt Pintor DCG BP 221 Armees France.

16. *16:1* Dobell C. Antony van Leeuwenhoek and his "Little Animals". Amsterdam 1932. *16:2–16:4* the landmark publication #16 (Volume IV). *16:5* and *16:6* reference 16.4. *16:7* reference 16.6. *16:8* Spallanzani L. Saggio di osservazioni microscopiche ... Bari 1914. Reprint of reference 50.3.

17. *17:1* the landmark publication #17. *17:2* detail from a painting by Thomas Hudson. National Portrait Gallery, London. From Clark-Kennedy A. Stephen Hales D.D.,F.R.S. Cambridge 1929. *17:3* the landmark publication #17. *17:4* the French translation of the landmark publication #17 by Compte de Buffon Paris 1735. *17:5* landmark publication #17. *17:6* the Medical Times 1944;72:11.

18. *18:1* and *18:2* from the landmark publication #18 Chapter XII. *18:3* Wolf A. A history of science technology, and philosophy in the eighteenth century. London 1952. *18:4* and *18:5* the landmark publication #18. *18:6* and *18:7* from Universitätsbibliothek Basel, Handschriftenabteilung. Lla 753, fol.328r/v. Courtesy of Dominik Hunger. Translated from the German translation in reference 18.1. *18:8* and *18:9* reference 18.9.

19. *19:1–19:3* the landmark publication #19. *19:5* reference 19.9. *19:6* from reference 19.4. *19:7* engraving by A.Marchi from reference 19.5. *19:8* Robinson V. Pathfinders in medicine. New York 1929. *19:9* and *19:10* reference 19.8. *19:11* engraving by Luigi Schiavonetti from reference 19.5. *19:12* and *19:13* reference 19.11. *19:14* Album de la science. Savants illustres. Grandes découvertes. Paris 1896. *19:15* and *19:17* de Boulogne D. Physiologie des mouvements ... Paris 1867. *19:16* reference 38.7.

20. *20:1* the British Library London. *20:2* and *20:3* the landmark publication #20. *20:4* Engraving by James Heath Wolf A. A history of science technology, and philosophy in the eighteenth century. London 1952. *20:5* and *20:6* the landmark publication #20.

21. *21:1* the landmark publication #21. Kungl.Tekniska Högskolan Biblioteket. Stockholm. *21:2* xylography by Evald Hansen. From Svenska Familj-Journalen

1881;20:197. *21:3* the portrait collection at Jernkontoret Stockholm. *21:4* Zekert O. Carl Wilhelm Scheele Gedenkschrift zum 150. Todestage Wien 1936. *21:5* the landmark publication #21. *21:6* reference 21.6. *21:7* reference 21.6 pages 138–139 and 178–179.

22. *22:1* the Science & Society Picture Library of the Science Museum London. *22:2* reference 24.3. *22:3* engraving by W. Holl. *22:4* from reference 22.6. *22:5* and *22:6* the landmark publication #22.

23. *23:1* and *23:2* the landmark publication #23. *23:4* reference 23.3. *23:5* and *23:6* 1767–1917 Geschiedkundig Overzicht van de Maatschappij tot Redding van Drenkelingen te Amsterdam 1917. *23:7* and *23:9* the landmark publication #23. *23:8* the Science & Society Picture Library of the Science Museum London. *23:10* reference 23.5.

24. *24:1* and *24:2* reference 24.2. *24:3* reference 24.3. *24:4* and *24:7* from reference 24.8. *24:5* and *24:6* from reference 24.8. Detail from a painting by Jacques-Louis David 1788, the Metropolitan Museum of Art. New York.

25. *25:1* and *25:2* from the landmark publication #25. *25:3* and *25:4* from Deutsches Museum Munich. *25:5* Deutsches Museum Munich. *25:6* reference 25.3. *25:7* landmark publication #25. *25:8* Deutsches Museum Munich. *25:9–25:11* the landmark publication #25. *25:12* reference 25.6. *25:13* and *25:14* reference 25.9.

26. *26:1* The Philosophical Transactions of the Royal Society 1800 part 2. (the landmark publication #26 is an English translation of this paper) *26:2* the Science & Society Picture Library of the Science Museum London. *26:3* Portraits berühmter Naturforscher. Wien. Leipzig n.d. Bibliotheca Walleriana No. 16169. *26:4* Album de la science. Grandes découvertes. Paris 1896. *26:5* drawing by Joséphine Ducollet. *26:6* painting by D.Hvidt. *26:7* Faraday M.Experimental researches in chemistry and physics. London 1859. *26:8* Dibner B. Oersted and the discovery of electromagnetism. Norwalk 1961. Courtesy Danmarks Tekniske Højskole. *26:9* reference 26.3. *26:10* reference 26.4. *26:11* Killian H. Gustav Killian sein Leben sein Werk. Remscheid-Lennep 1958. *26:12* and *26:13* the Medical Photographic Library of the Wellcome Trust. London. *26:14* The Electrician (London) Obituary. 1900. *26:15* and *26:17* reference 26.9. *26:16*, *26:18* and *26:19* Courtesy of Cochlear Limited. Lane Cove Australia.

27. *27:1* and *27:2* the landmark publication #27. *27:3* engraving by E.Scriven. *27:4–27:6* the landmark publication #27. *27:7* and *27:8* from reference 27.9. *27:9* Cade C. High-speed thermography. Ann.N.Y.Acad.Sci. 1964;121:71. *27:10–27:16* Flir Systems AB. Danderyd Sweden. Courtesy of Jan-Åke Andersson.

28. *28:1* and *28:2* the landmark publication #28. *28:3* painting by Henry Howard. National Portrait Gallery. London.

28:4–28:7 reference 28.3 and 28.6. *28:8* Gwathmey J. Anesthesia. New York 1914. *28:9* and *28:11* reference 28.8 and Rottenstein J. Traité d'anésthèsie chirurgical. Paris 1880. *28:10* reference 28.8.

29. *29:1* and *29:2* the landmark publication #29 and reference 29.7. *29:3* reference 29.4. *29:4* reference 3.1. *29:5* Ioannes Sambucus. Veterum aliquot ac recentium Medicorum Philosophorumque Icones 1574. *29:6* and *29:7* http://www.muslimphilosophy.com/sina/default.htm with permission and the text translation from Gruner C. A treatise on The Canon of Medicine of Avicenna. London 1930. *29:8* Médecins et chirurgiens célèbres,... Paris 1842. *29:9* reference 29.9.

30. *30:1* the landmark publication #30. *30:2* Wolf A. A history of science technology, and philosophy in the eighteenth century. London 1952. *30:3* the landmark publication #30 and a translation by H.A.Ruger and H.M. Walker Teachers College Columbia University. New York. *30:4* reference 30.4. *30:5* Tucker R. Carl Friedrich Gauss. Nature 1877; 15:533. *30:6* and *30:7* reference 30.7. *30:8* Galerie hervorragender Ärzte und Naturforscher. Beilage zur Münchener medizinischen Wochenschrift. *30:9* and *30:10* reference 30.8.

31. *31:1* the landmark publication #31. *31:2* the Science & Society Picture Library of the Science Museum London. *31:3* painting by T. Chartran from the National Library of Medicine Bethesda.MD. *31:4* the National Library of Medicine Bethesda. MD. *31:5* Forbes J. On percussion of the chest. Being a translation of Auenbrugger's original treatise. (London 1824) Baltimore 1936. *31:6* reference 31.2. *31:7* Sigerist H. Grosse Ärzte. München 1932. *31:8* Galerie hervorragender Ärzte und Naturforscher. Beilage zur Münchener medizinischen Wochenschrift. *31:9* National Library of Medicine Bethesda. MD. *31:11* Alex Peck Medical Antiques. Charleston. SC. *31:12* reference 31.6.

32. *32:1* and *32:2* the landmark publication #32. *32:3* Fourier J. Recherches expérimentales sur la Faculté conductrice des corps mince... Ann.Chem.Phys. 1828;37:291. *32:4* lithography by Julien Boilly. Archives de l'Académie des sciences. *32:5* reference 32.10. *32:6–32:8* Hodgkin D et.al. The structure of vitamin B12. Proc.Roy.Soc. A 1957;242:228.

33. *33:1* and *33:2* the landmark publication #33. *33:3* the Bibliothèque de l'Académie national de Médecine Paris. Courtesy of Marie Davaine. *33:4–33:6* reference 33.4. *33:7* and *33:8* Semmelweis' Gesammelte Werke Ed. Dr T von Györy. Jena 1905.

34. *34:1* and *34:2* landmark publication #34. *34:3* Médecins et chirurgiens célèbre,... Paris 1842. *34:4* and *34:6* the landmark publication #2. *34:5* the Dittrick Medical History Center, Case Western Reserve University. Cleveland. OH. *34:7* Deutsches Museum. Bonn. *34:8* courtesy of HMT High Medical Technologies AG. Lengwil Switzerland.

35. *35:1* and *35:2* the landmark publication

#35. *35:3* Brillouin M. Jean Léonard Poiseuille. J.Rheology 1930;1:345. *35:4* reference 35.5. *35:5* and *35:6* reference 35.7.

36. *36:1* and *36:2* the landmark publication #36. *36:3* Album de la science. Savants illustres. Grandes découvertes. Paris 1896. *36:4* reference 36.7. *36:5* reference 36.6. *36:6* the Bibliothèque de l'Académie national de Médecine Paris. Courtesy of Marie Davaine. *36:7* Pawling J. Dr. Samuel Guthrie Discoverer of Chloroform. Watertown 1947. *36:8* Portraits berühmter Naturforscher. Wien. Leipzig n.d. Bibliotheca Walleriana No. 16169. *36:9* lithography by A.Lemoine after a photography by André Disdéri. *36:10* reference 36.8. *36:11* and *36:12* reference 36.9.

37. *37:1* and *37:2* the landmark publication #37. *37:3* Söderbaum H. Jac.Berzelius Band 2. Uppsala 1929. *37:4* Gaule J. Die Kohlensäurespannung im Blut, im Serum und in der Lymphe. Arch.Physiol. 1878;5–6:469. *37:5* Portraits berühmter Naturforscher. Wien. Leipzig n.d. Bibliotheca Walleriana No. 16169. *37:6* reference 14.8. *37:7* reference 37.10. *37:8* reference 56.5. *37:9* Krogh A. On the Oxygen-Metabolism of the Blood. Skand.Arch.Physiol. 1910;23:193. *37:10* reference 37.7. *37:11* and *37:12* reference 14.8.

38. *38:1* and *38:3* the landmark publication #38. *38:2* Album de la science. Savants illustres. Grandes découvertes. Paris 1896. *38:4* Portraits berühmter Naturforscher. Wien. Leipzig n.d. Bibliotheca Walleriana No 16169. *38:5* the landmark publication #38. *38:6* reference 38.3. *38:7* the landmark publication #38. *38:8* reference 38.4. *38:9* reference 38.6. *38:10* reference 38.7. *38:11* reference 38.8. *38:12* Galerie hervorragender Ärzte und Naturforscher. Beilage zur Münchener medizinischen Wochenschrift. *38:13–38:15* reference 38.9.

39. *39:1* the landmark publication #39. *39:2* the Liebig-Museum Giessen. Courtesy of Dr Magnus Mueller. *39:3* Engraving by Johann Bankel after a painting by Wilhelm Trautschold 1875. Courtesy of Antiquariat Gerhard Gruber Heilbronn. Germany. *39:4* the Liebig-Museum. Giessen. Courtesy of Dr Magnus Mueller.

40. *40:1* Album de la science. Savants illustres. Grandes découvertes. Paris 1896. *40:2* Cohen E. Jacobus Henricus van't Hoff Sein Leben und Wirken. p.95 Leipzig 1912. *40:3* the landmark publication #40. *40:4* the University of St.Andrews Scotland. *40:5* and *40:6* reference 40.5. *40:7* courtesy of Perimed AB Järfälla Sweden. *40:8* courtesy of Perimed KB Sweden. *40:9* and *40:10* courtesy of Lisca AB Linköping Sweden. *40:11* and *40:12* Medical Diagnostic Ultrasound: A retrospective on its 40th Anniversary Eds. B.B.Goldberg, B.A.Kimmelman. Eastman Kodak Co.1988. Courtesy of Dr Eric Blackwell. *40:13* and *40:14* reference 40.8. *40:15–40:17* reference 40.9.

41. *41:1* and *41:2* the landmark publication #41. *41:3* reference 41.1. *41:4–41:6* the landmark publication #41. *41:7* reference 41.5. *41:8* and *41:9* reference 41.6. *41:10–41:13* reference 41.6 and 41.7.

42. *42:1* and *42:2* the landmark publication #42. *42:3* Galerie hervorragender Ärzte und Naturforscher. Beilage zur Münchener medizinischen Wochenschrift. *42:4* reference 42.1. *42:5* Galerie hervorragender Ärzte und Naturforscher. Beilage zur Münchener medizinischen Wochenschrift. *42:6* http://chem.ch.huji.ac.il/~eugeniik/history/matteucci.html *42:7–42:9* the landmark publication #42.

43. *43:1* the Dibner Library of the History of Science and Technology. *43:2* the landmark publication #43. *43:3* see 45:2. *43:4* and *43:5* reference 43.6.

44. *44:1* Voit M. Bildnisse Göttinger Professoren aus zwei Jahrhunderten (1737–1937) Göttingen 1937. *44:2* the landmark publication #44. *44:3* Spamer O. Illustriertes Konversationslexikon für das Volk. Leipzig 1870–1882. *44:4* Pettigrew T. Medical portrait gallery.Vol.1–4 London, 1838–40. *44:5–44:7* reference 44.8.

45. *45:1* the landmark publication #45. *45:2* Galerie hervorragender Ärzte und Naturforscher. Beilage zur Münchener medizinischen Wochenschrift. *45:3–45:5* reference 5.7. 45:6 Galerie hervorragender Ärzte und Naturforscher. Beilage zur Münchener medizinischen Wochenschrift. *45:7* reference 45.7. *45:8–45:10* reference 5.13. *45:11* the Medical Photographic Library of the Wellcome Trust. London. *45:12* and *45:13* Carl Zeiss Archiv Jena. Courtesy of Dr Wolfgang Wimmer.

46. *46:1* the landmark publication #46. *46:2* reference 46.7. *46:3* reference 46.4. Vol. IV. *46:4* and *46:8* the Science & Society Picture Library of the Science Museum London. *46:5–46:7* reference 63.4. *46:9* and *46:10* reference 46.8.

47. *47:1* Snow J. On the inhalation of the vapour of ether. London Medical Gazette 1847. *47:2* and *47:3* the landmark publication #47. *47:4* the Bibliothèque de l'Académie national de Médecine Paris. Courtesy of Marie Davaine. *47:5* the landmark publication #47. *47:6* reference 47.8. *47:7* and *47:9* Bryn Thomas K. The Development of Anaesthetic Apparatus. London 1975. *47:8* and *47:10* reference 47.9. *47:11* Siemens-Elema AB Solna Sweden. *47:13* reference A.7.9. *47:12* courtesy of Dr Jeffrey Cooper *47:14* reference 47.11. *47:15–47:17* Datex-Ohmeda Inc (now General Electric Healthcare) Bromma Sweden. Courtesy of Brian Högman.

48. *48:1* reference 48.8. *48:2* reference 48.6. *48:3* Moure E.Revue hebdomadaire de laryngologie, d'otologie et de rhinologie. Bordeaux 1908. *48:4* reference 48.4. *48:5* Turck L. Klinik der Krankheiten des Kehlkopfes und der Luftröhre.Wien 1866. *48:6* and *48:7* Moure E.Revue hebdomadaire de laryngologie, d'otologie et de rhinologie. Bordeaux 1908. *48:8* and *48:9* reference 48.8.

49. *49:1* and *49:2* the landmark publication #49. *49:3* Portraits berühmter Naturforscher. Wien Leipzig n.d. Bibliotecha Walleriana No 16169. *49:4* Pinder U. Epiphanie Medicorum Nurenberg 1506. Courtesy of Jonathan A Hill. Bookseller New York, NY. *49:5* courtesy of the Chemical Heritage Foundation Image Archives. Philadelphia, PA. *49:6* Portraits berühmter Naturforscher. Wien Leipzig n.d. Bibliotecha Walleriana No 16169. *49:7* reference 51.8. *49:8* reference 49.3. *49:10* reference 49.8. *49:11* reference 49.7. *49:12* Fysikum, Uppsala University. Uppsala. Photo courtesy Teddy Thörnlund. *49:13* courtesy of the Chemical Heritage Foundation Image Archives. Philadelphia, PA.

50. *50:1* and *50:2* the landmark publication #50. *50:3* Portraits berühmter Naturforscher. Wien Leipzig n.d. Bibliotecha Walleriana No. 16169. *50:4–50:6* reference 50.2 *50:7* and *50:8* reference 50.3.

51. *51:1* reference 51.8. *51:2* Zeitschrift für Physikalische Chemie 1895. *51:3* Galerie hervorragender Ärzte und Naturforscher. Beilage zur Münchener medizinischen Wochenschrift. *51:4* reference 51.10. *51:5* and *51:8* Haemoglobin BioNet. *51:6, 51:7* and *51:10* courtesy of HemoCue AB. Ängelholm Sweden. *51:9* reference 76.9.

52. *52:1* the landmark publication #52. *52:2* Christie's South Kensington MSI-8246 1998. *52:3* reference 52.1. *52:4* Galerie hervorragender Ärzte und Naturforscher. Beilage zur Münchener medizinischen Wochenschrift. *52:5* and *52:6* reference 52.1. *52:7* the landmark publication #52. *52:8* and *52:9* the landmark publication #52. *52:10* reference 52.1. *52:11* and *52:12* Marey E. La circulation du sang. Paris 1881.

53. *53:1* reference 53.1. *53:2* the landmark publication #53. *53:3* reference 53.1 Vol. 1. *53:4* reference 53.6. *53:5–53:7* Iconographia Mendeliana Brno 1965. *53:8* reference 53.6.

54. *54:1* after a painting by Jean Rixens, from the Medical Photographic Library of the Wellcome Trust. London. *54:2* reference 54.6. *54:3* reference 54.6 Vol.2. *54:4* reference 54.6. *54:5–54:8* the Medical Photographic Library of the Wellcome Trust. London.

55. *55:1* the landmark publication #55. *55:2* reference 55.2. *55:3–55:5* St.Jude Medical AB. Järfälla Sweden. Courtesy of Lars Forsmark. *55:6* courtesy of Smiths Medical UK. *55:9* reference 55.9. 55:10 Vakkuri A.et.al. Time-frequency balanced spectral entropy as a measure of anaesthetic drug effect in the central nervous system during sevoflurane, propofol, and thiopental anaesthesia. Acta.Anaesth.Scand. 2004;48:145. Courtesy of Pia Talja GE Healthcare Finland.

56. *56:1* the landmark publication #56. *56:2* reference 46.4 Vol. I. *56:3* and *56:4* reference 56.5. *56:5–56:7* reference 56.7.

57. *57:1* the landmark publication #57. *57:2* the Science & Society Picture Library of the Science Museum London. *57:3* Galerie hervorragender Ärzte und Naturforscher. Beilage zur Münchener medizinischen Wochenschrift. *57:4* reference 57.3. *57:5* reference 57.2. *57:6* and *57:8* Kuhn F. Die Perorale Intubation. Berlin 1911. *57:7* the Collection of the Instrument Maker Carl Reiner Vienna. *57:9* reference 57.9. *57:10* reference 57.11. *57:11* reference 57.10. *57:12* reference 57.11.

58. *58:1* and *58:2* the landmark publication #58. *58:3* Galerie hervorragender Ärzte und Naturforscher. Beilage zur Münchener medizinischen Wochenschrift. *58:4* reference 58.3. *58:5* Galerie hervorragender Ärzte und Naturforscher. Beilage zur Münchener medizinischen Wochenschrift. *58:6* reference 58.2. *58:7* and *58:8* reference 58.4.

59. *59:1* and *59:2* the landmark publication #59. *59:3* Berillon P. L'Oeuvre Scientific de Paul Bert. Paris 1887. *59:4* the landmark publication #59. *59:5* Duncum B. The Development of Inhalation Anaesthesia London 1947. *59:6* reference 28.8 and Rottenstein J. Traité d'anésthisie chirurgical. Paris 1880. *59:7–59:11* the landmark publication #59.

60. *60:1–60:8* reference 60.1. *60:9* and *60:11* the Hagströmer Medico-Historical Library Stockholm. *60:10* Wiener Medizinische Wochenschrift 42 Spalte 641–642 1892 and the Institut für Geschichte der Medizin der Universität Wien Vienna. Courtesy of Brigitte Maurer. *60:12* and *60:13* the Institut für Geschichte der Medizin der Universität Wien. Courtesy of Brigitte Maurer. *60:14* reference 60.10. *60:15* Sjövall A.Laparascopy. Kungl.Fysiografiska Sällskapets i Lund Förhandlingar 1962;32:130. *60:16–60:18* Killian H.G Killian Sein Leben Sein Werk. Remscheid-Lennep 1958.

61. *61:1* Carl Zeiss Archiv Jena. Courtesy of Dr. Wolfgang Wimmer. *61:2* the landmark publication #61. *61:3* Galerie hervorragender Ärzte und Naturforscher. Beilage zur Münchener medizinischen Wochenschrift. *61:4* reference 61.2. *61:5* Catalog 60 F.& M. Lautenschläger Berlin. *61:6* reference 61.9. *61:7* Dr. Robert Muencke Abteilung für Bacteriologie, Microscopie, Hygiene Berlin 1882. *61:8* Portraits berühmter Naturforscher. Wien. Leipzig n.d. Bibliotheca Walleriana No. 16169. *61:9* D.G.Schley R.K.Hoffman and C.R. Phillips. Simple Improvised chamber for Gas Sterilization with Ethylene Oxide. Appl.Microbiol. 1960;8:15.

62. *62:1* and *62:2* the landmark publication #62. *62:3* Cohen E. Jacobus Henricus van't Hoff Sein Leben und Wirken. Leipzig 1912. *62:4* Kohlrausch F. Einfache Methode und Instrumente zur Wiederstandsmessung inbesondere in Electrolyten. Ann.Phys. Chem.1880; 11:653. *62:5* the exhibition 200 years of Experimental Physics at the University of Innsbruck. 1997. *62:6* reference 62.8. *62:7* Cohen E.Jacobus Henricus van't Hoff Sein Leben und Wirken. Leipzig 1912.

63. *63:1* Cohen E.Jacobus Henricus van't Hoff Sein Leben und Wirken. Leipzig

1912. *63:2* reference 62.8. *63:3* the landmark publication #63. *63:4* Cohen E.Jacobus Henricus van't Hoff Sein Leben und Wirken. Leipzig 1912. *63:5* the landmark publication #63. *63:6* reference 62.8. *63:7* Cohen E.Jacobus Henricus van't Hoff Sein Leben und Wirken. Leipzig 1912. *63:8* reference 62.8. *63:9* detail from portrait in Svante Arrhenius till 100-årsminnet av hans födelse. K.Sv. Vetenskapsakademins Årsbok 1959.

64. *64:1* reference 64.5. *64:2* Carl Zeiss Archiv Jena. Courtesy of Dr. Wolfgang Wimmer. *64:3* Carl Zeiss Jena, Optische Werkstätte; 32. Ausgabe; 1902. *64:4* reference 64.5. *64:5* and *64:14* the Hagströmer Medico-Historical Library Stockholm. *64:6* Carl Zeiss Jena, Optische Werkstätte; 32. Ausgabe; 1902. *64:7* Carl Zeiss Jena, Optische Werkstätte; 27. Ausgabe; 1885. *64:8* Carl Zeiss Jena, Optische Werkstätte; 27. Ausgabe; 1885. *64:9* reference 64.2. *64:10* Carl Zeiss Archiv Jena. Courtesy of Dr. Wolfgang Wimmer. *6:11* reference 64.2. *64:12* von Rohr M.Ernst Abbes Apochromate Leipzig 1936. *64:13* Carl Zeiss Archiv Jena. Courtesy of Dr. Wolfgang Wimmer. *64:15* reference 64.2. *64:16* Carl Zeiss Optische Werkstätte Jena, Optische Messinstrumente 1893.

65. *65:1* and *65:2* the Medical Photographic Library of the Wellcome Trust. London. *65:3* and *65:4* the landmark publication #65. *65:5* the Medical Photographic Library of the Wellcome Trust. London. *65:6* reference 65.10. *65:7* and *65:8* Galerie hervorragender Ärzte und Naturforscher. Beilage zur Münchener medizinischen Wochenschrift. *65:9* the Medical Photographic Library of the Wellcome Trust. London. *65:10* reference 65.10.

66. *66:1–66:3* the landmark publication #66. *66:4* reference 66.1. *66:5* reference 66.3. *66:6* reference 66.2. *66:7* and *66:8* reference 66.6. *66:9* Krebs J.Ultraschalltherapie. Osnabruck 1950. *66:10* Kratochwil A. Geschichte der Ultraschalldiagnostik. Ultraschall 1981; 2:108. *66:11* and *66:12* reference 66.5. *66:13* and *66:14* courtesy of Engström Medical AB Bromma Sweden. (Now GE Healthcare). *66:15* and *66:16* Rohdahl M. On the frequency and Q factor response of the quartz crystal microbalance to liquid overlays. Thesis. Dept.Appl. Phys. Chalmers Univ Techn Göteborg 1995.

67. *67:1, 67:2* and *67:3* Über eine neue Art von Strahlen Neudruck Würzburg 1941. *67:4* Röntgen's second publication ("Mittheilungen") on X-rays following the landmark publication #67, The Hagströmer Medico-Historical Library, Stockholm. *67:5* Galerie hervorragender Ärzte und Naturforscher. Beilage zur Münchener medizinischen Wochenschrift. *67:6* Miller J.Yankee Scientist William David Coolidge. Schenectady 1963. *67:7* Christie's catalogue MSI-9426 London 2002. *67:8* courtesy of Siemens Medical Solutions Archives, Erlangen Germany. *67:9–67:12* Grossmann G. Einführung in die Röntgentechnik. Siemens & Haske A.-G. Berlin 1912. *67:13* Fortschritte auf dem Gebiete der Röntgenstrahlen 1933;47:VI. *67:14* courtesy of Siemens Medical Solutions Archives, Erlangen Germany. *67:15* and *67:16* AB Elema-Järnhs, Solna. Sweden. Courtesy of Bengt Stånge.

68. *68:1* http://www.unipv.it/webped/Scienze%20Pediatriche/cenni-storici.htm. *68:2* reference 68.7. *68:3* the Science & Society Picture Library of the Science Museum London. *68:4* Ruskin A.Classics in arterial hypertension Springfield 1956. *68:5* reference 68.5. *68:6* Galerie hervorragender Ärzte und Naturforscher. Beilage zur Münchener medizinischen Wochenschrift. *68:7* reference 68.1. *68:8* the Science & Society Picture Library of the Science Museum London. *68:9* reproduces reference 68.6. *68:10* and *68:11* von Recklinghausen H. Ueber Blutdrucksmessung beim Menschen. Arch.exp.Path.Pharm. 1901;46:69. *68:12* Galerie hervorragender Ärzte und Naturforscher. Beilage zur Münchener medizinischen Wochenschrift. *68:13–68:15* reference 68.7.

69. *69:1–69:3* the landmark publication #69. *69:4* after an engraving by E. Walker. *69:5* and *69:6* the landmark publication #79. *69:8* reference 69.7. *69:9* courtesy of Dr Anna-Liisa Brownell. *69:10–69:12* the Svedberg Laboratory Uppsala. Courtesy of Teddy Thörnlund. *69:13–69:15* the Hyogo Ion Beam Medical Center, Harima Science Garden City, Hyogo.Courtesy of Dr Takashi Akagi.

70. *70:1, 70:2* and *70:4* reference 66.1. *70:3* reference 70.4. *70:5* Galerie hervorragender Ärzte und Naturforscher. Beilage zur Münchener medizinischen Wochenschrift. *70:6* detail photolithography after N.S.Kay Manchester. A.Eckstein Berlin 1910. *70:7* and *70:8* reference 70.4. *70:9* reference 70.9. *70:10* Elekta Instrument AB, Stockholm Sweden. Courtesy of Nina Westerlind.

71. *71:1* the landmark publication #71. *71:2–71:6* de Waart A. Het levenswerk van Willem Einthoven 1860–1827. Haarlem 1957. *71:7* Directions in Cardiovascular Medicine. Svenska Hoechst AB Stockholm 1978. *71:8* the Science & Society Picture Library of the Science Museum London. *71:9* Dagens Nyheter 1930 from Grewin K, Thulesius O. Elektrokardiografins historia i Sverige. Läkartidningen 1972;69:613. *71:10–71:13* Elema-Schönander Solna. Sweden. Courtesy of Bengt Stånge. *71:14* Siemens-Elema AB Solna. Sweden. Courtesy of professor Håkan Elmqvist.

72. *72:1* Galerie hervorragender Ärzte und Naturforscher. Beilage zur Münchener medizinischen Wochenschrift. *72:2* the landmark publication #72. *72:3* reference 74.5. *72:4* and *72:5* the landmark publication #72. *72:6–72:7* Merck KGaA Darmstadt Germany. Courtesy of Katja Glock.

73. *73:1* and *73:3* reference 73.1. *73:2* and *73:4* reference 73.2. *73:5* reference 73.1. *73:6* the Edgar Fahs Smiths Collection, University of Pennsylvania Library. Philadelphia PA. *73:7* Eicher O. Das Chemische Wappen, Einbeck 1955. *73:8, 73:9* and *73:10* reference 73.5 and the British Library London. *73:11* Universitätsbibliothek Basel. Courtesy of Dominik Hunger. *73:12* and *73:14* reference 73.7. *73:13* Westphal O.Richard Kuhn zum Gedächtnis. Angew Chem 1968;80:501. *73:15* and *73:16* reference 73.10.

74. *74:1* and *74:2* reference 74.3. *74:3* reference 74.5. *74:4* Archives for the History of the Max Planck Society, Berlin-Dahlem. *74:5–74:7* reference 74.5.

75. *75:1* and *75:2* reference 75.4. *75:3* the landmark publication #75. *75:4* Galerie hervorragender Ärzte und Naturforscher. Beilage zur Münchener medizinischen Wochenschrift. *75:5–75:8* the landmark publication #75.

76. *76:1* and *76:2* the landmark publication #76. *76:3* Archives for the History of the Max Planck Society, Berlin-Dahlem. *76:4* and *76:6* reference 76.6. *76:5* the Edgar Fahs Smiths Collection, University of Pennsylvania Library. Philadelphia PA. *76:7* and *76:8* reference 76.7. *76:9* the Cold Spring Harbor Laboratory Archives. Courtesy of Teresa Kruger. *76:10* the The Ava Helen and Linus Pauling Papers. Special Collections of Oregon State University Libraries. Corvallis. Courtesy of Chris Petersen.

77. *77:1* and *77:2* the landmark publication #77. *77:3* reference 77.1. *77:4* Universitätsbibliothek Basel. Courtesy of Dominik Hunger. *77:5* the landmark publication #77. *77:6–77:8* 375 Jahre Medizin in Giessen. Benedum J. and Giese C. Katalog zur Ausstellung anlässlich der 375-Jahrfeier. Giessen 1983.

78. *78:1* the landmark publication #78. *78:2* Das Wissenschaftliche Werk von Hermann Staudinger Ed. M Staudinger Band I Basel 1969. *78:3* and *78:4* Staudinger H. Über Isopren und Kautschuk. Das Wissenschaftliche Werk von Hermann Staudinger Ed. M Staudinger Band I p22. Basel 1969. *78:5–78:7* Staudinger H et.al. Der Polymere Formaldehyd, ein Modell der Zellulose. Das Wissenschaftliche Werk von Hermann Staudinger Ed. M Staudinger Band II/1 p3. Basel 1972. *78:8* Museum Gustavianum Uppsala University Uppsala. *78:9* reference 78.4. *78:10* reference 78.9. *78:11* Corning Inc. Archives. Corning. Courtesy of Kristine Gable. *78:12* reference 78.7.

79. *79:1* and *79:2* the landmark publication #79. *79:3* the Edgar Fahs Smiths Collection, University of Pennsylvania Library. Philadelphia PA. *79:4* and *79:5* the landmark publication #79. *79:6* the Edgar Fahs Smiths Collection, University of Pennsylvania Library. Philadelphia PA. *79:7* the landmark publication #79. *79:8* reference 79.9. *79:9* and *79:10* courtesy of Ann-Charlotte Ryhage.

80. *80:1* the landmark publication #80. *80:2* courtesy of the Chemical Heritage Foundation Collections, Philadelphia,

PA. Reproduced with the permission of Helen Carothers. *80:3* and *80:5* reference 78.7. Courtesy of Imperial Chemical Industries Plc. London England. *80:4* and *80:6* reference 80.5. *80:7* Courtesy of National Museum of American History, Smithsonian Institution Washington D.C. *80:8* the Williams Haynes Portrait Collection, Chemists' Club Archives, Courtesy of the Chemical Heritage Foundation Image Archives. Philadelphia, PA. *80:9* the Science & Society Picture Library of the Science Museum London. *80:10* and *80:11* Courtesy of the Chemical Heritage Foundation Image Archives. Philadelphia, PA. *80:12* the Science & Society Picture Library of the Science Museum London. *80:13* Du Pont Co. "nylon: The First 25 Years"(1963) *80:14* courtesy of Hagley Museum and Library. Wilmington DE. *80:15* Du Pont Magazine November 1939. Courtesy of Hagley Museum and Library. Wilmington. DE.

81. *81:1–81:3* the landmark publication #81. *81:4* the Edgar Fahs Smiths Collection, University of Pennsylvania Library. Philadelphia, PA. *81:5* and *81:6* reference 81.6. *81:7* photo by Gregory Tobia. *81:8* Courtesy of the Chemical Heritage Foundation Image Archives. Philadelphia, PA. *81:9* Galerie hervorragender Ärzte und Naturforscher. Beilage zur Münchener medizinischen Wochenschrift. *81:10–81:12* reference 14.8. *81:12* and *81:12* Courtesy of Maj-Britt Blikdal Radiometer A/S Copenhagen. Denmark. *81:13* URL: http://poohbah.cem.msu.edu/ Portraits/ PortraitsHH_Detail.asp *81:14* reference 81.9. *81:15* reference 81.10.

82. *82:1–82:3* the landmark publication #82. *82:4* Proc IRE Sept. 1939 p620. *82:5* From Semaphore to Satellite ITU 1865–965 Geneva 1965. *82:6* reference 82.1. *82:7* http://philotfarnsworth.com/ page2.html. *82:8* reference 85.6. *82:9* and *82:10* the landmark publication #82. *82:11–82:14* reference 82.9. *82:15–82:17* reference 82.10.

83. *83:1–83:3* the landmark publication #83. *83:4* a private collection. *83:6* reference 64.9. *83:5, 83:7–83:10* reference 83.5. *83:11–83:13* reference 83.7. *83:14* and *83:16* reference 83.5. *83:15* Stewart A, Snelling M. A new scanning electron microscope. Proc 3rd Eur Reg Conf Electron Microscopy. Prague. 1964;A:55. *83:17* http://www2.eng.cam.ac.uk/~bcb/cw01.htm.

84. *84:1* the landmark publication #84. *84:2* courtesy of Mr Godfrey Argent London and the Royal Society London. *84:3* and *84:4* reference 84.2. *84:5* the Science & Society Picture Library of the Science Museum London. *84:6* the Chemical Heritage Foundation Image Archives Philadelphia. F&M 700 Gas chromatograph—photo by Gregory Tobias.

85. *85:1* photograph from the Eckert papers in a private collection. *85:2* reference 85.6. *85:3* and *85:4* the University of Pennsylvania Library Philadelphia.PA. *85:5* and *85:7* reference 85.2. *85:6* and *85:8* reference 85.3. *85:9* and *85:11* reference 85.6. *85:10* The origins of digital computers. Ed. B Randell 2nd ed. Springer–Verlag Berlin 1975. *85:12* and *85:14* reference 85.6 (Iowa State University Library/ Special Collections Department). *85:13* reference 85.6. *85:15* and *85:16* reference 85.6. *85:17* reference 85.8. *85:18* reference 85.9. *85:19, 85:21, 85:22* http://www.intel4004.com/ *85:20* Cochlear Limited Lane Cove. Australia. Courtesy of Bern Ferraz. *85:23* St. Jude Medical AB Järfälla. Sweden. Courtesy of Lars Forsmark.

86. *86:1–86:3* the landmark publication #86. *86:4* Institute for biomedical engineering, some of its projects some of its people. University of Utah 1973. *86:5* and *86:7* Gambro – en företagshistorik. Lund 1998. Courtesy of Gittan Holmström Gambro, Lund. Sweden. *86:6, 86:8–86:10* Romaine-Davis A. John Gibbon and His Heart-Lung Machine University of Pennsylvania Press Philadelphia 1991. *86:11* the Science & Society Picture Library of the Science Museum London. *86:12* Report of the Workshop on Diffusion of ECMO Technology. Ed. L Wright US Department of Health and Human Services NIH Publication No 93-3399 1993. *86:13* courtesy of professor Robert H Bartlett. *86:14* Institute for biomedical engineering, some of its projects some of its people. University of Utah 1973. *86:15* and *86:12* courtesy of ABIOMED Inc. Danvers Mass. TX *86:16* courtesy of Texas Heart Institute. Houston (©2000 Texas Heart Institute). *86:17* reference 86.11.

87. *87:1* All about ENGSTRÖM Engström Medical AB. Bromma Sweden 1982. *87:2* the landmark publication #87. *87:3* and *87:4* Datex-Ohmeda Inc (now General Electric Healthcare) Bromma. Sweden. Courtesy of Brian Högman. *87:5* All about ENGSTRÖM Engström Medical AB Bromma. Sweden 1982. *87:6* reference 87.6. *87:7* reference 87.7. *87:8* reference 87.2. *87:9* reference 87.11. *87:10* and *87:12* The Servo Ventilator Concept Siemens-Elema AB Bromma Sweden. *87:11* courtesy of Sven-Gunnar Olsson. *87:13* Gambro-Engström AB Bromma Sweden.

88. *88:1* the landmark publication #88. *88:2* and *88:3* courtesy of the James D.Watson Collection, Cold Spring Harbor Laboratory Archives, Cold Spring Harbor. Photo credit:David Micklos. *88:4* courtesy of the James D.Watson Collection, Cold Spring Harbor Laboratory Archives, Cold Spring Harbor. *88:5* reference 88.1. *88:6* courtesy of Bjørn Pedersen Kjemisk institutt, University of Oslo. *88:7* courtesy of L.Barry Hetherington/Broad Institute and Michelle Nhuch Cambridge, MA. *88:8* courtesy of the Archives, California Institute of Technology. Passadena.CA. *88:9* reference 88.10.

89. *89:1* mambo.ucsc.edu/psl/smus/ smus.html *89:2* the landmark publication #89. *89:3* Fant G. Talforskning-teknik och vetenskap. Ericsson Rev 1985;3:100. *89:4–89:6* reference 89.4. *89:7* reference 89.5. *89:8* mambo.ucsc.edu/psl/smus/ smus.html *89:9* Haskins Laboratories New Haven, CT. Courtesy of Anders Löfqvist. *89:10–89:12* Dudley H. PEDRO the VODER A Machine That Talks. Bell Lab Rec 1939;17(VI):170 *89:13–89:15* reference 89.1. *89:16* Kurzweil Technologies, Inc. Wellesley Hills, MA Courtesy of Mr Ray Kurzweil.

90. *90:1–90:3* the landmark publication #90. *90:4* courtesy of professor Lars Edler. *90:5* courtesy of professor em. Birgit Hertz. *90:6* and *90:7* reference 90.4. *90:8* and *90:9* Medical Diagnostic Ultrasound: A retrospective on its 40th Anniversary Eds. B.B.Goldberg, B.A.Kimmelman. Eastman Kodak Co.1988. Courtesy of Dr Eric Blackwell. *90:10* reference 90.11.

91. *91:1* the landmark publication #91. *91:2* St. Jude Medical AB Järfälla, Sweden. Courtesy of Susanne Jarl. *91:3* courtesy of professor Håkan Elmqvist. *91:4* reference 91.5. Courtesy of Medtronic Inc. Minneapolis. *91:5* and *91:6* reference 91.4. *91:7–91:12* reference 91.5. Courtesy of Medtronic Inc. Minneapolis. MN. *91:13* St. Jude Medical AB Järfälla, Sweden. Courtesy of Susanne Jarl.

92. *92:1* the landmark publication #92. *92:2* Schawlow A. Optical Masers. In Lasers and Light Readings from Scientific American. W H Freedman and Co, San Francisco 1969. *92:3* and *92:4* Maiman T. The Laser Odyssey. Laser Press, Blaine 2000. *92:5* reference 92.3. *92:6* and *92:7* Schawlow A. Optical Masers. In Lasers and Light Readings from Scientific American. W H Freedman and Co, San Francisco 1969. *92:8* courtesy of professor William R Bennett Jr. *92:9* and *92:11* courtesy of Nidek Co, Ltd Aichi Japan. *92:10* and *92:12* Alcon Laboratories Inc, Fort Worth, TX. Courtesy of Jonas Lübcke. *92:13* af Klintberg C. On the use of light for the characterisation and treatment of malignant tumours. Dissertation, Department of Physics Lund Institute of Technology, Lund 1999. *92:14* Wang I. et al. Superficial blood flow following photodynamic therapy of malignant and non-melanoma skin tumours measured by laser Doppler perfusion imaging. Brit J Derm 1997;136:184.

93. *93:1* and *93:2* the landmark publication #93. *93:3* courtesy of professor Per-Ingvar Brånemark. *93:4–93:6* reference 93.1. *93:7* and *93:8* reference 93.6. *93:9* and *93:10* Bragge U, Braide M. Blood—a mobile tissue. In Osseointegration From Molecule to Man. The Institute for Applied Biotechnology, Göteborg 1999. *93:11–93:16* Brånemark P-I. Osseointegration—a method of anchoring prostheses. The Söderberg Prize in Medicine 1992.

94. *94:1* and *94:3* the landmark publication #94. *94:2* and *93:4* courtesy of Dr Raymond Damadian. *94:5* reference 94.1. *94:6* reference 94.3. *94:7* the cover of Science (AAAS) 24 December 1976. Volume 194 No 4272. *94:8* and *94:9* courtesy of Dr Raymond Damadian.

94:10 reference 94.8. *94:11* reference 94.1.

95. *95:1* the landmark publication #95. *95:2* from a private collection. *95:3* reference 95.2. *95:4* and *95:5* du Boulay G. Help. Brit J Radiol 1973;46:783. *95:6* and *95:7* the landmark publication #95. *95:8–95:11* reference 95.6 (the second, clinical application, part following the landmark publication #95).

96. *96:1* and *96:2* the landmark publication #96. *96:3* courtesy of professor Paul Lauterbur. *96:4* and *96:5* the landmark publication #96. *96:6* General Electric Healthcare courtesy Ulf Degrell. *96:7–96:9* reference 96.9. *96:10* and *96:11* Ebbers T. Cardiovascular Fluid Dynamics. Method for flow and Pressure Field Analysis from Magnetic Resonance Imaging. Dissertation No 690 Departments of Biomedical Engineering & Medicine and Care, Linköping 2001. *96:12–96:15* courtesy of assistant professor Mitchell Albert. *96:16* courtesy of assistant professor Mitchell Albert and Dr Mary Mazzanti The Hyperpolarized Noble Gas MRI Laboratory. Harvard Medical School, Boston Mass.

97. *97:1* the landmark publication #97. *97:2* Illustration by Jörgen Gedeon after a sketch of professor Göran Hedenstierna. *97:3* courtesy of professor Peter Wagner. *97:4* courtesy of professor John West. *97:5* and *97:6* the landmark publication #97. *97:7* reference 97.6. *97:8* Klingstedt C. Lung function during anaesthesia: Effects of the lateral position. J Opuscula Medica Society Suppl. LXXV Stockholm 1990.

98. *98:1–98:4* ©1974 IEEE Reprinted with permission, the landmark publication #98. *98:5* courtesy of Dr Vinton Cerf. *98:6* courtesy of Dr Robert Kahn. *98:7* reference 98.3. *98:8* and *98:9* reference 38.3. *98:10* From Semaphore to Satellite ITU 1865–1965. Geneva 1965. *98:11* reference 98.3. *98:11, 98:13* and *98:14* From Semaphore to Satellite ITU 1865–1965. Geneva 1965. *98:15* reference 85.6. *98:16* courtesy of professor Leonard Kleinrock. *98:17–98:19* courtesy of professor Jacques Marescaux, IRCAD/EITS Institute and France Télécom.

99. *99:1–99:4* the landmark publication #99. *99:5* courtesy of professor Michael Phelps. *99:6* and *99:7* courtesy of professor Anna-Liisa Brownell. *99:8* courtesy of professor Michael Phelps. *99:9–99:11* reference 99.8 courtesy of professor Michael Phelps. *99:12* reference 99.7 courtesy of CPS INNOVATIONS Knoxville. TN (Siemens Medical Systems).

A, Å

A Century of Separation Science. Issaq HJ. editor. New York: M. Dekker; 2002. (#84)

AARC Clinical Guideline 949: Metabolic Measurement using Indirect Calorimetry during Mechnical Ventilation. *Resp Care* 1994; 39(12):1170. (#58)

Abel JJ. *Chemistry in relation to biology & medicine with especial reference to insulin & other hormones.* The Willard Gibbs Lecture 1927. Baltimore; 1939. (#77)

Adams G (the younger). *Essays on the Microscope* ... London; 1787. (#9)

Adell R, et al. Intra-osseous anchorage of the dental prostheses. II Review of Clinical Approaches. *Scand J Plast Reconstr Surg* 1970; 4:19. (#93)

Airy G. On the Diffraction of an Annual Aperture. *Phil Mag* 1841; XVIII:1. (#9)

Albert MS, et al.:Biological magnetic resonance imaging using laser-polarized 129Xe. *Nature* 1994; 370:199. (#96)

Aldini J. *Essai théorique et expérimental sur la galvanisme* Vol. 1,2. Paris; 1804. (#19)

Alhazen-Witelo. *Opticae thesaurus.* Basel; 1572 (#5)

Alonso JR. *Review of ion beam therapy: present and future* Proc EPAC 2000. p235 (#69)

Ambrose J. Computerized transverse axial scanning (tomography): Part 2. Clinical application. *Br J Radiol* 1973; 46:1023. (#95)

Andrews E. *The oxygen mixture, a new anaesthetic combination.* Chicago Med.Exam. 1868; 9:656. (#28)

Arago DF. *Rapport de M Arago sur la Daguerréotype.* Lu à la séance de la Chambre des Députés le 3 juillet 1839 Paris; 1839. (#38)

von Ardenne M. Das Elektronen-Rastermikroskop. *Z Phys* 1938; 109:553. (#83)

Aristotle. *Opera* ... *Venice*; 1482. Collected scientific writings printed in Augsburg 1518. (#4)

Arrhenius S. *Immunochemistry.* New York; 1907. (#62)

—— *The Life of the Universe, as conceived by Man from the Earliest Ages to the Present time.* London: Harper; 1909. (#62)

—— Über die Dissociation der in Wasser gelösten Stoffe. *Zeit Phys Chem* 1887; 1:631. (#62)

—— Ueber den Einfluss des Atmosphärischen Kohlensäuregehalts auf die Temperatur der Erdoberfläche. *Bihang K Sv Vet-Akad Handl* 22, Avd. I No. 1 Stockholm; 1896. (#62)

d'Arsonval A. Action physiologique des courant alternatifs ... *Arch Physiol Norm.Path.* 1893;5:401. (#2)

d'Arsonval JA, Deprez M. Galvanomètre apériodique. *C R Acad Sci* 1882; 94:1347. (#71)

Åsberg AG. Ultrasonic cinematography of the living heart. *Ultrasonics* 1967; 5:113. (#90)

Aschenbrandt T. *Die Bedeutung der Nase für die Athmung.* Würzburg; 1886. (#6)

Askanazi J, et al. Nutrition for the patient with respiratory failure: glucose vs fat. *Anesth* 1981; 54:373. (#58)

Astrup P, Severinghaus JW. *The history of blood gases, acids and bases.* Copenhagen: Munsgaard; 1986. (#14)

Auenbrugger L. *Inventum novum ex percussione humani ut signo abstrusos interni pectoris morbos detengendi.* Wien; 1761. (#31)

—— *Nouvelle méthode pour reconnaître les maladies internes de la poitrine par la percussion de cette cavité.* Ouvrage traduit du latin et commenté par J.N.Corvisart Paris; 1808. (#31)

Avery OT, MacLeod CM, McCarty M. Studies on the Chemical Nature of the Substance Inducing Transformation of Pneumococcal Types: Induction of Transformation by a Desoxyribonucleic Acid Fraction Isolated from Pneumococcus Type III. *J Exp Med* 1944; 79(1):137. (#88)

Avicenna: *Canon medicinae.* Milan; 1473.(#29)

Avogadro A. Essai d'une manière de déterminer les masses relatives des molécule élémentaires des corps ... *Journal de physique* 1811; 73:58. (#18)

B

Bacon R. *Perspectiva* ... Frankfurt; 1614. (#5)

Baeyer A. *Gesammelte Werke.* Brunswick; 1905. (#72)

Ballot B. Akustische Versuche auf der Niederländischen Eisenbahn nebst gelegentlichen Bemerkungen zur theorie des Hrn Prof Doppler. *Ann Phys Chem* 1845; 66:321. (#40)

Bang I. *Methoden zur mikrobestimmung einiger blutesandteile.* Wiesbaden: J.F.Bergman; 1916. (#81)

Barcroft J. *The respiratory function of the blood.* Cambridge University Press; 1913. (#37)

—— *The respiratory function of the blood.* Cambridge; 1913. (#37)

Bardeen J, Brattain WH. The Transistor, A Semi-Conductor Triode. *Phys Rev* 1948; 74(2):230. (#55)

Barron SL. *The development of the electrocardiograph.* Cambridge Monogr.5 London; 1952. (#71)

Bartelink DL. Röntgenschnitte. *Forschr Röntgenstr* 1933; 47:399. (#95)

Barthélemy M, Dufour. L'anesthésie dans la chirugie de la face. *La Presse Médicale* 27 Juillet 1907. p475. (#57)

Bartisch G. *Ophthalmoduleia. Das ist, Augendienst.* Dresden; 1583. (#5)

Bartlett RH, et al. Exctracorporeal membrane oxygenation (ECMO) cardiopulmonary support in infancy. *Trans Am Soc* Artif Intern Organs 1976; 22:80. (#86)

von Basch SS. Ueber die Messung des Blutdrucks am Menschen. *Z Klin Med* 1881; 2:79. (#68)

Bateson W. *Mendel's principles of Heredity.* Cambridge; 1909. (#40)

Bauber CD, Clark RG, Howlett P. Insensible water loss in operative patients. *Br J Surg.* 1972;59:300. (#6)

Becquerel H. Émission de radiation nouvelles par l'uranium métallique. *C R Acad Sci* 1896; 122:1086. (#70)

Beddoes T, Watt J. *Considerations on the Medicinal Use of Factitious Airs, and on the Manner of Obtaining Them in Large Quatities In two Parts.* Bristol; 1794. (#28)

Beiträge zur Geschichte der Brille. Carl Zeiss Oberkochen, Marwitz & Hauser Brillenmacher: Stuttgart; 1958. (#5)

Bell AG. *Telegraphy.* US Patent 174.465 March 1876. (#31)

Bell C. Of the Organs of the Human Voice. *Phil Trans Roy Soc* part II 1832. p299. (#25)

Benguigui I. *Théories électriques du XVIIe siècle. Isis* 1985; 76:442. (#19)

Bennett Jr WR. Background of an Inversion: The first gas laser. *IEEE J.Selected Topics in Quant. Electr.* 2000; 6(6):869. (#92)

Bennett Jr WR, et al. Superradiance, Excitation Mechanism, and Quasi-CW oscillations in the Visible Ar+ laser. *Appl Phys Lett* 1964; 4(10):180. (#92)

Bente PF, Zenner EH, Dandeneau RD. *Silica chromatographic column.* US Patent 4,293, 415 1981. (#84)

Bergman T.Tillägning Om Blåse-stenen. *Kungl Vet Handl* 1776; 37:333. (#72)

Bergström S. *The prostaglandins: from the laboratory to the clinic.* Nobel Lecture Stockholm; 1982. (#79)

Bernard C. *Introduction à l'étude de la médecine expérimetale.* Paris; 1865. (#4)

—— *Lecons sur la physiologie et la pathologie du système nerveux.* Paris; 1858. (#47)

—— *Lecons sur les anesthésiques et sur l'asphyxie.* Paris; 1875. (#55)

Bernoulli D. *Oratio physiologica de vita* 1737. Reprint of original and German translation Spiess O, Vezár F. Verhandlungen der Naturforschenden Gesellschaft in Basel 1940/1941; 52:189. (#18)

Berson SA, Yalow RS. Isotopic tracers in the study of diabetes. In: *Adv Biol Med Phys* Tobias CA, Lawrence JH. Editors. Vol.VI New York:Academic Press; 1958. p349. (#81)

Bert P. Sur la possibilité d'obtenir, à l'aide du protoxyde d'azote, une insensibilité de long durée et sur l'innocuité de cet anesthésieque. *C R Acad Sci* 1878; 87:728. See also ref. 28.8 p318–323. (#59)

Berzelius JJ. *Föreläsningar i djurkemien* Vol. I, Stockholm; 1806. p130–131. (#14)

—— *Lärobok i kemien.* Vol. 1–6 Stockholm; 1812–1830. (#36)

Beyer T, et al. A combined PET/CT scanner for clinical oncology. *J Nucl Med* 2000; 41:1369. (#99)

Bichat X. *Recherches physiologiques sur la vie et la mort.* Paris; 1800 and ref. 19.8 Vol.1 p153. (#23)

Bidloo G. *Anatomia humanis corporis & quinque tabulis, per artificiossis.* Amsterdam; 1685. (#1)

Bigelow HJ. Insensibility during surgical operations produced by inhalation. *Bost Med Surg J.* 1846; 35(16): 309 (#3)

—— Lithotrity by a single operation. *Am J med Sci* 1878; 75:117. (#34)

Bischoff T, von Voit C. *Die Gesetze der Ernährung des Fleischfresserers durch neue Untersuchungen festgestellt.* Leipzig; 1860. (#38)

Bitzer DL, Slottow HG. *Principles and Applications of the Plasma Display Panel.* Proc.1968 Microelectr. Symp.IEEE. St Louis; 1968. (#82)

Black HS. Stabilized feedback amplifiers. *Bell Syst Tech J* 1934; 13:1. (#55)

Black J. *Dissertatio medica inauguralis De Humore Acido a Cibis orto et Magnesia Alba.* Edinburg; 1754. (#20)

Bloch F. Nuclear induction. *Phys Rev* 1946; 70:478. (#94)

du Bois-Reymond E. *Reden* 2 vols. Leipzig (1912) (#42)

—— Ueber den sogennanten Froschstrom. *Ann Phys* 1843; 58:1. (#42)

Boklund U. Carl Wilhelm Scheele *Bruna Boken.* (brown book) Stockholm; 1961. (#21)

Boltzmann L. *Über die Beziehung zwischen dem zweiten Hauptsatze,* ... Sitzung d Kaiserl Akad Wiss LXXVI, Oktober 1877 Wien; 1878. (#55)

Boole G. *An investigation of the laws of thought, on which are founded the mathematical theories of logic and probabilities*. London; 1854. (#85)

Booth AD. *Fourier technique in X-ray organic structure analysis*. Cambridge: Cambridge University Press; 1948. (#32)

Borelli GA. *De motu animalium Ed novissima. Johannis Bernouilli meditationes mathematicae de motu musculorum*. Lugduni Bat; 1710. (#12)

Born M, Wolf E. *Principles of Optics*. Chapt. 8 and Chapt. 11. 7th ed. Cambridge: Cambridge University Press; 1999. (#76)

Boyle R. *New experiments physico-mechanical, touching the spring of the air and its effects*. Oxford; 1662. (#8)

—— *New experiments physico-mechanical, touching the spring of the air and its effects*. Oxford; 1662. p174: A Digression containing some Doubts touching Respiration (#11)

—— *The sceptical chymist or chymico-physical Doubts & Paradoxes*. London; 1661. (#4)

Bragg WH. X-rays and Crystals. *Nature* 1913; 90:360. and p572. (#76)

Bragg WH, Bragg WL. *X-rays and crystal structure*. G Bell and Sons; 1915. (#76)

Bragg WL. X-ray Crystallograpy. *Readings from Scientific American. Lasers and Light*. San Francisco: W.H. Freeman and Co; 1969. p161. (#76)

Braun F. Ueber ein Verfahren zur Demonstration und zum Studium des zeitlichen Verlaufes variabler Ströme. *Ann Phys Chem* 1897; 60:552. (#82)

Bravais A. Mémoire sur les systèmes formés par des points distribué régulièrement sur un plan ou dans l'espace. *J École Pol* 1850; 19:1. (#76)

Brenner R. *Untersuchungen und Beobachtungen auf die Gebiete der Elektrotherapie*. Vol I, II Leipzig; 1868. (#26)

de Broglie L. *Recherches sur la theorie des quanta*. These Paris: Masson & Cie; 1924. (#83)

Brownell GL, Sweet WH. Localisation of brain tumors with positron emitters. *Nucleonics* 1953; 11:40. (#99)

Bruche E, Johansson H. Elektronenoptik und Elektronenmikroskop. *Die Naturwissen*. 1932; 20(21):353. (#64)

Brücke E. Über das Leuchten der menschlichen Augen. *Anat Phys wiss Med* 1847. p225. (#45)

Brunette DM, et al. editors. *Titanium in Medicine*. Springer Verlag; 2001. (#93)

Brunschwig H. *Chirurgia*. Strassburg; 1497 (#2)

Brånemark P-I. Vital microscopy of bone marrow in rabbit. *Scand J Lab Invest* 1959; 11(Suppl. 38):1. (#93)

Brånemark P-I, et al. Regeneration of bone marrow. A clinical and experimental study following removal of bone marrow by curettage. *Acta Anat* (Basel) 1964; 59:1. (#93)

Brånemark P-I, Zarb GA, Albrektsson T. editors. *Tissue-Integrated Prosthesis: Osseointegration in clinical Dentistry*. Chicago: Quintessence Publ. Inc.; 1985. (#93)

Bunsen R. *Gesammelte Abhandlungen*. Bd. 1–3 Leipzig; 1904. (#49)

Burdon Sanderson J. Page FJ. Experimental Results relating to the Rythmical and Excitatory Motions of the Ventricle of the Heart of the Frog, and of the Electrical Phenomena which accompany them. *Proc Roy Soc* 1878; 27:410. (#65)

Burnham CA, Brownell GL. A multi-crystal positron camera. *IEEE Trans Nucl Sci* 1972; NS-19(3):201. (#99)

Bursztein S. editor. *Energy Metabolism, Indirect Calorimetry and Nutrition*. Baltimore: Williams and Wilkins; 1989. (#58)

Buxton RB. *An Introduction to Functional Magnetic Resonance Imaging*. Cambridge University Press; 2002. (#96)

C

Cade J. Lithium salts in the treatment of psychotic excitement. *Med J Austral* 1949; 36:349. (#75)

Callaghan JC, Bigelow WG. An electrical artificial pacemaker for standstill of the heart. *Ann Surg* 1951; 134:8. (#91)

Cambell-Swinton AA. Distant Electrical Vision. *Nature* 1908; 78:151. (#82)

Carlens E, et al. New method for atrial-triggered pacemaker treatment without thoracotomy. *J Thorac Cardiov Surg* 1965; 50:229. (#91)

Carlson R, Granström B. *A text-to-speech system based on a phonetically oriented programming language—Speech Transmission Laboratory report* QPSR1, 1 1975. (#89)

Carothers WH. Studies on polymerization and ring formation. I An introduction to the general theory of condensation polymers. *J Am Chem Soc* 1929; 51(8):2548. (#80)

Casserius J. *De vocis auditusque organis historia anatomica, tractatibus duobus explicata*. Ferrara; 1600. (#25)

Cater JP. *Electronically Speaking: Computer Speech Generation*. H.M.Sams & Co.; 1983. (#25)

Cavallo T. Some Discoveries Made by Mr Galvani of Bologna with Experiments and Observations on Them. *Phil Trans Roy Soc*. 1793; 10:83. (#19)

Cavendish H. Experiments on air. *Phil Trans Roy Soc* 1784; 74:119. (#24)

Celsus C. *De medicina* Florence; 1478. (#29)

Cesalpino A. *Peripateticarum Quationum Libri Quinque*. Venice; 1571. (#16)

Chagraff E, et al. The composition of the desoxyribonucleic acid of salmon sperm. *J Biol Chem* 1951; 192:223. (#88)

Chappe I. *Histoire de la télégraphie*. Paris: chez l'auteur; 1824. (#98)

Charch DH. *Moistureproof Material*. US Patent 1,737,187 1929. (Filed 1927) (#86)

Charcot J-M. I*conographie Photographique de la Salpetriere* 3 vols. Paris; 1877–1880. (#38)

—— *Nouvelle Iconographie de la Salpetriere* 28 vols. Paris; 1888–1918. (#38)

Chaussy C, Brendel W, Schmiedt E. Extracorporeally induced destruction of kidney stones by shock waves. *Lancet* 1980; 2:1265. (#34)

Chaussy C, et al. The use of chock waves for the destruction of renal calculi without direct contact. *Urol Res* 1976; 4:175. (#34)

Chauveau JB, Marey E-J. Appareils et expériences cardiographiques. *Mém Acad imp de Méd* 1863; 26:268. (#52)

Chesler DA. Positron tomography and three dimensional reconstruction techniques. In Freedman GS. Editor. *Tomographic Imaging in Nuclear Medicine*. New York: Society of Nuclear Medicine; 1973. p176. (#99)

Cheung AK, Leypoldt JK. *The Hemodialysis Membranes: A Historical Perspective, Current State, and future Prospect*. Seminars in Nephrology. 1997; 17(3):196. (#86)

Chilowsky C, Langvin P. *Procédés et appareils pour la production de signaux sous-marins dirigés et pour la localisation à distance d'obstacles sous-marins*. Brevet d'invention No 502.913 1920. Application 1916. (#66)

Chladni EF. *Die Akustik*. Leipzig; 1802. (#13)

Clark GM, Tong YC, Patrick JF. *Cochlear Protheses*. Melbourne: Churchill Livingstone; 1990. (#26)

—— Cochlear implants in the third millennium. *Am J Otol* 1999; 20:4. (#85)

Cleyer A. *Specimen Medicinae Sinicac, sive Opuscula Medica ad Mentem Sinensium,...* Frankfurt am Main; 1682. (#68)

Connes J. Reserches sur la spectroscopie par la transformation de Fourier. *Rev d'Optique Théor Exp* 1961; 40:41 and p116, p171, p231. (#32)

Conrad M, Guthzeit M. Ueber Barbitursäurederivate. *Ber Deutsch Chem Gesell* 1882; 15(2):2845. (#72)

Consden R, Gordon AH, Martin AJP. Quantitative Analysis of Proteins: A Partition Chromatographic Method Using Paper. *Biochem J* 1944; 38:224. (#84)

Cooke ED, Pilcher MF. Thermography in diagnosis of deep venous thrombosis. *Br Med J* 1973; 2:523. (#27)

Cooley JW, Tukey JW: An algorithm for machine calculation of complex Fourier series. *Mathematical Computation* 1965; 19:297. (#32)

Coolidge WD. *Improved x-ray tube*. US Patent 1,203,495 1916. (#67)

Cooper FS, et al. Some Experiments on the Perception of Synthetic Speech Sounds. *J Acoust Soc Am* 1952; 24:597. (#89)

Cooper JB et al. A new anesthesia delivery system. *Anesthesiology* 1978; 49:310. (#47)

Cormack AM. *Early two-dimensional reconstruction and recent topics stemming from it*. Nobel Lecture Stockholm; 1979. (#95)

—— Reconstruction of densities from their projections, with applications in radiological physics. *Physics in Medicine and Biology* 1973; 18:195. (#95)

—— Representation of a function by its line integrals, with some radiological applications. *J Appl Phys* 1963; 34:2722. (#95)

Correns C. G Mendel's Regel über das Verhalten der Nachkommenschaft der Rassenbastarde. *Ber dtsch bot Ges* 1900; 18:158. (#53)

Cotter RJ. Time of Fligt Mass Spectrometry: Instrumentation and Applications in biological research. *Am Chem Soc* Washington DC 1997; p13. (#79)

Coulomb C-A. Construction et usage d'une balance électrique,... *Mém de l'Acad Sci*. 1785. p569 (#15)

Craafoord C, Norberg B, Senning Å. Clinical studies in extracorporeal circulation with a heart-lung machine *Acta Chir Scand* 1957; 112:220. See also #86 Kolff page 444 ref. 86.7 and ref. 86.8. (#91)

Crooks W. Contributions to molecular physics in high vacua. *Phil Trans Roy Soc* 1879; 170:641. (#67)

Cumming W. On a luminous appearance of the human eye, and its application to the detection of disease of the retina and psoterior part of the eye. *Med.-Chir Trans Med Chir Soc* London. 1846; 29:283. (#45)

Currie J. *Medical reports, on the effect of water, cold and warm, as a remedy in fever and febrile diseases.* Liverpool; 1797. (#7)

Czermak J. *Der Kehlkopfspiegel und seine Verwerthung für Physiologie und Medicin.* Leipzig; 1860. (#48)

Czermak J. *Gesammelte Schriften.* Bd. I,II Leipzig; 1879. (#48)

—— Populäre physiologische Vorträge III Gesammelte Schriften Bd II, Leipzig; 1879. p60. (#48)

D

Dakin HD. On the use of certain antiseptic substances in the treatment of infected wounds. *Br Med J* 1915; 2:318. (#33)

Dalton J. *A New System of Chemical Philosophy.* Manchester; 1827. (#18)

—— Experimental essays on the constitution of mixed gases; ... *Mem Lit Phil Soc* Manchester 1802; 5:535. (#8)

Daly JW, Manganiello V, Jacobson KA. *Purines in Cellular Signalling: Target for New Drugs.* Springer Verlag; 1990. (#72)

Damadian RV. *Apparatus and method for detecting cancer in tissue.* US Patent 3,789,832 1974. (#94)

—— Field Focusing Nuclear Magnetic Resonance (FONAR): Visualization of a Tumor in a Live Animal. *Science* 1976; 194:1430. (#94)

Damadian RV, Goldsmith M, Minkoff L. NMR in cancer: XVI Fonar image of the live human body. *Physiol Chem Phys* 1977; 194:1430. (#94)

Daniel WG, Mugge A. Transesophageal Echocardiography. *The New England J Med* May 1995. p1268. (#90)

Darrigol O. *Electrodynamics from Ampere to Einstein.* Oxford University Press; 2000. Chapt.7. (#69)

Darwin C, Wallace AR. On the Tendency of Species to form Varieties; and on the Perpetuation of Varieties and Species by Natural Means of Selection. *J Proc Linnean Soc* 1858; 3(9):45. (#53)

—— *On the Origin of Species by Means of Natural Selection.* London; 1859. (#53)

—— *The expression of emotions in man and animals.* London; 1872. (#38)

Davies JWL, Lamke L-O, Liljedahl S-O. A guide to the rate of non-renal water loss from patients with burns. *Br J Plast Surg.* 1974; 27:325. (#6)

Daza de Valdes B. *Uso de los Antoios para todo genero de vistas:* ... Sevilla: por Diego Perez (1623). (#5)

Delay J, Deniker P, Harl JM. Traitment des états d'excitation et d'agitation par une méthode médicamenteuse derivée de l'hibernothérapie (part 2) *Ann Med-psychol* 1952; 110:267. (#75)

Dempster AJ. A new method of positive ray analysis. *Phys Rev* 1918; 11:316. (#79)

Denis J. A letter concerning a new way of curing sundry diseases by transfusion of blood. *Phil. Trans Roy Soc* 1667; 2:489. (#10)

Der Wiener Dioscorides. *Codex Medicus* 1,2 Akademische Druck- u Verlagsanstalt: Graz; 1998–1999. (#3)

Derham W. *Philosophical Experiments and Observations of the late Eminent Dr Robert Hooke* London; 1726. p295. (#38)

Derosne C. Mémoires sur l'opium. *Ann.Chim.* 1803; 45:257. (#29)

Desault PJ. *Oevres chirurgicales.* 3 vols. Paris; 1798–1803. (#57)

Descartes R. *De homine figuris.* Leyden; 1662. (#4)

—— *Discours de la méthod ... La Dioptrique.* Leyden; 1637. (#5)

Desormeaux AJ. *De l'endoscope et de ses applications au diagnostic et au traitement des affections de l'urèthre et de la vessie.* Paris; 1865. (#60)

Dibner B. *Early electrical machines.* Norwalk; 1957. (#15)

—— Galvani-Volta *A Controversy that led to the Discovery of Useful Electricity.* Norwalk; 1952. (#19)

Dictionary of Scientific Biography IV New York; 1970–1990. p258. (#1)

Dictionary of Scientific Biography Vol. II. New York; 1970–1990. p305 (#9)

Dinsdale A. *Television.* London: Sir I.Pitman & Sons; 1926. (#82)

Dioscorides P. *De materia medica.* Johannes of Medemblick Colle; 1478. (#3)

Dirac P. The Quantum Theory of the Electron. *Proc Roy Soc A* 1928; 117:610. (#69)

Djourno A, Eyries Ch. Prothèse auditive par excitation électrique a distance du nerf sensoriel a l'aide d'un bobinage inclus a demeure. *La Presse Medicale* 1957; 35:1431. (#26)

Dobelle WmH. Artificial Vision for the Blind by Connecting a Television Camera to the Visual Cortex. *ASAIO J* 2000; 46:3. (#85)

Donald I, Brown TG. Demonstration of tissue interfaces within the body by ultrasonic echo sounding. *British J Radiol* 1961; 34:539. (#90)

Donne A, Foucault L. *Cours de Microscopie complémentaire des études médicales* ... Paris; 1844–1845. (#38)

—— *Description du microscope photo-électrique. Extrait du bulletin de la société d'encouragement pour l'industrie nationale.* Paris; 1845 (#9)

Dorsch JA, Dorsch SE. *Understanding Anesthesia Equipment.* Baltimore: Williams & Wilkins; 1994. (#47)

Drinker P, Shaw LA. An apparatus for prolonged administration of artificial respiration. I. A design for adults and children. *J Clin Invest* 1929; 7:229. (#87)

Dubbleman CP. Attempts to Design an Artificial Heart-Lung Apparatus for the Human Adult (thesis). *Acta Physiol Parm Neerlandica* 1953; 2:1. (#86)

Duchenne de Boulogne G. *De l'électrisation localisée et de son application a la physiologie, a la pathologie et a la thérapeutique.* Paris; 1855. (#19)

—— *Mécanisme de la physionomie humaine, ...* Paris; 1862. (#38)

Dudley H, Reiss RR, Watkins SSA. A Synthetic Speaker. *J Franklin Inst* 1939; 227:739. (#89)

Dudley H. *The Vocoder.* Bell Lab. Records. December 1939. p122. (#25)

Dürer A. *Underweysung der messung ... zu nutz allen kunstlieb haben.* Nuremberg; 1525. (#1)

Dussik KTh, Dussik F, Wyt L. Auf dem Wege zur Hyperphonographie des Gehirnes. *Wiener Med Wsch* 1947; 38/39:425. (#66)

Dutrochet RJ. Nouvelles Recherches sur l'Endosmose et l'Endosmose. *Ann Chim Phys* 1828; 37:191. (#63)

E

Edison TA. *Electric-Lamp* U.S. Patent 223,898 January 27 1880. (#60)

Edler I. Ultrasoundcardiography. *Acta Med Scand Suppl.* 1961; 170. (#90)

Edler I, Lindström K. Ultrasonic doppler techniques in heart disease: Clinical applications. In: *Proc first World Congress on Ultrasonic Diagnostics in Medicine.* Vienna 1969. Bock J, Ossonig K. editors. 1971. p455. (#90)

Efron N, Pearson RM. Centenary Celebration of Fick's Eine Contactbrille. *Arch Ophtalmol.* 1988; 106: p1370, p1373 (#5)

Eichengrun A. 50 Jahre Aspirin. *Pharmazie* 1949; 4:582. (#75)

Einstein A. Zur Quantentheorie der Strahlung. *Physik Zeitschr* 1917; 18:121. (#92)

Einthoven W. Lippmann's Capillar-Electrometer zur Messung schnell wechselnder Potentialunterschiede *Pfluger's Arch ges Physiol* 1894; 56:528. (#71)

—— *The string galvanometer and the measurement of the action current of the heart.* The Nobel Lecture Stockholm; 1925. (#71)

—— Un nouveau galvanomètre. *Arch N Sc Ex Nat* 1901; 6:625. (#71)

Eisenmenger R. Therapeutic application of supra-abdominal suction and compressed air in relation to respiration and circulation. *Wien med Wochenschr* 1939; 89:1032. (#87)

Eisenmenger W. Eine elektromagnetische Impulsschallquelle zur Erzeugung von Druckstössen in Flussigkeiten und Festkörpern. In: *Proc. 3-rd Int.Congr. Acoustics*; 1961 Amsterdam: Elsevier; 1961 p326. (#34)

Electron Microscopy in Medicine and Biology. Gupta PD, Yamamoto H. editors. Science Publ. Inc; 2000. (#83)

Ellis H. *A History of Bladders Stone.* London: Blackwell Scientific Publications; 1969. (#34)

Elsberg CA. Zur Narkose beim Menschen mittelst der kontinuerlichen intratracheal Insufflation von Meltzer. *Berl klin Wschr* 1910; 47(21):957. (#57)

Elsholtz JS. *Clysmatica nova; oder newe Clystier-Kunst.* Berlin; 1665. (#10)

Engström C-G. *Dubbelverkande respirator.* Svensk Patent 141554 1953. (Filed 1950). (#87)

—— The clinical application of prolonged controlled ventilation: with special reference to a method developed by the author. *Acta Anaesth Scand Suppl* 13 1963. (#87)

Engström C-G, Svanborg NA. *The Importance of CO_2 Retension by Respiratory Insufficiency Caused by Poliomyelitis.* Same reference as the major paper cited p431. (#87)

Ettre LS. Evolution of Liquid Chromatography: A Historical Overview. In: Horváth C. editor. *High-Performance Liquid Chromatography* Vol.I. New York: Academic Press; 1980. (#84)

Ettre LS, Kalász H. *The Story of Thin-layer Chromatography.* LC*GC North America 2001; 19:712. (#84)

Ettre LS. M.S. *Tswett and the Invention of Chromatography.* LC-GC Europe 1, September 2003. (#83)

Euclid. *Elementa geometriae.* Venice; 1482. (#1)

—— *Optica & Catoptrica*. Paris; 1557. (#5)

Everhart TE, Thornley RF. Wide-band detector for micro-microampere low-energy electron currents. *J Sci Instrum* 1960; 37:246. (#83)

F

Fant G. *Acoustic Analysis and Synthesis of Speech with Applications to Swedish*. Ericsson Technics 1959; 1:3. (#89)

Faraday M. Experimental Researches in Electricity. *Phil Trans Roy.Soc* Part I, 1832. p125. (#26)

Farhi LE. Elimination of inert gas by the lung. *Resp Phys* 1967; 3:1. (#97)

Farnsworth PT. *Television system*. US Patent 1,773,980 1930. (filed 1927). (#82)

Fenn JB. *Electrospray for molecular elephants*. Nobel Lecture Stockhlm; 2002. (#79)

Fick A, Wislicenus J. Ueber die Entstehung der Muskelkraft. *Vierteljahresschrift Zurch Natur Gesell* Vol.X 1865. (#46)

—— *Die Alkoholfrage*. (Vortrag Würzburg am 16 März 1892) Würzburg; 1892. (#46)

—— *Die Geschwindigkeitskurve in der Arterie des lebenden Menschen*. Untersuchungen aus dem physiologischen Laboratorium der Züricher Hochschule Wien; 1869. (#46)

—— Experimenteller Beitrag zur Lehre von der Erhaltung der Kraft bei der Muskelzusammenziehung. Untersuchungen aus dem physiologischen Laboratorium der Züricher Hochschule. Wien; 1869. (#46)

—— *Gesammelte Schriften*. Band I-IV Würzburg; 1903-1905. (#46)

—— Ueber Diffusion. *Ann Phys Chem* 1855; 94:59. (#46)

—— Ueber Endosmose. *Wiener med Wochenschrift* 1857; 45:809/810. (#46)

—— Ueber Messung des Druckes im Auge. *Pfluger's Arch ges Physiol* 1888; 42:86. (#46)

Firestone FA. The Supersonic Reflectoscope, an Instrument for Inspecting the Interior of Solid Parts by Means of Sound Waves. *J Acoust Soc Am* 1946; 17(3):287. (#66)

Fischer E, Abderhalden E. Über das Verhalten verschiedener Polypeptide gegen Pankreasferment. *Sitzb d K Pr Akad Wiss* 1905; I:290. (#74)

—— Isomerie der Polypeptide. *Sitz d k Pr Akad Wiss* 1916; II:990. (#74)

—— Über phosphorsäureester des Methylglucosides und Theophyllinglucosids. *Sitz d k Pr Akad Wiss* 1914; II:905. (#74)

—— *Untersuchungen über Kohlenhydrate und Fermente* (1884-1908) Berlin: Springer; 1909. (#74)

Fischer EW, Dalton RG. Cardiac Output in Horses. *Nature* 1959; 184:2020. (#56)

Fizeau MH. Sur le hypothèses relatives a l'éther lumineux. *Ann Chim Phys* 3ser. 1859; 33:385. (#40)

Flanagan J. *Speech Analysis, Synthesis and Perception*. Berlin: Springer Verlag; 1972. (#25)

Flory PJ. Phase Equilibria in Solutions of Rod-like Particles. *Proc Roy Soc A* 1956; 234: 60. (#80)

—— *Spatial Configuration of Macromolecular Chains*. Nobel Lecture Stockholm; 1974. (#80)

Flourens P. Chloro-forme. *Arch Gen de Med* 4 ser. 1847; 13:549. (#36)

de Forest L. *Cautery*. U.S.Patent 874,178 Dec. 17; 1907. (#2)

Fothergill J. *An Account of the Sore Throat*. London; 1748. (#48)

—— Observation on a Case … of Recovering a Man Dead in Appearance, by distending the Lungs with Air. *Phil Trans Roy Soc*. 1744-1745. p275. (#23)

Franklin RE, Gosling RG. Molecular Configuration in Sodium Thymonucleate. *Nature* 1953; 171:740. (#88)

Frauenhofer J. Bestimmung des Brechungs- und Farbenzerstreuungs-Vermögens verschiedener Glasarten … *Denkschriften der k. Akad. d. Wiss. zu München*. 1817; Bd.V. (#9)

Friedenwald H. The History of the Invention and of the Development of the Ophthalmoscope. *JAMA* 1902; 38(9):549 (#45)

Frizot M. *La Chronophotographie*. Beaune (Cote-d'Or); 1984. (#12)

Furberg SV. On the Structure of Nucleic Acids. *Acta Chem Scand* 1952; 6:634. (#88)

G

Galambos R. The Avoidance of Obstacles by flying Bats: Spallanzani's Ideas (1794) and Later Theories. *Isis* 1942; 34:132. (#66)

Galenus C. *Omnia quae extant opera*. Venice; 1550. (#4)

Galilei G. *Discorsi e demonsrazioni matematiche, intorno a due nuoue scienze,* … Leiden; 1638. (#66)

le Gallois J. *Expériences sur le principe de la vie, notamment sur celui des movemens du coer,* … Paris; 1812. (#23)

Galton F. Typical laws of heredity. *Nature* 1877; 15:492, 512, 532. (#30)

Galvani L. *De viribus electricitatis in motu musculari*. Bologna; 1791. (#12)

Gandevia B. John Hutchinson in Australia and Fiji. *Med.History* 1977; 21:365. (#41)

Ganz W, et al. A new technique for measurement of cardiac output by thermodilution in man. *Am J Cardiol* 1971; 17:392. (#56)

Garcia M. Observations on the Human Voice. *Phil Mag* 1855; 10:218. (#48)

Gauss CF. Nachlass, Theoria Interpolationis Methodo Nova Tractata. In: *Carl Friedrich Gauss Werke* 3 Göttingen; 1866. p265. (#32)

—— *Theoria Motus Corporum Coelestium*. Hamburg; 1809. (#30)

Gay-Lussac JL. Mémoire sur la combinaison des substances gazeuses, les unes avec les autres. *Mém phys chim Soc d'Arcueil* 1809; 2:207. (#18)

—— Sur la dilatation des gaz et des vapeurs. *Ann de chimie* 1802; 43:137. (#7)

Geddes LA. *Handbook of Blood Pressure Measurements*. Clifton NJ: Humana Press; 1991. (#68)

Gedeon A. Anesthetic Agent Analysis Using Piezoelectric Microbalance. *Biom Instr Tech* Nov/Dec 1989. (#66)

Gedeon A, et al. A new method for noninvasive bedside determination of pulmonary blood flow. *Med. & Bio Eng & Comp* 1980; 18:411. (#56)

Gedeon A, Mebius C. The Hygroscopic Condenser Humidifier. *Anaesthesia* 1979; 34:1043. (#6)

Gedeon A, Olsson SG. *A new type of anaesthetic vaporizer*. In: 30-th Ann Conf Eng Med Biol 1977; 19: 203. (#47)

Gehrke CW, Wixom RL, Bayer E. Editors. *Chromatography—a Century of Discovery*

1900–2000. Amsterdam: Elsevier; 2001. (#73)

Gernsheim H. *The History of Photography*. London: Thames Hudson; 1969. (#38)

von Gersdorff H. *Feldbuch der wundarztney*. Strassburg; 1517. (#2)

Gesammelte Abhandlungen von Ernst Abbe. 5vols. Jena; 1904-1940. (#64)

Gesner C. *Annotationes in Pedacij Dioscoridis … De Medica Materia. De artificiosis extractionibus*. Strassburg; 1561. (#3)

Geusic JE, Marcos HM, Van Uitern LG. Laser Oscillation in Nd:doped yttrium aluminium, yttrium gallium and gadolinium garnets. *Appl Phys Lett* 1964; 4:182. (#92)

Gibbon JH. An oxygenator with a large surface-volume ratio. *J Lab Clin Med* 1939; 24:1192. (#86)

Gilbert W. *De magnete, magneticisque corporibus, et de mango magnete tellure*. London; 1600. (#15)

Goodwyn E. *The connection of Life with Respiration* … London; 1788. (#23)

Goppelsroeder F. *Studien über die anwendung der Capillaranalyse*. I. Bei Harnuntersuchungen. II. Bei vitalen Tinktionsversuchen. Basel: E.Birkhäuser; 1904. (#73)

—— *Über Capillar-Analyse und ihre verschienenen Anwendung sowie über das Emporsteigen der Farbstoffe in den Pflanzen*. Wien: Selbstvlg; 1888. (#73)

Gosling RG, King DH. Arterial assessment by Dopplershift ultrasound. *Proc Roy Soc Med* 1974; 67:447. (#40)

Gould G. *Light amplifying apparatus*. US Patent Application 804504 1959. Approved as US Patent 4,053,845 Optically pumped laser amplifiers 1977. (#92)

Graham T. The Bakerian Lecture: On Osmotic Force. *Phil Trans Roy Soc* 1854; 144:177. (#63)

Greatbatch W, Chardack WM. A transistorized implantable pacemaker for the longterm correction of complete atrioventricular block. *M Electron NEREM* 1959; 48:643. (#91)

Green T. On death from chloroform; its prevention by galvanism. *Brit Med J*. 1872; 1:552. (#23)

Gregor W. Beobachtungen und Versuche über den Menakanite, einen in Corwall (Kierchspiel Menaccan bei Falmouth) gefundenen magnetischen Sand. *Chem Ann*. (L von Crell) 1791; Bd.1. (#93)

Gréhant N. *Recherches physiques sur la respiration de l'homme*. Paris; 1864. (#6)

Gréhant N, Quinquaud CE. Recherches expérimentales sur la mesure du volume de sang qui traverse les poumons en un temps donné. *C R Séance et Mém d Soc biol* 1886; 38:159. (#56)

Grimaux E. *Lavoisier 1743-1794* Paris; 1888. (#24)

Guericke O. *Experimenta Nova (ut vocantur) Magdeburgica De Vacuo Spatio* … Amsterdam; 1672. (#8)

Guerlac H. *Lavoisier in Dictionary of Scientific Biography* VIII New York; 1973. p66. (#24)

Gullstrand A. Die reflexlose Ophtalmoskopie. *Arch Augenheilkunde* 1911; 68:101. (#45)

Günther RT. *Early science in Oxford* Vol.VI The life and work of Robert Hooke (Part I) Oxford; 1930. (#43)

Guthrie S. New mode of preparing a spiritu-

ous solution of Chloric Ether. *Am J Sci and Arts* 1832; 21:64, and p405. (#36)
—— On pure Chloric Ether. *Am J Sci and Arts* 1832; 22:105. (#36)
Gwathmey JT. *Anesthesia*. Chapter X. New York: D.Appleton and Co; 1914. (#57)

H

Haas G. Über Blutauswaschung. *Klin Wochenschr.* 1928; 7(29):1356. (#77)
—— Versuche der Blutauswaschung am Lebenden mit Hilfe der Dialyse. *Klin. Wochenschr.* 1925; 4(1): 13. (#77)
Haeusler E, Kiefer W. Anregung von stosswellen in flussigkeiten durch hochgeschwindigkeitswassertropfen. *Verh D Physikal Gesell* 1971; 6:786. (#34)
Hagen GH. Ueber die Bewegung des Wassers in engen cylindrischen Rohren. *Ann Phys Chem* 1839; 46:423. (#35)
Hahn EL. Spin echoes. *Phys Rev* 1950; 80:580. (#94)
Haldane JB. *The causes of evolution*. London; 1932. (#53)
Haldane JC. *Respiration*. New Haven: Yale University Press; 1922. (#59)
Haldane JS. *Methods of Air Analysis*. 2nd ed. London; 1918. (#37)
Hall RN, et al. Coherent light emission from GaAs junctions. *Phys Rev Lett* 1962; 9:366. (#92)
Haller Av. *Elementa physiologiae corporis humani*. Lausanne Berne Leiden; 1757–1766. (#12)
Hamburger HJ. *Osmotische Druck und Ionenlehre in den Medicinischen Wissenschaften*. 3 Bde Wiesbaden; 1902–1904. (#62)
Hamilton WF, et al. Comparison of the Fick and dye injection methods of measuring the cardiac output in man. *Am J Physiol* 1948; 153:309. (#56)
Harris JA, Benedict FG. *A Biometric Study of Basal Metabolism in Man*. Publ.279 Washington DC: Carnegie Institute of Washington; 1919. (#58)
Hartmann A. Ueber eine neue Methode der Hörprufung mit Hulfe elektrischer Ströme. *Arch Physiol Leipzig*; 1878. p155. (#26)
Harvey W. *Excercitation Anatomica de motu Cordis et Sanguinis in Animalibus*. Frankfurt am Main; 1628. (#12)
—— *Exercitationes de Generatione Animalium*. London; 1651. (#16)
Hazlewood CF, Nichols BL, Chamberlain NF. Evidence for existence of a minimum of two phases of ordered water in skeletal muscle. *Nature* 1969; 222:747. (#94)
Heideman MT, Johnson DH, Burrus CS. Gauss and the History of Fast Fourier Transform. *Arch Hist Exact Sci* 1985; 34:265. (#32)
Heister L. *Chirurgie in welcher alles was zur Wund-Artzney gehöret, nach der neuesten und besten Art*. Nurnberg; 1718. (#57)
von Helmholtz H. *Das Denken in der Medizin*. Berlin; 1877. (#4)
—— *Die Lehre von den Tonempfindungen als physiologische Grundlage für die Theorie der Musik*. Braunschweig; 1863. (#13)
—— *Die Thatsachen in der Wahrnehmung*. Berlin; 1879. (#43)
—— Handbuch der physiologischen Optik. *Allgemeine Encyclopädie der Physik* IX Bd. Leipzig; 1867. (#5)

—— Messungen über Fortpfanzungsgeschwindigkeit der Reizung in den Nerven. *Arch Ant Physiol Berlin*; 1852. p199. (#43)
—— *Über die Erhaltung der Kraft, eine physikalische Abhandlung vorgetragen in der Sitzung der physikalisches Gesellschaft zu Berlin am 23sten juli 1847*. Berlin; 1847. (#43)
Henderson LJ. Das Gleichgewicht zwischen Basen und Säuren im tierischen Organismus. *Ergebn Physiol* 1909; 8:254. (#62)
—— *Blood*. New Haven: Yale University Press; 1928. (#81)
Herholdt JD, Rafn CG. *Forsög til en historisk udsikt over redningsanstalter for drunknede, og underretning om de bedste midler ved hvilke de igen kunne bringes til live*. Copenhagen; 1796. (#23)
Herman L. Ueber die Wirkungen des Stickstoffoxydgases auf das Blut. *Arch Anat Physiol wiss Med* 1865. p469. (#51)
Herschel JF. On the chemical action of the rays of the solar spectrum on preparations of silver and other substances,... *Phil Trans* 1840; 1:1. (#38)
Herschel W. Experiments on the Refrangibility of the invisible Rays of the Sun. Experiments on the solar, and on the terrestrial Rays that occasion Heat. *Phil Trans Roy Soc* Part I 1800. p284, p293 (#27)
Hertwig O. *Beiträge zur Kentniss der Bildung Befruchtung und Theilung des tierischen Eies*. Leipzig; 1875. (#16)
Herzog RO, Jancke W, Polanyi M. Röntgen spectrographische Beobachtungen an Zellulose. *Z Phys* 1920; 3:343. (#78)
Hesse G, Weil H. *Michael Tswett's first paper on chromatography*. M.Woelm Eschwege; 1954, a translation and reprint of the Russian publication. (#73)
Hevesy G. Applications of isotopes in biology. *J Chem Soc* 1939; 39(2):1213. (#70)
Hewson W. *An experimental inquiry into the properties of the blood*. London; 1771. (#14)
Hickman H. *A letter on suspended animation, containing experiments showing that it may be safely employed during operations on animals,...* Ironbridge; 1824. (#59)
Hill L, Barnard H. A simple and accurate form of sphygmomanometer or arterial pressure gauge contrived for clinical use. *Brit med J* 1897; 2:904. (#68)
Himmelweit F. editor. *The Collected Papers of Paul Ehrlich* 3 vols. London: Pergamon Press; 1956–1960. (#75)
Hittorf W. Über die Elektricitätsleitumg der Gase. Erste Mitteilungen. *Ann Phys Chem* 1869; 136:1. (#67)
Hoesch K. Emil Fischer Sein Leben und sein Werk. *Ber Dtsch Chem Ges* 1921:54 (#74)
Hoff HE, Geddes LA. Ballistics and the Instrumentation of Physiology: The Velocity of the Projectile and of the Nerve Impulse. *J Hist Med* 1960; 15:133. (#43)
Holter NJ. Radioelectrocardiography: A New Technique for Cardiovascular Studies. *Ann N Y Acad Sci* 1957; 65:913. (#71)
Holzmann GJ, Pehrson B. *The Early History of Data Networks*. IEEE Computer Society Press; 1995. (#98)
Hooke DH, Norman JM. *Origins of Cyberspace. A Library on the History of Computing, Networking, and Telecommunications*. Novato: historyofscience.com; 2001. (#85)

Hooke R: *Micrographia: or some Physiological Descriptions of Minute Bodies ...* London; 1665. (#9)
Hoppe-Seyler EF. Ueber den chemischen und optischen Eigenschaften des Blutfarbstoffs. *Virchows Arch Pathol Anat* 1864; 29:233 and p597. (#51)
—— *Handbuch der physiologisch-und pathologisch-Chemischen Analyse für Ärtzte und Studirenden*. Berlin; 1865. p201. (#51)
Horbaczewski J. Synthese der Harnsäure. *Ber Deutsch Chem Gesell* 1882; 15(2):2678. (#72)
Hubbell J. Biomaterials in tissue engineering. *Biotechnology*. 1995; 13:565. (#93)
Hufner CG. Neue Versuche zur Bestimmung der Sauerstoffkapazität des Blutfarbstoffs. *Arch Pat Anat. Physiol* 1894. p130. (#51)
von Humboldt A. *Versuche über die gereizte Muskel-und Nervenfaser ...* Vol. 1,2 Berlin; 1797. (#19)
Hyatt JW, Hyatt IS. *Improvement in Treating and Moulding Pyroxyline*. US Patent 105,338 1870. (#77)
Hyde JF, DeLong RC. Condensation Products of the Organo-silane Diols. *J Am Chem Soc* 1941; 63(5):1194. (#78)
Hyman AS. Resuscitation of the stopped heart by intracardial therapy. *Arch Int Med* 1930; 46:553. (#91)
Höök F, et al. Structural changes in hemoglobin during adsorption to solid surfaces: Effects of pH, ionic strength and ligand Binding. *Proc Natl Acad Sci* 1998; 95:12271. (#66)

I

Ingelstedt S. Studies on the conditioning of air in the respiratory tract. *Acta Oto-laryng.* 1956; Suppl.131 (#6)
Ingen-Housz J. *Experiments upon Vegetables, discovering their great Power of Purifying the common Air in the Sun-shine ...* London; 1779. (#22)

J

Jackson ChT. *A Manual of Etherization*. Boston; 1861. (#3)
Jacobaeus HC. Ueber die Möglichkeit die Zystoscopie bei Untersuchungen seröser Höhlungen anzuwenden. *Münch med Wschr* 1910; 57:2090. (#60)
Jarvik RK. The Total Artificial Heart. *Scientific American* 1981; 244 (1):74. (#86)
Jaszczak RJ. Tomographic radiopharmaceutical imaging. *Proc IEEE* 1988; 76(9):1079. (#97)
Javan A, Bennett Jr WR, Herriott DR. Population inversion and continuous optical maser oscillation in a gas discharge containing a He-Ne mixture. *Phys Rev Lett* 1961; 6:106. (#92)
Jobsis FF. Noninvasive, infrared monitoring of cerebral and myocardial oxygen sufficiency and circulatory parameters. *Science*, 1977; 198:1264. (#27)
Johnsson WL, et al. Detection of Fetal Life in Early Pregnancy with an Ultrasonic Doppler Flowmeter *Obst Gyn* 1965; 26:305. (#40)
Judson HF. *The Eigth Day of Creation*. New York: Simon & Schuster; 1979. (#88)

K

Kanazawa KK, Gordon III JG. Frequency of quartz microbalance in contact with liquid. *Anal.Chem.* 1985; 57:1770. (#66)

Kanel WB, et al. The value of measuring vital capacity for prognostic purposes. *Trans Assoc Life Insur Med Dir Am* 1980; 64:66. (#41)

Kapany NS, et al. Fiber Optics. Part I-IV. *J.O.S.A* 1957; 47:413. p423, p594 and p1109. (#60)

Karass Th. *Geschichte der Telegraphie.* Teil 1. Braunschweig: F.Vieweg & Sohn; 1909. p27. (#98)

Kaufmann M. The Internet: A reliable source? *Washington Post* February 16 1999. pZ17. (#98)

Kelling G. Über die Besichtigung der Speiseröhre und des Magens mit biegsamen Instrumente. *Verh Gesell Dtsch Naturf u Ärzte* 1901; 73:117. (#60)

Kepler J. *Dioptrice seu demonstratio eorum quae visui & visibilibus propter conspicilla.* Augsburg; 1611. (#5)

von Kern V. *Bemerkung über die neue, von Civiale und le Roy verubte Methode, die Steine in der Harnblase zu zermalen und auszuziehen.* Wien; 1826. (#34)

Kety SS. Measurement of regional circulation by the local clearance of radioactive sodium. *Am Heart J* 1949; 38:321. (#70)

Keys TE. The Early Pneumatic Chemists and Physicians: Their influence on the Developement of Surgical Anesthesia. *Anesthesiology* 1969; 30:447. (#20)

—— *The History of Surgical Anesthesia.* Schuman's New York; 1945. p24. (#28)

Keyserlingk JR et al. Infrared imaging of the breast. *The Breast Journal* 1998; 4:245. (#27)

Killian G. Ueber directe Bronchoskopie. *Münch med Wschr* 1898; 45:844. (#60)

Kipping FS. Organic derivatives of silicon. *Proc Roy Soc A* 1937; 159:139. (#78)

Kilby JS. *Turning potential into realities: The invention of the integrated circuit.* Nobel Lecture Stockholm; 2000. (#85)

Kircher A. *Scrutinium physico-medicum contagiosae luis, quae pestis dicitur.* Romae; 1658. (#13)

—— *Magnes, sive, de Arte magnetica opus tripartium . . .* Cologne; 1643. (#13)

Kirchhoff G, Bunsen R. Analyse chimique fondée sur les observations du spectre. *Ann Chim Phys* 1862; 64:257. (#49)

—— Chemische Analyse durch Spectralbeobachtungen. *Ann Phys Chem* 1860; 60:161. (#49)

Kisch F, Schwarz H. Das Herzschlagvolumen und die Methodik seiner Bestimmung. *Erg Inner Med u Kinderh* 1925; 27:169. (#56)

Klarreich E. Take a deep breath. *Nature* 2003; 424:873. (#96)

Klatt D. Review of Text-to-Speech Conversion for English. *J Acoust Soc Am* 1987; 82(3): 737. (#25)

Kläsi J. Ueber die therapeutische anwendung der "dauernarkose" mittels somnifens bei schizophrenen *Zeitsch Gesamt.Neurol Psych* 1922; 74:557. (#75)

Knoll M, Ruska E. Beitrag zur geometerischen Elektronenoptik I und II. *Ann Phys* 1932; 12:607. and p641. (#83)

Knowles Middleton WE. *A History of the Thermometer.* Baltimore; 1966. (#7)

Koch H, et al. A method for humidifying inspired air in posttracheotomy care. *Ann Oto Rhin Laryng.* 1958; 76:991. (#6)

Koch R. Die Aetilogie der Tuberkulose. *Berl Klin Wschr* 1882; 19:221. (#61)

—— Ueber Desinfection. *Mittheil kais Gesundheitsamt* 1881; 1:234. (#54)

—— *Verfahren zur Untersuchung, zum Conservieren und Photografieren der Bakterien.* Beitr Biol. Pflanz 1876. p399. (#61)

—— Zur Aetiologie des Milzbrandes. *Mitthei d Kais Gesundheitsamte* 1881; 1:49. (#61)

Koch R, Gaffky G, Loeffler F. Versuche über die Verwerthbarkeit heisser Wasserdämpfe zu Desinfectionszwecke. *Mitthei d Kais Gesundheitsamte* 1881; 1:322. (#61)

Kohlrausch F. Das elektrische Leitungsvermögen der wässerigen Lösungen von den Hydraten und Salzen der leichte Metallen . . . *Ann Phys Chem* 1879; 6:167. p1. and p145. (#62)

Kolff WJ. *Artificial Organs.* New York: John Wiley & Sons; 1976. (#86)

—— *New Ways of Treating Uraemia.* London: J & A Churchill Ltd; 1947. (#86)

—— The Artificial Heart. *Encyclopedia of Human Biology.* Vol.I Academic Press Inc; 1991. p386. (#86)

Kolff WJ, Berk HJ. The Artificial Kidney: A Dialyzer with a Great Area. *Acta med Scand* 1944; 117:121. (#86)

Korotkoff NC. To the question of methods of determining the blood pressure. *Reports Imp mil med Acad* 1905; 11:365. (#68)

Kratzenstein ChT. Sur la naissance de la formation des voyelles. *Journal de Physique* 1782; 21:358. (#25)

Kreill J(ames). *Tentamina medico-physica, ad quasdam quastiones,quae oeconomiam animalem spectant, accommodata.* London; 1718. (#35)

Krogh A. On the mechanism of the Gas-Exchange in the Lungs. *Skand Arch Physiol* 1910; 23:248. (#37)

—— *The respiratory exchange of animals and man.* London:Longmans Green & Co; 1916. Chapter 2 (#58)

Krogh A, Krogh M. On the tension of gases in the arterial blood. *Skand Arch Physiol* 1910; 23:179. (#37)

Kruta V. *J. E.Purkyne (1787–1869) Physiologist. A Short Account of His Contributions to the Progress of Physiology With a Bibliography of His Works.* Prag; 1969. (#48)

Krömeke F. *Friedrich Wilh. Sertürner, der Entdecker des Morphiums.* Jena; 1925. p5. (#29)

Kuhn F. Die perorale Intubation. *Zbl Chir* 28/52 Leipzig; 1901. (#57)

—— Perorale Tubagen mit und ohne Druck. *Dtsch Z Chir* 1905; 76:148. (#57)

Kuhn R. Über die Behandlung depressives Zustande mit einem Iminodibenzylderivat (G22355) *Schweiz Med Wschr* 1957; 87:1135. (#75)

Kuhn R, Lederer E. Zerlegung des Carotins in seine Komponente. *Dt Chem Ges* 1931; 64B:1349. (#73)

Kumar A, Welti D, Ernst RR. NMR Fourier Zeugmatography. *J Magn Res* 1975; 18:69. (#96)

Kurzweil R. The Kurzweil Reading Machine: a technical overview.In: Science, Technology and the Handicapped. Redden MR, Schwandt W. editors. *AAAS Report* 76-R-11 1976;3. (#89)

Kwolek SL. *Wholly aromatic carbocyclic polycarbonate fiber having orientation angle of less than about 45 degrees.* US Patent 3,819,587 1974. (#80)

von Kölliker R, Müller H. Nachweis der negativer Schwankung des Muskelstroms am naturlich sich contrahirenden Muskel. *Verh phys-med Ges Würzburg* 1856; 6:528. (#65)

L

Labarraque AG. *Ordonance du préfet de police, en date du 19 octobre 1823, prescrivant l'emploi de chlorure de chaux . . .* Paris; 1825. (#33)

Landmarks of the plastics industry 1862–1962 ICI Plastics Division 1962. (#78)

Landriani M. *Richerche fisiche intorno alla salubrità dell'aria.* Milano; 1775. (#22)

Lane TH, Burns SA. Silica, silicon and silicones . . . unraveling the mystery. In: *Immunology of Silicones Current Topics in Microbiology and Immunology.* Potter M, Rose NR. editors. Berlin: Springer-Verlag; 1996. p210. (#78)

Laplace P. *Oevres completes de Laplace (1878–1912)* Vol 12 Paris; 1898. p349. (#30)

Larsson B, et al. Lessons From the First Patient with an Implanted Pacemaker: 1958–2001. *PACE* 2003; 26(1):114. (#91)

Lassen HCA. *Management of Life-Threatening Poliomyelitis Copenhagen 1952–1956.* London: E & S Livinstone Ltd.; 1956. (#87)

Laue M. Eine quantitative Prufung der Theorie fur die Interferenzerscheinungen bei Röntgenstrahlen. *Ann d Phys* 1913; 41:989. (#76)

Lauterbur PC, et al. Zeumatographic high-resolution nuclear magnetic resonance spectroscopy of chemical inhomogeneity within macroscopic objects. *J Am Chem Soc* 1975; 97:6866. (#96)

Lavoisier A-L. *Traité élémentaire de chimie, présenté dans un ordre nouveau et d'après les découvertes modernes.* Paris; 1789. (#24)

Lavoisier AL, et al. *Mémoires de Chimie.* Paris; 1803–1805. (#24)

—— *Méthode de Nomenclature Chimique.* Paris; 1787. (#24)

Lawrence W. The synthesis of speech from signals which have a low information rate. In: *Communication Theory.* Jackson W. editor. Symposium on "applications of Communication Theory" London September 1952. London: Butterworth Scientific Publications; 1953. p460. (#89)

Lawson RN. Implication of surface temperatures in the diagnosis of breast cancer. *Can Med Assoc J* 1956; 75:309. (#27)

Leared A. On the self-adjusting double stethoscope. *Lancet* 1856; 2:138. and p202. (#68)

LeCanu LR. De l'Hematosine, au Matière Colorante du Sang. *Ann Chim Phys* 1830; 45:5. (#51)

Lehmann HE, Ban TA. The History of Psychopharmacology of Schizophrenia. *Can J Psych* 1997; 42:152. (#75)

Leibniz GW. *Opera Omnia* 6 vols. 1768. Explication de l'arithmétique binaire. Vol.III 1703. p390. (#85)

Leiter J. *Instrumente und Apparate zur direkten Beleuchtung Menschlicher Körperhöhlen durch Elektrischen Glühlicht.* Wien; 1880. (#60)

Leksell L. Echoencephalography. I Detection

of Intracranial Complications following Head Injury. *Acta Chir Scand* 1956; 110:301. (#90)

Lenard P. Über die Absoption der Kathodenstrahlen *Ann phys Chem* 1895; 56:255. (#69)

Lenfant C, Okubo T. Distribution function of pulmonary blood flow and ventilation-perfusion ratio in man. *J Appl Physiol* 1968; 24:668. (#97)

Lenz HF. Ueber das galvanische Leitungsvermögen alcoholischer Lösungen. *Mém l'Acad Imp Sci* St. Petersbourg VIII:e Sér. 1882; 30(9). (#62)

Leonardo da Vinci: *Leonardo on the human body*. Drawing 39 New York:Dover Publications Inc.; 1983. (#25)

Leroy d'Etoilles JJ. *Histoire de la lithotritie, précédée de réflexions sur la dissolution des calculs urinaires*. Paris; 1839. (#34)

—— Reserches sur l'asphyxie. *J Physiol* 1827; 7:45. (#87)

Levine SZ, Kelly M, Wilson JR. The insensible perspiration in infancy and in childhood II. Proposed basal standards for infants. *Am J Dis Child*. 1930; 39:917. (#6)

Levitt GM. *The Turk, Chess Automaton*. Jefferson: McFarland & Co; 2000. (#25)

von Liebig J, Wöhler F. Untersuchung über die Natur der Harnsäure. *Ann Pharm* 1838; 26:241. (#72)

—— *Die Organische chemie in ihrer Anwendung auf Agricultur und Physiologie*. Braunschweig; 1840. (#38)

—— Ueber die Erscheinungen der Gährung, Fäulniss und Verwesung und ihre Ursache. *Ann d. Pharm* 1839; 30(31):38. (#54)

—— Ueber die Verbindungen welche durch die Einwirkung des chlors auf Alkohol, Aether, ölbildendes Gas und Essiggeist entstehen. *Ann der Pharm* 1832; 1:182. (#36)

Lippmann G. Relation entre les phénomènes électriques et capillaires. *C R Acad Sci* 1873. p1407 (#65)

Lister J. An Address on the present Position of Antiseptic Surgery, delivered before the International Medical Congress Berlin; 1890. In: *Brit Med J* 1890; II:377. (#54)

——On the Effects of the Antiseptic System of Treatment upon the Salubrity of a Surgical Hospital. *Lancet* 1870; I p4. and p40. (#54)

Lister JH. *The Purines*. John Wiley & Sons; 1996. (#72)

Lister JJ. On some properties in achromatic object glasses . . . *Phil Trans* 1830; 120:187. (#9)

Long CW. An Account of the First Use of sulphuric Ether . . . *Southern Med Surg J*. 1849;5(12):705 (#3)

Longet F-A. *Expériences relatives aux effects de l'inhalation de l'éther sulphurique sur le système nerveux*. Paris; 1847. (#47)

Lord Rayleigh (Strutt JW). *The theory of sound*. London; 1878. (#13)

Loudon R, Murphy RLH. Lung sounds (state of the art). *Am Rev Respir Dis* 1984; 130: 663. (#31)

Lower R. The method observed in transfusing the blood out of one animal into another. *Phil Trans* 1666; 1:353. (#10)

Lower R, King E. An account of the experiment of transfusion, practiced upon a man in London. *Phil. Trans Roy Soc* 1667; 2:557. (#10)

Lube M, Safarov YuD, Yakimenkov LI. Ultra-sonic Detection of the Motions of Cardiac Valves and Muscles. *Sov Phys Acoust* 1967; 13:59. (#40)

Ludwig C. Beiträge zur Kentniss des Einflusses der Respirationsbewegung auf den Blutlauf im Aortensysteme. *Arch Anat Phys wiss Med*. 1847. p242. (#35)

——Zusammenstellung der Untersuchungen über Blutgase. *Z k k Ges Ärtzte in Wien* 1865; 1:145. (#37)

Lummer O, Reiche F. editors. E Abbe. *Die Lehre von der Bildentstehung im Mikroskop*. Brauschweig; 1910. (#64)

Lyman HM. *Artificial Anaesthesia and Anaesthetics* New York: William Wood & Co.; 1881. p309. (#28)

Lynch DC. Historical Evolution. In: Lynch DC, Rose MT. editors. *Internet System Handbook*. Reading: Addison-Wesley Comp.; 1993. (#98)

Lyonet P. *Traité anatomique de la chenille,. . .* La Haye; 1762. (#16)

Löwy A, Schrötter Hv. Untersuchungen über die Blutcirculation beim Menschen. *Zeit f exp Pathol u Therapie* 1905; 1:197. (#56)

M

MacInnis HF. The Clinical Application of Radioelectrocardiography. *Ca Med Assoc J* 1954; 70:574. (#71)

Mackenzie M. *Essays on Growths in the Larynx*. London; 1871. (#48)

Magendie F. *Formulaire pour la préparation et l'emploi de plusieurs nouveaux médicaments, tels que la noix vomique, la morphine . . .* Paris; 1821. (#29)

—— *Précis élémentaire de physiologie* 2 vols. Paris; 1816–1817. (#38)

—— *De pulmonibus observationes anatomicae*. Bologna; 1661. (#16)

—— *Opera Omnia*. London; 1686. (#16)

Mansfield P, Maudsley AA. Planar spin imaging by NMR. *J Phys C: Solid State Phys* 1976; 9:L409. (#96)

Mansfield P, Maudsley AA, Bains T. Fast scan proton density imaging by NMR. *J Phys E: Sci Instr* 1976; 9:271. (#96)

Marescaux J, et al.: Transatlantic robot-assisted telesurgery. *Nature* 2001; 413:379. (#98)

Marey E-J. *La machine animale, locomotion terreste et aérienne*. Paris; 1873. (#12)

—— *La méthod graphique dans les sciences expérimentales et particulièrement en physiologie et en médecine* Paris; 1878. (#52)

—— *Le Vol des Oiseaux*. (Physiologie du Mouvement) Paris; 1890. (#52)

—— *Recherches sur le pouls au moyen d'un nouvel appareil enregistreur le spyghmographe*. Paris; 1860. (#52)

Marey E-T. Inscription photographique des indications de l'électromètre de Lippmann. *C R Acad Sci* 1876. p278. (#65)

Markwart F. Untersuchungen über Hirudin. *Naturwissenschaften* 1955; 42:537. (#77)

Marquardt M. *Paul Ehrlich*. London: William Heinemann Medical books Ltd; 1949. (#75)

Martin AJP. *The development of partition chromatography*. Nobel Lecture Stockholm; 1952. (#84)

Martine G. *Essays Medical and Philosophical*. London; 1740. (#7)

Marton L. Electron microscopy of biological objects. *Phys Rev* 1934; 46(2):527. (#83)

von Marum M. *Description d'une Très Grande Machine Électric . . .* Haarlem; 1785–1787. (#15)

Matteucci C. *Essai sur la phénomènes électrique des animaux*. Paris; 1840. (#42)

—— Sur un phenomene physiologique produit par les muscles en contraction. *Ann Chim Phys* 1842; 6:339. (#65)

Mattson J, Simon M. *The pioneers of NMR and magnetic resonance in medicine. The Story of MRI*. New York: Dean Books Co.; 1966. Chapt. 6 and Chapt. 3. (#94)

Mauchly JW. The use of high speed vacuum tube devices for calculating. In: *The Origins of digital Computers: Selected Papers*. Randell B. editor. Berlin: Springer; 1973. p329. (#85)

Maupertuis P. *Oeuvres*.Vol.1–4 Lyon; 1756. particularly Vol.2 p139 Systeme de la Nature. (#53)

Maxwell JC. *Treatise on Electricity and Magnetism*. Vol.1,2 Oxford; 1873. (#55)

Mayow J. *Tractatus quinque medico-physici*. Oxford; 1674. (#11)

McGhee NJ, et al. editors. *Excimer Lasers in Ophthalmology, Principles and Practice*. Butterworth-Heinemann Medical; 1997. (#92)

McRobbie DW, et al. *MRI From Picture to Proton* Cambridge University Press; 2003. (#96)

McWilliam JA. Electrical stimulation of the heart in man. *Brit Med J* 1889; 1:348. and ref. 23.10, 23.11. (#91)

Meijer P. Bekendmaaking, *Philosooph* N.86, N.88, N.94 Aug–Oct. Amsterdam; 1767. (#23)

Melbye H. Bronchial airflow limitation and chest findings in audults with respiratory infection. *Scand J Prim Health Care* 1995; 13:261. (#31)

Menabrea LF. *Sketch of the Analytical Engine invented by Charles Babbage*. London; 1843. (#85)

Menghini V. De ferrearum particularum sede in sanguine. Bonon. *Sci Art Inst Acad Comment* 1746; 2(2):244. (#51)

Mesmer FA. *Memoire sur la Decouverte du Magnetisme Animal*. Geneva & Paris; 1779. (#8)

Meyer L. *Die Gase der blutes*. Inauguraldissertation Medicinische Fakultät Würzburg. Göttingen; 1857. (#37)

Middeldorpf AT. *Die Galvanokaustik*. Breslau; 1854. (#2)

von Mikulicz-Radecki J. Ueber Gastroscopie und Oesophagoskopie. *Wien med Presse* 1881; 22:1405. p1437, p1473, p1505, p1537, p1573 and p1629. (#60)

Milne JS. *Surgical Instruments in Greek and Roman times*. Oxford; 1907. (#2)

Mitchill SL. *Remarks on the Gaseous Oxyd of Azote or of Nitrogene,. . .* New York; 1795. (#28)

Mitscherlich E. Analyse kohlenstoffhaltige Verbindungen. *Ann Phys* 1834; 33:331. (#72)

Morris PJ. Polymer Pioneers. *A popular history of the science and technology of large molecules*. Philadelphia: Center for the History of Chemistry; 1986. p39. Also see ref. 78.7 p13. (#80)

Morton W. *Remarks on the Proper Mode of Administering Sulphuric Ether by Inhalation*. (#3)

de Morveau G. *Traité des moyens de désinfecter l'air, de prévenir la contagion, et d'en arrêter les progrès*. Paris; 1805. (#33)

Müller J. *Ueber die Compensation der physischen Kräfte am menschlichen Stimmorgan,...* Berlin; 1839. (#25)

Murdoch CA. *Means for use in the administering of drugs, medicines and the like to animals.* US Patent 3,207,157 1965. (appl.1962) (#10)

Murray DWG, et al. Heparin and the thrombosis of veins following injury. *Surgery* 1937; 2:163. (#86)

N

Natelson S, Lugovoy JK, Pincus JB. Determination of micro quatities of citric acid in biological fluids. *J Biol Chem* 1947; 170:597. (#81)

Natta G. *From the Stereospecific Polymerisation to the Assymetric Autocatalytic Synthesis.* Nobel Lecture Stockholm; 1963. (#80)

Newton I. *Philosophia Naturalis Principia Mathematica.* London; 1687. (#4)

Nilsson GE. *On the measurement of evaporative water loss, methods and clinical applications.* Linköping Studies in Science and Technology Dissertations No 11 Linköping; 1977. (#7)

Nitze M. *Kystophotographischer Atlas.* Wiesbaden; 1894. (#60)

—— *Lehrbuch der Kystoskopie ihre Technik und klinische Bedeutung.* Wiesbaden; 1907. (#60)

Niven WD editor. *The Scientific Papers of James Clerk Maxwell.* Vol.1,2 Cambridge; 1890. Vol.1 p377 Illustrations of the Dynamic theory of Gases. 1860. Vol.2 p26 On the dynamic Theory of Gases. 1866. (#55)

Nixon DW, et al. *Resting energy expenditure in lung and colon cancer.* Metabolism 1988; 37:1059. (#58)

Nollet JA. *Essai sur l'Électricité des Corps.* Paris; 1746. (#15)

Nordström L. On automatic ventilation. *Acta Anaesth Scand* Suppl 47 1972. (#87)

Norlander OP. The use of respirators in anaesthesia and surgery. *Acta Anaesth Scand* Suppl 30 1968. (#87)

Norris AC. *Essentials of Telemedicine and Telecare.* John Wiley & Sons; 2002. (#98)

Nutt R. The History of Positron Emission Tomography. *Molecular Imaging and Biology* 2002; 4(1):11. (#99)

Nyquist H. Regeneration theory. *Bell Syst Tech J* 1932; 11:126. (#55)

—— Thermal agitation of electric charge in conductors. *Phys Rev* 1928; 32:110. (#55)

O, Ö

Oatley CW. *The Scanning Electron Microscope.* Cambridge: Cambridge University Press; 1972. (#83)

Öberg PÅ, Shepherd AP, editors. *Laser-Doppler Blood Flowmetry* (Developments in Cardiovascular Medicine DICM 107) Kluwer Academic Publisher; 1990. (#40)

Odeblad E. Nuclear magnetic resonance in biology and medicine. *Ztschr f med Isotopenforsch* 1956; 1:25. (#94)

Oersted HC. *Experimenta circa effectum conflictus electrici in acum magneticam.* Copenhagen; 1820. (#26)

—— *Laeresaetninger af den nyere Chemie.* Copenhagen; 1820. p15. (#26)

Oevres de Pierre Curie. Société Francaise de Physique. Paris: Gauthier-Villars; 1908. (#66)

Ohm GS. *Die galvanische Kette, mathematisch bearbeitet.* Berlin; 1827. (#32)

—— Über die Definition des Tones ... *Ann Phys Chem* 1843; 59:513. (#32)

Oksala A, Lehtinen A. Diagnosis of Detachment of the Retina by Means of Ultrasound. *Acta Ophth* 1957; 35:461. (#90)

Okubo T, Lenfant C. Distribution function of lung volume and ventilation determined by lung N2 washout. *J Appl Physiol* 1968; 24:658. (#97)

Olby R, Posner E. An early reference to genetic coding. *Nature* 1967; 215:556. (#51)

Oldendorf WH. Isolated flying spot detection of radiodensity discontinuities-displaying the internal structural pattern of a complex object. *IRE Trans Bio-medical Electr* 1961; 8:68. (#95)

Oré PC. *Études cliniques sur l'anesthésie chirurgicale par la méthode des injections de chloral dans les veines.* Paris; 1875. (#10)

Osmer JC, Cole BK. The stethoscope and roentgenogram in acute pneumonia. *South Med J* 1966; 59:75. (#31)

Ostwald WF. Die dissociation des Wassers. *Z phys Chem* 1893; 11:521. (#81)

P

Pacioli L. *De divina Proportione.* Venice; 1509. (#1)

Paracelsus. *Der Buecher und Schriften.* Vol.VII; 1590. p172 (#3)

—— *Von der frantzösischen kranckheit drey Bücher.* Franckfurt a.M.; 1553. (#75)

Paré A. *The Collected Works of Ambroise Paré Lib.*17 chapt. 34–44 Transl. T. Johnson London; 1634. (#34)

Partington JR. *A History of Chemistry.* Vol. III Mansfield Centre; 1999. p135. Reprint of Ed. 1961–1979 (#21)

—— *A History of Chemistry.* Vol. III Chapter X. Mansfield Centre: Martino Fine Books; 1999. (#36, #38)

—— *A History of Chemistry.* Vol. IV Mansfield Centre: Martino Fine Books; 1999. p195 (#77), p775 (#72), p497, p557 (#33)

Pascal B. *Oeures* 5 vols. 1779. Machine Arithmétique. Vol.4 1645. p7. (#85)

—— *Traitez de l'équilbre des liqueurs, et de la pesanteur de la masse de l'air.* Paris; 1663. (#8)

Paskalev DN. Georg Haas (1886–1971) The forgotten hemodialysis pioneer. *Dialysis &Transplantation.* 2001; 30(12):828. (#77)

Pauling L, Corey RB. Atomic Coordinates and Structure Factors for Two Helical Configurations of Polypeptide Chains. *Proc Nat Acad Sci* 1951; 37(5):235. and also p251, p256, p272 and p282. (#88)

Pawley JB editor. *Handbook of Biological Confocal Microscopy.* New York: Plenum Press; 1995. (#9)

Pavlov IP. *Physiology of Digestion.* Nobel Lecture Stockholm; 1904. (#74)

Perutz MF. *X-ray Analysis of Haemoglobin.* Nobel Lecture. Stockholm; 1962. (#51)

Pettenkofer M. *Ueber einen neuen Respirations-Apparat.* Abh d k b Akad d Wiss 1861. p231. (#58)

Pettenkofer MJ, Voit Cv. Untersuchungen über die Respiration. *Ann Chem Pharm* 1862/1863; Suppl 2:52. (#38)

Petty TL. John Hutchinson's mysterious machine revisited. *Chest* 2002; 121:219S. (#41)

Pfeffer W. *Osmotische Untersuchungen.* Leipzig; 1877. (#63)

Pfluger E. Zur Gasometrie des Blutes. *Zbl Med Wiss* 1866; 4(20):305. (#37)

Phelps ME. Positron emission tomography provides molecular imaging of biological processes. *PNAS* 2000; 97(16):9226. (#99)

Pinder U. *Epiphanie Medicorum.* Nurenberg; 1506. (#49)

Piorry PA. *De la percussion médiate et des signes obtenue à l'aide de ce nouveau moyen d'exploration, dans les maladies des organes thoraciques et abdominaux.* Paris; 1828. (#31)

Plücker J. Über die Einwirkung des Magneten auf die elektrischen Entladungen in verdünnten Gasen. *Ann Phys Chem* 1858; 103:88. p151, p113. (#67)

Pohlman R, Richter R, Parow E. Über die Ausbreitung und Absorption des Ultraschalls im menschlichen Gewebe und seine therapeutische Wirkung in Ischias und Plexusneuralgie. *Dtsch Med Wschr* 1939; 52(7):251. (#66)

Poiseuille JL. Recherches expérimentales sur le mouvement des liquides dans les tubes de très-petits diamètres. *C R Acad Sci* 1840; 11:961, p1041, p1841 and *C R Acad Sci* 1841; 12:112. (#35)

—— Recherches expérimentales sur le mouvement des liquides dans les tubes de très petits diamètres *Mém Acad Roy Sci.* 1846; 9:433. (#18)

Polanyi M. Das Röntgen-Faserdiagramm. *Z Phys* 1921; 7:149. (#78)

Porath J, Flodin P. Gel filtration: A method for desalting and group separation. *Nature* 1959; 183:1657. (#84)

Potter RK, Kopp GA, Green HC. *Visible Speech.* New York: D.Van Nostrand Co.; 1947. (#41)

Pouillet CS. Note sur un moyen de mésurer des intervalles de temps extrémement courts,... *C R Acad Sci* 1844; 19:1384. (#43)

Pravaz CG. Sur un nouveau moyen d'opérer la coagulation du sang dans les artères. *C R Acad Sci* 1853; 36:88. (#10)

Priestley J. *Experiments and Observations on different kinds of Air.* Vol. III London; 1774. p380. (#22)

—— *Experiments and Observations on different kinds of Air.* Vol.II London; 1774. p304. (#22)

—— Observations of different kinds of air. *Phil Trans Roy Soc* 1772; 62:147. (#22)

Purcell EM, Torrey HC, Pound RV. Resonance absorption by nuclear magnetic moments in a solid. *Phys Rev* 1946; 69:37. (#94)

R

Rabi II, et al. A new method of measuring nuclear magnetic moment. *Phys Rev* 1938; 53:318. (#94)

Ramsey NF, Purcell EM. Interactions between nuclear spins in molecules. *Phys Rev* 1952; 85:143. (#96)

Raoult F-M. Loi de congélation des solutions acqueuses des matières organiques. *C R l'Acad Sci* 1882; 94: 1517. (#63)

von Recklinghausen H. Ueber Blutdruckmessung beim Menschen. *Arch exp Path Pharm.* 1901; 46:78. (#68)

Redi F. *Esperienze intorno alla generazione degl'insetti.* Firenze; 1668. (#50)

Regnault HV, Reiset J. Recherches Chimique sur la Respiration des Animaux des Diverses Classes. *Ann chim phys* 1849; 26:299. (#58)

Reiser SJ. *Medicine and the reign of technology.* Cambridge University Press: Cambridge; 1978. (#4)

Reivich M, et al. The (18F) fluorodeoxyglucose method for the measurement of local cerebral glucose utilization in man. *Circulation Research* 1979; 44:127. (#99)

Report of the committee, appointed to inquire into the uses and the physiological, therapeutical and toxical effects of chloroform. *Medico-Chirurgical Trans The Roy.Med Chir Soc London*; 1864. (#47)

Riley RL, Cournand A. Analysis of factors affecting partial pressures of oxygen and carbon dioxide in gas and blood of lungs: theory (methods). *J Appl Physiol* 1951; 4:77 and p102. (#97)

Riva C, Ross B, Benedek GB. Laser Doppler measurements of blood flow in capillary tubes and retinal arteries. *Invest Ophtalmol* 1972; 11:936. (#40)

Robertson JI, Birkenhäger WH. Editors. *Cardiac Output Measurement* London: Saunders; 1991. (#56)

Robinson J. *Lectures on the elements of chemistry.* Edinburgh; 1803. (#20)

Rochow EG. *An introduction to the chemistry of the silicones.* New York: J Wiley & Sons, Inc.; 1946. (#78)

—— *Silicon and Silicones.* New York: Springer-Verlag; 1987. (#78)

Roehr ZM. *Hypodermic syringe.* US Patent 2,728,341 1955. (appl.1951) and *Disposable needle assembly.* US Patent 2,953,243 1960. (appl. 1957) (#10)

Rosenbaum G, Homles KC, Witz J. Synchroton radiation as a source for x-ray diffraction. *Nature* 1971; 230:434. (#76)

Rosenfeld L. *Four Centuries of Clinical Chemistry.* G & B Science Pub; 1999. (#81)

Rothschuh C. *History of Physiology.* New York: R.E.Krieger; 1978. (#44)

Runge F. Ueber einige Produkte der Steinkohlendestillation. *Ann Phys* 1834; 31:65 and p513 and *Ann Phys* 1834; 32:308. (#73)

Runge F. *Zur Farbenchemie.* München; 1850. (#73)

Rushmer FF, Baker DW, Stegall HF. Transcutaneous Doppler flow detection as a non-invasive technique *J Appl Physiol* 1966; 21:554. (#40)

Ruska E, Knoll M. Die Magnetische Sammelspule fuer schnellen Elektronenstrahlen. *Z techn Phys* 1931; 12:389. and p448. (#83)

Rusovick RM, Warner DJ. The globalization of interventional informatics through Internet mediated distributed medical intelligence. *New Medicine* 1998; 2:155. (#98)

Rutherford D. *Dissertatio Inauguralis de Aere Fixo dicto, Aut Mephitico.* Edinburgh; 1772. (#17)

Rutherford E. Collision of alfa Particles with Light Atoms IV. An Anomalous Effect in Nitrogen. *Phil Mag 6ser.* 1919; 37:581. (#70)

—— *Radio-activity.* Cambridge At the University Press; 1904. (#70)

—— The Scattering of alfa and beta Particles by Matter and the Structure of the Atom. *Phil Mag 6ser.* 1911; 21:669. (#70)

Ryhage R. Efficiency of molecule separators used in gas chromatograph-mass spectrometer applications. *Arkiv Kemi* 1967; 26:305. (#79)

S

Saggi di natura esperienze fatte nell'Accademia del Cimento. Florence; 1667. (#7)

Sakodynskii KI. J *Chromatogr* 1981; 220:1. (#73)

—— *Michael Tswett Life and work.* Carlo Erba Instrumentazione Milano; 1983. (#73)

Sanger F. *The chemistry of insulin.* Nobel Lecture Stockholm; 1958. for the importance of IEC and paper chromatography in the determination of the amino acid sequence of insulin. (#84)

Santorio S. *Medica Statica: Beeing the Aphorism of Sanctorius.* Translated by J Quincy London; 1720. (#6)

Satomura S. Ultrasonic Doppler Method for the Inspection of Cardiac Functions. *J Acoust Soc Am* 1957; 29:1181 (#40)

Sauerbrey G. Verwendung von Schwingquartzen zur Wägung dünner Schichten und zur Mikrowägung. *Z Phys* 1959; 155:206. (#66)

Saussure HB. *Essais sur l'Hygrométrie.* Neuchatel; 1783. (#7)

Savart F. Sur la sensibilité de l'organe de l'ouie. *Ann Chim Phys* 1830; 44:337. (#26)

Schawlow AI, Townes CH. Infrared and optical masers. *Phys Rev* 1958; 112:1940. (#92)

Schechter DC. *Exploring the origins of electrical cardiac stimulation.* Minneapolis: Medtronic Inc.; 1983. and ref. 65.2, 65.3, 65.7 (#91)

Scheele CW. *Sämmtliche physische und chemische Werke...* Vol. I,II Berlin; 1793. (#1)

—— Undersökning om Blåse-stenen. *Kungl Vet Handl* 1776; 37:327. (#72)

Scheiner C. *Oculus hoc est: fundamentum octicum,...* Oeniponti, D. Agricola; 1619. (#5)

Schmidt-Nielsen K. Countercurrent Systems in Animals. *Scientific American* 1981; 244 (5):118. (#6)

Scholander PF, Irving L. Micro blood gas analysis in fractions of a cubic millimeter of blood. *J Biol Chem* 1947; 169:561. and p551. (#81)

Schrödinger E. *What is life?* Cambridge; 1944. (#4)

Schuitmaker JJ, et al. Photodynamic therapy: a promising new modality for the treatment of cancer. *J Photochem Photobiol B Biology* 1996; 34(1):3. (#92)

Segall HN. Nicolai S Korotkoff. *Experiments for determining the efficiency of arterial collaterals (translation of thesis 1910) with preface and biographical notes.* Montreal; 1980. (#68)

Seldinger SI. Catheter replacement of the needle in percutaneous angiography. A new technique. *Acta radiol* 1953; 39:368. (#67)

Semmelweis IP. *Die Aetiologie, der Begriff und die Profylaxis des Kindbettfiebers.* Pest; 1861. (#33)

Sertürner FW. Säure im Opium, Nachtrag zur Charakteristik der Säure im Opium. Auszuge aus Briefen an den Herausgeber. *J der Pharm* 1805; 13:229. (#29)

—— Über das Opium und dessen kristallisirbare Substanz. *J der Pharm* 1811; 20:99. (#29)

—— Ueber eins der furchterlichsten Gifte der

Pflanzwelt,... *Ann. der Phys* 1817; 27:192. (#29)

Sérullas GS. Mémoire sur l'iodure de potassium l'acid hydriodique et sur un composé nouveau de carbone, d'iode et d'hydrogène. *Ann Chim Phys* 2 sér. 1822; 20:163. (#33)

Severinghaus JW. History and recent developments in pulse oximetry. *Scand J Clin Lab Invest* 1993; Suppl. 214:105. (#27)

Severinghaus JW, Astrup P, Murray JF. Blood Gas Analysis and Critical Care Medicine. *Am J Respir Crit Care Med* 1998; 157:S114. (#37)

Sevick-Muraca E, Benaron D, editors. Biomedical Optical Spectroscopy & Diagnostics (*Trends in Optics & Photonics* Vol. 3) Optical Society of America; 1996. (#49)

Shanon C, Weaver W. *The Mathematical Theory of Communication.* Urbana; 1949. (#55)

Shtilman MI. *Polymeric Biomaterials* Part I Polymer Implants. Brill Academic Publishers; 2003. (#93)

Silberg WM, Lundberg GD, Musacchio RA. Assessing, controlling and assuring the quality of medical information on the Internet. *JAMA* 1997; 277:1244. (#98)

Simmons HA, Stone TW. *Purines: Basic and Clinical Aspects.* Kluwer Academic Publisher; 1991. (#72)

Simpson JY. Account of a New Anaesthetic Agent as substitute for sulphuric Ether in Surgery and Midwifery. *Comm Medico-Chirurgical Soc Edin.* Edinburgh; 1847. 10th November. (#36)

Sircus W, Flisk E, Craigs B. Milestones in the evolution of endoscopy: A short history. *J Roy Coll Physicians Edinb* 2003; 33:124. (#60)

Sjögren TA. *Fall af epiteliom behandladt med Röntgenstrålar.* Förh Sv Läkare-Sällsk Sammank Stockholm; 1899. p208. (#67)

Skeehan Jr RA, King Jr JH, Kaye S. Ethylene oxide sterilization in opthalmology. *Am J Opthalmol.* 1956; 42:424. (#61)

Skeggs LT. Principles of automatic chemical analysis. *Stand Methods Clin Chem* 1965; 5:31. (#81)

Skoda J. *Abhandlung über Perkussion und Auskultation.* Vienna; 1839. (#31)

—— Ueber die von Dr Semmelweis entdeckte wahre Ursache... *Sitz.d.kaiserl.Akad. Wiss. math. nat* 1849; 8:168. (#33)

Sohn JH, et al. Current status of the anticoagulant hirudin: its biotechnological production and clinical practice. *Appl.Microb. Biotech.* 2001; 57:606. (#77)

Sokolov SY. Ultrasonic oscillations and their applications. *Tech Phys* 1935; 2:1. (#90)

Sommerfeld A. Über der Beugung der Röntgenstrahlen. *Ann d Phys* 1912; 38:473. (#76)

Soubeiran E. Recherches sur quelques Combinaisons du Chlore. *Ann Chim Phys* 1831; 48:113. (#36)

Spallanzani L. *De' Fenomeni della Circolazione...* Modena; 1773. (#16)

—— *Lettere sopra il sospetto di un nuovo senso nei pipistrelli.* Torino; 1794. (#66)

—— *Mémoires sur la respiration...* traduits en Francais, d'après son manuscrit inédit, par J. Senebier Geneva; 1803. (#11)

—— *Saggio di osservazioni microscopiche concernenti il sistema della generazione. In Dissertazioni due...* Modena; 1765. (#50)

Speck C. Untersuchungen über Sauerstoffverbrauch und Kohlensäureausathmung der Menschen. *Schriften Ges Beförd.gesam Naturwiss zu Marburg Cassel*; 1871:10. (#41)

Spielberg AR. On call and online: Sociohistorical, legal and ethical implications of email for the patient- physician relationship. *JAMA* 1998; 280. (#98)

Spink MS, Lewis IL. *Albucasis on surgery and instruments*. London: Wellcome Institute of the History of Medicine; 1973. (#34)

Spriggs EA. John Hutchinson, the inventor of the spirometer—his North Country background, life in London and scientific achievements. *Med History* 1977; 21:357. (#41)

Stahl G. *Theoria Medica*. Vera Halle; 1708. (#4)

Stannius FH. Zwei Reihen physiologischer Versuche. *Arch Anat Physiol wiss Med*. 1852. p85. 23.10 (#23)

Staudinger H, Fritschi J. Über Isopren und Kautschuks. 5.Mitt.: Über die Hydrierung des Kautschuks und über seine Konstitution. *Helv chim Acta* 1922; 5:285. (#78)

—— Ueber die Makromolekulare Chemie. *Angew Chem*. 1936; 49:801. (#78)

Stein STh. Das Sphygmophone, ein neuer electro-telephonischer Apparat zur diagnose der Herz- und Pulsbewegungen. *Berl Klin Wochsch* 1878; 49:723. (#23)

Steiner F. Über die Electropunctur des Herzens als Wiederbelebungsmittel in der Chloroformsyncope. *Arch.klin.Chir*. 1871; 12:748. (#23)

Stephens WE. A Pulsed Mass Spectrometer with Time dispersion. *Phys Rev* 1946; 69:691. (#79)

Stern MD. In vivo evaluation of microcirculation by coherent light scattering. *Nature* 1975; 254:56. (#40)

Stewart AD, Snelling MA. *A new scanning electron microscope*. Proc 3rd Eur Conf Electron Microscopy Prague; 1965. p55. (#83)

Stevens SS, Jones RC. The Mechanism of Hearing by Electrical Stimulation. *J Acoust Soc Am* 1939; 10:261. (#26)

Stevenson LW, Perloff JK. The limited reliability of physical signs for estimating hemodynamics in chronic heart failure. *JAMA* 1989; 261:884. (#31)

Stevenson RC, Guthrie G. *A History of Oto-Laryngology*. Edinburgh; 1949. (#48)

Stiegler SM. *The History of Statistics The Measurement of Uncertainty before 1900*. Cambridge: The Beknap Press Harvard University Press; 1998. (#30)

Stoelting RK. *Pharmacology and Physiology of Anesthetic Practice*. Chapter 4 Lippincott Williams & Wilkins Publ.; 1999. (#72)

Stuart A. *Dissertatio de Structura et Motu Musculari*. London; 1738. (#19)

Svanberg S. Time-Resolved spectroscopic Techniques in Laser Medicine. In: *Ultrafast Spectroscopy* G. Mourou et al. Editors. Springer; 1994. (#49)

Svedberg T, Fåhraeus R. A New Method for the Determination of the Molecular Weight of the Proteins. *J Am Chem Soc* 1926; 48:430. (#78)

Svedberg T, Rinde H. The Ultra-Centrifuge, a new instrument for the determination of the size particle in amicroscopic colloids. *J Am Chem Soc* 1924; 46:2677. (#78)

Swedish Special Apparatus for heart clinics.

Electrocardiograph-Elmquist system. AB Elema-Järnhs 1952. (#71)

Sykes WS. *Essays on the first hundred years of anaesthesia.* Vol. I Chap.7 Churchill Livingstone; 1982. (#59)

T

Tanaka K. *The origin of macromolecule ionization by laser irradiation.* Nobel Lecture Stockholm; 2002. (#79)

The Beginnings of Electron Microscopy. In: *Advances in Electronics and Electron Physics.* Hawkes PW. Editor. Academic Press; 1985. p167, and p43. (#83)

The birth of molecular biology. *New Scientist.* Special issue 1987) 114 (No 1561):38. (#76)

The Collected Papers of Joseph, Baron Lister. Vol.1,2 Oxford; 1909. Vol.2 part III The antiseptic system. (#54)

The International Human Genome Mapping Consortium: A physical map of the human genome. *Nature* 2001; 409:934. The Celera Genomics Sequencing Team: The sequence of the human genome. *Science* February 16 2001. p1304. (#88)

Theophrastus: *De Plantis, De causis plantarum.* Venice; 1465. (#29)

Thiele FAJ, Senden KG. Relation between skin temperature and the insensible perspiration of the human skin *J Invest Dermatol.* 1966; 47:307. (#6)

Thompson T. *History of Chemistry* I Chapter 9 London; 1830. (#20)

Thomson JJ. Rays of positive electricity. *Proc Roy Soc A* 1913; 89:I. (#69)

Tissot J. Nouvelle méthode de mesure et d'inscription du débit et des mouvements respiratoires. *J Physiol Path Gén* 1904; 6:688. (#41)

—— Nouvelle méthode de mesure et d'inscription du débit et des movements respiratoires de l'homme et des animaux. Trav l'Assoc Inst Marey Vol II 1910. p231. (#41)

Townes CH. *Production of coherent radiation by atoms and molecules.* Nobel Lecture Stockholm; 1964. (#92)

von Tschermak-Seysenegg E. Über kunstliche Kreuzung von Pisum sativum. *Z landwirtsch Versuchsw in Österreich* 1900; 3:465. (#53)

Tswett MS. *Chromofilli v Rastitelnom i Zhivotnom Mire (Chromophylls in the Plant and Animal Kingdom)* Warsaw: Karbasnikov Publishers; 1910. (#73)

—— Physical chemical studies on chlorophyll adsorption (translated from Ber Dt Bot Ges. 1906; 24: 316. and p384. In: Strain HH, Sherma J. *J Chem Ed* 1967; 44:235. (#73)

Turk L. Der Kehlkopfrachenspiegel und die Methode seines Gebrauchs. *Zeit k k Ges Aertzte zu Wien* 1858; 1:401. (#48)

—— Praktische Anleitung zur Laryngoskopie. Wien; 1860. (#48)

Turner M. *An Account of the extraordinary medical fluid called Aether.* Liverpool; 1761.

Tyndall J. *Essays on the floating-matter of the air in relation to putrefaction and infection.* London: Longmans, Green and Co; 1881. p210. (#61)

Tyrell HJ. The Origin and Present Status of Fick's Diffusion Law. *J Chem Ed.* 1964; 41(7):397. (#46)

V W

Wagner PD, Naumann PF, Laravuso RB. Simultaneous measurement of eight foreign gases in blood by gas chromatography. *J Appl Physiol* 1974; 36(5):600. (#97)

Waller AD. Introductory Address on The Electromotive Properties of the Human Heart. *Brit Med J* 1888; 2: 751. (#65)

—— *The signs of life from their electrical aspekt.* New York: E.P.Dutton & Co; 1903. (#65)

Van Slyke DD, Sendroy Jr J. Manometric analysis of gas mixtures. I. The determination, by simple absorption, of carbon dioxide, oxygen and nitrogen in mixtures of these gases. *J Biol Chem.* 1932; 95:509. (#81)

Van't Hoff J. Une propriété générale de la matière diluée. *Kungl Sv Vet Akad Handl* Stockholm; 1886; 21 (17):42. (#63)

Washington CM, Leaver D. Editors. *Principles and Practice of Radiation Therapy.* Mosby; 2003. (#70)

Watson JD, Crick FH. Genetic implications of the structure of deoxyribonucleic acid. *Nature* 1953; 171:964. (#88)

Watson W. *Expériences et Observations pour servir a l'Explication de la Nature et des Propriétés de l'Électricité.* Paris; 1748. (#15)

Weber E, Weber EH. Experimenta, quibus probaturnervos vagos … *Ann Univ Med.* (Milano) 3ser. 1845; 20:227. (#44)

—— *Wellenlehre auf Experimente gegrundet …* Leipzig; 1825. (#18)

Weber EH. Der Tastsinn und das Gemeingefühl. *R. Wagner Handwörterbuch Physiol* III part 2 1850. p481. (#44)

—— Programma, Pulsum arteriarum non in omnibus arteriis simul,… *Annot anat physiol.* 1 Leipzig; 1827. (#44)

Weber W, Weber E. *Mechanik der menschlichen Gehwerkzeuge Eine anathomisch-physiologische Untersuchung.* Göttingen; 1836. (#12)

Weiger J. *Über Ether und Chloroform.* Wien; 1850. (#47)

de Weir JB. New methods to calculating metabolic rate with special reference to protein metabolism. *J Physiol* 1949; 109:1. (#58)

Wells H. The discovery of etheral inhalation. *The Boston Med. Surg. J.* 1847; 36(15): 298. (#28)

Wells PN. A range-gated ultrasonic Doppler system. *Med.&Biol.Eng* 1969; 7:641. (#40)

Werkö L. The influence of positive pressure breathing on the circulation in man. *Acta med Scand.* 1947; 193:1. (#97)

Vesalius A.*De humani corporis fabrica libri septem.* Basel; 1543. (#1)

West JB, et al. Measurement of the ventilation perfusion ratio inequality in the lung by the analysis of a single expirate. *Clin Sci Lond* 1957; 16:529. (#97)

West JB, Dollery CT. Distribution of blood flow and ventilation-perfusion ratio in the lung, measured with radioactive CO_2. *J Appl Physiol* 1960; 15:405. (#97)

Wiener N. *Cybernetics or control and communication in the Animal and the Machine.* MIT Press; 1961. (#55)

Vierordt K. *Die anwendung des Spectralapparates zur Photometrie der Absortionsspectren und zur quantitativen chemischen Analyse.* Tubingen; 1873. (#49)

—— *Die Lehre vom Arterienpuls in gesunden und*

kranken Zustände, gegrundet auf eine neue Methode der bildlichen Darstellung des menschlichen Pulses. Braunschweig; 1855. (#17)
—— *Die Quantitative Spectralanalyse in ihrer Anwendung auf Physiologie, Physik, Chemie und Technologie.* Tubingen; 1876. (#49)

Viertiö-Olja HE, et al. Entropy of EEG signal is a robust index for depth of hypnosis. *Anesthesiology* 2000; 93:1369. (#55)

Wild JJ. The Use of Ultrasonic Pulses for the Measurement of Biological Tissue and the Detection of Tissue Density Changes. *Surgery* 1950; 27:183. (#90)

Wild JJ, Reid JM. The Effects of Biological Tissues on 15-mc Pulsed Ultrasound. *J Acoust Soc Am* 1953; 25(2): 270. (#90)

Wilkins MHF, Stokes AR, Wilson HR. Molecular Structure of Deoxypentose Nucleic Acid. *Nature* 1953; 171:738. (#88)

Williams E, Rydevik B, Brånemark P-I. editors. *From Molecule to Man; Facts and Hypotheses—Options and Opportunities.* Göteborg: The Institute of Applied Biology; 2000.

Williams E. *A Matter of Balance.* Akademiförlaget; 1992. (#93)

Wilson G. *The Life of the Honourable Henry Cavendish.* Chapter III London; 1851. (#21)

Wilson RR. Radiological use of fast protons. *Radiology* 1946; 47:487. (#69)

Winkler JH. *Die Stärke der Electrischen Kraft des Wassers in gläsernen Gefässen, welche durch den Musschenbroekischen Versuch bekannt geworden.* Leipzig; 1746. (#15)

Vitruvius Pollio M. *De architectura.* Rome; 1486. (#1)

Woillez E. Sur le spirophore, appareil de sauvetage pour les asphyxiés principalement pour les noyés et les enfants nouveau-nés. *C R Acad Sci* 1876; 82:1447. Also see *Scientific American* 1876; XXXV(25). (#87)

Volkmann H. *Carl Zeiss und Ernst Abbe ihr Leben und ihr Werk.* Deutsches Museum 34 Heft 2 1966. (#64)

Volta A. Lettera a Priestley sull'elettroforo perpetuo. *Scelta di Opusculi* 1775; 9:91. (#15)

Wong DT, Bymaster FP, Engleman EA. Prozac (Fluoxetine Lilly 110140) the first selective serotonine uptake inhibitor and an antidepressant drug: twenty years since its first publication. *Life Sciences* 1995; 57:411. (#75)

Wood A. New method of treating neuralgia by the direct application of opiates to the painful joints. *Edinb Med Surg J* 1855; 82:265. (#10)

Woolston J. Irradiation Sterilization of Medical Devices. *Medical Device Technology* 1990; 1(4):25. (#61)

Wrenn Jr FR, Good ML, Handler P. The use of positron emitting radioisotopes for localization of brain tumors. *Science* 1951; 113:525. (#99)

deVries H. Das Spaltungsgesetz der Bastarde. *Ber dtsch bot Ges* 1900; 18:83. (#53)
—— *Die Muthationstheorie.* Vol. 1,2 Leipzig; 1901–1903. (#53)

Wunderlich C. *Das Verhalten der Eigenwärme in Krankheiten.* Leipzig; 1868. (#7)

Y

Yalow RS, Berson SA. Assay of Plasma Insulin in human subjects by Immunological Methods. *Nature* 1959; 184:1648. (#70)

Yeh Y, Cummins HZ. Localized fluid flow measurements with an He-Ne laser spectrometer. *Appl Phys Letters* 1964; 4:176. (#40)

Young T. *A course of lectures on natural philosophy and the mechanical arts.* London; 1807. (#5)
—— On the function of the heart and arteries. *Phil. Trans.* 1809; I:12. (#44)
—— On the theory of light and colours. *Phil Trans Part 1*; 1802. p12. (#5)
—— Outlines of Experiments and Inquiries respecting Sound and Light. *Phil Trans Roy Soc.* 1800; Jan.16 (#13)

Z

Zernike F. Das Phasenkontrastverfahren b.d. microscopischen Beobachtung. *Phys Z* 1935; 36:848. (#9)

Ziegler K. *Consequences and Development of an Invention.* Nobel Lecture Stockholm; 1963. (#80)

Zoll PM. Resuscitation of the heart in ventricular standstill by external electric stimulation. *New Engl J Med* 1952; 247:768. (#91)

Zuntz N, Hagemann O. *Untersuchungen über den Stoffwechsel des Pferdes bei Ruhe und Arbeit.* Berlin; 1898. (#56)

Zworykin VK. Description of an experimental television system and the kinescope. *Proc IRE* 1933; 21(12): 1655. (#82)
—— *Television system.* US Patent 2,141,059 1938. (filed 1923) (#82)
—— Television techniques in biology and medicine. In: *Adv Biol Med Phys* Vol.V Lawrence JH, Tobias CA. editors. New York: Academic Press; 1957. (#82)

Zworykin VK, Hillier J, Snyder RL. A scanning electron microscope. *ASTM Bull* 1942; 117:15. (#83)

Zworykin VK, Flory LE, Pike WS. *Research on reading aids for the blind.* J Frankl Inst May 1949. p483. (#82)

Zworykin VK, Morton GA. *Television. The electronics of image transmission.* New York: J Wiley; 1940. (#82)